Lecture Notes in Electrical Engineering

Volume 841

The book series *Lecture Notes in Electrical Engineering* (LNEE) publishes the latest developments in Electrical Engineering - quickly, informally and in high quality. While original research reported in proceedings and monographs has traditionally formed the core of LNEE, we also encourage authors to submit books devoted to supporting student education and professional training in the various fields and applications areas of electrical engineering. The series cover classical and emerging topics concerning:

- Communication Engineering, Information Theory and Networks
- Electronics Engineering and Microelectronics
- Signal, Image and Speech Processing
- Wireless and Mobile Communication
- Circuits and Systems
- Energy Systems, Power Electronics and Electrical Machines
- Electro-optical Engineering
- Instrumentation Engineering
- Avionics Engineering
- Control Systems
- Internet-of-Things and Cybersecurity
- Biomedical Devices, MEMS and NEMS

For general information about this book series, comments or suggestions, please contact leontina.dicecco@springer.com.

To submit a proposal or request further information, please contact the Publishing Editor in your country:

China

Jasmine Dou, Editor (jasmine.dou@springer.com)

India, Japan, Rest of Asia

Swati Meherishi, Editorial Director (Swati.Meherishi@springer.com)

Southeast Asia, Australia, New Zealand

Ramesh Nath Premnath, Editor (ramesh.premnath@springernature.com)

USA, Canada:

Michael Luby, Senior Editor (michael.luby@springer.com)

All other Countries:

Leontina Di Cecco, Senior Editor (leontina.dicecco@springer.com)

**** This series is indexed by EI Compendex and Scopus databases.****

More information about this series at https://link.springer.com/bookseries/7818

N. Marriwala · C. C. Tripathi · Shruti Jain ·
Shivakumar Mathapathi
Editors

Emergent Converging Technologies and Biomedical Systems

Select Proceedings of ETBS 2021

Springer

Editors
N. Marriwala
Department of Electronics
and Communication Engineering
University Institute of Engineering
and Technology
Kurukshetra, Haryana, India

Shruti Jain
Department of Electronic
and Communication Engineering
Jaypee University of Information
Technology
Solan, Himachal Pradesh, India

C. C. Tripathi
Dean Engineering and Technology
Kurukshetra University
Kurukshetra, Haryana, India

Shivakumar Mathapathi
Co-Founder of Dew Mobility
Santa Clara University
Santa Clara, CA, USA

ISSN 1876-1100 ISSN 1876-1119 (electronic)
Lecture Notes in Electrical Engineering
ISBN 978-981-16-8773-0 ISBN 978-981-16-8774-7 (eBook)
https://doi.org/10.1007/978-981-16-8774-7

This Springer imprint is published by the registered company Springer Nature Singapore Pte Ltd.
The registered company address is: 152 Beach Road, #21-01/04 Gateway East, Singapore 189721, Singapore

Preface: Emergent Converging Technologies and Biomedical Systems

This book will provide a platform and aid to the researchers involved in designing systems that will permit the societal acceptance of ambient intelligence. The overall goal of this book is to present the latest snapshot of the ongoing research as well as to shed further light on future directions in this space. The aim of publishing the book is to serve educators, researchers, and developers working in the area of recent advances and upcoming technologies utilizing computational sciences in signal processing, imaging, computing, instrumentation, artificial intelligence, and their applications. As the book includes recent trends in research issues and applications, the contents will be beneficial to professors, researchers, and engineers. This book will provide support and aid to the researchers involved in designing the latest advancements in communication and intelligent systems that will permit the societal acceptance of ambient intelligence. The "Next Generation Technology: Artificial Intelligence in Healthcare and Cyber Intelligent Systems" book encompasses all branches of artificial intelligence, computational sciences and machine learning which are based on computation at some level such as AI-based Internet of things, sensor networks, robotics, intelligent diabetic retinopathy, intelligent cancer genes analysis using computer vision, evolutionary algorithms, fuzzy systems, medical automatic identification intelligence system and applications in agriculture, healthcare, smart grid, instrumentation systems, etc. It presents the latest research being conducted on diverse topics in intelligence technologies with the goal of advancing knowledge and applications in this rapidly evolving field. Authors are invited to submit papers presenting novel technical studies as well as position and vision papers comprising hypothetical/speculative scenarios.

The overall goal of this conference is to present the latest snapshot of the ongoing research in convergent technologies and biomedical systems as well as to shed further light on future directions in this area. Authors were invited to submit papers presenting novel technical studies as well as position and vision papers comprising hypothetical/speculative scenarios. The objective of the International Conference on Emergent Converging Technologies and Biomedical Systems, (ETBS-2021) is to provide a platform for researchers, engineers, and academicians as well as industrial professionals from all over the world to present their research results and development activities on biomedical engineering and applications.

ETBS-2021 tries to investigate, simulate, and analyze very complex issues and phenomena in a real-life situation. ETBS-2021 aims to,

- Bring the research fraternity together in the field of biomedical engineering and converging technologies.
- Investigate the future prospective directives by employing recent advances.
- Encourage practitioners/researchers to enhance their ability for problem-solving in optimization.

More complex systems arising in biology, medicine, and management systems remain intractable to conventional mathematical and analytical methods. The conference deals with various topics such as imprecision, uncertainty, partial truth, and approximation to achieve tractability, robustness, and low solution cost. It extends its application to various disciplines of engineering and science.

For the proper review of each manuscript, every received manuscript was first checked for plagiarism, and then, the manuscript was sent to three reviewers. In this process, the committee members were involved, and the whole process was monitored and coordinated by the general chair. The technical program committee involved senior academicians and researchers from various reputed institutes. The members were from India as well as abroad. The technical program mainly involves the review of the paper. An overwhelming response was received from the researchers, academicians, and industry from all over the globe. A total of **325** research papers were received, out of which 60 papers were accepted and registered and presented during the three-day conference; acceptance ratio is **18.4%**.

The papers were from PAN India covering all the states like Maharashtra, Uttar Pradesh, Haryana, Punjab, Rajasthan, Sikkim, West Bengal, Tamil Nadu, Kerela, Andhra Pradesh, Madhya Pradesh Delhi, etc. and many international countries like Finland, Siberia, Oman, Bangladesh, USA, etc. The authors are from premium institutes IITs, NITs, Central Universities, PU, and many other reputed institutes.

The editors would like to express their sincere gratitude to general chairs, plenary speakers, invited speakers, reviewers, technical program committee members, international advisory committee members, and local organizing, committee members of ETBS-2021, without whose support, the quality and standards of the conference could not be maintained. Editors would like to express their deepest sense of gratitude to the Patron and Presiding Chair of the conference ETBS-2021 **Prof. (Dr.) Som Nath Sachdeva**, Honorable Vice-Chancellor, Kurukshetra University, Kurukshetra; Chief Guest **Prof. Rajive Kumar**, Member Secretary, AICTE; Guest of Honor "**Ms. Kamiya Khatter**," Editor at Springer Nature, Applied Sciences and Engineering; and Keynote Speakers **Dr. Ahmed A. Elngar**, Associate Professor of Computer Science Beni-Suef University, Faculty of Computers and Artificial Intelligence, Egypt; **Dr. Utku Kose**, Associate Professor, in Suleyman Demirel University, Turkey; and **Dr. Celia Shahnaz**, Professor, Department of EEE, BUET, Bangladesh. A special thanks to the Springer and its team for their valuable support in publication of the proceedings of the confernce ETBS-2021.

Kurukshetra, India N. Marriwala
Kurukshetra, India C. C. Tripathi
Solan, India Shruti Jain
Santa Clara, USA Shivakumar Mathapathi

Contents

About the Editors

Dr. N. Marriwala is working as Assistant Professor and Head of the Department Electronics and Communication Engineering Department, UIET, Kurukshetra University, Kurukshetra. He did his PhD from National Institute of Technology (NIT), Kurukshetra, in the Department of Electronics and Communication Engineering. He did his post-graduation (M-Tech) in Electronics and Communication Engineering from Institute of Advanced Studies in Education (IASE) University and did his B-Tech in Electronics and Instrumentation from MMEC, Mullana, Kurukshetra University, Kurukshetra. He has more than 19 years of experience in teaching graduate and postgraduate students. More than 31 students have completed their M-Tech dissertation under his guidance. He has filed seven patents out of which six patents have been granted with two Indian patents and four international patents. He has published more than five book chapters in different international books, has authored more than ten books with Pearson, Wiley, etc., and has more than 40 publications to his credit in reputed international journals (SCI, SCIE, ESCI, and Scopus) and 20 papers in international/national conferences. He has been Chairman of Special Sessions in more than 20 international/national conferences and has delivered a keynote address at more than seven international conferences. He has also acted as an organizing secretary for more than five international conferences and one national conference. He has delivered more than 70 invited talks/guest lectures in leading Universities/Colleges PAN India. His areas of interests are SDRs, CRs, soft computing, blockchain, wireless communications, WSNs, fuzzy system design, and advanced microprocessors.

C. C. Tripathi completed his Ph.D. in electronics from Kurukshetra University, Kurukshetra. Since 2016, he is working as a Director of the University Institute of Engineering Technology (an autonomous institute), Kurukshetra University, Kurukshetra. His research areas are microelectronics, RF MEMS for communication, and industrial consultancy. He has filled 1 patent and published over 80 papers journals and conference proceedings. Prof. Tripathi is an experienced professor with a demonstrated history of working in the higher education industry. He has been working extensively on graphene-based flexible electronics devices, sensors, etc.

Shruti Jain is an Associate Professor in the Department of Electronics and Communication Engineering at the Jaypee University of Information Technology, Waknaghat, India. Dr. Jain received her Doctor of Science (D. Sc.) in electronics and communication engineering. She has 16 years of teaching experience with three filed patents, over 120 journal publications, and 15 book chapters. She has also published nine books. Her research interests are image and signal processing, soft computing, bio-inspired computing, and computer-aided design of FPGA and VLSI circuits.

Shivakumar Mathapathi is an adjunct faculty member at multiple universities including the University of California San Diego, Sonoma State University, Santa Clara University, and he is also teaching at regional community academia including ethnically diverse institutions such as Ohlone and De-Anza College in California. Prof. Mathapathi has been a passionate educator for nearly 25 years of industry experience with a strong desire to help students recognize the connection between learning and Industry needs. His teaching and research areas include the internet of things, machine learning, artificial intelligence, cybersecurity, and Blockchain. He has also authored numerous articles published in prestigious journals. Prof. Mathapathi is also a team leader of the education cluster at the Global City Team Challenge project in collaboration with the National Institute of Standards and Technology (NIST), under the U.S Department of Commerce. He is the key contributor in creating tutorials, workshops, and practice use cases for smart cities. The workshop also discusses IoT standards and protocol which would help; community partners and city/municipality staff to get familiar with national as well as international IoT standards.

Performance and Security Issues of Integrating Cloud Computing with IoT

Rubika Walia and Prachi Garg

Abstract Internet of things (IoT) empowers different gadgets to interface with one another by means of web. This guarantees the gadgets to be brilliant and send the data to an incorporated framework, which will at that point screen and take activities as per the undertaking given to it. IoT can be utilized in numerous areas such human services, transportation, amusement, power lattices, and keen structures. IoT is required to go about as a motivation for the future developments, and its utilization is relied upon to rise exponentially over the coming years. As indicated by security point of view, the IoT will be challenged with more extreme difficulties. Subsequently, the new security and protection issues will emerge.

Keywords Internet of things · Destination-oriented directed acyclic graph · Queue utilization · Service level agreement · Routing protocol for low power and lossy network

1 Introduction

Internet of things is a kind of setup of several physical entities or stuffs. This setup comprises software, microelectronics, and sensors to achieve superior facility through exchanging facts with makers, operatives, and several other associated devices. In direction to build mobile devices more capable, a combination of cloud work out expertise and mobile devices is used. Mobile cloud combination is helpful to increase computational supremacy and storing of mobile devices as in Fig. 1. In direction to realize the complete distribution, permitted transmission, on-demand use, and ideal distribution of several built-up assets and competences, the uses of the services of IoT and cloud work out in engineering are considered. Through the combination of IoT and cloud, we have the prospect to enlarge the use of the existing

R. Walia (✉)
MMEC, MMICT & BM, M. M. (Deemed to be University), Mullana, Ambala, Haryana, India

P. Garg
MMEC, M. M. (Deemed to be University), Mullana, Ambala, Haryana, India

N. Marriwala et al. (eds.), *Emergent Converging Technologies and Biomedical Systems*, Lecture Notes in Electrical Engineering 841,
https://doi.org/10.1007/978-981-16-8774-7_1

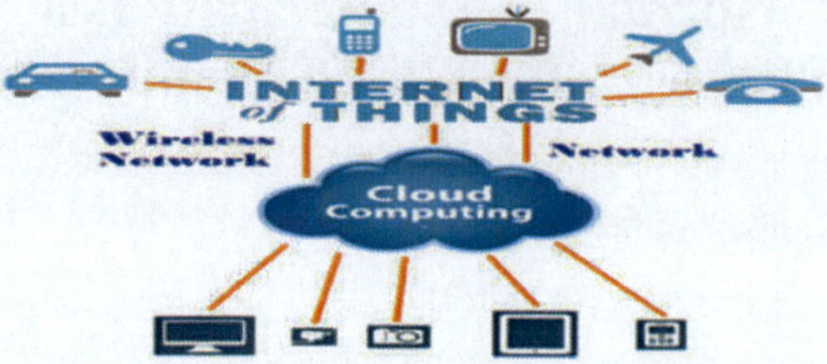

Fig. 1 IoT and cloud computing integration

expertise which is available in cloud settings. This integration can provide cloud storage to IoT applications [1].

But integrating IoT with cloud arise new problems such as latency, bandwidth requirements, reliability, security, etc. All of these problems motivated to investigate, fog computing, as new distributing computing paradigms, to see the necessities of latency-sensitive IoT submissions. Most of the IoT devices are available with lowest level of security. Some of these devices do not get enough updates during its usage. These devices having obsolete hardware and software open to probable attack for their trusted customers [2]. The world is experiencing key changes or high-tech progresses with the arrival of PC "things," main on the web and then in cloud computing [3]. The fundamental problem here is safety which is not reflected in product plan because networking devices and other entities are comparatively fresh. Usually, IoT products are available with outdated operational system and software which cannot be easily patched. Another problem is usually buyers use smart devices with default passwords which are weak and often fail to modify adequately tough secret word as password. Encryption procedure shows a key role to deliver safe transmission above network [1].

1.1 Cryptography

From last few years, network security has grown considerable importance because it provides security mechanism for web-based applications. In order to mitigate modern attacks, protection is very necessary. Mitigation of attacks, confidentiality uncertainties is solitary the important traits of present attacks. Cryptography encodes information, and the individual having the key can decodes this. Cryptography makes sure that the data being communicated has not been transformed in transfer. A cryptographic procedure, or cryptogram, is a scientific task castoff for encryption and decryption process. Cryptography procedure along with a key (combination of numbers, alphabets or special symbols) is used to encode plaintext. The identical plaintext can be encoded to unique encrypted content with dissimilar keys. The security strength of encryption statistics depends on the power of set of rules of encryption procedure and secrecy of the key. In order to put on encryption procedures for IoT, it is required to make additional work to more investigation to guarantee how these procedures can be effectively applied for IoT with restricted storage and small speed processor.

1.2 Trust Models

Nowadays, documents are isolated in various data hubs, and faraway hosts contain the applications. This separate data and remote applications are fetched by the cloud to consumer's PC in simulated form. Cloud customers get computation and storing from cloud regardless of time and locality. But for the better commercialization of this cloud technology, there must have the reliance by the cloud users for the cloud providers that they complete their requested work as per the provision level contracts; thus, the data of the cloud users after processing the data will be secured as shown in Fig. 2. To achieve all these necessities, trust management can be an important portion of marketable traits of cloud tools. There are three kinds of provision transfer prototypes provided by the cloud infrastructure. They are such as "Software as a Service (SaaS), Infrastructure as a Service (IaaS), and Platform as a Service (PaaS)." Cloud service providers provide infrastructure, platform and software to consumers in a cost-effective and truthful manner. Firms like Google and Amazon grounded on the trust running system have implemented reputation and helped the customers to find the reliable source providers to perform e-business trades in a safe and assured way [4]. Now, the question arises how trust is computed. Trust can be measured in two ways:

(a) By checking the current abilities of the supplier whether it can offer worthy service to users.
(b) By checking previous credentials of the supplier. Previous credentials of cloud source define the past repute and facility archives of the assets. It comprises

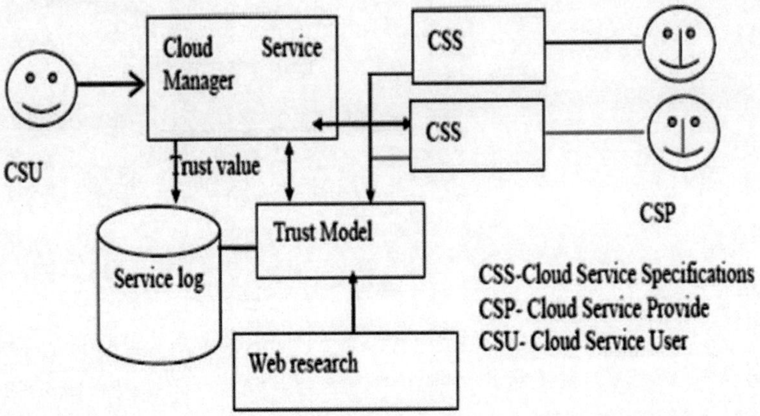

Fig. 2 Architecture of trust evaluation in cloud environment

consistency, obtain ability, turnaround time, and data truthfulness, safety level of the location, bandwidth and expectancy of the assets [4].

1.3 Load Balancing Based on Routing Protocol for Low Power and Lossy Networks (RPL)

One of the most well-known issues in WSNs is the manner by which to advance the information broadcast whereas augmenting the system lifespan. In this unique circumstance, the IPv6 Routing Protocol for low power and lossy networks (RPL) was suggested by the IETF. The IETF IPv6 Routing Protocol for low power and lossy networks (RPL) is extensively used to provide routing among sensor nodes as presented in Fig. 3. In most setups, a mainstay network of intermediate nodes is set up, which is likely to be fixed. RPL practices a hierarchical routing method for the static backbone network. Key characteristic of movement is an extremely self-motivated topology which marks in recurrent interruptions with neighboring nodes. As of these interruptions, data packets directed to a movable device can be directed to edges (parents) even then the mobile device is currently out of reach of these parents [5]. The practice of this protocol could become public and standard in IPv6 sensor networks in the future, even though some obstacles slow acceptance today [6].

Load Balancing

Load-balancing mechanism can benefit an IoT network between its sensor nodes in twofold methods: firstly, link to determine all possible routes available for routing can be enabled and secondly, the network can be distributed evenly to make finest practice of the system life span [6].

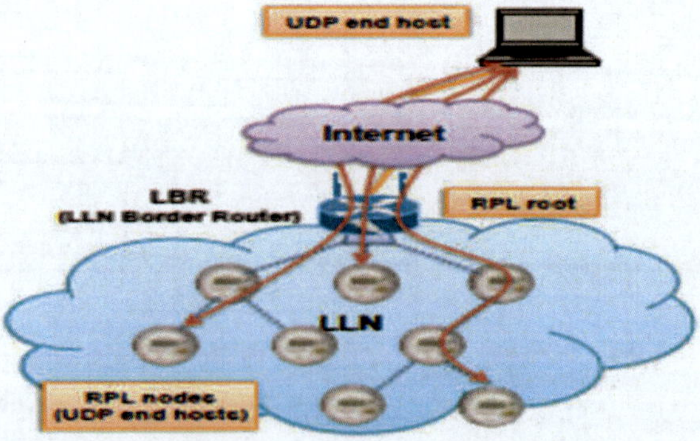

Fig. 3 Illustration of an IOT multi-hop LLN scenario

2 Related Work

2.1 Security and Privacy of IoT

Nie et al. [5] reviewed the base functions of two algorithm (DES and Blowfish)), examined the safety of procedures, and assessed encryption function speed grounded on altered memory bulks. Patil et al. [7] applied and investigated price tag and enactment of widely used cryptography algorithms (DES, 3DES, AES, RSA and Blowfish). It is concluded that based on the entropy Blowfish scores highest among all these procedures and is top appropriate against guessing attack. Poonia et al. [8] enhanced and evaluated the Blowfish procedure on the base of dissimilar constraints. Suresh et al. [9] analyzed several safety mechanisms for IoT and the importance of encryption in IoT. After several comparisons, "Blowfish" as a capable encryption procedure is designated. Bruschi et al. [10] proposed an intercommunication layer which allows isolating the physical assets but managing the migration of facility instances according to the operator's location. Mota et al. [11] compared commonly used cryptography procedure such as symmetric algorithms (DES, Blowfish, AES) and asymmetric algorithms (ECC, RSA). It is concluded that Blowfish is finest in footings of finishing time, memory used, throughput, power intake, safety, and is fit for IOT. Stergiou et al. [12] presented a review of IoT and cloud computing with an emphasis on the safety concerns of both skills. The author joints the two above-mentioned skills to inspect the shared topographies and reported the profits of their combination. Nandy et al. [13] reported on IoT safety mainly on validation mechanisms. The author emphasized massive attacks and real methodologies on the IoT verification mechanism and argued current safety authentication procedures and assessment systems of IoT validation. Kamgueu et al. [14] reviewed latest workings on RPL and highlights key offerings to its enhancement, particularly those associated to topology optimization, safety, and movement. Donno et al. [15] presented the current and well-structured investigation of the safety problems of integrating cloud computing with IoT. A clear picture of various security issues and their potential impact was presented. It is concluded that securing IoT devices is not enough, as many cyber-storms come from clouds also. Malge and Singh [16] state that IoT has four main modules comprising recognizing, data handling, applications and facilities, diverse access and supplementary modules, e.g., safety and confidentiality. The author offered safety view from the viewpoint of layers that covers IoT. Adamou et al. [17] focused on safety and confidentiality thoughts by examining selected probable challenges and threats that must to be fixed. The author examined the IoT design and present uses to complete this and talk over safety as well as confidentiality worries and problems. Kutzias et al. [2] derived general integration design as a supporting tool for the suggestion of the different integration contests. Vijayalakshmi et al. [18] discussed about the motive, investigation carried out in this field, diverse skills, and the future progress of edge computing background. Kaur et al. [19] focused on cloud providers to offer a pay-as-you-use prototypical where clients pay for the particular assets used. Similarly, cloud accommodating by worth of a facility adds value to IoT startups by providing cost-cutting of scale to lessen their total cost configuration.

2.2 Trust Models

Li et al. [20] examined some trust prototypes castoff in big and scattered location and then presented a new cloud trust prototype to resolve safety problems in cross-clouds setting in which cloud client can select dissimilar suppliers' facilities and assets in dissimilar fields. Manue et al. [21] presented a unique trust prototype established on previous credentials and existing aptitudes of a cloud source supplier. Trust assessment is done using four constraints such as obtain capability, consistency, turnaround competence, and data reliability. Kaur et al. [22] discussed several constraints and reliance prototypical structure for particular web service and a number of constraints used by them for computing reliance. Xu et al. [23] provided a categorized trust demonstrating technique to consumer to expand safety situational consciousness in the cloud computing situations. Kaur et al. [19] focused on cloud providers to offer a pay-as-you-use model where clients pay for the particular resources used. Also, cloud hosting as a facility adds value to IoT startups by providing cost-cutting of scale to lessen their total cost configuration.

2.3 Load Balancing

Kim et al. [24] proposed QU-RPL (an effective queue utilization which is based on RPL) that significantly improved the performance of e2e packet distribution as compared to the regular RPL. It is planned to choose the parental node for each node by considering their hop distances to an LBR as well as the queue consumption of its nearby nodes. Zhou et al. [25] proposed a context-aware unburdening decision procedure targeting to deliver code offloading choices at runtime on picking wireless intermediate and which probable cloud resources as the offloading place established on the device situation. Zhu et al. [6] proposed a routing protocol with an energy equalization to make the most of the living time of the constrained nodes. Also based on the cache utilization, a multi-path advancing path is suggested. Qasem et al. [26] proposed a protracted objective function that set of scales the count of kid's nodes of the parent nodes to escape the congestion problem and guarantee node life span expansion in RPL. The usual OFs are castoff to figure a destination-oriented directed acyclic graph (DODAG) where the traffic jam nodes may suffer from unbalanced traffic burden. Tarak Nandy et al. [13] reported on IoT safety mainly on validation mechanisms. The author emphasized massive attacks and useful methodologies on the IoT verification mechanism and argued current safety authentication procedures and assessment systems of IoT validation. Kaur et al. [19] focused on cloud providers to offer a pay-as-you-use model where clients pay for the particular resources used.

Also, cloud hosting as a facility adds value to IoT startups by providing cost-cutting of scale to lessen their total cost configuration.

2.4 Cloud Computing

Gonzalez et al. [27] reported that cloudlet idea is a subclass of edge computing useful to mobile systems, and the fog idea is a subclass of edge computing practical to Internet of things (IoT). The author delivered a detailed investigation of associated issues, classifying the focal study areas associated to edge computing concerning the state of the art and the prospect of edge computing. Singh et al. [28] depict a comprehensive systematic works investigation of resource administration in the area of cloud in broad and cloud resource planning. Wazir et al. [29] present the various models projected for SLA in cloud computing, to beat on the challenges exists in SLA. Challenges associated with performance, client level fulfillment, safety, profit, and SLA Defilement and additionally discuss SLA design in cloud computing, existing models projected for SLA in several cloud service models like SaaS, PaaS, and IaaS or the benefits and restrictions of present models with the assistance of tables. Padmaja et al. [30] to increment the proficiency of the work load of cloud computing application, programming is the tasks performed to urge most extreme profit. Author mentioned concerning reasons to adopt programming, programming phases, programming sorts, and a few of the programming algorithms utilized in differing kinds of clouds (Table 1).

Table 1 Findings and research gaps

Author	Year	Approach/technique	Findings	Research gaps
Wenjuan Li and Lingdi Ping	2009	Trust model in cross-clouds environment to solve security issues	Experimental results showed the suggested model can competently and securely build trust association in cross-clouds setting	In reality entities behaviors are more complex and there are many other potential security risks
Paul Manue	2014	Trust model built on previous credentials and current abilities of a cloud resource supplier	Showed in what way a facility level arrangement is organized joining excellence of facility necessities of consumer and abilities of cloud store supplier	However, there are some more attributes such as Honesty, Return on Investments and Utilization of Resources to measure trust

(continued)

Table 1 (continued)

Author	Year	Approach/technique	Findings	Research gaps
Rizwana Shaikh and M. Sasi Kumar	2015	Trust model to measure the security strength	Competence of the model is also confirmed by estimating trust worth for present cloud services	
Usvir Kaur and Dheerendra Singh	2015	Trust model for web services	Majority of trust models focused on reviews provided by consumers and providers	
Hyung-Sin Kim	2015	Queue utilization-based RPL (QU-RPL)	Improved the performance of end-to-end packet delivery as compared to the standard RPL significantly	
Bowen Zhou	2015	Context-aware offloading decision algorithm	Proficiency of mobile policies has been upgraded in latest years	Performance of the decision making algorithm can be improved by considering more context parameters, e.g., context of public cloud to provide an optimal solution for code offloading decision making process
Gokulnath and Rhymendthari araj	2016	Analyzed available solutions for cloud trust	Any safety negotiation toward lessening the cost is highly unbearable	As cloud is dynamic and hence needs sophisticated approaches to solve the problem of cloud trust dynamism
Nelson Mimura Gonzalez	2016	Analysis of edge computing concerning the state of the art and the coming of edge work out	Fog computing is quickly moving toward mobile networks and mobile technologies	
Manju Suresh and Neema M	2016	An efficient cryptographic algorithm "Blowfish."	Enhancements in footings of encryption time by 16.9% and output by 18.7%	Implementation of modified Blowfish algorithm in an IoT environment

(continued)

Table 1 (continued)

Author	Year	Approach/technique	Findings	Research gaps
Licai Zhu	2017	Routing protocol with energy equalization	Surviving time of restricted nodes has improved	To make the most of the persistence time of the nodes around the sink, they can be further optimized
Xu W	2018	Hierarchical trust modeling method	Proposed method reduces the complexity of trust computing and assists cloud computing participants to make good trust decisions	
Christos Stergiou	2018	Surveyed various security issues related with the integration of IoT and cloud computing	Benefits of integration of IoT and cloud have discovered	
Ado Adamou	2019	Security and privacy considerations	All records in a CoT system cannot have the similar level of sensitivity. Particular statistics as medicinal or economic data are more delicate than others, and then prerequisite additional care and more care should be reserved for it	The IoT entity secretes large quantity of statistics. So to accomplish the objective of competently handling the huge volume of produced data; the present cloud design needs to be secure. This enhancement is essential to be more effectual and useful for the IoT-based real-time facilities in footings of energy ingesting, safety, confidentiality, and end-to-end delays
Sunil Kumar Malge	2019	Highlights the research status in this field from encryption mechanism, communication safety, protecting sensor data, and encryption procedure		Expansion of the IoT will bring additional thoughtful safety glitches, which are constantly the attention and the key undertaking of the investigation

(continued)

Table 1 (continued)

Author	Year	Approach/technique	Findings	Research gaps
Michele De Donno	2019	Provides an up-to-date and well-structured review of the safety matters of cloud computing in the IoT era	Massive common of attacks presently directed to IoT devices are fueled by trivial faults, such as absence of validation procedures	Formal approaches and rigorous semantics have also not been considered in this work despite their importance for cloud and distributed concurrent systems in general

3 Findings and Research Gaps

4 Conclusion and Future Scope

Hybrid encryption for security of IOT devices can be used for safety in multi-clouds, at user level (to improve the safety of IoT devices) and at sever side (to secure the data before sending to cloud. Attaining good performance at server is conditional and depends on an optimal division of the application mechanism among the IoT devices and cloud platforms that depends on runtime conditions. Implementation of framework consisting of hybrid encryption before uploading the customer records to cloud in vision to safely distribute data among several clouds by trust evaluation is our immediate future work.

References

1. Bonomi F, Milito R, Zhu J, Addepalli S (2012) Fog computing and its role in the internet of things. In: MCC'12, August 17, 2012, ACM 978-1-4503-1519-7/12/08
2. Kutzias D, Falkner J, Kett H (2019) On the complexity of cloud and IoT integration: architectures, challenges and solution approaches. In: Proceedings of the 4th international conference on internet of things, big data and security, pp 376–384
3. Fotouhi H, Moreira D, Alves M, Yomsi PM (2017) mRPL+: a mobility management framework in RPL/6LoWPAN. Comput Commun 104(2017):34–54
4. Dillon T, Wu C, Chang E (2010) Cloud computing: issues and challenges. In: 24th IEEE international conference on advanced information networking and applications
5. Nie T, Zhang T (2009) A study of DES and blowfish encryption algorithm. In: IEEE Reg. 10 Annu. Int. Conf. Proceedings/TENCON, pp 1–4. https://doi.org/10.1109/TENCON.2009.5396115
6. Zhu L, Wang R, Yang H (2017) Multi-path data distribution mechanism based on RPL for energyconsumption and time delay. Information 8(4):1–19. https://doi.org/10.3390/info8040124
7. Patil P, Narayankar P, Narayan DG, Meena SM (2016) A comprehensive evaluation of cryptographic algorithms: DES, 3DES, AES, RSA and Blowfish. Procedia Comput Sci 78:617–624. https://doi.org/10.1016/j.procs.2016.02.108

8. Poonia V, Yadav NS (2015) Analysis of modified Blowfish algorithm in different cases with various parameters. In: ICACCS 2015 - Proceeding 2nd international conference on advanced computing and communication systems, pp 5–9. https://doi.org/10.1109/ICACCS.2015.7324114
9. Suresh M, Neema M (2016) Hardware implementation of blish algorithm for the secure data transmission in internet of things. Procedia Technol 25(Raerest):248–255. https://doi.org/10.1016/j.protcy.2016.08.104.
10. Bruschi R et al (2017) Open stack extension for fog-powered personal services deployment. In: Proceeding of 29th international teletraffic congress ITC 2017, vol 2, pp 19–23. https://doi.org/10.23919/ITC.2017.8065705.
11. Mota AV, Azam S, Shanmugam B, Yeo KC, Kannoorpatti K (2018) Comparative analysis of different techniques of encryption for secured data transmission. In: IEEE International conference on power, control, signals and instrumentation engineering ICPCSI 2017, pp 231–237. https://doi.org/10.1109/ICPCSI.2017.8392158.
12. Stergiou C, Psannis KE, Kim BG, Gupta B (2018) Secure integration of IoT and cloud computing. Futur Gener Comput Syst 78(December 2017), 964–975. https://doi.org/10.1016/j.future.2016.11.031
13. Nandy T et al (2019) Review on security of internet of things authentication mechanism. IEEE Access 7(October):151054–151089
14. Kamgueu PO, Nataf E, Ndie TD (2018) Survey on RPL enhancements: a focus on topology, security and mobility. Comput Commun 120(July 2017):10–21
15. De Donno M, Giaretta A, Dragoni N, Bucchiarone A, Mazzara M (2019) Cyber-storms come fromclouds: security of cloud computing in the IoT era. Futur Internet 11(6), 1–30. https://doi.org/10.3390/fi11060127.
16. Malge S, Singh P (2019) Internet of things IoT: security perspective. Int J Trend Sci Res Dev 3(4):1041–1043. https://doi.org/10.31142/ijtsrd24010
17. Ari AAA et al (2019) Enabling privacy and security in cloud of things: architecture, applications, security and privacy challenges. Appl Comput Inf xxxx. https://doi.org/10.1016/j.aci.2019.11.005
18. Vijayalakshmi V, Vimal S (2019) A new edge computing based cloud system for IoT applications. Int J Recent Technol Eng (IJRTE) 8(2)
19. Kaur C (2020) The cloud computing and internet of things (IoT). Int J Sci Res Sci Eng Technol 7(1) (www.ijsrset.com)
20. Li W, Ping L (2009) Trust model to enhance security and interoperability of cloud environment. Lect. Notes Comput. Sci. (including Subser. Lect. Notes Artif. Intell. Lect. Notes Bioinformatics) 5931:69–79. https://doi.org/10.1007/978-3-642-10665-1_7
21. Manuel P (2015) A trust model of cloud computing based on quality of service. Ann Oper Res 233(1):281–292. https://doi.org/10.1007/s10479-013-1380-x
22. Kaur U, Singh D (2015) Trust: models and architecture in cloud computing. Int J Comput Sci Inf Secur 13(12):150–155
23. Xu W (2018) Study on trust model for multi-users in cloud computing. Int J Netw Secur 20(4), 674–682
24. Kim HS, Paek J, Bahk S (2015) QU-RPL: queue utilization based RPL for load balancing in largescale industrial applications. In: 2015 12th Annu. IEEE Int. Conf. Sensing, Commun. Networking, SECON2015, pp 265–273. https://doi.org/10.1109/SAHCN.2015.7338325
25. Zhou B, Dastjerdi AV, Calheiros RN, Srirama SN, Buyya R (2015) A context sensitive off loading scheme for mobile cloud computing service. In: Proc.—2015 IEEE 8th Int. Conf. Cloud Comput. CLOUD2015, pp 869–876. https://doi.org/10.1109/CLOUD.2015.119
26. Qasem M et al (2018) Load balancing objective function in RPL draft-qasem-roll-rpl-load-balancing-01. Stand Track October:1–10
27. Gonzalez NM, et al. (2016) Fog computing: data analytics and cloud distributed processing on the network edges. In: Proc.—Int. Conf. Chil. Comput. Sci. Soc. SCCC. https://doi.org/10.1109/SCCC.2016.7836028

28. Singh S, Chana I (2015) Q-aware: quality of service based cloud resource provisioning. Computers and electrical engineering. Elsevier Ltd, Amsterdam
29. Wazir U, Khan F, Shah S (2016) Service level agreement in cloud computing: a survey. Int J Comput Sci Inf Secur (IJCSIS) 14(6)
30. Padmaja K, Seshadri R, Anusha P (2016) Different scheduling algorithms in types of clouds. Int J Comput Sci Trends Technol (IJCST) 4(5)

Social Cloud Computing: Architecture and Application

Santosh Kumar and Sandip Kumar Goyal

Abstract With the increase in the use of social networks and cloud computing, users have started a new way to interact with people, including their friends, colleagues, etc. Social networks reflect real-world relationships, which allows users to share information and establish connections with each other, thereby creating dynamic virtual organizations. Cloud applications need to provide a large number of heterogeneous, geographically distributed resources, which are managed and shared by many stakeholders who may or may not know earlier. Online relationships in social networks are usually based on real-world relationships, so they can be used to infer the degree of trust between users. Due to this, many security issues are arising, which, if not addressed carefully, may affect the adoption of this promising computing model. Apt response to these threats is of special significance in the social cloud environment. In the social cloud environment, computing resources are provided by users themselves. We believe that considering trust and reputation requirements can take advantage of security by incorporating the concepts of trust relationship and reputation into these schemes. In this paper, a survey is presented on the social cloud. The article includes its architecture, application on Facebook as a social networking site, and other usages. At last, the relation between trust and reputation is presented that is essential while sharing cloud resources in the social cloud environment.

Keywords Cloud computing · Social networking · Social cloud · Trust · And reputation

S. Kumar (✉) · S. K. Goyal
CSE Department, MMEC, MM (DU), Mullana, Ambala, Haryana, India

N. Marriwala et al. (eds.), *Emergent Converging Technologies and Biomedical Systems*, Lecture Notes in Electrical Engineering 841,
https://doi.org/10.1007/978-981-16-8774-7_2

1 Introduction

Social networks provide individuals with new ways to communicate and share information. For scientists, multiagency collaboration is widespread, but face-to-face meetings usually only happen occasionally in conferences and seminars, so communication is often difficult. Social networks can provide a higher level of scientific co-operation to enhance communication and facilitate the discovery of other scientists working on the same projects. However, scientific co-operation usually also has resources that are expected to be dynamically shared during the course of the project. Currently, this is a difficult process, requiring manual (peer-to-peer) user account registration, and creation, etc. [1].

In this digital lifestyle, social networks play an important role in communicating with friends, family, and colleagues. The rapid and continuous growth of social networking platforms has proved this. For example, Facebook has more than 500 million active users, of which 50% log in every day. A platform for information sharing is provided by social networks so that a real-time model can be established [2]. For example, there are many integrated applications, and some organizations even use users' Facebook credentials for authentication instead of requiring their own credentials (e.g., Calgary Airport Authority, Canada, uses authentication protocol to authenticate users for granting access to its WiFi network).

A social network is a dynamic virtual organization that is structured based on the trust between social users. We recommend that based on this trust, social users can share resources like information, hardware, and services through a social cloud. Cloud system is used to provide services to their users by sharing virtual services rather than accessing physical products. To offer better services to cloud users, cloud providers used an efficient storage cloud. These clouds offered a high level of services to their users. These clouds are also used to enhance the workability of limited storage devices like mobile phones, laptops, and many more and provide data access from anywhere. There are a number of small scales (Nimbus [3], and Eucalyptus [4]) and large-scale (Amazon EC2/S3) cloud providers are available [5]. Access to scalable virtualized resources such as computing, storage, and applications is provided by storage cloud providers through the pre-posted cost-based mechanism. Therefore, the social cloud provides a scalable computing environment in which virtualized resources are contributed by users that is dynamically past participated among a group of friends. The use of compensation is optional because users may wish to share resources without paying but instead use a model based on mutual credit (or bartering) [6]. Before registering users into the cloud environment, the service-level agreement (SLA) is signed. It is an agreement between the service provider and the service users that the services are provided in a quality and cost-efficient manner. Similarly, in the social cloud, SLA is signed between both parties (user and service providers).

Thaufeeg et al. (2011) have believed that the combination of cloud structure with social network offered the following benefits to the scientific community. These include:

(1) During the collaboration, the resources can be shared among scientists. Therefore, scientists who do not have enough computing resources are allowed to make requests to other members of their social cloud. Furthermore, even if other parties do not belong to a specific research group, they can share computing resources through the trust established by the social network.
(2) Social networks can make more effective use of available resources because scientists with the same projects will be encouraged to integrate resources to achieve common goals. In turn, this helps to reduce research costs and save time.
(3) Most importantly, it uses the familiar tools, publicity, and networking opportunities provided by social networks to promote greater collaboration between the scientific communities. In this way, social networking is not only an additional function but is actually the main function of the social cloud.

Like any community, each user of a social network is constrained by limited abilities and capacities. However, in many cases, members like friends in the social cloud may have redundant abilities, and if shared, they can be used to meet changing needs. The social cloud utilizes the pre-established trust relationship between users to realize mutually beneficial sharing in the perspectives of social networks. In the social cloud, data is exchanged between users not only point to point basis but can be shared among the entire social community group.

Chard et al. (2011) have stated that "a social cloud is a resource and service sharing platform that uses the relationship established between members of a social network [7]."

In Sect. 2, the state of the art related to the social cloud is presented. In Sect. 3, the social cloud, along with an example, is explained. Social cloud architecture that includes extra work performed by the social site (Fb) and registration process is discussed in Sect. 4. In Sect. 5, trust and reputation toward the social cloud are discussed. The application Scenario is presented in Sect. 6. The conclusion is presented in Sect. 7, followed by references.

2 Related Work

In this section, the work related to the social cloud, preferably related to trust management, is discussed. The concept of trust and reputation takes advantage of cloud security that can be studied in multiple research articles. Generally, trust and reputation can be utilized to help cloud users to make decisions about the services they want to interact with.

Habib et al. (2014) have explored how these concepts were support users in choosing a trusted cloud provider [8], while **Limam and Butaba (2010)** have proposed a reputation system to enhance the process of selecting external services that can be integrated to the project for further development [9].

Abawajy (2009) has achieved a similar goal by developing a model that suggests cloud users determine the trusted cloud environment [10].

Xiao et al. (2010) have proposed a reputation-based quality of service (QoS) supply model. As far as we know, no proposal aims to establish a unified framework that allows developers to implement existing or new trust models in the social cloud platform. However, there are other platforms or models, the aim of which is to build a trust model for different applications [11].

Singh et al. (2020) have been presented a trust model for e-government to monitor and control government policies using a social cloud environment. The researchers have used the pragmatic scheme to integrate the abilities of both cloud computing and social media platforms. The results show better results while tested to analyze Goods and Services Tax (GST) [12].

Suryanarayana et al. (2006) have presented a 4C framework, in which a trust model is described, which consists of four sub-models that are a content sub-model, communication sub-model, computation sub-model, and reaction sub-model. For all sub-models, the authors have recognized the main building block similar to the pre-existing reputation model. Finally, the researchers have used a Java-based editor and followed a personalized XML mechanism to create an XML document in which the trust model was described based on these components. Then, a PACE support generator has been used to design a software component, which can be merged into the PACE structure [13]. Later on, in the same research article, **Suryanarayana et al. (2006)** have described it further. In this research article, the authors have discussed the feasibility of an event-based structure with full guidelines on how a user can use the trust model in a decentralized app [14].

Huynh (2009) have proposed a personalized trust management model with the goal to replicate the process of trust evaluation that was performed by humans in a computing environment. People have the ability to find out the environment in which to perform a trust assessment, but this is a challenge for computers. To overcome this challenge, the researchers have proposed a policy-based system, which has been designed using semantic technology. Using this concept, the knowledge from different contexts has been gathered, and after applying the semantic approach, the most appropriate trust model based on these contexts has been determined. Although this is an interesting contribution, it focuses only on resolving the perspective dependence of trust. It lacks a framework-oriented scheme because it does not provide guidelines or any application interface to create a new trust model [15].

Yew (2011) has proposed a computational-based trust model and a middleware known by SCOUT. The middleware is composed of three services that have been used to implement the model: evidence collection service, belief formation service, and emotional trust service. Although this is a comprehensive trust model that considers many aspects of human trust, it is not created as an enhanced framework of existing research, and it is not even clear how developers implement the proposed trust models [16].

Encalada and Sequera (2017) have proposed social cloud architecture to provide experimental skills for information technology, which are called Massive Open Online Courses (MOOC). The purpose of this research is to establish a virtual community through various services and resources on the basis of trust, sharing and collaboration, and conduct large-scale, ubiquitous, and open access according to demand. The proposed framework mainly combines three important key aspects, like content, guiding principles, and technology [17].

Adelmeyer et al. (2018) have analyzed the key role of trust and replication, that is, to obtain a certain degree of trust from the directly established trustworthy relationship between a single customer and an intermediary and between online service providers and thereby obtain a certain degree of trust. The results show that there is no large amount of evidence to prove the transfer of trust, that is, the complete distribution of trust among participants in the cloud computing trust chain. The confidence of each customer is distributed between middlemen and cloud service providers. This evidence is important to providers because it can minimize direct trust issues by providing indirect services [18].

Ruan and Durresi (2019) developed a trust management method to defend cloud providers and customers from large-scale attacks. In the link or flow level, the trust level of the node and the task has been considered as a novel security parameter to determine the trust degree and hence calculate the level of security. Here, trustworthiness is used to measure the trust of a system that can be trusted under a specific attack vector. It can be used to reveal the design space of resource allocation so that it can choose the correctness between trustworthiness and the resources used [19].

Ghazvini et al. (2020) proposed a novel multilevel trust management model, which improves the existing method by defining new components to enhance the data quality of feedback storage. In the method proposed here, a new component can solve the inefficiency and sparseness of feedback storage. Some restrictions are deducted; for example, the number of existing feedback levels is invalid because some suspicious cloud users (CU) transmit unfair feedback to modify the trust evaluation value. Choosing a trusted cloud service provider (CSP) is the main challenge for CU because many CSP provides cloud services with the same functions [20].

3 Social Cloud

An individual can be a part of the social network, which is called a "friend." He/she can be added to the social network based on some understanding between the individuals. This kind of connectivity between individuals can be utilized to understand a trust relationship between them. On the other hand, it does not describe the context of trust levels or relationships. For example, "friends" can be family members, colleagues, college friends, sports or dance club members, etc. Presently, FB has created different groups in order to distinguish friends and other communities like colleagues, sports club friends, friend members, etc. The group in the social cloud is created based on the level of trust. For example, users can restrict sharing information with close friends, friends in the same community or group, and other friends [21].

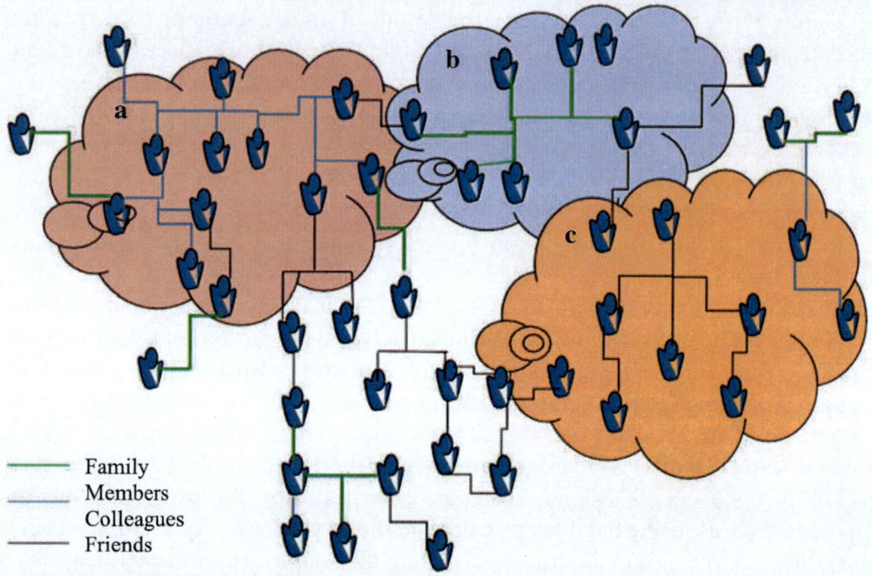

Fig. 1 Example of social cloud Chard et al. [7]

Another way to think about social clouds is to consider social network groups that are similar to dynamic virtual organizations (VO). Like VO, the created groups have some set of rules that define group intent, group membership, and group sharing policies. The related social model is shown in Fig. 1. The example considered three communities that are divided into three groups Group A (colleagues), Group B (family members), and Group C (friends). It is clear that the level of trust between colleagues, friends, and family members is different for all groups.

From Fig. 1, it is seen that the social network users may be a member of any community. For example, in group A, which is considered as the community of colleagues but instead of consisting of colleagues, the group also consists of few family members. Therefore, one can say that social clouds are not mutually exclusive. The group lasts longer and can be used for multiple applications.

4 Social Cloud Architecture

The social cloud structure designed for the Facebook application is shown in Fig. 2.

Social cloud is accessed by the user through Facebook logos by following some set of policies. For example, a user can restrict his or her trade with close friends in the same community and in the same country or region. A dedicated banking component manages credit transfers between users and also stores information related to current reservations.

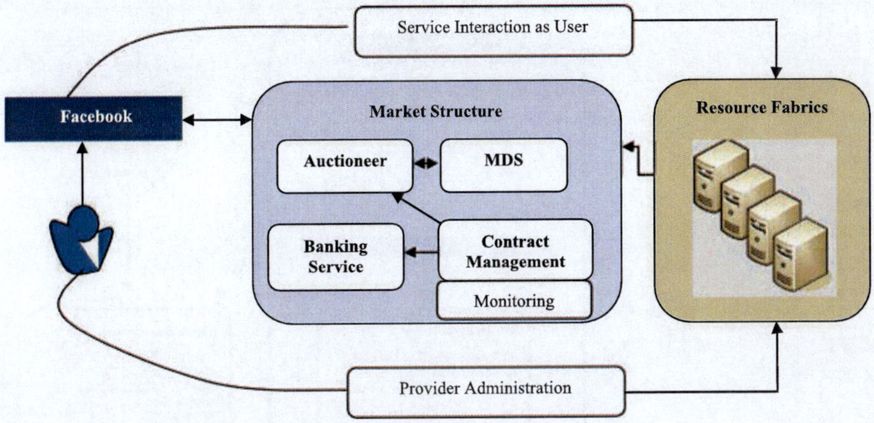

Fig. 2 Social cloud: architecture Chard et al. [22]

4.1 Extra Work Performed by FB

In this section, additional work that has to be performed by the Facebook Application Program Interface (API) in order to discuss its relation with the cloud has been discussed. The outside application can run in the Fb as a user interface; an API-based Fb graph is used to retrieve information and present it as social information. Both users and applications should use the OAuth protocol on Fb for authentication to access the Graph API. This permits the Graph API to display a basic social graph that consists of users along with their interconnections to other nodes in the social graph. This means that people, photos, events, videos, and pages can be accessed visually as well as in the form of a graph. Combining the use of Graph API with a large number of users on Fb can properly demonstrate the concept of social cloud [23]. The Facebook application is hosted independently and outside the Fb environment. An image-based Facebook URL is created for users to access, which is mapped to a remotely hosted user-defined callback URL. The process of accessing the application page is illustrated in Fig. 3. Initially, the user sends a request to the social cloud through the Fb interface that is by login his/her ID and password. The accepted request is then forwarded to the called URL. The application creates a page as per user request and returns it to the Facebook account of the user.

4.2 Registration Process of Social Cloud

The registration process for the user in the social cloud is shown in Fig. 4.

Firstly, the user has to register him/her and then select the services he/she want to access from the social cloud as the user is registered through their FB ID (login and password); therefore, during banking services, user instances can be created transparently by using his/her Fb ID.

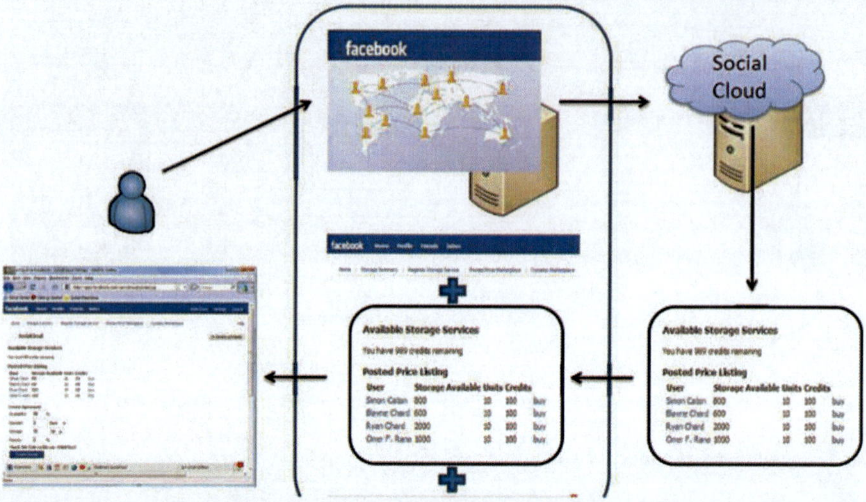

Fig. 3 Page deliver process requested by the social cloud user Chard et al. [22]

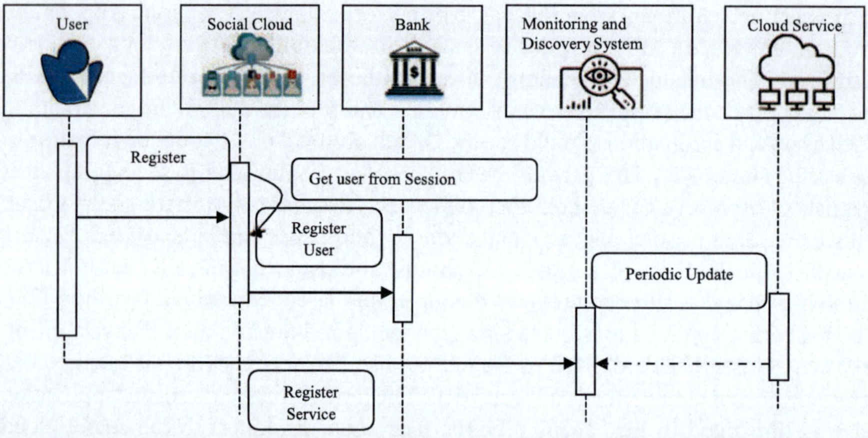

Fig. 4 Social cloud registration process Chard et al. [22]

5 Exploiting Trust in the Cloud: Toward the Social Cloud

To enhance the cloud model in collaborative network environments (such as social networks), trust and reputation are the major issues. Chard et al. (2010) have proposed architecture for the social cloud that basically uses traditional social networks to create a trusted cloud environment, where social cloud users can effortlessly share storage resources of the cloud. The researchers have implemented the prototype by utilizing an API that is provided by Facebook, which allows the use of pre-established trust relationships between friends.

We believe that although this method is interesting and new, it also has a disadvantage: it assumes that the trust relationship completely depends upon the relationship between friends, which is far from the truth. The reason behind this is that social networking users accept friend's requests from known as well as unknown persons who ask for friendship. Moreover, when any of the user's friends start an annoying behavior, the user tried to not finish the relationship because it can be considered as an impolite reaction. On the other hand, due to the status and quality of the services provided, the author does not consider changes in reputation or trust relationships.

For the above reasons, we observed that the need for a more comprehensive approach that considers both trust and reputation requirements from the beginning, and a framework to help developers to build this environment from scratch is required [24].

5.1 Scenario Description of Social Cloud

Developers need to implement social networking sites for cloud providers. Next, briefly explain the purpose and operation of the site to figure out a real situation that requires trust and reputation considerations. To access the services, cloud users have to register on the site. After registration, the web services are published on their sites, and the entire detail related to the web service can be obtained by calling the API app. Web services can find out by the cloud providers based on their needs. Then, these services are used to create larger and mixed web services. After utilizing the services offered by the cloud providers, cloud users have to pay as per the complexity and the type of services. Therefore, the websites are acting as a "software-as-a-service" market among CSP. In the end, each CSP will use its own infrastructure to deliver the final service to its cloud users, although this is beyond the scope of the solution [24].

5.2 Trust and Reputation Requirements

For cloud providers, the core framework should apply trust and reputation requirements to avoid risks and increase site trust.

There are two main influential people in this scenario: Cloud providers and web service providers. The reputation of each provider depends upon the personal opinion or can be obtained from the providers of another site. For example, if the services provided by the CSP are not up to mark, then the user rates it negatively, which affects the reputation of the CSP negatively.

As shown in Fig. 5, when a service holder demands or searches or aims to buy things up for the processing, the cloud service provider looks for the reputation

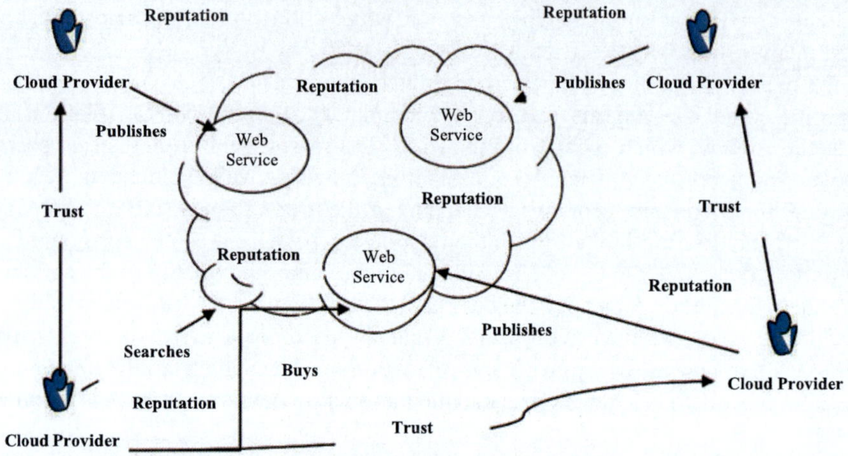

Fig. 5 Trust and reputation scenario Moyano et al. [25]

holders for the selection of the provider. There are various ways through which the reputation can be evaluated and are discussed in the proceeding sections.

In addition to reputation, cloud providers can also establish trust relationships with each other. Although there is a significant relationship exists between trust and reputation, both should be required to be established on the website. The relationship between trust and reputation is shown in Fig. 5. The way to calculate trust and reputation depends on the model being implemented and should provide a mechanism for accessing cloud services to decide which model the user should use while accessing services.

Trust plays a vital role in the selection of a service-oriented architecture for the process of user demand. There are many ways through which trust can be evaluated in the cloud network. There are some of the foremost application architectures and independent evaluation bodies that have already given evaluation methods and architecture [26]. In the trust evaluation, there are certain aspects that have been discussed and are illustrated as follows in Fig. 6.

There are several factors that are responsible for the evaluation of trust in the real-time network. Some of the parameters are well known, whereas some of the parameters are strictly performance-oriented. As shown in Fig. 6, trust has four evaluation factors, namely co-work, co-location, co-operations, and performance. Two people are said to be in work relation if they work together. Co-operations are similar to co-work with the difference that two people should have worked at least once in order to come under co-operations, including the fact that the produced outcome should be positive. If all the aspects are combined, it will form an equation as follows

$$T = \mu \times W1 + \rho \times W2 + \epsilon \times W3 \qquad (1)$$

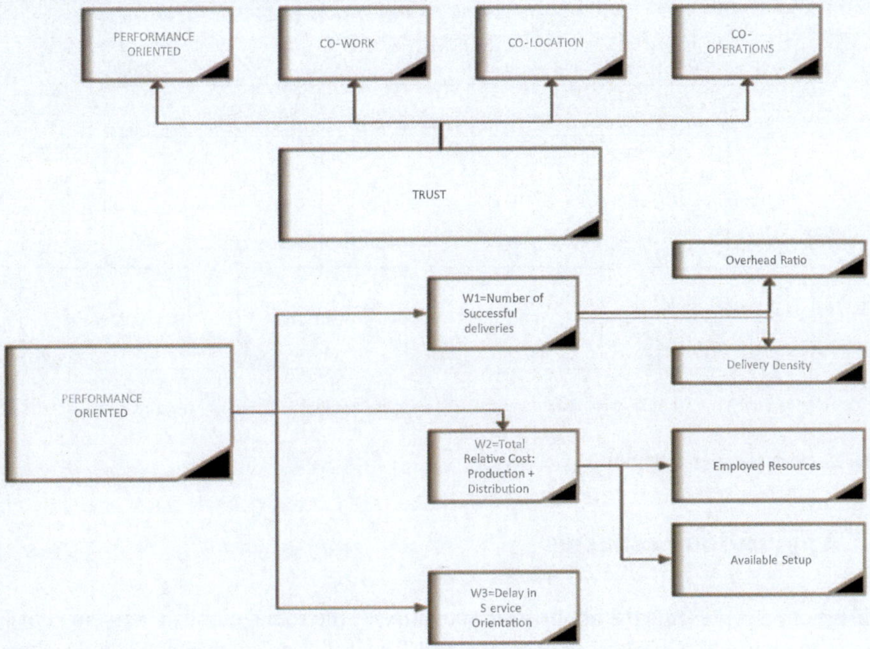

Fig. 6 Trust evaluation and factors

where $W1$, $W2$, and $W3$ are converted factors attained from the trust model, and μ, ρ and €are coefficients that may increase with the increase in the factors affecting the trust model. This paper takes the service contrast in action and analyzes how reputation can be generated using the service factor. It is not necessary that if a user is associated with another user in any term of work, the second user will provide the best facilities for the desired work. Hence, an analytical model evaluation is required based on the services provided by the user in the past.

Based on the service orientation, two feedback architectures have been studied and used in the modern frame. The first one is called direct feedback, and another one is called transactional feedback. Direct feedback is attained when a person demands work from another user and develop a feedback mechanism on his own based on the type of service he/she gets. The transitional feedback involves a lot of other processing that the user exhibits in the current network. All the work areas are different, and their attained potentials are also different, and hence to use them, it has to be bring brought to one scale. There are different methods of normalization and scaling, as shown in Fig. 7 [27].

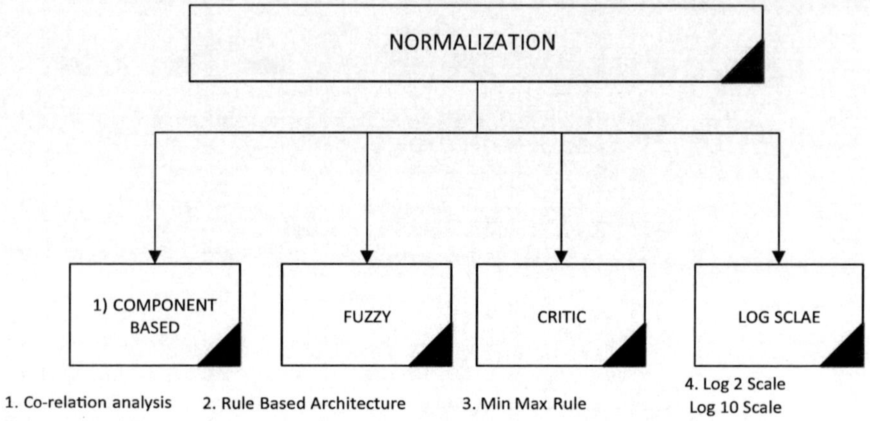

Fig. 7 Normalization methods

6 Application Scenarios

This section represents the application scenarios of the social cloud. There are enormous benefits while one uses the social cloud. The difference with social cloud is that applications can use user relationships to provide or shared resources and services.

A social computation cloud: It is common for personal computers not to use large amounts of computing power. Using the social cloud, an infrastructure is provided where users can easily share computing resources among friends or groups.

A social storage cloud: Storage is one of the simplest and easiest ways to share resource whenever cloud user needs in a social cloud environment. Online storage is mostly used by cloud users to save, backup, and to create a duplicate copy of the data. An open use for social storage cloud is to store and share multimedia data such as photos. Although most social networks like Facebook, Twitter, Instagram, etc., already save photos, to balance the load, these photos can be moved from the service providers to their members so that the scalability can be increased with the reduction in infrastructure cost.

A collaborative social cloud: Increasingly, collaborations are turning the concept of social networking that can be used to share information as well as resources within diverse user communities. The usefulness of the social cloud can be realized by hosting it in the existing social networks. Storage services can be utilized to save or share data (e.g., academic papers, scientific workflows, databases, and analysis, etc.).

A social cloud for public science: Social cloud provides a platform for a scientist to solve complex problems by using communities of social networks. There are a number of projects that are working as volunteer computing to solve the problem; one such project is Berkeley Open Infrastructure for Network Computing (BOINC) [28]. This project requires a large amount of computing power from the available resources. Using the social cloud, resources of social networking sites are utilized in an efficient manner with the aim to provide services to the social users with high service-level agreement (SLA).

An enterprise Social Cloud: Depending on the community social cloud serves, the configuration of it may vary. For all organizations, it is mainly common for all; for example, educational institutes like schools, colleges, and universities all have a public cloud. This offers great opportunities for a professional organization with the social cloud. The users get double benefits. That is, one is from the available sources, and the other is from the shared resources [7].

7 Conclusion

This article introduced social cloud computing, which the integration of cloud is computing and social networks. The uniqueness of the social cloud is that it provides heterogeneous resource transactions based on the inherent social motivation in social networks and the external real-world relationship. The architecture and registration process of social clouds and extra work performed by Fb has been discussed. The trust relationship established by the face book user to discover and use cloud storage space with their friends and communities has been discussed. Also, a trust framework that can help developers to implement applications that need to consider trust and reputation requirements has been presented. Such applications are appearing steadily in response to users' growing needs eager to share their information in collaborative environments. With the increase in blogging and social networking sites, social cloud applications take a step forward by turning users into service providers, which raises a lot of security and trust issues. This requires a holistic approach to solve these problems. We believe that trust and reputation requirements have become particularly important elements to take advantage of the security and promote the adoption of such applications.

References

1. Thaufeeg AM, Bubendorfer K, Chard K (2011) Collaborative eresearch in a social cloud. In: 7th international conference on eScience. IEEE, pp 224–231
2. Foster I, Kesselman C, Tuecke S (2001) The anatomy of the grid: enabling scalable virtual organizations. Int J High Perform Comput Appl 15(3):200–222
3. Keahey K, Foster I, Freeman T, Zhang X (2005) Virtual workspaces: achieving quality of service and quality of life in the grid. Sci Program 13
4. Nurmi D, Wolski R, Grzegorczyk C, Obertelli G, Soman S, Youseff L, Zagorodnov D (2009) The eucalyptus open-source cloud-computing system. In: 9th IEEE/ACM international symposium on cluster computing and the grid. IEEE, pp 124–131
5. Cutillo LA, Molva R, Strufe T (2009) Safebook: a privacy-preserving online social network leveraging on real-life trust. IEEE Commun Mag 47(12):94–101

6. Andrade N, Brasileiro F, Mowbray M, Cirne W, Buyya R, Bubendorfer K (2009) A reciprocation-based economy for multiple services in a computational grid. In: Market oriented grid and utility computing. Wiley Press, Hoboken, pp 357–370
7. Chard K, Bubendorfer K, Caton S, Rana OF (2011) Social cloud computing: a vision for socially motivated resource sharing. IEEE Trans Serv Comput 5(4):551–563
8. Habib SM, Ries S, Muhlhauser M (2010) Cloud computing landscape and research challenges regarding trust and reputation. In: 7th international conference on ubiquitous intelligence and computing and 7th international conference on autonomic and trusted computing. IEEE, pp 410–415
9. Limam N, Boutaba R (2010) Assessing software service quality and trustworthiness at selection time. IEEE Trans Software Eng 36(4):559–574
10. Abawajy J (2009) Determining service trustworthiness in intercloud computing environments. In: 10th international symposium on pervasive systems, algorithms, and networks. IEEE, pp 784–788
11. Xiao Y, Lin C, Jiang Y, Chu X, Shen X (2010) Reputation-based QoS provisioning in cloud computing via dirichlet multinomial model. In: International conference on communications. IEEE, pp 1–5
12. Singh P, Dwivedi YK, Kahlon KS, Sawhney RS, Alalwan AA, Rana NP (2020) Smart monitoring and controlling of government policies using social media and cloud computing. Inf Syst Front 22(2):315–337
13. Suryanarayana G, Diallo M, Taylor RN (2006) A generic framework for modeling decentralized reputation-based trust models. In: 14th ACM SigSoft symposium on foundations of software engineering
14. Suryanarayana G, Diallo MH, Erenkrantz JR, Taylor RN (2006) Architectural support for trust models in decentralized applications. In: 28th international conference on software engineering, pp 52–61
15. Huynh TD (2009) A personalized framework for trust assessment. In: Proceedings of the 2009 ACM symposium on applied computing, pp 1302–1307
16. Yew CH (2011) Architecture supporting computational trust formation
17. Encalada WL, Sequera JLC (2017) Social cloud for information technology skills: an experience with Universities in Ecuador. IEEE Revista Iberoamericana de Tecnologias del Aprendizaje 12(2):76–85
18. Adelmeyer M, Walterbusch M, Biermanski P, Teuteberg F (2018) Trust transitivity and trust propagation in cloud computing ecosystems
19. Ruan Y, Durresi A (2019) A trust management framework for clouds. Comput Commun 144:124–131
20. Ghazvini GA, Mohsenzadeh M, Nasiri R, Rahmani AM (2020) A new multi-level trust management framework (MLTM) for solving the invalidity and sparse problems of user feedback ratings in cloud environments. J Supercomput 1–29
21. Lin N (2002) Social capital: a theory of social structure and action. Cambridge University Press, Cambridge
22. Chard K, Caton S, Rana O, Bubendorfer K (2010) Social cloud: cloud computing in social networks. In: 3rd international conference on cloud computing. IEEE, pp 99–106
23. Chang V (2017) A cybernetics social cloud. J Syst Softw 124:195–211
24. Moyano F, Fernandez-Gago C, Lopez J (2021) A conceptual framework for trust models. In: International conference on trust, privacy and security in digital business. Springer, Berlin, Heidelberg, pp 93–104
25. Moyano F, Fernandez-Gago C, Lopez J (2013) A framework for enabling trust requirements in social cloud applications. Requirements Eng 18(4):321–341
26. Chahal RK, Kumar N, Batra S (2020) Trust management in social internet of things: a taxonomy, open issues, and challenges. Comput Commun 150:13–46

27. Žižović M, Miljković B, Marinković D (2020) Objective methods for determining criteria weight coefficients: a modification of the CRITIC method. Decis Mak Appl Manag Eng 3(2):149–161
28. Anderson DP (2004) Boinc: a system for public-resource computing and storage. In: Fifth IEEE/ACM international workshop on grid computing. IEEE, pp 4–10

A Systematic Approach for Evading Antiviruses Using Malware Obfuscation

Keshav Kaushik, Harshpreet Singh Sandhu, Neelesh Kumar Gupta, Naman Sharma, and Rohit Tanwar

Abstract Investigators and malware creators are getting neck to neck in the competition and thinking of new deadly implements in their fields. Normally, malware such as viruses and others are detected by looking for a string of bits, which is present in the virus or malware. These strings are considered as the "fingerprint" of the malware. Malware creators are utilizing novel modern methods like metamorphosis to foil recognition instruments while security experts are sprouting better approaches to defy them. Today, virus scholars regularly cover their viruses by utilizing code confusion procedures with an end goal to defeat signature-based discovery plans. Metamorphic viruses are those in which their uses are slightly similar but they differentiate in their inner structure. Both metamorphic viruses and polymorphic viruses are different in the technique they use to concealing the mark. While metamorphic viruses conceal their mark by manipulating their own code, polymorphic viruses principally depend on encryption for signature confusion. In this paper, we have shown that we can bypass virus detection on different platforms (operating system). The authors have compared the three methods for bypassing the antivirus Veil–Evasion, Graffiti, code obfuscation and have uncovered their results. Eventually, we give our methodology to make any virus imperceptible utilizing various procedures.

Keywords Obfuscation · Antivirus · Veil–Evasion · Malware · Malicious · Graffiti · Virus total · Antivirus bypass

K. Kaushik (✉) · R. Tanwar (✉)
Department of Systemics School of Computer Science, University of Petroleum and Energy Studies, Dehradun, India

H. S. Sandhu · N. K. Gupta · N. Sharma
Bachelors of Technology in Computer Science, University of Petroleum & Energy Studies Dehradun, India

K. Kaushik · H. S. Sandhu · N. K. Gupta · N. Sharma · R. Tanwar
School of Computer Science, University of Petroleum and Energy Studies, Dehradun, Uttarakhand, India

N. Marriwala et al. (eds.), *Emergent Converging Technologies and Biomedical Systems*, Lecture Notes in Electrical Engineering 841,
https://doi.org/10.1007/978-981-16-8774-7_3

1 Introduction

In the present age, where a greater part of the exchanges including delicate data access occurs on systems and over the network, it is first thing to consider data security as a worry of fundamental significance. Malware and system viruses are there from the very starting of the computer systems and consider as a regular threat to home and undertaking clients the same. A computer virus is a pernicious bit of programming that adjusts different records to infuse its code. A code of virus varies from virus to virus. Virus identification is a dubious measure. As against virus advancements developed to battle these viruses, the virus developers keep on changing their strategies and method of activity so that virus prediction and identification become more complex, and the battle between them continues forever. Antivirus frameworks utilize different location methods including signature recognition what is more, code copying to identify malware. Signature-based tools tries to found the specific signature while code emulators execute virus in a virtual atmosphere for recognizable proof. The most mainstream virus discovery procedure utilized today is signature-based technique, which includes searching for a fingerprint—bits taken out from a known example of the virus in the speculate record. To dodge code imitating strategies, different strategies of copying methods have been created by the malware creators. These incorporate, Entry Point Obscuring (EPO) strategies, unscrambling and executing code piece by lump, utilizing odd guidelines those bamboozle an impersonator, irregular disguising of unscrambling, and wide circling through dead code, numerous encryption layers. Veil-Framework is an assortment of tools that help with data assembling and post-exploitation. One such tool is Veil–Evasion which is utilized for making payloads that can undoubtedly sidestep antivirus utilizing known and archived procedures. This is done through a variety of encoding plans that change the marks of records significantly enough to dodge standard recognition methods. Graffiti is a tool that can create obfuscated payloads utilizing a wide range of encoding methods. It offers a variety of one-liners and shells in languages, for example, Python, Perl, PHP, Batch, PowerShell, and Bash. Payloads can be encoded utilizing base64, hex, and AES256, among others. It additionally includes two methods of activity: command-line mode and interactive mode. Other valuable highlights of Graffiti incorporate the capacity to make your own payload records, terminal history, and the choice to run local OS commands, and tab-completion in interactive mode. Graffiti should work out of the case on Linux, Mac, and Windows, and it tends to be introduced to the framework as an executable on both Linux and Mac. We will utilize Kali Linux to investigate the tool beneath.

2 Related Work

Unique dispute is that the payload is encoded into different choices like Xor, Base64, Hex, ROT13, and Raw. Fundamental thought behind it is we are attempting to change the signature of the payload as to sidestep the generally present signatures of payloads in the database of the antivirus. From a virus identification perspective, it is significantly harder to distinguish viruses which do not convey their own signatures. After the payload is produced, it is then encoded making it imperceptible for the antivirus. Once the code is divided into blocks, the request for code blocks should be haphazardly rearranged. Later we rearranged blocks; spitted blocks of dead code (also called trash code) must be embedded between blocks of unique code. Dead code happens to be square of code, which is linguistically right yet semantically immaterial to the set of instructions being executed. When dead code is added in the code, the right progression of the infectious code is constrained by the outcome accomplished from a numerical condition that consistently registers to equivalent system. The main objective is to utilize a condition that consistently brings about a similar outcome (condition continuously obvious or in every case bogus) and yet is an adequately unpredictable articulation that it is troublesome break down from assembly code. Evading antivirus is regularly overlooked craftsmanship that can represent the moment of truth a penetration test. Current antivirus items can recognize meterpreter payloads effectively and can leave a pen-tester dishonestly accepting a framework is not exploitable. Antivirus has a troublesome work; it needs to sort out if a document is malicious in an amazingly short measure of time to not affect the client experience. It is critical to comprehend antivirus sidestep strategies to plan all-encompassing security that ensures your association. Two normal techniques utilized by antivirus answers to look for malicious programming are heuristic and signature-based scans. Signature-based filtering checks the type of a document, searching for strings and capacities that coordinate a known bit of malware. Heuristic-based filtering takes a gander at the capacity of a document, utilizing calculations and examples to attempt to decide whether the product is accomplishing something dubious.

From a defense point of view, most antivirus arrangements are signature-based. Disentangled, these frameworks looks for executables and different records for different kind of characters, known to happen in explicit bits of malware/payload. On the off chance that a record contains precisely the same set of bits as one of the strings in the antivirus's saved database, the document is distinguished as malware [1]; else it will not. From the hacking point of view, considers had demonstrated that approx. 22k new strains of malware show up consistently [2]. For an antivirus based on signature, to precisely recognize every one of these strains, it would require information on each and every strain delivered. By and by, this seems, to be a nearly impossible task—unquestionably some payloads or malware will undoubtedly be missed. First analyzing whether bits of payload or malware will be distinguished by different antivirus systems and later by matching empirical studies about detection rates later on will outline such difficult task.

A Payload.dll containing an insignificant to recognize Windows, shellcode, (e.g., a totally un-encoded or decoded payload) at that point Windows Defender can be produced that will positively distinguish your DLL as harmful and quarantine the document. As such, you should even now encode your shellcode that will be stacked from the DLL to guarantee that it bypasses signature-based recognition. Graffiti currently underpins producing scrambled payloads that permits to make a payload scrambled with RC4, AES256 or encoded yield utilizing Base64 or XOR. It happens that basically XOR encoding your payload routine is adequate and utilizing the implicit "x86/xor dynamic" encoder is everything necessary to create a sans signature DLL. Regardless of Windows Defender offering critical improved recognition recently for basic schedules and created parallels, it is as yet unimportant to sidestep and offers little security against meterpreter. Anyway, all things considered, this will get identified soon and as such a variety of this ought to be adjusted for your own employments. We strongly suggest utilizing Windows CryptoAPI and utilizing an AES256 encoded payload to additionally hinder recognition of shellcode inside a payload.dll, left as an activity to the reader, anyway XOR appears to be entirely adequate as of now.

We can simply alter and execute these scripts or codes into OS like Linux and Windows. There is least probability to get contracted by antivirus arrangements, and this is the most successful technique to dodge antivirus in the event that you can't compose malware without anyone else. Antivirus avoidance toolboxes work for brief timeframe, until unless they are not leaked to antivirus sellers. Later, when antiviruses companies improve their system's databases and strategies, organizations can without much of a stretch perceive malware produced by toolboxes. That is the reason minor changes in the already available shell codes on the net always help. We can discover many payloads or reverse shell codes on the web, just simply change IP address and the associated port number and we can pass through majority of the defense systems of antivirus systems in less than an hour without composing a single line of code.

3 Working Methodology

3.1 *Obfuscate with Graffiti*

It is energizing to get that reverse shell or execute a payload, yet some of the time these things do not function true to form when there are sure protections in play. One approach to get around that issue is by obfuscating the payload, and encoding it utilizing various procedures will typically bring differing levels of accomplishment. Graffiti can get that going. Graffiti is a tool that can produce obfuscated payloads utilizing a wide range of encoding strategies. It offers a variety of jokes and shells in dialects, for example, Python, Perl, PHP, Batch, PowerShell, and Bash. Payloads

	Veil evasion	Graffiti
Output Format	.py , .bat, .exe	Text format
Server	RPC server	Local
Supported Operating system	Windows, Linux	Windows, Linux

Fig. 1 Obfuscating with Graffiti

can be encoded utilizing base64, hex, and AES256, among others. It additionally includes two methods of activity: command-line mode and interactive mode.

Other helpful highlights of Graffiti [3] incorporate the capacity to make your own payload documents, terminal history, and the choice to run local OS commands, and tab-fulfillment in intelligent mode. Graffiti should work out of the crate on Linux, Mac, and Windows, and it tends to be introduced to the framework as an executable on both Linux and Mac (Fig. 1).

3.2 Obfuscate with Code

The sequence of changes performed by our code obfuscation engine is appeared in Fig. 2. The payload is right off the bat created in the bat record organization and this code is recognized by a large portion of the antivirus so we need to transform it. We can change the.bat record into a.exe document and around then we can change the code. Here, we have eliminated the if-else proclamation, and it works for me. It will bring about the detours of the antivirus.

If-else Deletion: We need to see which portion of code is required, and as indicated by this, we can kill the if-else explanation so the code can vary from the genuine payload document.

Dead Code Insertion: We can add some important code to the payload with the goal that it will contrast with the real payload. Much the same as we added some additional alternatives of PowerShell code; however, they are redundant for the execution of the payload. We can add to vary the payload from the genuine.

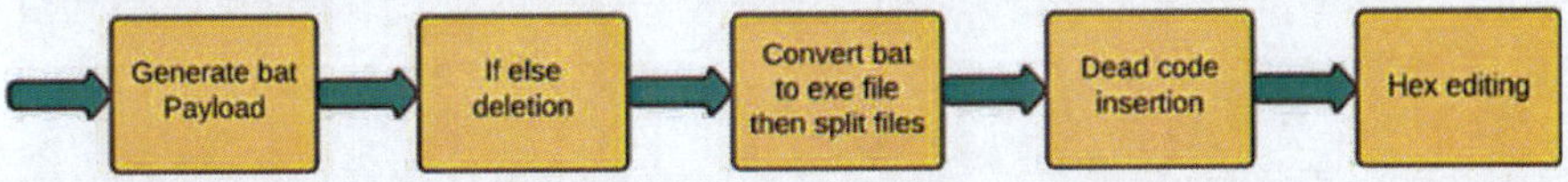

Fig. 2 Code obfuscation measure in our metamorphic engine

4 Results and Comparison

These are the payloads Graffiti have, and we can use any of them to evade the antivirus. These payloads can be encoded in different algorithms to not catch by the antivirus. Most of time, they can be caught by antivirus, so then we have to manipulate or make some changes to them. Graffiti is not as much effective to evade the antivirus, it is detected by most of the antivirus. Like see the image below, PowerShell is not running the base64 encoded payload. Therefore, we need to edit this or try some other way to bypass it (Fig. 3).

Obfuscate with Veil–Evasion: Veil–Evasion is another famous framework written in python. We can utilize this framework to produce payloads that can sidestep most of AVs. The Evasion device is utilized to create a scope of various payloads with the capacity to evade [4] standard endpoint antivirus. Like polymorphic malware [5], Veil-Evasion makes a remarkable payload for which no mark should exist and can, subsequently dodge against antivirus. This gives it an unmistakable bit of leeway over other payload generators. We have generated a payload, which is a reverse tcp meterpreter [6] PowerShell payload by using Veil as shown in image below (Fig. 4).

This payload is also detectable by most of the antivirus. Therefore, it is required to convert it into exe file, and at this time, there is a need to change some part of code to make it undetectable.

The below is PowerShell code in which there is two conditions with if and else. One is if processor architecture is x86, and the other is else part which will run in any other case. So, it is deleted the x86 part because the system has 64-bit processor architecture. This will result as image below (Figs. 5 and 6).

After this, the Windows 10 defender is successfully bypassed and the payload work smoothly. This new code with the meterpreter implanted inside will move beyond most AV programming and security gadgets. Like whatever else, the AV developers will probably figure out how to identify even the above payload, so be inventive and attempt other payload muddling techniques in Veil–Evasion until you discover one that shrouds your payload. Evading security programming and gadgets are among the main errands of the hacker, and Veil–Evasion is another tool in our munitions stockpile. Remember, however, that there will never be a single, last solution. The hacker should be persevering and innovative in discovering ways past these gadgets, so in the event that one strategy comes up short, attempt another, at that point attempt another, until you discover one that works.

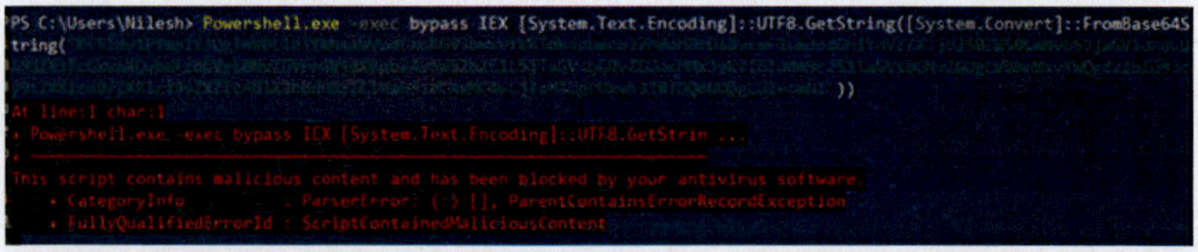

Fig. 3 Executing PowerShell

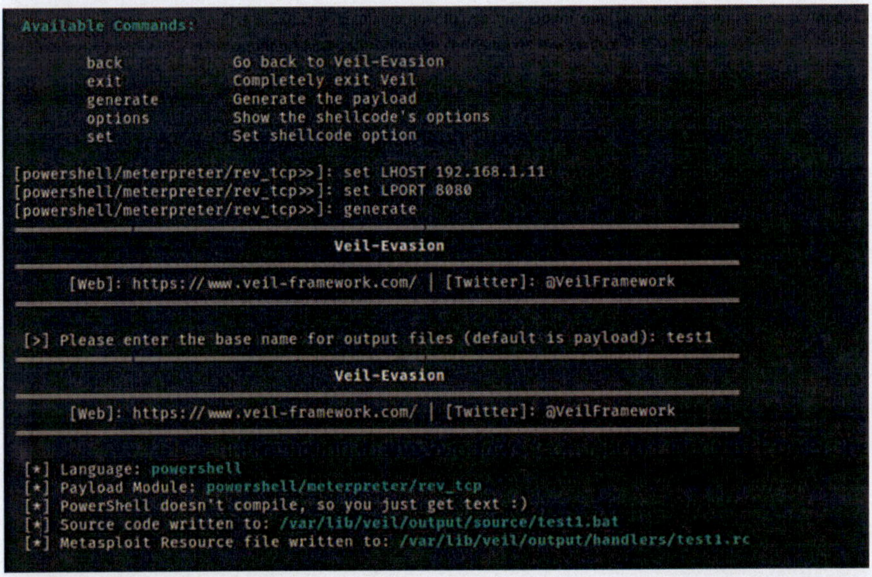

Fig. 4 Executing Veil-Evasion

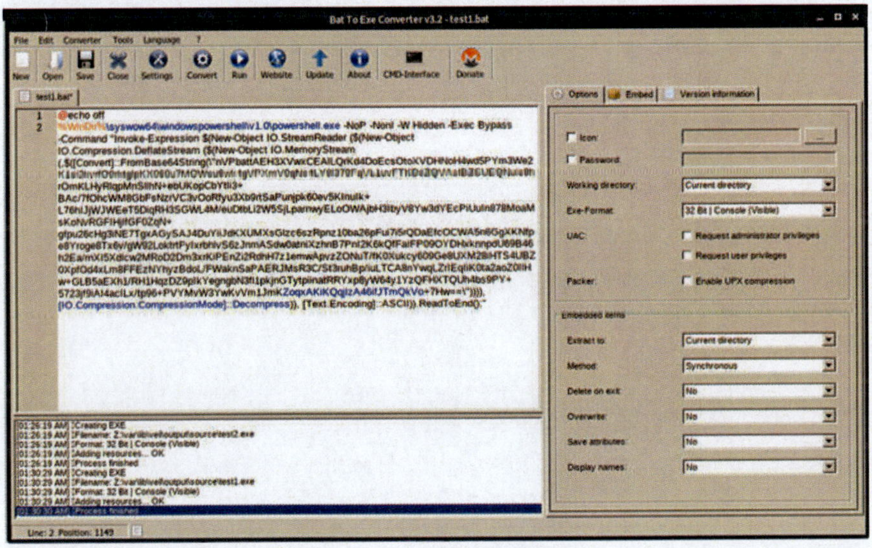

Fig. 5 Output of Veil-Evasion

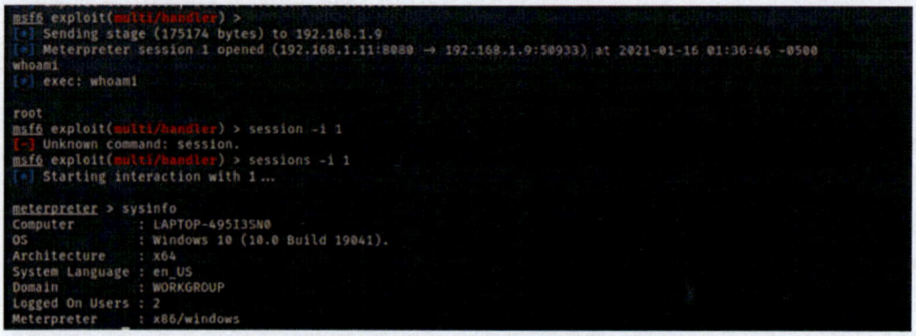

Fig. 6 Malicious payload

Comparison: Graffiti offers us numerous highlights like making own payload documents to run local orders. It likewise offers to encode payloads utilizing base64, hex and Aes256, and so forth still it does not come out as a solid method to change signature of the virus to bypass against virus. There are some different devices for performing comparative sort of errand like Veil invasion and Shellter yet both offer better payloads for bypassing the counter virus. As of now examined technique for bypassing, it came out that we can utilize Shellter to make payload and gap it into blocks; at last getting a more modest square to modify bits. Finally, it will go through antivirus without disturbing any notices. At the point, when checked at VirusTotal just barely any enemy of virus had the option to distinguish the first signature of the payload (Fig. 7).

Fig. 7 Virus total comparison of Veil–Evasion and Graffiti

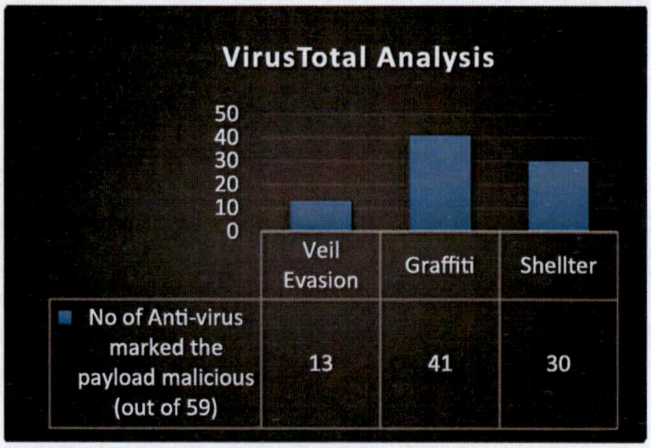

5 Conclusion

We have shown effectively that we can easily make a malware undetectable utilizing code obfuscation strategies implementing insignificant changes by finding the particular signature. A big challenge for the antivirus companies to cook this improved set of malware or virus that are based on metamorphic methods. Code obfuscation utilization also demonstrated that size of the malware or payload was not changed much. Each virus has its specific size, and after implementation, it still remained unnoticeable. Indeed, we were able to achieve same usefulness as of the first virus while accomplishing its untraceable behavior. Hence, we suggest a technique for creating transformed duplicates of an easily available payload or virus that have a similar usefulness as the available payload or virus and have negligible size difference of the transformed duplicates. At last, we conclude that code obfuscation can be applied where signature of the payload or malware is distinguished in the available payload or virus. In the future, we can work on building a metamorphic system that mechanizes this cycle. The best system to dodge protector is to make your own obfuscate tools whether that be with a custom obfuscator or transforming them physically by hand. There is a major obfuscation local area with way bigger obfuscation projects then this one, so another conceivable course is to alter one of those tools barely enough as to not get captured by their old signatures.

References

1. Infinity.wecabrio.com (2021) Download learning malware analysis. explore the concepts, tools, and techniques to analyze and investigate windows malware. http://infinity.wecabrio.com/1788392507-learning-malware-analysis-explore-the-concepts-to.pdf. Accessed 19 Jan 2021
2. Panda Security (2008) Creation of new malware increases by 26 percent to reach more than 73,000 samples every day, PandaLabs reports—Panda Security Mediacenter. https://www.pandasecurity.com/en/mediacenter/press-releases/creation-of-new-malware-increases-by-26-percent-to-reach-more-than-73000-samples-everyday-pandalabs-reports/ (accessed Dec. 29, 2021)
3. WonderHowTo (2021) Bypass antivirus software by obfuscating your payloads with graffiti. https://null-byte.wonderhowto.com/how-to/bypass-antivirus-software-by-obfuscating-your-payloads-with-graffiti-0215787/. Accessed 19 Jan 2021
4. WonderHowTo (2021) Hack like a Pro: how to evade AV software with Shellter. https://null-byte.wonderhowto.com/how-to/hack-like-pro-evade-av-software-with-shellter-0168504/. Accessed 19 Jan 2021
5. En.wikipedia.org (2021) Polymorphic code. https://en.wikipedia.org/wiki/Polymorphic_code. Accessed 19 Jan 2021
6. Scriptjunkie.us (2021) Why encoding does not matter and how Metasploit generates EXE'S. Thoughts on Security. https://www.scriptjunkie.us/2011/04/why-encoding-does-not-matter-and-how-metasploit-generates-exes/. Accessed 19 Jan 2021

Development of Wi-Fi-Based Weather Station WSN-Node for Precision Irrigation in Agriculture 4.0

Dushyant Kumar Singh and Rajeev Sobti

Abstract Agriculture sector utilizes almost 80% of the available fresh water for irrigation. Conventional irrigation practices are very inefficient and add to fresh water scarcity drastically. Agriculture 4.0 is the technology that can be adopted for precision irrigation. Evapotranspiration, soil and crop transpiration are the major factors that decides the demand of irrigation. To estimate the evapotranspiration, soil and crop transpiration local weather condition needs to be gathered, for which local weather station are required. The development of Internet of things (IoT)-based weather station wireless senor network node (WSN) is discussed in the present work. The weather station node developed gathers the air temperature, humidity, wind conditions and provides the data to the IoT cloud server. In the end, challenges in front of WSN Agriculture 4.0 are discussed.

Keywords Air temperature · Crop transpiration · Evapotranspiration · Internet of things · Relative humidity · Soil transpiration · Weather station · Wind direction · Wind speed · WSN

1 Introduction

Precision agriculture (PA) and Agriculture 4.0 aim to modernize agriculture sector by focusing on farmer's behavior and operation management. IoT is one of the main elements of Agriculture 4.0. Various researchers have highlighted the potentials of Agriculture 4.0 as shown in Fig. 1.

Along with discussing the various IoT sensing technologies, including weather station, the article has also highlighted that little research is available for Agriculture 4.0, and the pace of adoption of PA is quite slow. Weather stations are used to capture

D. K. Singh (✉) · R. Sobti
Lovely Professional University, Phagwara, Punjab, India

R. Sobti
e-mail: rajeev.sobti@lpu.co.in

N. Marriwala et al. (eds.), *Emergent Converging Technologies and Biomedical Systems*, Lecture Notes in Electrical Engineering 841,
https://doi.org/10.1007/978-981-16-8774-7_4

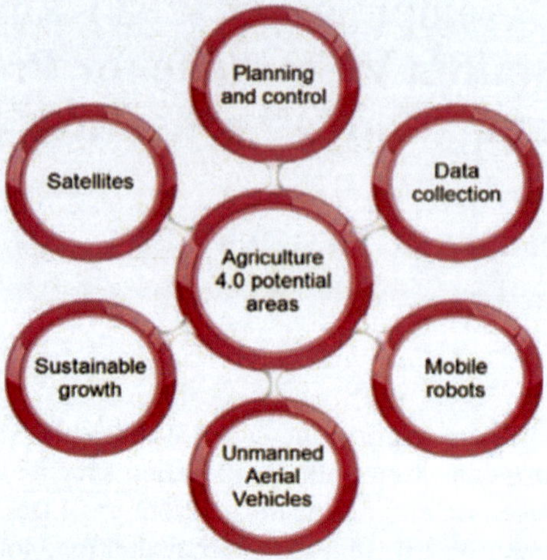

Fig. 1 Potentials of agriculture 4.0

relative humidity, temperature for evaluating evapotranspiration. Evapotranspiration plays an important role in irrigation planning [1].

PA uses information technology, proximity data collection and remote sensing for farm management. With these technologies, the article has analyzed different industrial/agricultural facilities to propose new functionalities in agriculture. IoT has also opened various opportunities in soil cultivation (with low-cost sensors and actuators) and communication technologies. The different opportunities highlighted in papers provided by Agriculture 4.0 are shown in Fig. 2.

2 Literature Review

In the recent times, environment conditions are unpredictable and make framer's life miserable. Farmers are not able to take proper decision time. In such situations, local weather stations with real-time data monitoring and reporting are the need of time. They keep the farmers informed about the local weather conditions. The important weather parameters considered are air humidity, air temperature, wind speed, wind direction, rainfall, and precipitation [2, 3].

In [4], design of intelligent weather station is discussed capable of capturing solar radiations, air temperature, relative humidity, and wind speed and wind direction. The proposed design exploits artificial neural networks (ANN) to make the system intelligent.

Temperature measured by the weather stations is used to forecast the electricity demand. Proposed framework for the selection of weather stations, number of weather stations, and type of weather stations for a particular territory is discussed. The proposed framework is implemented in seven steps [5].

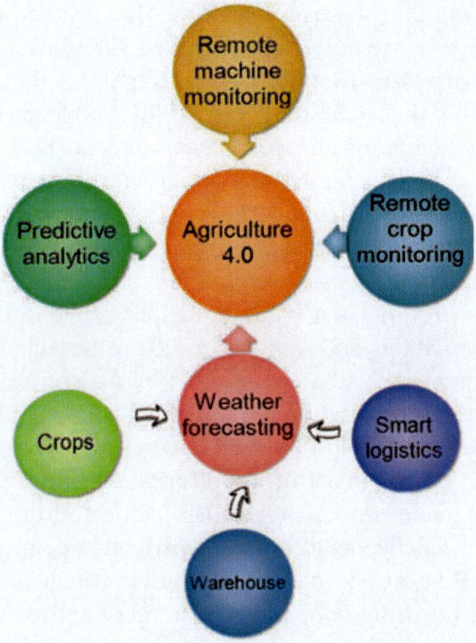

Fig. 2 IoT opportunities in precision agriculture

Temporal convolution neural (TCN), a better approach for weather forecasting, is proposed. The proposed TCN is claimed to be better than the conventional long short-term memory method. The article also highlights the main component of local weather stations as shown in Fig. 3 [6].

The design of weather station over the time has changed due to advancement in technology and lesson learned from past experience in the field. The article discusses design of weather station developed by Geological Survey of Denmark and Greenland. The paper also provides the different weather parameters being monitored along with the height of each sensor at which they are installed [7].

Weather station data of April 2014 Mount Everest avalanche has been provided and discussed. The data reveals approximately 0.8 °C warming of Mount Everest.

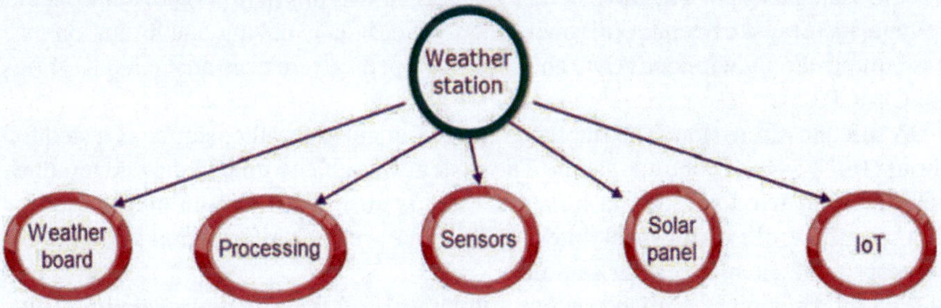

Fig. 3 Main components of local weather stations

Warming of the Mount Everest has resulted 100–300 m rise in height of permanently frozen ground and thinning of the glacier. The weather station data observed is situated in Khumbu valley, Nepal, height of about 140 m above the valley floor. This shows the important of local weather stations in observing and analyzing the behavior and changes in environment [8].

Water is an important and with time becoming a limited resource, not in India but at world level. Many organizations including World Health Organization raises concern over the depleting resources of fresh water mainly underground. In India, dependency on underground water for irrigation is very high such as in Punjab, it is 79%, in Uttar Pradesh, it is 80%, and in Uttarakhand, it is 67% [9, 10]. Precision agriculture and Agriculture 4.0 are the technologies which can improve the irrigation efficiency and are confirmed by many researches and literature published. Various researches and literature published, as per Table 1, have shown that IoT, weather parameters, and weather forecasting play an important role in irrigation planning.

Development of weather station: From the different research and literature, the extracted important weather parameters are shown in Fig. 4 [1–5, 7, 11, 12].

The factors affecting the irrigation demand of crops are evapotranspiration along with soil and crop transpiration which in turn are affected by weather parameters mainly temperature, humidity and wind conditions [13–16]. For the purpose of evaluating evapotranspiration, soil and crop transpiration, local weather condition is required through local weather station. Many weather stations are developed some with IoT and some without IoT. Table 2 gives the detail and comparison of the developed state-of-the-art weather station with the previous developed weather stations.

Investigation of Table 2 discloses that Raspberry Pi, Arduino, and NodeMCU are the common processing units used in weather stations. Raspberry Pi is a costly selection, and if we compare the cost and power consumption of Arduino Uno and NodeMCU, as shown in Table 3 and Fig. 5, NodeMCU becomes a better selection.

Weather station developed uses wind speed, wind direction, and DHT22 (temperature and humidity) sensors sensing weather conditions. NodeMCU is used as central processing unit and also uploads the weather details on IoT cloud. Thingspeak IoT cloud is selected being free to some extent, graphical representation of uploaded information for easy interpretation of weather trends and provided capability for weather data analysis. The developed system is shown in Fig. 6. Figure 7 shows the voltage and drawn current at full operation. NodeMCU is having one limitation that it is equipped only with one ADC and the developed system uses dual channel serial ADC MCP3202.

Result and discussion: The implemented IoT enabled weather station is tested for about 10–12 days of continuous run. The system was able to upload the temperature, humidity and wind speed data on clouds and is successfully monitored remotely. Figure 8 shows the Thingspeak interface with the weather information uploaded by developed IoT enable weather station.

The information is available which can be utilized for irrigation planning. With suitable machine learning computational tools, with the available data, irrigation demand can also be predicted.

Table 1 Role of IoT, weather parameters, and weather forecasting in irrigation scheduling

Ref/year	Title	Description
[11]/2021	Challenges and opportunities in precision irrigation decision support systems for center pivots	The paper focuses on the major challenges faced toward irrigation planning in precision agriculture. Different opportunities for the discussed challenges are also mentioned and discussed
[1]/2020	Exploring the adoption of precision agriculture for irrigation in the context of Agriculture 4.0: the key role of Internet Things	The paper has highlighted about the little research in agriculture and slower pace of precision agriculture adoption. Different factors involved in irrigation planning are discussed along with the importance of weather monitoring
[12]/2020	Advanced IoT-based smart irrigation	The paper heighted that evapotranspiration is the main irrigation water consumption along with soil and plant transpiration. For estimating evapotranspiration, soil and plant transpiration, gathering of local weather conditions is important
[13]/2020	Daily evapotranspiration prediction using boost regression model for irrigation planning	Machine learning model is proposed to predict evapotranspiration for irrigation requirement. System uses weather data along with soil condition to predict the evapotranspiration and accordingly the irrigation is planned
[14]/2019	Cost-effective smart irrigation controller using automatic weather stations	The work proposes a real-time irrigation control system based on local weather conditions. Automatic weather stations are used for gathering the local weather conditions. Here, evapotranspiration and soil moisture content are utilized for irrigation planning
[15]/2019	A real-time fuzzy decision support system for alfalfa irrigation	An irrigation decisive support system is developed for irrigation management. The proposed model takes soil and weather condition as input for irrigation planning
[16]/2018	Precision agriculture design methods using a distributed computing architecture on Internet of Things context	Various agricultural related facilities are analyzed with farmers and growers to outline the new facilities based on IoT. Along with other parameters of precision agriculture, irrigation planning is also discussed

(continued)

Table 1 (continued)

Ref/year	Title	Description
[17]/2016	Development and assessment of a smartphone application for irrigation scheduling in cotton	Mobile application is developed for irrigation planning of cotton. Application uses various data including data from weather stations for estimating root zone soil deficiency

Fig. 4 Weather parameters for precision agriculture

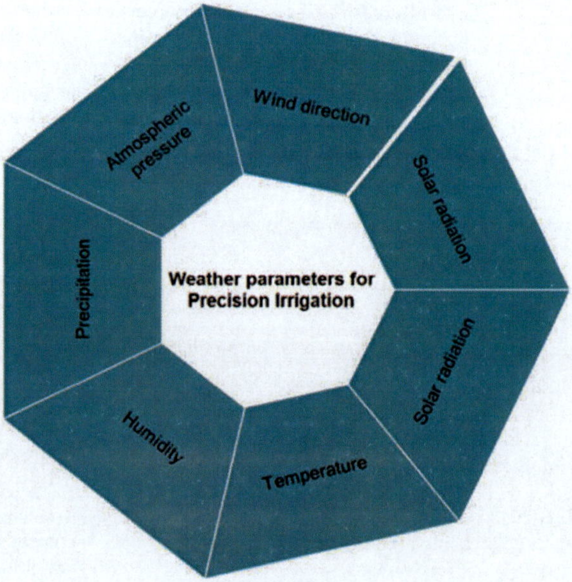

Precision irrigation systems, supported by weather stations, so developed and published in different literatures offer feasible and workable solution to efficient utilization of irrigation water in agriculture. Apart from offering the advantages, Agriculture 4.0 poses some challenges in front of researches, as shown in Fig. 9 [17].

Table 2 Comparison of developed weather station with previous art

Ref/year	Parameters	Technologies	Processing	Data visualization	Application	Improvement /advancement in proposed system
[18]/2020	Temperature Precipitation Wind speed Wind direction	Wi-Fi Fog computing Cloud computing	NodeMCU	Information to different devices	Urban area	Standalone weather station with IoT Relative humidity For agrometeorological application Thingspeak IoT cloud for data storage and visualization Low cost
[19]/2020	Temperature Humidity Rain	LTE Zigbee	Not mentioned	HTML-based web page	Smart agriculture	Wind speed and direction Thingspeak IoT cloud for data storage and visualization NodeMCU as processing board Low cost
[2]/2018	Air pressure Rain Light intensity Humidity	Wi-Fi	NodeMCU	OLED Thingspeak	Precision agriculture	Wind speed and direction Weather station with IoT technology Thingspeak IoT cloud for data storage and visualization No local display for power efficiency Low cost
[3]/2019	Temperature Humidity Solar radiation Wind speed and direction	SD card Wi-Fi	Arduino Mega	Mobile application	Agriculture	NodeMCU as processing board Thingspeak IoT cloud for data storage and visualization Low cost No local display and storage media

Table 3 Comparison of Arduino Uno and NodeMCU

Board	Analog I/O	Digital I/O	Average power (mW)	Cost ($)	Best Application	Source of Information
Arduino Uno	6	14	0.734	3.7	Desktop prototyping and use with Arduino shields	https://maker.pro/arduino/tutorial/a-comparison-of-popular-arduino-boards
Node-MCU	1	16	0.7	2.31	Suitable for Wi-Fi-based applications	https://www.elprocus.com/an-overview-of-arduino-nano-board/

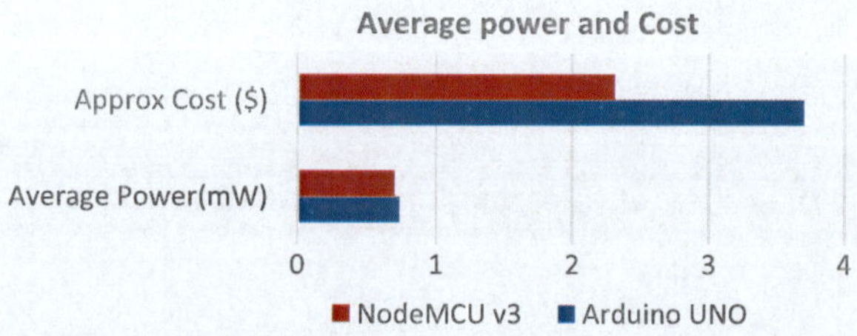

Fig. 5 Average power consumption and cost of NodeMCU and Arduino Uno

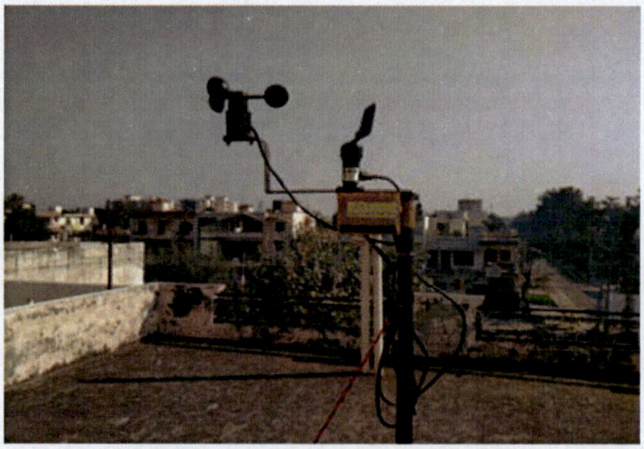

Fig. 6 Weather station installed

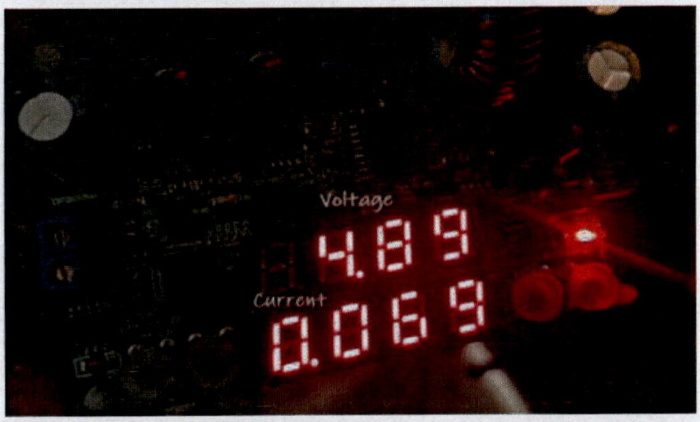

Fig. 7 Voltage and current at full operation

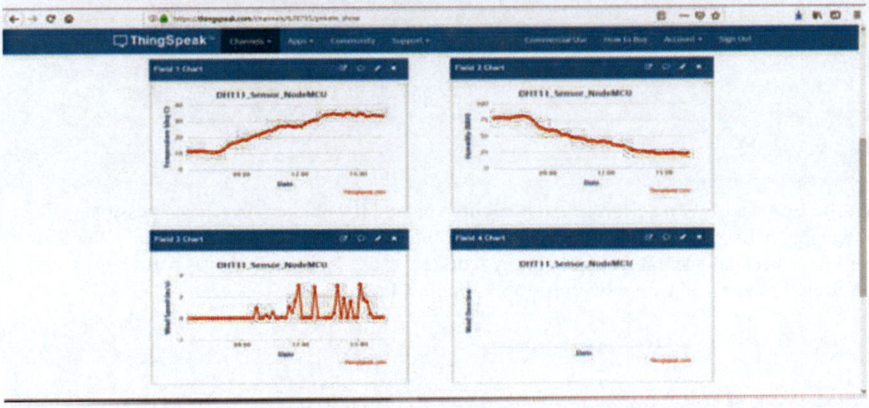

Fig. 8 Thingspeak visualization of weather station data

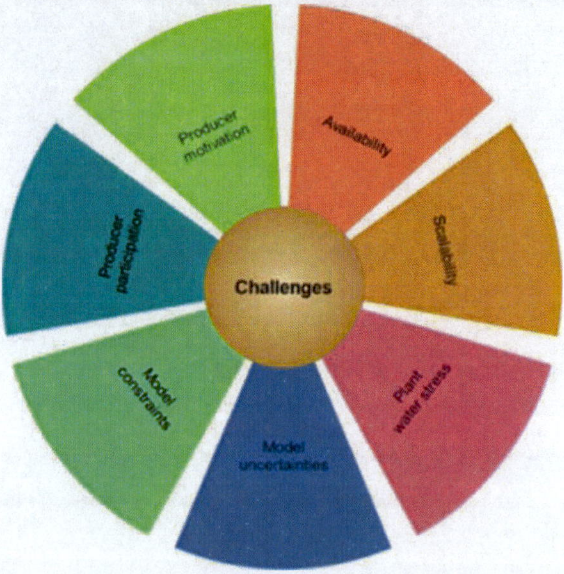

Fig. 9 Agriculture 4.0 challenges

Acknowledgements This paper and the research behind it would not have been possible without the exceptional support of my supervisor. His enthusiasm, knowledge, and exacting attention to detail have been an inspiration and kept my work on track. This research was partially supported by Lovely Professional University, Phagwara, Punjab, India.

References

1. Monteleone S, Moraes EAD, Tondato de Faria B, Aquino Junior PT, Maia RF, Neto AT, Toscano A (2020) Exploring the adoption of precision agriculture for irrigation in the context of agriculture 4.0: the key role of internet of things. Sensors 20(24):7091
2. Math RKM, Dharwadkar NV (2018) IoT based low-cost weather station and monitoring system for precision agriculture in India. In: 2018 2nd international conference on I-SMAC (IoT in social, mobile, analytics and cloud)(I-SMAC) I-SMAC (IoT in social, mobile, analytics and cloud)(I-SMAC), 2018 2nd international conference on 2018 August. IEEE, pp 81–86
3. El-magrous AA, Sternhagen JD, Hatfield G, Qiao Q (2019). Internet of things based weather-soil sensor station for precision agriculture. In: 2019 IEEE international conference on electro information technology (EIT). IEEE, pp 092–097
4. Mestre G, Ruano A, Duarte H, Silva S, Khosravani H, Pesteh S, Ferreira PM, Horta R (2015) An intelligent weather station. Sensors 15(12):31005–31022
5. Hong T, Wang P, White L (2015) Weather station selection for electric load forecasting. Int J Forecast 31(2):286–295
6. Hewage P, Behera A, Trovati M, Pereira E, Ghahremani M, Palmieri F, Liu Y (2020) Temporal convolutional neural (TCN) network for an effective weather forecasting using time-series data from the local weather station. Soft Comput 24(21):16453–16482
7. Citterio M, van As D, Ahlstrøm AP, Andersen ML, Andersen SB, Box JE, Charalampidis C, Colgan WT, Fausto RS, Nielsen S, Veicherts M (2015) Automatic weather stations for basic and applied glaciological research. Geol Surv Den Greenl Bull 69–72

8. Moore GWK, Cristofanelli P, Bonasoni P, Verza GP, Semple JL (2017) Automatic weather station observations of the April 2014 Mount Everest avalanche. Arct Antarct Alp Res 49(2):321–330
9. Department of Agriculture, Cooperation & Farmers Welfare Ministry of Agriculture & Farmers Welfare Government of India (2018) Krishi report 2017–2018, New Delhi. http://www.agricoop.nic. Accessed 19 Aug 2019
10. Federal Ministry of Food and agriculture (2017) Water and agriculture in India, Germany
11. Ferrández-Pastor FJ, García-Chamizo JM, Nieto-Hidalgo M, Mora-Martínez J (2018) Precision agriculture design method using a distributed computing architecture on internet of things context. Sensors 18(6):1731
12. Buchholz M, Musshoff O (2014) The role of weather derivatives and portfolio effects in agricultural water management. Agric Water Manag 146:34–44
13. Togneri R, Kamienski C, Dantas R, Prati R, Toscano A, Soininen JP, Conic TS (2019) Advancing IoT-based smart irrigation. IEEE Internet Things Mag 2(4):20–25
14. Ponraj AS, Vigneswaran T (2019) Daily evapotranspiration prediction using gradient boost regression model for irrigation planning. J Supercomput 1–13
15. Hema N, Kant K (2019) Cost-effective smart irrigation controller using automatic weather stations. Int J Hydrol Sci Technol 9(1):1–27
16. Sarkar I, Pal B, Datta A, Roy S (2020) Wi-Fi-based portable weather station for monitoring temperature, relative humidity, pressure, precipitation, wind speed, and direction. In: Information and communication technology for sustainable development. Springer, Singapore, pp 399–404
17. Zhang J, Guan K, Peng B, Jiang C, Zhou W, Yang Y, Pan M, Franz TE, Heeren DM, Rudnick DR, Abimbola O (2021) Challenges and opportunities in precision irrigation decision-support systems for center pivots. Environ Res Lett
18. Vellidis G, Liakos V, Andreis JH, Perry CD, Porter WM, Barnes EM, Morgan KT, Fraisse C, Migliaccio KW (2016) Development and assessment of a smartphone application for irrigation scheduling in cotton. Comput Electron Agric 127:249–259
19. Marwa C, Othman SB, Sakli H (2020) IoT based low-cost weather station and monitoring system for smart agriculture. In: 2020 20th international conference on sciences and techniques of automatic control and computer engineering (STA). IEEE, pp 349–354

An Intelligent Weather Station Design for Machine Learning in Precisions Irrigation Scheduling

Dushyant Kumar Singh and Rajeev Sobti

Abstract Agriculture 4.0 has taken a big trend in society focusing on precision irrigation based on Internet of Things and machine learning techniques. Agriculture 4.0 is intended as the demand increases, due to the rise of population and climate changes. So, focusing on precision water management, an innovative model is required to provide better functionality. A weather station is set to collect precise data from the atmosphere. The collected data, which is of paramount importance in crop water demand and prediction, is transmitted over an Internet of Things (IoT) cloud server. The received data from the weather station for local weather conditions is in ready to use format by various machine learning algorithms to predict irrigation requirements. The system design provides a cost-effective solution to Agriculture 4.0 in comparison with commercial weather stations.

Keywords Agriculture 4.0 · Irrigation system · Machine learning · Precision irrigation · Sustainable development · Weather station

Abbreviations

IoT	Internet of Things
CWSI	Crop Water Stress Index
ELM	Extreme Learning Machine
ANN	Artificial Neural Network
MARS	Multivariate Adaptive Regression Splines
GRNN	Generalized Regression Neural Network

D. K. Singh (✉) · R. Sobti
Lovely Professional University, Phagwara, Punjab, India

R. Sobti
e-mail: rajeev.sobti@lpu.co.in

N. Marriwala et al. (eds.), *Emergent Converging Technologies and Biomedical Systems*, Lecture Notes in Electrical Engineering 841,
https://doi.org/10.1007/978-981-16-8774-7_5

1 Introduction

Agriculture is the backbone of India which has major crops cultivated based on seasons. The first and foremost part of growing and cultivating a plant is watering the plants. Not considering the season's water is a basic need of a plant. The efficient supply of water based on the need of the plant is a problem that is addressed, and an innovative solution based on IoT and ML is proposed. The agriculturist or a farmer needs a sustainable change, and this precise water management plays a major role. And speaking about majorly cultivated crop paddy, the water is the heart of the plant which makes it live and farmers provide water in excess to stay on the safe side. The management of water and automatic irrigation of water would help a farmer or an agriculturist in a better way. The existence of solutions and the proposed solution based on a critical review conducted is discussed.

Machine learning and IoT are the most advanced and proposed ideas in this paper. Machine learning is a special way of teaching the system or machine to learn things and make a wise decision later based on the learned data. The ML has a list of algorithms and classifiers that work based on the situation and data. For better efficiency of the system, one has to choose the appropriate algorithm and classifier. There lies the ways in improving the model performance. The collection of data and transmission of data are done through IoT technologies. Connecting the devices through Internet and the communication is held over the Internet in most of the cases in this new era. IoT has brought a great impact on society making people understand the need for technology in different fields. The IoT and ML have combined today in most of the fields in giving valuable and worthy solutions. The weather station and data transmission system are done using IoT, and the prediction system is done using ML in the proposed idea, which gives strength and value to the invention from a technology point of view.

Comparative study of different weather stations based on the prerequisites of the smart irrigation scheduling based on ML is elaborated. The irrigation scheduling based on ML is the motive of the paper. The paper is intended to find the list of parameters that an innovative irrigation system needs. The weather station is built with the parameters, and the value is logged into the cloud platform (ThingSpeak).

1.1 Motivation of This Paper

The need for improvement in precise water management has forced the authors to work on various technologies available to propose a uniquely effective solution. Agriculture 4.0 motivates the researchers to propose different futuristic ideas based on IoT and ML to improve the sector as the need increases day by day. The IoT-based weather station and ML-based prediction system to initiate an IoT-based irrigation system would cause an effective change in implementation which is predicted, and the work is carried out.

2 Related Work

Pressure on agriculture will be increasing as a result of the continuous increase in world population. Agriculture utilizes a technology called precision agriculture or also termed digital agriculture. For the efficiently using the agriculture resources like fertilizers, pesticides, and most importantly irrigation water. Now machine learning in agriculture has provided opportunities for understanding the data-intensive processes involved with the agricultural environment. Machine learning provided the machines with the capability to learn. The paper provides the different areas of agriculture which are benefitted from machine learning, as shown in Fig. 1. Figure 2 gives the different ML algorithms used for water management in agriculture based on parameters evapotranspiration and dew point temperature, as shown in Fig. 2. For

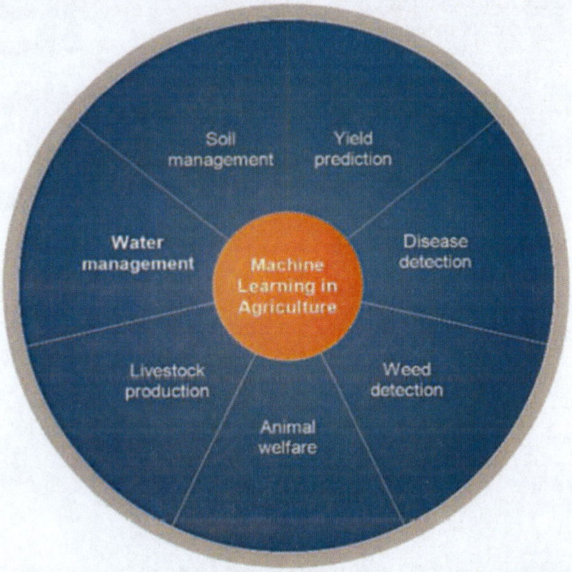

Fig. 1 Agricultural application utilizing machine learning

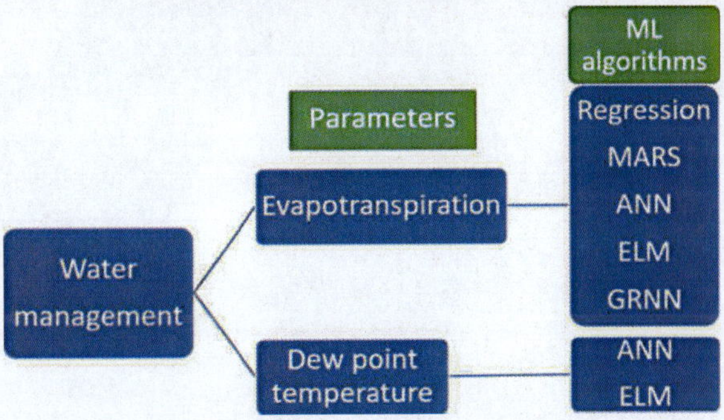

Fig. 2 Machine learning in water management

water management, the important weather parameters' measures are temperature, humidity, and wind conditions [1].

In [2], the application of machine learning algorithms used for water stress determination is reviewed. Various methods for crop water stress measurement as highlighted in the article are shown in Fig. 3.

Evapotranspiration is an important method to determine the demand for irrigation or in irrigation planning. The article has also provided the important machine learning algorithms which are employed in agriculture as shown in Fig. 4.

For estimating evapotranspiration, it is important to gather weather temperature, humidity, and wind condition information. A weather station is a setup used to collect weather data and provides the information to the user. The classification of weather stations present in various works of literature is provided in Tables 1 and 2.

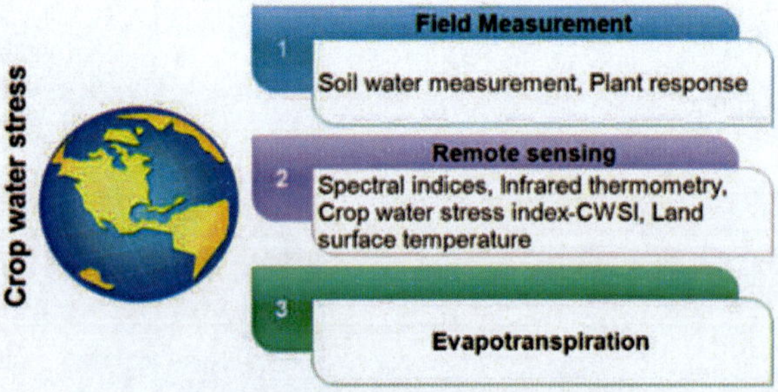

Fig. 3 Crop water stress measurement methods

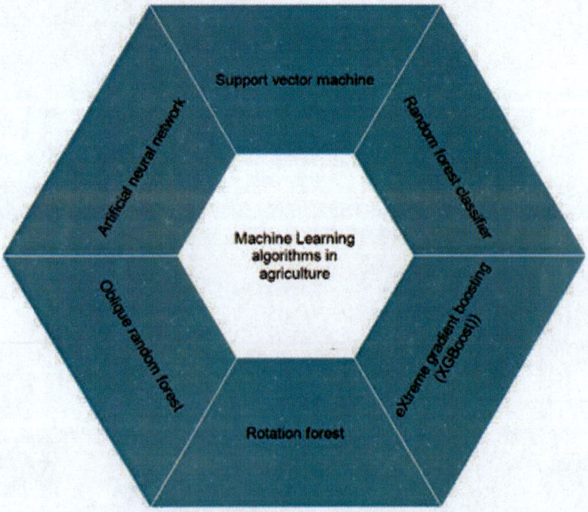

Fig. 4 Different machine learning algorithms for agriculture

Table 1 Classification of weather station

Classification	Functionalities	Reference papers	Key points	Conclusion
Data collection	Weather stations are built or data is taken from some online site and fed to the system	[3–13]	Data collection from the sensor node is proposed. The station is proposed to be Automatic Weather Station (AWS) where the system sends the data to the remote user	Data collection is done from a single node most of the time. The need for collection from multiple nodes for processing makes the system efficient
Transmission	The transmission of data from the sensor node to the central hub	[3, 5, 7–12, 19, 20]	NB IoT, ThingSpeak, Fog and Edge computing, ZigBee, Lora, Wi-Fi, cloud, email, and Twitter are different ways proposed	The efficient use of different systems was proposed. The work on Lo-Ra is not widely seen in the proposed application
ML	Predicting the functionality based on the received data	[4, 11, 14, 20–23]	ML-based predictions were done in a better way. The prediction accuracy was mentioned to be above 90 in these papers	Building a system with ML features with real-time data is proposed earlier. The actuator and sensor system connected to a single ML-based system where the actuator is actuated using ML decision is not widely seen in the research

(continued)

Table 1 (continued)

Classification	Functionalities	Reference papers	Key points	Conclusion
Irrigation scheduling	Scheduling the irrigation based on ML results and initiating IoT services to enable irrigation system	[10, 13, 19–28]	The irrigation system includes of the actuator based on the IoT signal which is proposed, and, in some cases, the decision from pre-loaded data is fed as a control signal	The real-time data that is used to evoke the ML system to predict and actuate the system is not seen in most of the studies. The complexity of merging up the technologies in giving an efficient solution is not seen in most cases

Table 2 Machine learning algorithms applied to weather data

Ref/year	Weather station measured parameters	Machine learning technique for irrigation scheduling
21/2020	Wind speed, wind direction, temperature, rain, humidity, light	TCN
22/2020	Temperature, humidity, solar radiation, wind speed	Boost regressing model
29/2020	Based on soil conditions	VAR and RNN-LSTM
30/2019	Air temperature, humidity, wind speed, precipitation, radiation	Fuzzy logic
3/2015	Temperature, humidity, wind velocity, atmospheric pressure, rain	NEN and ANN

2.1 Study on Various Irrigation Models

The ignition system of irrigation is automated through IoT and the decision taken using ML algorithms. The prediction is done using ML or a different process. Different models are developed for irrigation scheduling by using weather stations and machine learning algorithms. The weather station models developed in different researches/works of literature are discussed in Table 2. Most of the researches/works of literature have considered evapotranspiration prediction using machine learning for irrigation scheduling.

The system is designed to be low-cost, for which free IoT cloud server ThingSpeak has been selected for data storage and visualization. Figure 5 provides the developed weather station block diagram.

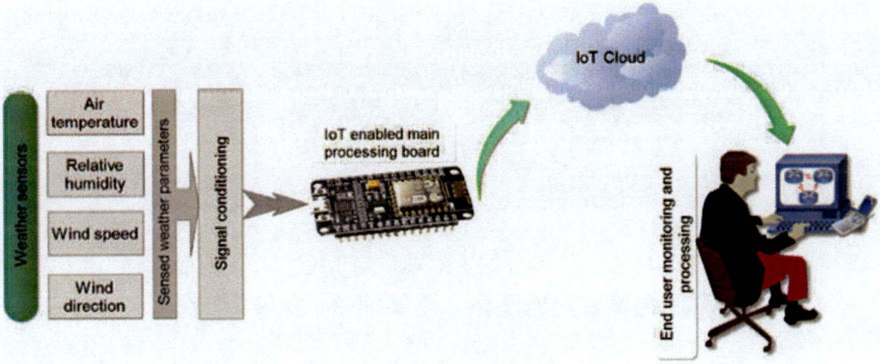

Fig. 5 Block diagram of developed weather station

3 Result and Discussion

The system so developed is tested, and the data is monitored for more than a month in November–December, 2020. Figure 6 shows the installed weather station for measuring weather conditions, and measured weather conditions' ThingSpeak visualization is shown in Fig. 7.

The weather station developed is a cost-effective system for efficient utilization of agricultural irrigation water. Along with the irrigation water efficient utilization, agricultural yield quality and quantity can also be increased through predictive irrigation by applying the machine learning algorithms to the provided weather information.

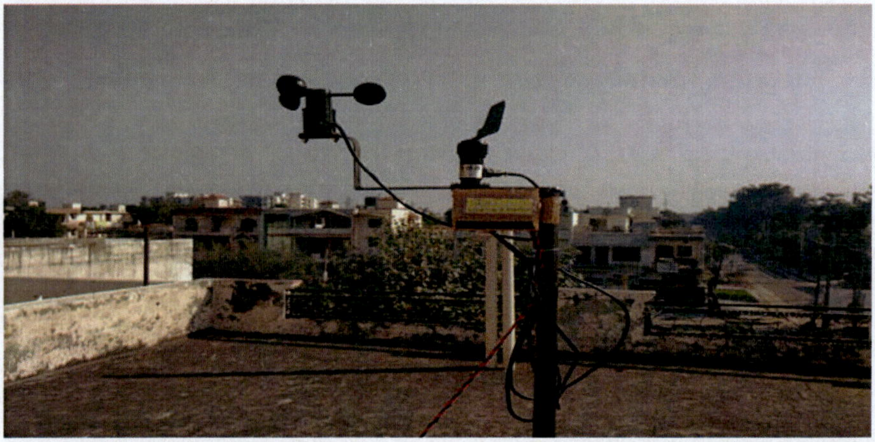

Fig. 6 Weather station

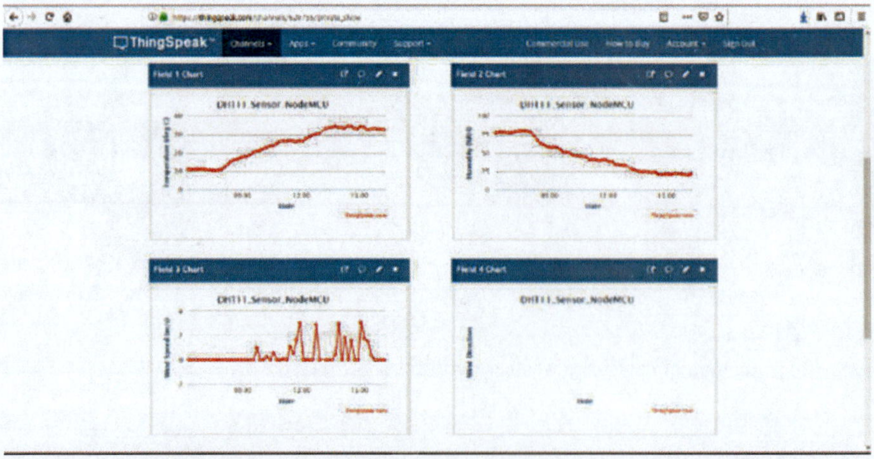

Fig. 7 ThingSpeak data visualization interface

Table 3 Cost comparison of commercial weather stations

S. No	Weather station product	Cost/unit	Make	IoT feature	Source
1	Automatic weather station for industrial: ATM1136	70,000	Advance Tech India Private Limited	No	https://www.indiamart.com/proddetail/automatic-weather-station-12477572848.html
2	V Tech ultrasonic weather station for agriculture: VT-UWS01	120,000	V TECH	No	https://www.indiamart.com/proddetail/ultrasoni-weather-station-19054403862.html
3	Portable weather station: 110-WS-18	325,000	Auro Electronics Private Limited	No	https://www.indiamart.com/proddetail/portable-weather-station-4539296991.html
4	Automatic weather station, usage: industrial: RK900-01	143,000	Infinity Enterprise Private Limited	No	https://www.indiamart.com/proddetail/automatic-weather-station-18244123933.html
5	Automatic weather station for official	500,000	Nevco Engineer Private Limited	No	https://www.indiamart.com/proddetail/automatic-weather-station-13513226588.html

The system developed is much cost effective (less than 50% of the commercially available weather stations without IoT) with IoT technology in comparison with most of the commercially available weather station. The commercially available weather station lacks in IoT technology. They either uses local display or GSM for data visualization and transmission that too at heavy cost addition. Table 3 provides the cost comparison (in INR) of different commercially available weather stations.

Acknowledgements This paper and the research behind it would not have been possible without the exceptional support of my supervisor. This research was partially supported by Lovely Professional University, Phagwara, Punjab, India.

References

1. Liakos KG, Busato P, Moshou D, Pearson S, Bochtis D (2018) Machine learning in agriculture: a review. Sensors 18(8):2674
2. Virnodkar SS, Pachghare VK, Patil VC, Jha SK (2020) Remote sensing and machine learning for crop water stress determination in various crops: a critical review. Precision Agric 21(5):1121–1155
3. Mestre G, Ruano A, Duarte H, Silva S, Khosravani H, Pesteh S, Ferreira PM, Horta R (2015) An intelligent weather station. Sensors 15(12):31005–31022
4. Lorite IJ, Ramírez-Cuesta JM, Cruz-Blanco M, Santos C (2015) Using weather forecast data for irrigation scheduling under semi-arid conditions. Irrig Sci 33(6):411–427
5. Citterio M, Van AD, Ahlstrøm AP, Andersen ML, Andersen SB, Box JE, Charalampidis C, Colgan WT, Fausto RS, Nielsen S, Veicherts M (2015) Automatic weather stations for basic and applied glaciological research. Geol Surv Den Greenl Bull 69–72
6. Moore GWK, Cristofanelli P, Bonasoni P, Verza GP, Semple JL (2017) Automatic weather station observations of the April 2014 Mount Everest avalanche. Arct Antarct Alp Res 49(2):321–330
7. Smeets PC, KuipersMunneke P, Van As D, van den Broeke MR, Boot W, Oerlemans H, Snellen H, Reijmer CH, van de Wal RS (2018) The K-transect in west Greenland: automatic weather station data (1993–2016). Arct Antarct Alp Res 50(1):S100002
8. Sarkar I, Pal B, Datta A, Roy S (2020) Wi-Fi-based portable weather station for monitoring temperature, relative humidity, pressure, precipitation, wind speed, and direction. In: Information and communication technology for sustainable development. Springer, Singapore, pp 399–404
9. Jianyun C, Yunfan S, Chunyan L (2017) Research on application of automatic weather station based on Internet of Things. In: Proceedings of IOP conference series: earth and environmental science, vol 104, no 1. IOP Publishing, Bristol, p 012015
10. Ferrández-Pastor FJ, García-Chamizo JM, Nieto-Hidalgo M, Mora-Martínez J (2018) Precision agriculture design method using a distributed computing architecture on internet of things context. Sensors 18(6):1731
11. Marwa C, Othman SB, Sakli H (2020) IoT based low-cost weather station and monitoring system for smart agriculture. In: Proceedings of 2020 20th international conference on sciences and techniques of automatic control and computer engineering (STA). IEEE, pp 349–354
12. Chebbi W, Benjemaa M, Kamoun A, Jabloun M, Sahli A (2011) Development of a WSN integrated weather station node for an irrigation alert program under Tunisian conditions. In: Proceedings of eighth international multi-conference on systems, signals and devices. IEEE, pp 1–6
13. Hema N, Kant K (2019) Cost-effective smart irrigation controller using automatic weather stations. Int J Hydrol Sci Technol 9(1):1–27
14. Kapoor P, Barbhuiya FA (2019) Cloud based weather station using IoT devices. In: Proceedings of TENCON 2019–2019 IEEE Region 10 conference (TENCON). IEEE, pp 2357–2362
15. Kodali RK, Sahu A (2016) An IoT based weather information prototype using WeMos. In: Proceedings of 2016 2nd international conference on contemporary computing and informatics (IC3I). IEEE, pp 612–616
16. Kodali RK, Mandal S (2016) IoT based weather station. In: Proceedings of 2016 international conference on control, instrumentation, communication and computational technologies (ICCICCT). IEEE, pp 680–683
17. El-magrous AA, Sternhagen JD, Hatfield G, Qiao Q (2019) Internet of things based weather-soil sensor station for precision agriculture. In: Proceedings of 2019 IEEE international conference on electro information technology (EIT). IEEE, pp 92–97
18. Bienvenido-Huertas D, Rubio-Bellido C, Pérez-Ordóñez JL, Martínez-Abella F (2019) Estimating adaptive setpoint temperatures using weather stations. Energies 12(7):1197

19. Fourati MA, Chebbi W, Kamoun A (2014) Development of a web-based weather station for irrigation scheduling. In: Proceedings of 2014 third IEEE international colloquium in information science and technology (CIST). IEEE, pp 37–42
20. Vellidis G, Liakos V, Andreis JH, Perry CD, Porter WM, Barnes EM, Morgan KT, Fraisse C, Migliaccio KW (2016) Development and assessment of a smartphone application for irrigation scheduling in cotton. Comput Electron Agric 127:249–259
21. Hewage P, Behera A, Trovati M, Pereira E, Ghahremani M, Palmieri F, Liu Y (2020) Temporal convolutional neural (TCN) network for an effective weather forecasting using time-series data from the local weather station. Soft Comput 24(21):16453–16482
22. Ponraj AS, Vigneswaran T (2019) Daily evapotranspiration prediction using gradient boost regression model for irrigation planning. J Supercomput 1–13
23. Zhang J, Guan K, Peng B, Jiang C, Zhou W, Yang Y, Pan M, Franz TE, Heeren DM, Rudnick DR, Abimbola O (2021) Challenges and opportunities in precision irrigation decision-support systems for center pivots. Environ Res Lett
24. Li M, Sui R, Meng Y, Yan H (2019) A real-time fuzzy decision support system for alfalfa irrigation. Comput Electron Agric 163:104870
25. Prasad AS, Umamahesh NV, Viswanath GK (2011) Optimal irrigation planning model for an existing storage based irrigation system in India. Irrig Drain Syst 25(1):19–38
26. Monteleone S, Moraes EAD, De Faria BT, Aquino Junior PT, Maia RF, Neto AT, Toscano A (2020) Exploring the adoption of precision agriculture for irrigation in the context of agriculture 4.0: the key role of internet of things. Sensors 20(24):7091
27. Togneri R, Kamienski C, Dantas R, Prati R, Toscano A, Soininen JP, Conic TS (2019) Advancing IoT-based smart irrigation. IEEE Internet Things Mag 2(4):20–25
28. Buchholz M, Musshoff O (2014) The role of weather derivatives and portfolio effects in agricultural water management. Agric Water Manag 146:34–44

Accelerating Polynomial-Based Image Secret Sharing Using Hadoop

Sonali Patil, Roshani Raut, Chaitrali Sorte, and Gauri Jha

Abstract Polynomial-based secret sharing techniques are most preferred in many applications. Image secret sharing techniques based on polynomial functions become computationally heavy if image size is large. Sequential operations are not that effective for construction and reconstruction algorithms on large size images. Parallel computing works efficiently when load and time reduction on a single machine is required. The concurrent execution of polynomial operations on image pixel values while applying steps of construction of shares and reconstruction of the secret makes the scheme more efficient. Hadoop-based concurrent approach is proposed for polynomial-based image secret sharing scheme. The experimental results show that Hadoop-based cluster speeds up the process up to 18% by one slave and up to 14% by adding two slave nodes. The addition in number of slave nodes accelerates the performance up to 50% for very large size images in the polynomial-based secret sharing algorithms.

Keywords Secret sharing · Image processing · Parallel computing · Hadoop · HDFS

1 Introduction

A polynomial-based secret sharing scheme is first time proposed by Shamir [1] in 1979. Later, Thein and Lin [2] put forward image secret sharing based on Shamir's [1] polynomial-based secret sharing on image pixel values. The approach reduces size of the image shares generated in construction phase, and also the generated secret image is of good quality (same as the original image). The wide ranges of applications are possible using extended capabilities [3] in secret sharing schemes.

S. Patil · R. Raut (✉) · C. Sorte
Department of Information Technology, Pimpri Chinchwad College of Engineering, Nigdi, Pune, India

G. Jha
Consultant, Advanced Delivery Consulting, Sydney, Australia

N. Marriwala et al. (eds.), *Emergent Converging Technologies and Biomedical Systems*, Lecture Notes in Electrical Engineering 841,
https://doi.org/10.1007/978-981-16-8774-7_6

A polynomial-based image secret sharing algorithms are highly secure but computationally heavy due to the requirement of polynomial operation on each pixel value. In large size of images, construction and reconstruction step computation is done on pixel-by-pixel for complete image. This is computationally meticulous as the database size to be processed is comparatively large. This results into large computational complexities of construction and reconstruction algorithms. In real life, these approaches need acceleration of processing of algorithms for use. The parallel advancements of image-based algorithms are suggested by few researchers [4, 5].

The Hadoop File System (HDFS) [6, 7] is implemented using distributed file system design. Hadoop File System is fault tolerant and can be implemented with minimal cost. It is able to accumulate the huge amount of data and also can provide access to that data at ease. Hadoop enables interface to HDFS through a command interface. It also provides streaming access to file system data. The clusters are formed by the integral servers, Name Node and Data Node [8, 9].

2 Related Work

2.1 Thein and Lin's Secret Sharing [2]

Thein and Lin [2] used polynomial-based Shamir secret sharing [1] for image threshold secret sharing. The secret image pixel values are used as coefficients to construct as polynomial used for constructing share images. The share image pixel values are used for reconstruction of the secret image using Lagrange's interpolation. This is very effective secret sharing method to distribute confidential images secretly. For very large size of images, it becomes inefficient due computationally heavy load.

2.2 Efficient Image Secret Sharing Using Parallel Processing for Row-Wise Encoding and Decoding [4]

A multithreading approach is implemented in [4] where it is observed that the concurrent approach is very effective and efficient to apply practically. In every algorithm, the multithreading logic needs to be implemented to achieve parallelism. The author demonstrated the use of parallel processing for efficient secret construction and reconstruction algorithms. The parallel approach is implemented using Unix platform. The more efficient parallel platforms can enhance the performance of image secret sharing methods.

2.3 Hadoop and HDFS [6–8]

Hadoop is basically an open-source framework which focuses on computations of distributed storage. Hadoop processes massive data on commodity hardware. A dedicated file system called Hadoop Distributed File System (HDFS) stores big data and supports distributed tasks estimations in Hadoop clusters. The conception of HDFS is implemented using Java. The Hadoop services may be characterized in terms of components such as storage component and processing component. Here, the HDFS works as storage component, whereas MapReduce works as processing component.

The HDFS grants dependable data storage. It also trails Master–Slave architecture. The Name Node is the master node. It only contains the metadata. The Name Node protects and maintains incoming data. The maintained information, i.e., metadata, is required for data retrieval as the data is distributed over numerous nodes. Data Node behaves as a slave node. It stores the actual data in the HDFS and interconnects with the files which are stored in that particular node along with the Name Node. The slave node is efficient enough to create new blocks of data along with manipulating and removing the blocks. It can also replicate the blocks if Name Node requires it to be done [9].

2.4 Hadoop-HDFS-Map Reduce [10]

The parallel processing of large amount of data is modeled through MapReduce. The main advantages are in effective storing of large images and effective accessing of large size images. Also, filtering of images and processing of images become effective.

2.5 Hadoop Image Processing Interface

A traditional Hadoop MapReduce program strives in presenting input image and output image data in a convenient format. The image library, "Hadoop Image Processing Interface" (HIPI) is built to be exercised with Apache Hadoop. HIPI is a solution to store a huge compilation of images on the dedicated file system of Hadoop. It also makes them available for effective distributed processing with few parallel programming components like MapReduce. A HIPI Image Bundle (HIB) is a collection of images characterized as a single file on HDFS.

3 Proposed Method

The proposed method is implemented for two steps—Formation of image shares from secret images and reformation of original secret from shares. The below section elaborates construction and reconstruction method of images for polynomial image secret sharing using Hadoop.

3.1 Image Secret Sharing

Construction and Reconstruction of Master–Slave Approach using Hadoop

The proposed parallel approach is based on master–slave model, as shown in Fig. 1 on Hadoop to achieve the parallel computation. It is implemented on one master and multiple slaves. The used approach is shown below.

As shown in Fig. 1, the intermediate results are produced using input records functional with Mapper. Reducer aggregates these generated results. The local summation is executed by combiners. The shuffling of intermediate data with reducer is performed by partitions.

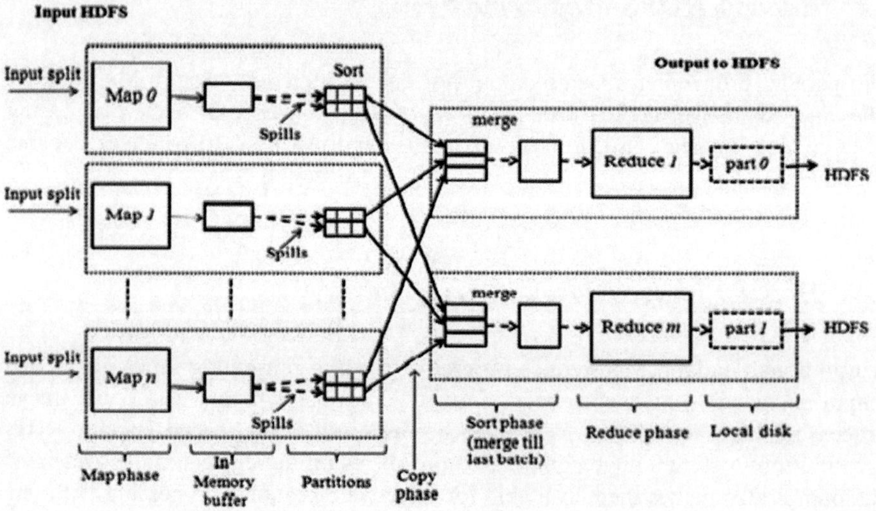

Fig. 1 HDFS framework

3.2 Construction of Shares

Figure 2 indicates construction of shares on Hadoop framework which consist of single Name Node (Master Node) and two Data Nodes (Slave Node). The Name Node distributes partition datasets to Data Nodes. The Data Nodes will compute polynomial computations of their respective pixel values of secret image.

The detailed illustration formation of shares of secret image using polynomial method is shown in Fig. 2.

Master node

i. Master will split the image row-wise into *k*-number of blocks (partitions) of fixed size.
ii. Master will transfer each partition to respective slaves.
iii. Each partition will contain parameters with row and column numbers.

Slave node

i. Each slave will apply Thein and Lin's method on every row of received partition to construct a $(k - 1)$ degree polynomial.
ii. Polynomials must be computed for each participant, starting from 1…n.
iii. No slaves will quit until the task is finished.
iv. All the computed values will be sent to master node.

Master node

i. Master node will collect all the values from all slaves and will create shares.
ii. These shares will be distributed to all the participants.

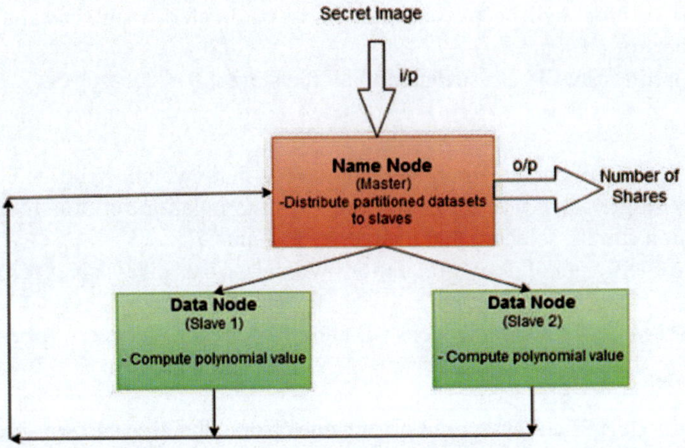

Fig. 2 Construction of shares

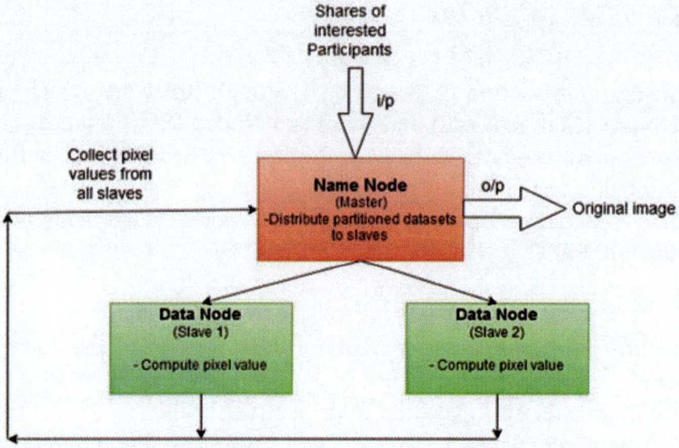

Fig. 3 Reconstruction of original secret

3.3 Reconstruction of Original Secret from Shares

Figure 3 indicates reconstruction of original secret on Hadoop framework with single Name Node (Master) and two Data Nodes (Slave).

Master node

i. *k*-shares will be given as input to master node collected from interested participants.
ii. Master node will decide *k*-partitions for slaves.
iii. Each partition will be passed containing parameters with row and column numbers of all shares.
iv. The partitions will be distributed to all the slaves.

Slave node

i. Each slave will choose first pixel from every share which is chosen.
ii. Every single slave will utilize Lagrange's interpolation formula to create an equation from *k*-selected pixel values of *k*-shares.
iii. Entire coefficient of derived equations will be used as pixel values for resultant image.
iv. Each slave will imitate the steps (ii) and (iii) for each and every specified row.

Master node

i. Master node will collect all the pixel values from all slaves and will present the reconstructed secret image.

The proposed method is implemented in HDFS with varying the number of slave nodes which results in better performance as compared to the traditional approach.

4 Result and Analysis

The proposed approach is implemented using Apache Hadoop on one master node and multiple slave nodes. The secret image of Leena, Baboon, Barbara, and Pepper of size 512 × 512 pixel are used from standard image dataset.

Tables 1 and 2 show the experimental results obtained with both approaches. The readings are observed for sequential approach (standalone machine) and using Hadoop cluster having one slave and Hadoop cluster having two slaves.

As it is observed from Table 1, the Hadoop cluster speeds up the process as we increase the number of slaves in the system for processing of large images as compared to sequential method.

The construction time is more as compared to reconstruction time as the number of shares, from which original image is to be generated are less than the shares needs to be created in the construction phase.

5 Conclusion

It is observed that the time required by the system on a Hadoop-based distributed platform is much less than that is required on a standalone machine for sequential approach. Compared to standalone machine, time requirement of system with one slave is 18% and the same with two slaves is 14%. This demonstrates

Table 1 Time comparison table for construction using sequential verses Hadoop approach

Secret image	Required time		
	Standalone machine (in s)	Single slave machine (in s)	Two-slave machine (in s)
Lena	1.012	0.182	0.142
Baboon	0.981	0.177	0.138
Barbara	0.962	0.173	0.135
Pepper	0.912	0.164	0.128
Average	0.9675	0.174	0.135

Table 2 Time comparison table for reconstruction using sequential verses Hadoop approach

Secret image	Required time		
	Standalone machine (in s)	Single slave machine (in s)	Two-slave machine (in s)
Lena	0.0683	0.0122	0.010
Baboon	0.0652	0.0117	0.0091
Barbara	0.0644	0.0115	0.0089
Pepper	0.0612	0.0110	0.00854
Average	0.0647	0.0116	0.0091

that on increasing number of slaves, the system will be more efficient and will construct/reconstruct in even less time, thus reducing load on single machine. Also for image of smaller sizes, sequential approach is proved to be better but as the size of image goes on increasing, time efficiency is observed. Hadoop accelerated the construction and reconstruction time for bigger images, for which computations are extra compared to smaller images by distributing the task to various slaves.

References

1. Shamir (1979) How to share a secret. Commun ACM 22(11):612–613
2. Thein CC, Lin JC (2002) Secret image sharing. Comput Graph 26:765–770
3. Patil S, Deshmuth P (2012) An explication of multifarious secret sharing schemes. Int J Comput Appl 46(19):0975–8887
4. Sonali P (2018) Efficient image secret sharing using parallel processing for row-wise encoding and decoding. In: International conference on intelligent computing and applications, advances in intelligent systems and computing. Springer Nature Singapore Pvt Ltd, Singapore, p 632
5. Sachdeva K, Kaur J, Singh G (2017) Image processing on multi node hadoop cluster. In: International conference on electrical, electronics, communication, computer and optimization techniques (ICEECCOT)
6. Premchaiswadi W, Romsaiyud W (2012) Optimizing and tuning map reduce jobs to improve the large-scale data analysis process. Int J Intell Syst
7. Arkan A, Al-Hamodi G, Songfeng LU (2016) MRFP: discovery frequent patterns using mapreduce frequent pattern growth. In: International conference on network and information systems for computer
8. Chen H, Lin TY, Zhibing Z, Zhong J (2013) Parallel mining frequent patterns over big transactional data in extended mapreduce. In: IEEE international conference on granular computing (GrC)
9. Archita B, Deipali G (2015) CFI mining using DAG based on MapReduce. Int J Emerg Trends Technol Comput Sci (IJETTCS) 4(3)
10. Mohamed HA (2012) Hadoop mapreduce for remote sensing image analysis. Int J Emerg Technol Adv Eng (IJETAE) 2(4)

A Computational Model for Detection of Lung Diseases Due to Forkhead Transcription Factors

Shruti Jain

Abstract Machine learning refers to the process of programming the machine in such a way that it performs tasks with initial coding or programming, and eventually learns through pattern recognition and makes decisions and conclusions on its own. The purpose of this study is to investigate the capability of various machine learning algorithms in predicting obstructive and restrictive disease which was classified using the artificial neural network (NN) technique that is due to deficiency of FOXO protein. Forkhead transcription factors of the O class (FOXO) deficiency lead to increased susceptibility to air space enlargement, or chronic obstructive pulmonary disease (COPD). COPD is an inflammatory lung syndrome that is characterized by the limitation of expiratory airflow that deteriorates over time. This research paper proposes a computational model for the detection of different lung diseases using ANN. The data preprocessing techniques and statistical analysis are applied to the raw data before developing a model. Different features were extracted which were selected using Principal Component Analysis (PCA). Accuracy is evaluated as the performance metric of the model developed using ANN consisting of multiple layer perceptron (MLP) and radial basis function (RBF). MLP outperforms the result as 96.5% of accuracy is achieved using MLP with zero error while RBF results in more training, testing, and validation error. The results indicate that the proposed model can be used as a tool in predicting different lung diseases and could be an effective method for decision makers.

Keywords Lung diseases · Artificial neural network · FOXO protein · Graphical analysis · Correlation

---

S. Jain (✉)
Jaypee University of Information Technology, Solan, Himachal Pradesh, India

N. Marriwala et al. (eds.), *Emergent Converging Technologies and Biomedical Systems*, Lecture Notes in Electrical Engineering 841,
https://doi.org/10.1007/978-981-16-8774-7_7

1 Introduction

Indian diet is high in carbs, and the lack of knowledge also adds to it. They fail to meet even the minimum requirement mostly because the vegetarian population is more than any other country [1]. Protein requires more energy to digest and is the key to losing weight. Protein is the building block of the human body, it is present in every cell in nature, and thus, proteins have multiple physiological functions including synthetic, regulatory, protective functions, etc. Also, it plays an essential role in all body tissues. Proteins are essential to muscle and tendon repair. On the contrary, there is a very common disease of the excess of carbohydrates called insulin resistance which has multiple symptoms that are generally grouped called metabolic syndrome. The body's ability to absorb protein and break down decreases with age, and also the protein requirements are different for different individuals based on their age, weight, and height [2, 3]. As the body cannot absorb protein in its original form, so it is very important to include protein with a carbohydrate source, acidic foods, and Vitamin B6 rich foods which improve bioavailability. The body is dependent on a daily supply of dietary proteins for its essential amino acids requirement. The RDA for protein for adult Indians is 1 g/kg desirable body weight. Protein deficiency may also occur because of diseases such as liver disease, mal-absorption diseases, and kidney diseases. Malnutrition is the cause of protein deficiency [4, 5]. The blood protein level drops, synthesis of enzymes for digestion of food, carrier proteins, etc., are also reduced. This in turn affects the digestion and absorption function which may slowly lead to the development of multiple nutrient deficiencies. FKHR protein deficiency leads to many diseases; one of them is a lung disease.

The forkhead transcription factor (FKHR) family is categorized by a forkhead domain [6, 7] and by a winged-helix DNA binding motif [8, 9]. FOXO1, FOXO3, FOXO4, and FOXO6 are the members of forkhead transcription factors of the O class (FOXOs). FOXO has important roles in cellular proliferation, metabolism, stress apoptosis, and resistance [10, 11]. FOXO1 and FOXO3 are uttered in all tissues; FOXO4 is highly expressed in colorectal tissue, muscle, and kidney, while FOXO6 is mainly articulated in the liver and brain [12, 13]. The activity of FOXOs is tightly regulated by posttranslational modification, including acetylation, phosphorylation, and ubiquitylation. FOXO3 is a member of the FOXO transcription factor subfamily that regulates the expression of target genes not only through DNA binding as a transcription factor but also through protein–protein interaction [14, 15]. FOXO3 deficiency guides to airspace enlargement, increased susceptibility to cigarette smoke-induced inflammation, and chronic obstructive pulmonary disease (COPD). The COPD patient is/was a heavy smoker [16, 17]. Typically, COPD consists of two components: 1) chronic bronchitis and 2) emphysema. The chronic bronchitis component is reversible to a certain extent if the patient stops smoking early enough. The emphysema component destroyed lungs and is not reversible [18, 19]. COPD is now occurring in nonsmokers who live in areas plagued by severe air pollution. It also occurs in cultures where poorly ventilated cooking is done via indoor fires. Interestingly, there are smokers whose COPD presents as almost pure chronic bronchitis or pure emphysema, the former can get dramatically better if they quit smoking, while the latter cannot expect improvement [20, 21]. For the majority of people with COPD, symptoms such as shortness of breath with mild exertion may not occur until they are living off their reserve lung capacity. Such patients have near end-stage disease, but may not realize it until it is too late.

Mutations in PTEN lead to an activation of phosphatidylinositol 3-kinase (PI3K) pathway and results in the loss of the FOXO family of FKHR. FOXO deficiency leads to increased susceptibility to air space enlargement and COPD. COPD is an inflammatory lung syndrome that is exemplified by the restriction of expiratory airflow that deteriorates over time. To detect the different lung diseases (obstructive and restrictive disease), this paper proposes a computational model that extracts different attributes, selection of attributes followed by a machine learning technique using ANN [22, 23]. The novelty of the paper lies in the detection of lung diseases that occurs due to deficiency of FOXO protein using ANN. ANN is networks of several processors or neurons working together, and every neuron has a few amounts of local memory. These neurons are small units and linked by numeric data (weights). This model exceeds other statistic models because of its robustness and ease of usage. The important advantage for ANN is the constraints on the local operation that overwhelm by other learning processes.

This paper comprises: Sect. 2 explains the methodology for detection of different lung diseases, Sect. 3 explains results and discussion followed by a conclusion and future work.

2 Proposed Methodology

Millions of people are suffering from lung diseases. Mainly infections, smoking, and genetics are more responsible for lung diseases. Lung diseases affecting the blood vessels, pleura, chest wall, airways, etc., give respiration problem and infections. It can be diagnosed by various methods like X-ray, CT scan, and echocardiogram which is used to visualize the heart. If find abnormal pressure in the heart, a pulmonary test, or lung tissues analysis is done. Lung disease refers to many disorders such as infections, asthma, COPD, lung cancer, tuberculosis, and pneumonia. This also consists distinctive between various lung conditions, like obstructive lung disease and restrictive lung disease. *Obstructive lung* diseases obstruct the flow of air out of the lungs. In other words, these genres of diseases cause a problem with the exhalation phase of the breathing cycle. The lung tissue loses its recoiling capabilities and thus finds it difficult to push air out during exhalation. "Air trapping" occurs, and the lungs appear like over-inflated balloons like asthma, emphysema, chronic bronchitis, etc. *Restrictive lung diseases* are quite the opposite. This type of disorder restricts the flow of air into the lungs. So, the problem is with the inhalation phase of the breathing cycle. The lung tissue develops scars. The scarring makes the lung unyielding to the incoming air. The total lung capacity reduces, and the lungs appear as rigid, under-inflated balloons. Any disease can cause the deposition of fibrous tissue in the lungs. Fibrous tissue forms scars, tuberculosis, pneumonitis, acute respiratory

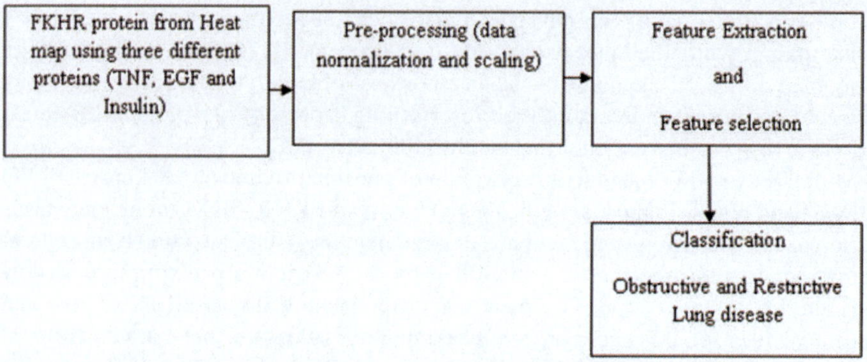

Fig. 1 Computational model for detection of different lung diseases

distress syndrome, etc. In this paper, the author has proposed a machine learning model for the detection of obstructive and restrictive lung diseases due to deficiency of FOXO protein [24–26]. The data is preprocessed by normality and scaling of data. Later, different attributes were extracted and selected which were classified using artificial neural network. (ANN) using multilayer perceptron (MLP) and radial basis function (RBF) as shown in Fig. 1.

Data cleaning is an important step for data preprocessing. Without data, machine learning is nothing. More useful data more will be the accuracy. The more the number of features, the more the chances of overfitting or the model becomes complex. Sometimes, misleading data (always noise) can lead to bad accuracy in predictive models. Different features were extracted [27, 28] which were selected using feature selection. The purpose of feature selection is to find the features that have a greater impact on the outcome of the predictive model while dimensionality reduction is about reducing the features without losing much genuine information and improve the performance [29]. Dimensionality reduction can be achieved by feature selection. Linear dimensionality reduction and nonlinear dimensionality reduction are two types of dimensionality reduction techniques. Principal component analysis (PCA), factor analysis, and linear discriminant analysis form linear techniques, while multidimensional scaling, isometric feature mapping, locally linear embedding, and spectral embedding form nonlinear techniques. Algorithm 1 shows the steps of feature selection.

Algorithm 1: Feature selection

1. Import all features of the dataset
2. Select the best subset
3. Apply algorithm like Backward Elimination, Forward Selection, Pearson Correlation, Recursive feature Elimination, Genetic Algorithm, Lasso, Simulated Annealing, Dalex

In this paper, the authors have used PCA for the selection of the best features. PCA is a dimension reduction technique used for a large number of variables, out of which some are correlated. To reduce cost complexity and computational time, PCA is used to transform original variables into the linear combination of variables. The selected features were classified using ANN. Activation functions are very crucial for an ANN in learning and making sense of something complicated. ANN uses nonlinear properties of the network, in ANN, conversion of the input signal of a node to an output signal took place. The output signal function as an input to the next layer. In ANN, products of input (x) and weight (w) are summed, and activation function is applied to get the output of that layer which further serves as input to another layer [30, 31].

3 Results and Discussion

Obstructive lung disease involves the blockage of the lung air passages (airways) by constriction or endogenous matter lodging in the airway lumen and generating inflammation and scarring, as well as the complete collapse of the lungs as in obstructive atelectasis and the invasion of the air sacs by foreign particles that generate inflammation or endogenous fluid such as mucus and endogenous solid matter or the degeneration in the integrity of the alveolar epithelium due to hyperplasia or scarring that prevents gaseous exchange. Air may not succeed to reach the alveoli, and this may result in suffocation or asphyxiation or it reaches but fails to go across the lung epithelium (in, for oxygen and out, for carbon dioxide). Restrictive lung disease is not a single disease but represents a kind of physiologic abnormality observed in multiple diseases of the lung or even neuromuscular breathing apparatus. It can range from various kinds of inflammatory/scarring lung diseases to respiratory difficulties inflating the chest because of muscle weakness or severe abnormalities of the thoracic spine. The treatment varies depending on the specific disease. It may also be caused by an incident out of the lungs (extrapulmonary or extrinsic) such as pleural effusion, breathing muscle paralysis, scoliosis, or be of lung parenchymal origin (intrinsic) that restricts lung expansion. Obesity, diaphragmatic hernia, and ascites can cause restrictive lung disease. Pneumoconiosis due to inhalation of dust particles such as in asbestosis is a common intrinsic cause. Other intrinsic causes are acute respiratory distress syndrome (ARDS) which leads to pneumonitis, eosinophilic pneumonia, and sarcoidosis. Usually, in all cases, some fibrosis makes the lungs stiff(er). The lung volume declines, and there is increased work of breathing with concomitant inadequacy in ventilation and/or oxygenation resulting in shortness of breath.

Before classification, the normality test has been performed that aims to test whether residual or confounding variables have a normal distribution and is known as t and F tests assuming the residual value follows a normal distribution. Graph analysis and statistical tests are two ways to detect whether the residuals are normally distributed or not. In this paper, Kolmogorov–Smirnov (K–S) test, P–P plot, and box whisker plot are used and are shown in Fig. 2. Residuals are normally distributed if they have a significant value >0.05.

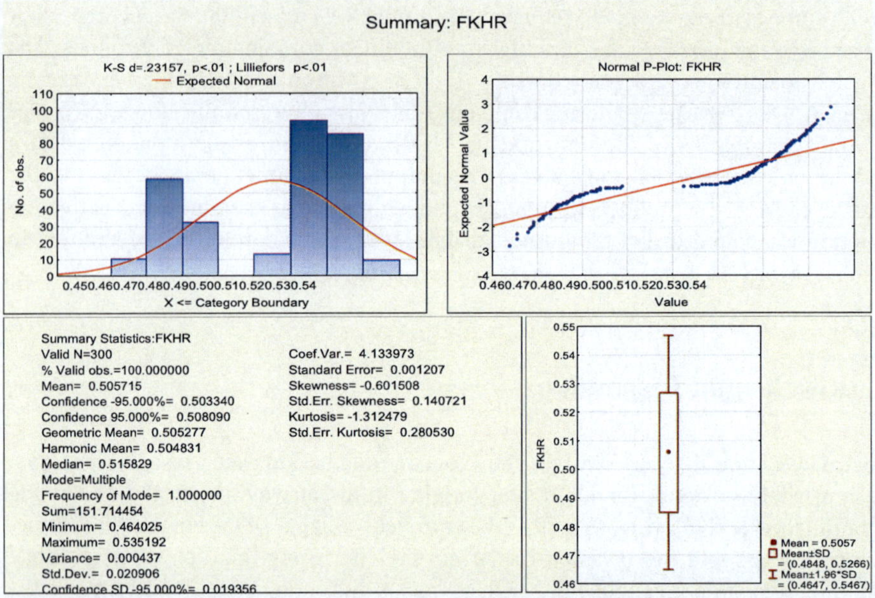

Fig. 2 K–S plot, *P–P* plot, and box whisker plot with different features

After graphical analysis, correlation analysis is done which is a statistical method used to measure the closeness of the relationship between two variables without paying attention to the variables that are influenced or the variables that affect it and how much influence a variable has on other variables. Table 1 shows the correlation matrix for FKHR protein. Table gives means, standard deviation, p-value, t-value, $r(X, Y)$, and coefficient of determination (r^2).

Different features were extracted which were selected using PCA as a feature selection technique. PCA involves extracting linear composites of observed variables. The selected features are classified using MLP and RBF. However, a neural network, along with learning a model for classification can select automatically useful features. Neural networks take in vectors or matrices (arrays) and perform either classification or function approximation (regression). Fundamentally, these two tasks are the same. In either case, training data is required. Image classification is the task of extracting information classes from a multiband image. It is the task that extracts information as classes from the image. In the classification method, data points into a certain class or category are classified. In other words, machine learning model training samples are labeled data points/observations with a label of the class belong to, and the ML model learns the association between features/independent variables and the target/response variable. In unsupervised (learning) classification (also known as clustering), training data does not have the class/category labels, and therefore, the model is trying to find/detect trends or clusters in the data (segment/cluster similar data points together). For verification, the authors use the available data and train

Table 1 Correlation matrix for FKHR protein

	Mean	Std. Dv	$r(X, Y)$	r^2	t	p
0-0-0	122.495	34.693				
FKHR	0.506	0.021	0.282	0.079	5.072	0.000
5-0-0	214.208	14.940				
FKHR	0.506	0.021	−0.814	0.663	−24.201	0.000
100-0-0	211.869	134.682				
FKHR	0.506	0.021	−0.157	0.025	−2.749	0.006
0-100-0	261.221	19.292				
FKHR	0.506	0.021	0.670	0.449	15.592	0.000
5-0-0.2	175.225	26.416				
FKHR	0.506	0.021	−0.939	0.882	−47.292	0.000
100-100-0	251.197	39.727				
FKHR	0.506	0.021	−0.007	0.000	−0.127	0.899
0-0-500	224.113	17.230				
FKHR	0.506	0.021	−0.038	0.001	−0.658	0.511
0.2-0-1	110.625	70.104				
FKHR	0.506	0.021	−0.713	0.508	−17.557	0.000
5-0-5	198.285	61.889				
FKHR	0.506	0.021	0.143	0.020	2.497	0.013
100-0-500	187.033	75.681				
FKHR	0.506	0.021	−0.661	0.437	−15.209	0.000

existing data to predict the available target. Depending on the size of data, 70–30 ratio is used. Generally, the distribution of the data also affects the performance of the classification model. So to make the performance independent of distribution, cross-validation is performed where the data in k-folds is distributed and test the performance over each fold. A cross-validation set is a third dataset next to the training and test set. It is used to pick the best values for certain parameters like lambda (when using regularization). Using the test set, train the model multiple times using different values for lambda and pick the value which has the highest accuracy on the cross-validation set. Table 2 gives the performance parameters in terms of training perfection, testing perfection, validation perfection, training error, testing error, and validation error using MLP and RBF. SOS is used as an error function.

In the table, MLP (12) signifies 12 hidden layers and RBF (25) signifies 25 hidden layers. In this paper, a type of ANN called "multilayer perceptron" is used, and due to comparison, both types of networks with various number neurons hidden layer and various activation function are set by STATISTICA toolbox. MLP shows better results than radial basic function ANN. The best results are obtained using MLP as 96.5% with zero errors, while RBF results in more training, testing, and

Table 2 Evaluation of performance parameters using MLP and RBF

S. no	Net. name	Training perf	Test perf	Validation perf	Training error	Test error	Validation error	Training algorithm	Hidden activation	Output activation
1	MLP (12)	96.50	95.90	96.20	0.00	0.00	0.00	BFGS 24	Tanh	Exponential
2	MLP (11)	96.50	96.00	96.10	0.00	0.00	0.00	BFGS 23	Tanh	Exponential
3	MLP (6)	96.60	96.30	96.00	0.00	0.00	0.00	BFGS 14	Exponential	Logistic
4	MLP (7)	96.50	96.10	96.10	0.00	0.00	0.00	BFGS 18	Exponential	Identity
5	MLP (10)	96.20	95.40	96.00	0.00	0.00	0.00	BFGS 13	Identity	Exponential
6	RBF (26)	33.2	31.5	37.8	26,079.178	19,037.691	3575.458	RBFT	Gaussian	Identity
7	RBF (23)	38.4	37.6	53.4	20,103.584	11,176.019	20,255.030	RBFT	Gaussian	Identity
8	RBF (25)	28.5	17.6	33.5	1160.301	322.488	1809.270	RBFT	Gaussian	Identity
9	RBF (24)	8.7	9.2	34.8	145,636.195	97,370.155	159,025.032	RBFT	Gaussian	Identity
10	RBF (21)	75.9	71.9	82.3	96.418	60.728	109.309	RBFT	Gaussian	Identity

validation error. MLP uses the sigmoid activation function and dot product between input and weights. The training is done using the backpropagation technique. RBF uses Gaussian activation function and Euclidean distance between input and weights which makes neurons more sensitive.

4 Conclusion

In this paper, researchers proposed a computational model for the detection of obstructive and restrictive lung disease. Different features were extracted which were selected using PCA and classified using the machine learning technique. A total of 96.5% accuracy has been observed using MLP, while the training, testing, and validation error is more in the case of RBF. The results using MLP outperform the result of RBF. MLP-ANN is not self-organizing model; therefore, a number of the nodes in each layer and number of the hidden layers is investigated via the user. When specifying the number of neurons in the hidden layer of the network, it could notice that if more nodes the hidden layer contains the more complex will be. Also, the larger the number of nodes in a neural network models the robust the model is; this means the increase in the ability of the network to figure out complex relationships between the input and the target variables. The main point for future work is introducing more input parameters that have not been investigated due to the lack of such information and the selecting optimum hyperparameters still needed to be achieving via enhancing the artificial intelligence model with further advanced meta-heuristic optimization algorithms which may provide a sufficiently good solution to an optimization problem.

References

1. World Health Organization (2006) Neurological disorders: public health challenges. WHO Library Cataloguing-in-Publication Data
2. Filley CM, Rollins YD, Alan Anderson C, et al (2007) The genetics of very early onset Alzheimer disease. Cogn Behav Neurol 20(3):149–156
3. Maiese K (2014) Driving neural regeneration through the mammalian target of rapamycin. Neural Regen Res 9(15):1413–1417
4. Nakka VP, Prakash-babu P, Vemuganti R (2014) Crosstalk between endoplasmic reticulum stress, oxidative stress, and autophagy: potential therapeutic targets for acute CNS injuries. Mol Neurobiol
5. Jain S (2012) Communication of signals and responses leading to cell survival/cell death using engineered regulatory networks. PhD Dissertation, Jaypee University of Information Technology, Solan, Himachal Pradesh, India
6. Weigel D, Jürgens G, Küttner F, Seifert E, Jäckle H (1989) The homeotic gene *fork head* encodes a nuclear protein and is expressed in the terminal regions of the Drosophila embryo. Cell 57(4):645–658
7. Cheng Z, White MF (2008) Targeting forkhead Box O1 from the concept to metabolic diseases: Lessons from mouse models. Antioxid Redox Signal 14(4):649–661; Maiese K, Chong ZZ,

Shang YC, Hou J (2008) Clever cancer strategies with FoxO transcription factors. Cell Cycle 7(24):3829–3839
8. Maiese K, Zhao ZC, Yan CS (2007) 'Sly as a FOXO': new paths with forkhead signaling in the brain. Curr Neurovasc Res 4(4):295–302
9. Maiese K, Hou J, Chong ZZ, Shang YC (2009) A fork in the path: developing therapeutic inroads with foxO proteins. Oxid Med Cell Longev 2(3):119–129
10. Maiese K, Chong ZZ, Shang YC, Hou J (2009) FoxO proteins: cunning concepts and considerations for the cardiovascular system. Clin Sci 116(3):191–203
11. Maiese K (2010) Forkhead transcription factors: vital elements in biology and medicine, vol 665. Advances in experimental medicine and biology. Springer Science+Business Media, Berlin
12. Clark KL, Halay ED, Lai E, Burley SK (1993) Co-crystal structure of the HNF-3/fork head DNA-recognition motif resembles histone H5. Nature 364(6436):412–420
13. Jin C, Marsden I, Chen X, Liao X (1998) Sequence specific collective motions in a winged helix DNA binding domain detected by 15N relaxation NMR. Biochemistry 37(17):6179–6187
14. Maiese K, Chong ZZ, Shang YC (2008) OutFOXOing disease and disability: the therapeutic potential of targeting FoxO proteins. Trends Mol Med 14(5):219–227
15. Larson ET, Eilers B, Menon S et al (2007) A winged-helix protein from sulfolobus turreted icosahedral virus points toward stabilizing disulfide bonds in the intracellular proteins of a hyperthermophilic virus. Virology 368(2):249–261
16. Biggs WH III, Cavenee WK, Arden KC (2001) Identification and characterization of members of the FKHR (FOX O) subclass of winged-helix transcription factors in the mouse. Mamm Genome 12(6):416–425
17. Huang H, Tindall DJ (2007) Dynamic FoxO transcription factors. J Cell Sci 120(15):2479–2487
18. Tsai KL, Sun YJ, Huang CY, Yang JY, Hung MC, Hsiao CD (2007) Crystal structure of the human FOXO3a-DBD/DNA complex suggests the effects of post-translational modification. Nucleic Acids Res 35(20):6984–6994
19. Maiese K, Chong ZZ, Hall J, Shang YC (2009) The 'O' class: crafting clinical care with FoxO transcription factors. Adv Exp Med Biol 665:242–260
20. Merkely B, Gara E, Lendvai Z et al (2015) Signaling via PI3K/FOXO1A pathway modulates formation and survival of human embryonic stem cell-derived endothelial cells. Stem Cells Dev 24(7):869–878
21. Zhao Y, Yu Y, Tian X, et al (2014) Association study to evaluate FoxO1 and FoxO3 gene in CHD in Han Chinese. PLoS ONE 9(1):e86252
22. Dogra J, Jain S, Sood M (2019) Glioma Classification of MR brain tumor employing machine learning. Int J Innov Technol Explor Eng (IJITEE) 8(8):2676–2682
23. Jain S (2021) Computer aided detection system for the classification of non small cell lung lesions using SVM. Curr Comput Aided Drug Des 16(6):833–840
24. Jain S, Salau AO (2019) An image feature selection approach for dimensionality reduction based on kNN and SVM for AkT proteins. Cogent Eng 6(1):1599537, 1–14
25. Amandeep, Jain S, Bhusri S (2017) CAD system for non small cell lung carcinoma using laws' mask analysis, March 1–3, 2017. In: Proceedings of the 11th INDIACom: 4th 2017 international conference on computing for sustainable global development, BVICAM, New Delhi, pp 6285–6288
26. Al-Jarrah OY, Yoo PD, Muhaidat S, Karagiannidis GK, Taha K (2015) Efficient machine learning for big data: a review. Big Data Res (Elsevier Inc.) 2(3):87–93. https://doi.org/10.1016/j.bdr.2015.04.001
27. Bhusri S, Jain S, Virmani J (2016) Classification of breast lesions using the difference of statistical features. Res J Pharm Biol Chem Sci (RJPBCS) 7(4):1365–1372
28. Rana S, Jain S, Virmani J (2016) SVM-based characterization of focal kidney lesions from B-mode ultrasound images. Res J Pharm Biol Chem Sci (RJPBCS) 7(4):837–846; Prashar N, Sood M, Jain S (2020) A novel cardiac arrhythmia processing using machine learning techniques. Int J Image Graph 20(3):2050023(17 pages)

29. Ayodeji Olalekan Salau, Shruti Jain, Adaptive Diagnostic Machine Learning Technique for Classification of Cell Decisions for AKT Protein, Informatics in Medicine Unlocked, 7 January 2021, 100511, B. Warner and M. Misra, "Understanding neural networks as statistical tools," *The American Statistician*, vol. 50, no. 4, pp. 284–293, 1996.
30. Microsoft time series algorithm technical reference | Microsoft Docs. https://docs.microsoft.com/en-gb/analysis-services/data-mining/microsoft-time-series-algorithm-technical-reference?redirectedfrom=MSDN&view=sql-server-ver15
31. Mosavi A, Salimi M, Ardabili SF, Rabczuk T, Shamshirband S, Varkonyi-Koczy AR (2019) State of the art of machine learning models in energy systems, a systematic review. Energies 12(7):https://doi.org/10.3390/en12071301

A Compact Planar Inverted F Antenna for 5G Applications in Biomedical Applications

Debarpita and Nikhil Marriwala

Abstract The aim of this paper is to structure a compact size Planar Inverted F Antenna (PIFA) for 5G applications in biomedical applications. The scale of the antenna is kept as small as possible; here, we have considered 18 × 15 × 2.7 mm and operating frequency of 11.2 GHz. The antenna designed here is probably going to own its applications in wireless communication system. The antenna designed in this project is structured in such a way that it is covering a good wide range of frequency from 10.2 to 12.3 GHz. The radiating patch of the designed antenna is having circular edge on both side of its patch to produce circular polarization. The antenna designed even has partial ground with slot which increases gain, reduces return loss, improves bandwidth, and offers improved VSWR. In this work various parameters like return loss, VSWR, gain, and radiation pattern are also discussed together with comparison of previous work.

Keywords Partial ground · Slot · PIFA · Circular edge · 5G · Return loss · VSWR · Radiation pattern

1 Introduction

The need for portable antenna in modern days are increasing gradually because the size of mobile phone is reducing day by day normal antennas have gotten replaced by PIFA due to its mini size and wide bandwidth [1–5].

The wireless communication is emerging nowadays, and frequencies below 6 GHz have gotten fully occupied due to which the requirement of 5G becomes it improve the speed of working within the hustle lifetime of today's generation. Everyone wants everything to be done at a one tip; thus, 5G comes to save us [6, 7]. 5G works for

Debarpita (✉) · N. Marriwala
Department of Electronics and Communication Engineering, University Institute of Engineering and Technology, Kurukshetra University, Kurukshetra, Haryana, India

N. Marriwala
e-mail: nmarriwala@kuk.ac.in

N. Marriwala et al. (eds.), *Emergent Converging Technologies and Biomedical Systems*, Lecture Notes in Electrical Engineering 841,
https://doi.org/10.1007/978-981-16-8774-7_8

frequency below and above 6 GHz for wireless applications [8]. Many works are still occurring for 5G devices; earlier many antennas are proposed already [9–11]. During this project, I have got tried to structure a compact antenna with improved bandwidth and reduce return loss. **Planar Inverted F Antenna (PIFA) is** basically one of the varieties of microstrip patch antenna. To boost performance of microstrip patch antenna, shorting pins at various locations are employed. It is nowadays widely being employed in mobile phone industry [3]. By doing shorting of pins underneath, advantages are obtained:

- Size is reduced
- Multi-frequency resonance
- Gain improvement
- Desired radiation pattern [3, 5, 11, 12]. During this project, the proposed antenna have a bandwidth of 2.1 GHz and have circular edge with lumped port. And also slot is introduced to boost up gain and reduce return loss as introduction of slot has underneath benefits [13]:
- Obtain broad impedance
- Stability of the radiation patterns
- Improved VSWR [2].

In this paper, partial ground is taken into consideration, which enhanced bandwidth, also improved gain, and helped in reduction of return loss [7].

Also truncated radiating patch is employed to produce circular polarization which provides constant electromagnetic field in all told direction [14].

The PIFA has reduced SAR rate (specific absorption rate) which makes it suitable to be used for biomedical applications as wearable device [5]. This 5G antenna can work as wearable device as it is using dielectric constant material, and it will be beneficial for telehealth where technology meeting healthcare sector for remote sensing as in current scenario people are often restricted to move from one place to another, so this kind of wearable device with 5G speed can help the chronically ill patients and doctors to keep track of those patients without any mobility and with faster speed [15].

The antenna is simulated and designed using the software named HFSS.

2 Antenna Design

The proposed antenna have partial ground plane of dimension 15 $\times$ 15 mm. Substrate used here is Rogers Duroid 5889 (Er = 2.2), and resonating frequency is 11.2 GHz. Height of the substrate is kept 0.8 mm. Radiating patch having width is 2.46 mm and length 7 mm with circular edge (truncation). (Circle radius is kept 1.54 mm to provide circular edge.) Feed line for exciting the antenna using lumped port has dimension of 2.7 $\times$ 3.5 mm. Shorting pin is kept close to the feed line as 50 ohm impedance is provided and has length and width of 2.7 and 2 mm, respectively. In

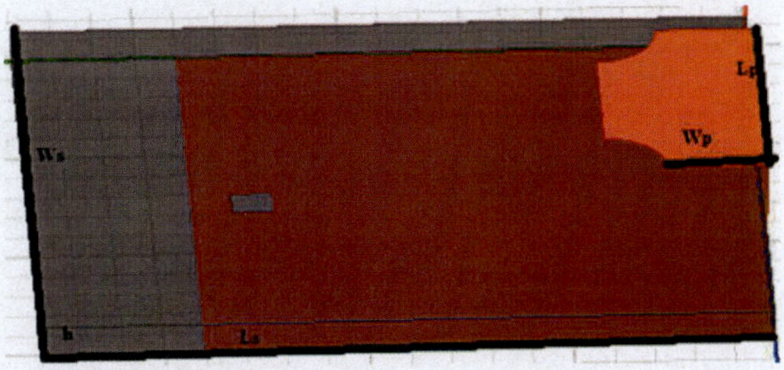

Fig. 1 Side view of antenna in HFSS

Table 1 Designing parameters of desired antenna

Parameter	Value (mm)
Lg	15
Wg	15
Ls	18
Ws	15
Wp	2.46
Lp	7
Lf	2.7
Wf	3.5
Wshort	2
Lshort	2.7
Lslot	1
Wslot	1
H	0.8

this paper, slot is additionally introduced to boost gain and reduce return loss. Slot dimension is (1 × 1) mm (Fig. 1).

Table 1 gives the dimension of the proposed antenna.

Figure 2 shows the feeding technique used for the proposed antenna. In this structure lumped port is used for exciting the antenna.

Figure 3 shows the ground plane structure with slot having dimension 1 × 1 mm, and material used for ground plane is copper which employs infinite conductivity.

3 Simulation Result

The desired antenna is designed using HFSS. The result is simulated keeping operating frequency as 11.2 GHz and certain important parameters like return loss which describes power loss by the antenna, VSWR shows how effectively antenna is working, gain, and radiation pattern as it is used as wearable device having %G characteristics it must be omnidirectional and safe for human body.

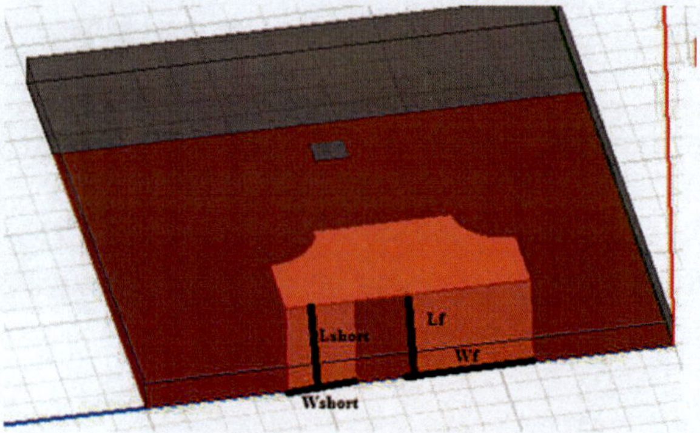

Fig. 2 Structure of feed line in HFSS

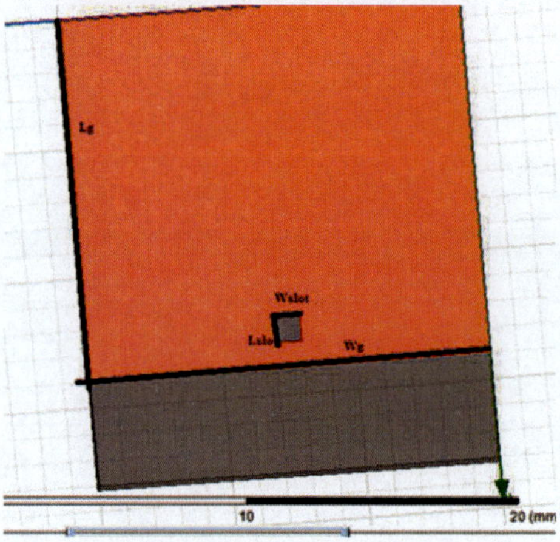

Fig. 3 Ground plane structure

3.1 Return Loss

S11 parameters are checked to observe antenna return loss, as lumped port method is used to excite the antenna, −10 dB is considered as base value for mobile communication. The proposed antenna is showing resonating frequency at 11.2 GHz having return loss of −24.7593 dB (with slot) and −21.7299 dB (without slot) and wider bandwidth of (10.2–12.3 GHz) 2.1 GHz after simulation. The simulation result is shown below in Fig. 4a, b.

3.2 Vswr

We know that for any antenna VSWR must not exceed 3; ideally, it should be 1. In this paper, the proposed antenna shows VSWR (with slot) of 1.0055 and VSWR

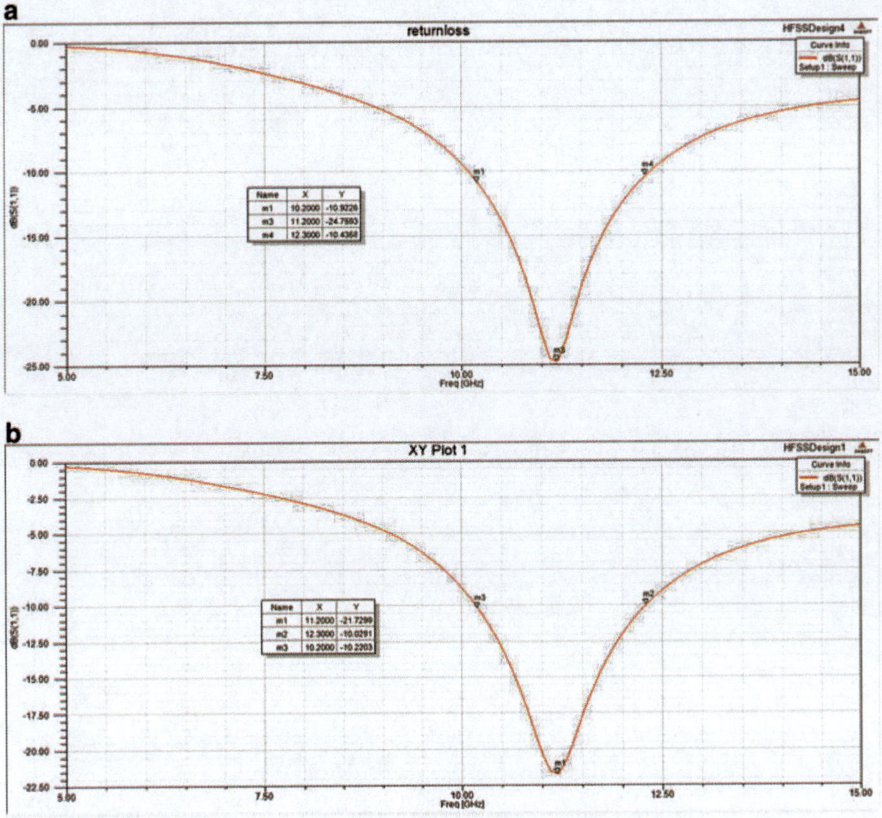

Fig. 4 **a** Return loss (S11) (with slot), **b** Return loss (S11) (without slot)

(without slot) of 1.42 which is close to 1 and is obtained at 11.2 GHz. The simulation result is shown below in Fig. 5a, b.

3.3 *Gain Pattern*

Efficiency of any antenna is determined by its gain parameter, and in proposed antenna design, gain of 5.0423 dB with slot and without slot 4.8404 dB is obtained well for Planar Inverted F Antenna (PIFA). The simulation result is shown in Fig. 6a, b.

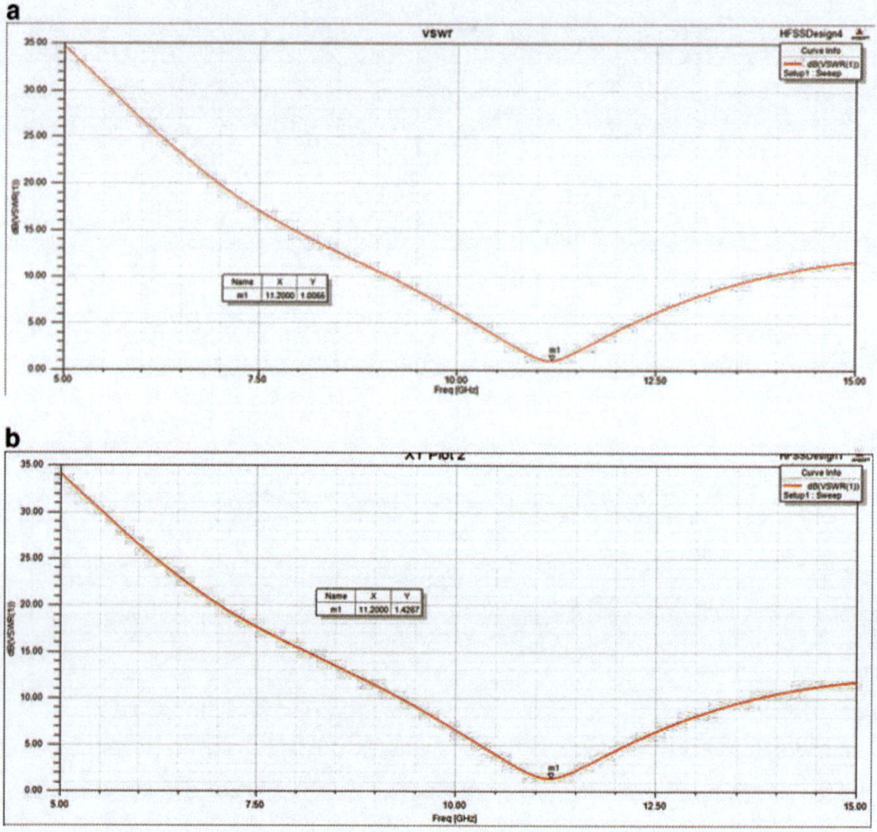

Fig. 5 **a** VSWR (with slot), **b** VSWR (without slot)

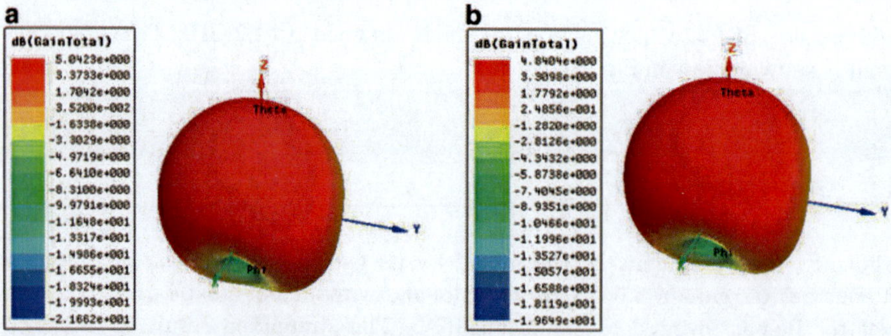

Fig. 6 **a** Gain (with slot), **b** Gain (without slot)

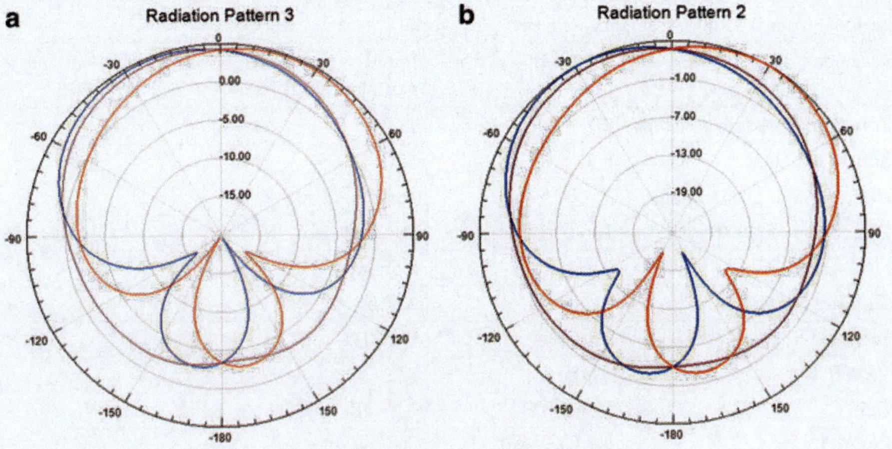

Fig. 7 **a** Radiation pattern (with slot), **b** Radiation pattern (without slot)

3.4 Radiation Pattern

The radiation pattern achieved shows that it is omnidirectional, has good radiation pattern of 2.1 GHz good for 5G applications, and has high-speed transmission. The simulation result is shown in Fig. 7a, b.

4 Comparison Table

This comparison is done in order to increase the bandwidth for our required purpose as form the previous work done the bandwidth is of 1.8 GHz which is improved in this project by employing partial ground and slot having bandwidth 2.1 GHz much greater and improvised version of previous one along with high gain and return loss is close to −30 dB which means less power loss during transmission. This comparison is given in Table 2.

In Table 3, the comparison of my proposed work is done on the basis of providing slot.

5 Conclusion

In this work, a compact edge fed Planar Inverted F Antenna has been proposed. The antenna resonates at 11.2 GHz with a return loss of −24.7593 dB which is often utilized in future 5G wireless devices and for healthcare devices too. The designed

Table 2 Comparison of my work with previous work [5]

Parameter	My proposed work	Previous researched work (without slot and partial ground)
Substrate dielectric constant	2.2	2.2
Substrate height	0.8	0.8
Dimension of ground plane	15 × 15 (mm)	18 × 10 (mm)
Dimension of substrate	18 × 15 (mm)	18 × 10 (mm)
Feed height	2.7 mm	3.5 mm
Shorting pin width	2 mm	2 mm
Bandwidth	2.1 GHz	1.8 GHz
VSWR	1.005	2.31
Gain	5.0423 dB	4.27 dB
Return loss	−24.7593 dB	−17.62 dB
Resonating frequency	11.2 GHz	10.61 GHz

Table 3 Comparison of my work with and without slot

Parameter	My proposed work	My proposed work (without slot)
Substrate dielectric constant	2.2	2.2
Substrate height	0.8	0.8
Dimension of ground plane	15 × 15 (mm)	15 × 15 (mm)
Dimension of substrate	18 × 15 (mm)	18 × 15 (mm)
Feed height	2.7 mm	2.7 mm
Shorting pin width	2 mm	2 mm
Bandwidth	2.1 GHz	2.1 GHz
VSWR	1.005	1.42
Gain	5.0423 dB	4.8404 dB
Return loss	−24.7593 dB	−21.7299 dB
Resonating frequency	GHz	11.2 GHz

antenna shows good radiation pattern and good gain of 5.0423 dB. The structure of the antenna is extremely compact, i.e., 18 × 15 × 2.7 mm, and can be easily placed in the housing of the wireless devices [5].

References

1. Wong H, Luk KM, Chan CH, Xue Q, So KK, Lai HW (2012) Small antennas in wireless communications. Proc IEEE 100(7):2109–2121. https://doi.org/10.1109/JPROC.2012.2188089
2. Sharma A (2017) Design and analysis of planer inverted-F antenna (PIFA) with electromagnetic bandgap structures
3. Rhee E (2020) Miniaturized PIFA for 5G communication networks. Appl Sci 10(4). https://doi.org/10.3390/app10041326
4. Rappaport TS et al (2013) Millimeter wave mobile communications for 5G cellular: It will work! IEEE Access 1:335–349. https://doi.org/10.1109/ACCESS.2013.2260813
5. Loharia A, Rana SB, Kumar N A novel miniature edge fed planar inverted-F antenna (PIFA) for future 5G wireless devices I. http://www.samsung.com/global/
6. Anouar M, Larbi S (2018) PIFA antenna for future mobile 5G. https://doi.org/10.1145/3286606.3286808
7. Aziz MAA, Seman N, Chua TH (2019) Microstrip antenna design with partial ground at frequencies above 20 GHz for 5G telecommunication systems. Indones J Electr Eng Comput Sci 15(3):1466–1473. https://doi.org/10.11591/ijeecs.v15.i3.pp1466-1473
8. Kaur A, Kaur B, Pasricha R (2019) Planar antenna covering sub-6 GHz for 5G enabled mobile devices worldwide. Int J Innov Technol Explor Eng 8(11):1549–1554. https://doi.org/10.35940/ijitee.K1817.0981119
9. Cheung CY, Yuen JSM, Mung SWY (2018) Miniaturized printed inverted-f antenna for internet of things: a design on PCB with a meandering line and shorting strip. Int J Antennas Propag 2018. https://doi.org/10.1155/2018/5172960
10. El Kilani S, El Abdellaoui L, Zbitou J, Errkik A, Latrach M (2019) A compact dual band PIFA antenna for GPS and ISM BAND applications. Indones J Electr Eng Comput Sci 14(3):1266–1271. https://doi.org/10.11591/ijeecs.v14.i3.pp1266-1271
11. Gao GP, Yang C, Hu B, Zhang RF, Wang SF (2019) A wide-bandwidth wearable all-textile PIFA with dual resonance modes for 5 GHz WLAN applications. IEEE Trans Antennas Propag 67(6). https://doi.org/10.1109/TAP.2019.2905976
12. Haraz OM, Ashraf M, Alshebeili S (2015) Single-band PIFA MIMO antenna system design for future 5G wireless communication applications. In: 2015 IEEE 11th international conference on wireless and mobile computing, networking and communications, WiMob 2015, pp 608–612. https://doi.org/10.1109/WiMOB.2015.7348018
13. Nasimuddin, Chen ZN, Qing X (2013) Slotted microstrip antennas for circular polarization with compact size. IEEE Antennas Propag Mag 55(2):124–137. https://doi.org/10.1109/MAP.2013.6529322
14. Mak KM, Lai HW, Luk KM, Chan CH (2014) Circularly polarized patch antenna for future 5G mobile phones. IEEE Access 2:1521–1529. https://doi.org/10.1109/ACCESS.2014.2382111
15. Ahad A, Tahir M, Sheikh MA, Ahmed KI, Mughees A, Numani A (2020) Technologies trend towards 5G network for smart health-care using IoT: a review. Sensors (Switzerland) 20(14):1–22. https://doi.org/10.3390/s20144047

AI-Powered Semantic Segmentation and Fluid Volume Calculation of Lung CT Images in COVID-19 Patients

Kokka Paramban Sabeerali, T. S. Saleena, P. Muhamed Ilyas, and Neha Mohan

Abstract COVID-19 pandemic is a deadly disease spreading very fast. People with the confronted immune system are susceptible to many health conditions. A highly significant condition is pneumonia, which is found to be the cause of death in the majority of patients. The main purpose of this study is to find the volume of GGO and consolidation of a COVID-19 patient, so that the physicians can prioritize the patients. Here, we used transfer learning techniques for segmentation of lung CTs with the latest libraries and techniques which reduces training time and increases the accuracy of the AI Model. This system is trained with DeepLabV3 + network architecture and model ResNet50 with ImageNet weights. We used different augmentation techniques like Gaussian noise, horizontal shift, color variation, etc., to get to the result. Intersection over Union *(IoU)* is used as the performance metrics. The IoU of lung masks is predicted as 99.78% and that of infected masks is as 89.01%. Our work effectively measures the volume of infected region by calculating the volume of infected and lung mask region of the patients.

Keywords COVID-19 · Transfer learning · DeepLabV3 + · ResNet50 · Albumentation · GGO volume calculation · IoU

K. P. Sabeerali (✉) · T. S. Saleena · P. Muhamed Ilyas
Sullamussalam Science College, Areekode, India
e-mail: sabeeralikp8@sscollege.ac.in

T. S. Saleena
e-mail: tssaleena@sscollege.ac.in

P. Muhamed Ilyas
e-mail: principal@sscollege.ac.in

Neha Mohan
Govt. Medical College, Manjeri, India
e-mail: radiologygmchmji@gmail.com

N. Marriwala et al. (eds.), *Emergent Converging Technologies and Biomedical Systems*, Lecture Notes in Electrical Engineering 841,
https://doi.org/10.1007/978-981-16-8774-7_9

1 Introduction

The corona virus disease 2019 (COVID-19) is an ongoing pandemic, gripping the world over and affecting millions of people ever since the first outbreak in December 2019 at Wuhan, China. It is an infectious disease caused by the novel RNA virus SARS-CoV-2 (severe acute respiratory syndrome coronavirus-2) mainly manifesting as respiratory illness of varying severity. Though the disease can be asymptomatic in healthy individuals, it can cause significant morbidity in others, especially in elderly patients and those with other co-morbidities where it can even be fatal.

As per WHO statistics, globally, there have been 11,36,95,296 confirmed cases of COVID-19 till March 1, 2021, including 25,26,007 deaths [1]. The rapid spread of COVID-19 to global level pandemic created the urgent need for a reliable and efficient way of diagnosing patients. Even though a positive RT-PCR test is required for definitive diagnosis of COVID-19, CT chest has a potential role in diagnosis, detection of complications, and most importantly prognostication of the disease. The presence and extent of abnormality in the lungs on CT is based on the stage and severity of the disease, and the most common abnormal findings are bilateral peripheral ground-glass opacity and/ or consolidation with predilection for lower lobes of lungs [2]. Ground glass opacity and consolidation are areas of increased attenuation/ density in lungs on CT and represent infected/ inflamed lungs in patients with COVID-19 pneumonia. Detecting these findings and assessing the severity of the involvement of lungs will help triage patients properly, so that the worst affected ones are quickly identified and addressed, leading to better patient care and treatment.

Usually, radiologists qualitatively evaluate the extent of lung volume infected in CT and issue reports. Manual CT image segmentation takes time and may have different hurdles like variation in shapes of ROI, difficulty in edge detection of ROI, clarity of image, noise inbuilt in the medical imaging devices, etc. [3]. Also, the ratio of the number of radiologists available to report to the number of CT images to be read is very much on the lower side. And as the number of patients increases exponentially, it further becomes a herculean task, affecting workflow. A fast auto-contouring computerized tool to accurately quantify the infection lung regions in COVID-19 infection will be a boon in this testing time and is a need of the hour. So we come up with a method to help radiologists in which a computer system can segment the lung CTs and quantify infected lung volumes, so that healthcare providers can prioritize patients who need critical care and can make the right treatment decisions. This will be done based on the severity of the disease which can be categorized using this system.

Chen [4] The semantic segmentation using fully convolutional neural networks may end up with fuzzy object boundaries and low-resolution images as it causes loss of information due to convolution and pooling. This has been overtaken by the DeepLab series that uses Atrous Spatial Pyramid Pooling. Among them, DeepLabV3 version onward, the required features are extracted from the pretrained networks like VGG, ResNet, DenseNet, etc. The proposed system uses ResNet50 as the backbone network along with DeepLabV3 + which is an extended version of DeepLabV3 [5].

The percentage of infected regions can be calculated from the total lung area.

$$\text{Percentage of the infected portion} = \\ (\text{volume of infection mask/volume of total lung mask}) * 100$$

This system can be used in collaboration with the CT scanner and set a threshold value, so that patients can be prioritized based on that value. The radiologist will be notified of this value and such patients will be treated with more care and attention and others will be discharged. This helps to utilize the hospital resources efficiently.

2 Related Works

Ali et al. [6] narrates the findings that a radiologist should identify from lung CT images in the case of COVID-19. The key infection indicators are ground-glass opacity (GGO) and consolidation. Feng Shi et al. [7] made a sail on different AI techniques that applied in X-ray and CT of COVID-19 patients, and they made a consolidation about AI-empowered contactless medical image acquisition workflows, segmentation, diagnosis, and follow-up studies. In all these cases, U-Net architecture is predominant. The laboratory tests, especially the RT-PCR test, are now considered as the gold standard for the diagnosis of COVID-19. But still, it may be inadequate in some situations. Ophir Gozes et al. [8] developed an AI-based automated CT image analysis tool that classifies the COVID-affected patients using thoracic CT and tracks the disease burden. The work showed 98.2% sensitivity and 92.2% specificity on datasets of Chinese control and infected patients. Shuai Wang et al. [9] used inception migration-learning model to set a deep learning model. The performance metrics of accuracy, specificity, and sensitivity of internal validation are 82.9%, 80.5%, and 84%, respectively, whereas the same of external testing is 73.1, 67, and 74% [10]. The DeepLab has been introduced by Liang-Chieh Chen et al. which was the state-of-the-art network in the competition of semantic image segmentation task using PASCAL VOC-2012. Its mIOU value has been measured as 79.7% [5]. A novel model DeepLabV3 + which is the extension of DeepLabV3 has been introduced by Liang-Chieh Chen in which DeepLabV3 acts as the encoder module and an additional decoder module to refine the segmentation process. This architecture along with ResNet101 and Xception as network backbone is used in which the Xception model results the best test set performance of 89%.

3 Methods

3.1 Data Preparation

Images have been downloaded from the site *radiopedia.org* and *coronacases.org*. This work has been implemented using the pytorch library. The Med2image library converts each slice of Nifti image and its mask into a corresponding.png file with the same dimension without any loss of data. The system used 512 X 512 X 3 and 512 X 512 images and masks, respectively. Preprocessing is not explicitly giving for this network, as it makes use of the same of the pretrained model. Each pretrained model will have its preprocessing steps. We just have to input the model name and its corresponding weight obtained from ImageNet, which will give preprocessed data as output.

The whole dataset has been divided into three sets: training set—1789 images and corresponding masks (82%), validation set—207(10%); testing set—176 images (8%).

3.2 Data Augmentation

Ter-Sarkisov [11] As the deep neural networks heavily rely on big data for better performance and medical image analysis has no access to the same, data augmentation is an inevitable factor in such cases. The augmentation using keras will change the pixel value of the image. But the semantic segmentation highly relies on the pixel, and it should not be changed during augmentation. In such cases, **Albumentation** is the right choice. In this system, the training data has been augmented using this library. Even though the library provides more than 70 augmentations, this system used horizontal flip, shift scale rotate, random crop, additive Gaussian noise, perspective, CLAHE, random brightness, sharpen, blur, motion blur, random contrast, and hue saturation (Fig. 1).

3.3 Semantic Segmentation

Segmentation is a process in which it not only identifies whether the disease present or not, but also contours the area which is affected by the disease. It helps in the localization of disease and quantization of the volume of disease, whereas semantic segmentation aims at the pixel-wise labeling of the image using the corresponding category to which it belongs [5, 12, 13]. Each pixel of the image is checking whether it belongs to fluid content or not. The segmentation task can be performed without explicitly coding with the help of segmentation models that provide preconfigured models and backbones. This backbone refers to any pretrained classification model without dense

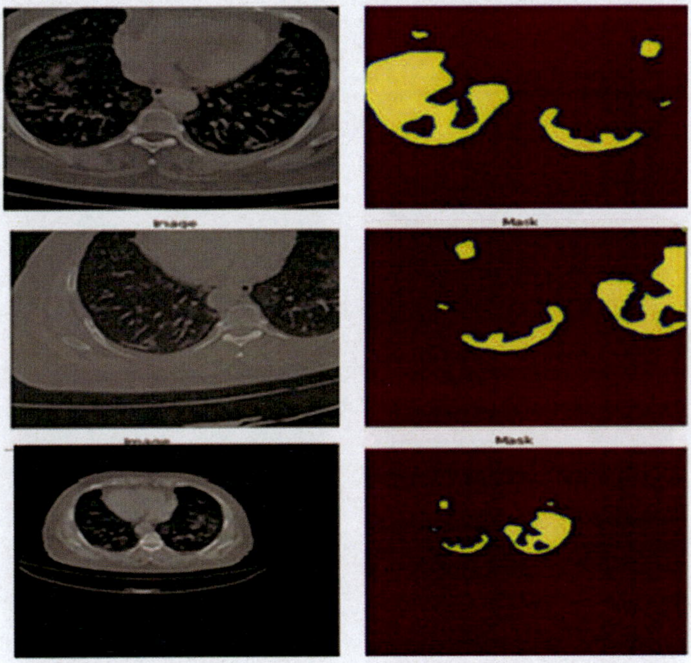

Fig. 1 Different augmentations done on a single CT image (left) and its masks at right

layer, which is used for feature extraction to build the model. Figure 2 depicts the workflow of the system that uses DeepLabV3 + architecture with ResNet50 as the feature provider.

DeepLabV3 + architecture: Wang et al. [14] DeepLabV3 + is the latest and the most effective architecture in the DeepLab series which is the invention of Google. The Atrous Spatial Pyramid Pooling or ASPP and the encoder–decoder architecture make this version capable of outperforming all other similar kinds. This makes it possible to create the output image of same size as the input image, as here occurs the pixel to pixel mapping in semantic segmentation [5]. This combination is leading to semantic image segmentation tasks [10]. ASPP enables the object and image context

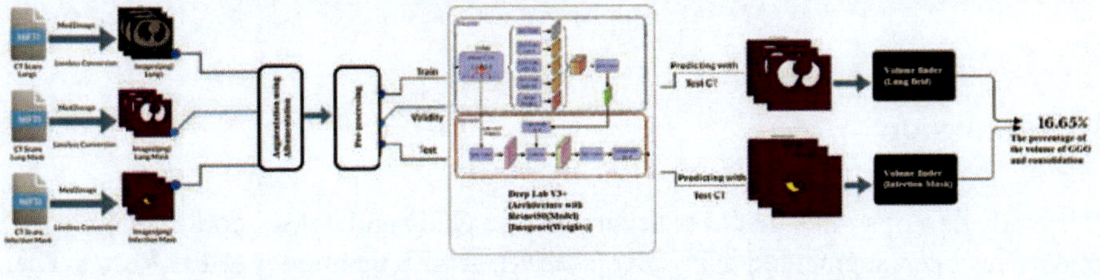

Fig. 2 Segmentation model using DeepLabV3 + and ResNet50 as backbone is finding the volume of affected part in lung CT

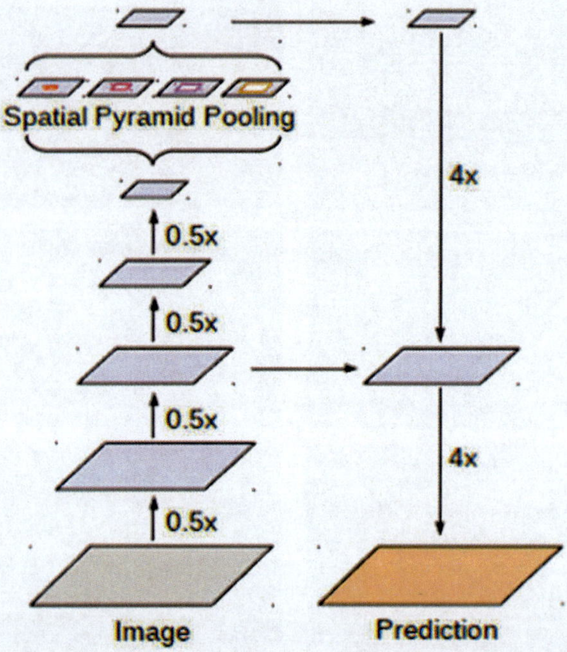

Fig. 3 Architecture of DeepLabV3 +

segmentation in multiple scales [15]. The encoder–decoder architecture consists of a contracting path that extracts the required features and an expanding path that will localize the affected region. Liang-Chieh Chen et al. [10] depicts the above-described features of DeepLabV3 + through Fig. 3.

ResNet50 as feature extractor pre-trained network: ResNet50 is used here as a network backbone for feature extraction. ResNet is one of the powerful classification networks that proved its excellence in the ***ILSVRC 2015*** classification challenge. It is pretrained on the ImageNet dataset. So we can load the predefined weights of the model, freeze the encoder part as it is, and need to begin with the decoder part only while training [16]. It has 48 convolution layer, 1 max-pooling, and 1 average pooling layer [17]. The figure shows the residual block of the deep residual network (Figs. 4 and 5).

4 Discussion

This study demonstrates that how accurately the GGO and consolidation in CT scan images has been segmented using DeepLabV3 + with the model of ResNet50. The Nifti images of original CT scan, lung mask, and infection mask have been losslessly converted to .png images and after augmentation and preprocessing they are fed into

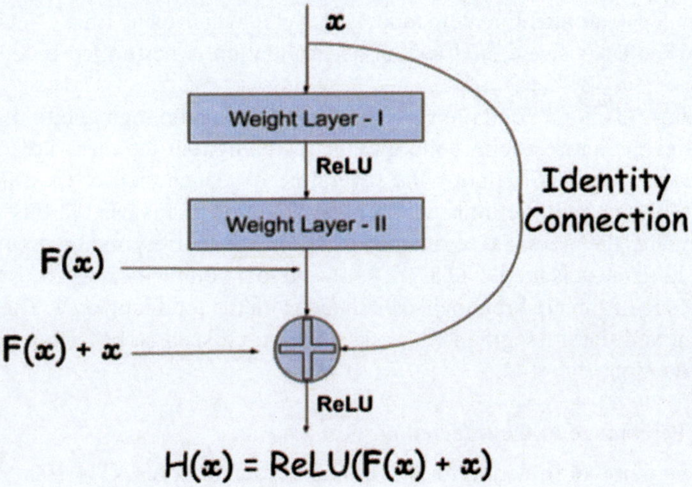

Fig. 4 Residual function block of ResNet

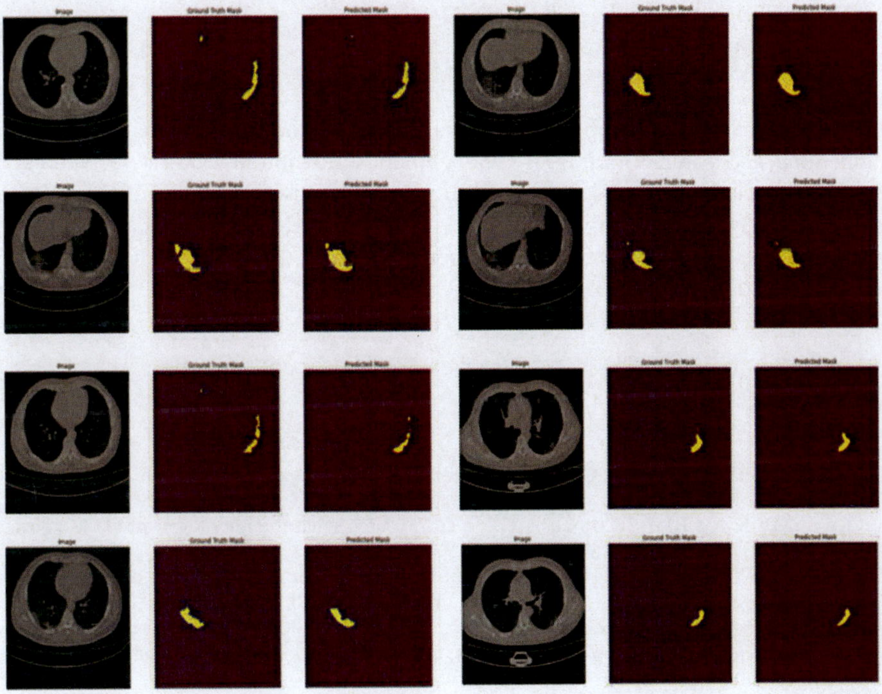

Fig. 5 CT image (from left), ground truth mask (middle), and predicted mask (output of the system)

the DeepLabV3 + architecture with model ResNet50 which using ImageNet weights. The trained model is saved, and testing and validation is performed based on that model.

The accuracy is not a good metric in the case of semantic segmentation, because in some cases the entire background may be matching, but the mask area may not be matching very well. So among the several performance metrics to evaluate the efficiency of the model, the Intersection over Union or IoU is used in this scenario [17]. It compares the predicted segmented mask with the corresponding ground truth. The IoU of lung mask is predicted as 99.78%, and IoU of infected mask is as 89.01%. The percentage of infected region is calculated from the total lung area. The volume of total lung and that of segmented mask is measured separately further part done using the equation,

$$\begin{aligned}&\text{Percentage of the infected portion } = \\ &(\text{volume of infection mask/volume of total lung mask}) \ * 100\end{aligned}$$

5 Conclusion

This study proves that deep learning is an effective tool to help radiologists in segmenting and volume finding of GGO and consolidation in COVID-19 patients. This can reduce the inter-observer variability and subjectivity of the radiologist. This will also greatly reduce their workload and reporting time. This system can prioritize the patients based on the volume of infection which can ensure that medical care can be given to those who are really in need.

References

1. WHO Coronavirus Disease (COVID-19) (2021) Dashboard https://covid19.who.int/. Accessed 1 Mar 2021
2. Kwee TC, Kwee RM (2020) Chest CT in COVID-19: what the radiologist needs to know. RadioGraph 40(7):1848–1865
3. Li C, Zhao C, Bao J, Tang B, Wang Y, Gu B (2020) Laboratory diagnosis of coronavirus disease-2019 (COVID-19). Clin Chim Acta. https://doi.org/10.1016/j.cca.2020.06.045
4. Chen LC, Papandreou G, Kokkinos I, Murphy K, Yuille AL (2016) DeepLab: semantic image segmentation with deep convolutional nets, atrous convolution, and fully connected CRFs. arXiv:1606.00915v2
5. Dai W, Zhang H, Yu J, Xu H, Chen H, Luo S, Zhang H, Liang L, Wu X, Lei Y, Lin F (2020) CT imaging and differential diagnosis of COVID-19. Canad Assoc Radiol J 71(2):195–200
6. Ronneberger O, Fischer P, Brox T (2015) U-Net: convolutional networks for biomedical image segmentation. In: MICCAI 2015: medical image computing and computer-assisted intervention (MICCAI 2015), pp 234–241
7. Shan F, Gao Y, Wang J, Shi W, Shi N, Han M, Xue Z, Shi Y (2020) Lung infection quantification of COVID-19 in CT images with deep learning. arXiv:2003.04655

8. Shorten C, Khoshgoftaar TM (2015) A survey on image data augmentation for deep learning. J Big Data
9. Gozes O, Frid-Adar M, Greenspan H, Browning PD, Zhang H, Ji W, Bernheim A, Siegel E (2020) Rapid AI development cycle for the coronavirus (COVID-19) pandemic: initial results for automated detection & patient monitoring using deep learning CT image analysis
10. Chen LC, Zhu Y, Papandreou G, Schroff F, Adam H (2018) Encoder-decoder with atrous separable convolution for semantic image segmentation
11. Ter-Sarkisov A (2020) Detection and segmentation of lesion areas in chest CT scans for the prediction of COVID-19. https://doi.org/10.1101/2020.10.23.20218461
12. https://developers.arcgis.com/python/guide/how-deeplabv3-works/
13. Ali TF, Tawab MA, ElHariri MA (2020) CT chest of COVID-19 patients: what should a radiologist know? Egypt J Radiol Nuclear Med 51:120
14. Wang S, Kang B, Ma J, Zeng X, Xiao M, Guo J, Cai M, Yang J, Li Y, Meng X (2020) A deep learning algorithm using CT images to screen for CoronaVirus Disease (COVID-19). https://doi.org/10.1101/2020.02.14.20023028
15. Review: DeepLabv3+—Atrous Separable Convolution (Semantic Segmentation)
16. Wang P; Chen P; Yuan Y, Liu D, Huang Z, Hou X, Cottrell G (2018) Understanding convolution for semantic segmentation. In: IEEE winter conference on applications of computer vision (WACV)
17. He K, Zhang X, Ren S, Sun J (2015) Deep residual learning for image recognition
18. F Shi J Wang J Shi Wu Ziyan Q Wang Z Tang K He Y Shi D Shen 2020 Review of artificial intelligence techniques in imaging data acquisition, segmentation and diagnosis for COVID-19 IEEE Rev Biomed Eng 1–1 https://doi.org/10.1109/rbme.2020.2987975
19. Koundal D, Gupta S (2020) Advances in computational techniques for biomedical image analysis methods and applications
20. Fang Y, Zhang H, Xie J, Lin M, Ying L, Pang P, Ji W (2020) Sensitivity of chest CT for COVID-19: comparison to RT-PCR
21. https://www.jeremyjordan.me/semantic-segmentation/
22. https://iq.opengenus.org/resnet50-architecture/
23. https://towardsdatascience.com/intersection-over-union-iou-calculation-for-evaluating-an-image-segmentation-model-8b22e2e84686
24. https://www.youtube.com/watch?v=J_XSd_u_Yew

WSN Based Health Monitoring System for COVID-19 Patients

Shaurya Sinha, Dheerika Pandey, and Garima Mahendru

Abstract The entire humankind is combating the COVID-19 pandemic since the onset of 2020. The increase in the cases has triggered an alarming situation all over the world. Doctors and hospital staff are working overtime in the COVID wards by putting their lives at risk. As the health line workers are in immediate contact with the patients, it causes a high risk of spreading the infection among them. To avoid immediate contact of the medical personnel with the patients, the work presented in this paper aims at devising wireless sensor network (WSN)-based COVID-19 patient health monitoring system, which is enabled with IoT and is useful in evaluating the patients, keeping a check on their vital/ health status without coming in contact with them, and eventually creating a feasible method of sending information related to the health of patients to the health staff. The doctors/nurses can keep an eye on the health stats and keep a check on the overall condition of the patients. In case hospital beds are not available, this system can also be used when the patient is home quarantined. The health personnel can take necessary action according to the parameters through mobile phone/desktop. The medical personnel may check these parameters through mobile phone or desktop and may take necessary action accordingly. Thus, the health monitoring system proposed in this paper helps monitor the data of patients remotely, and this decreases the need for contact between the health line workers and patients. This further lessens the possibility of infecting them.

Keywords Wireless sensor networks (WSN) · Internet of Things (IoT) · I2C communication · Wi-Fi

S. Sinha (✉) · D. Pandey · G. Mahendru
Amity University, Noida, Uttar Pradesh, India

G. Mahendru
e-mail: gmahendru@amity.edu

N. Marriwala et al. (eds.), *Emergent Converging Technologies and Biomedical Systems*, Lecture Notes in Electrical Engineering 841,
https://doi.org/10.1007/978-981-16-8774-7_10

1 Introduction

Since the very initial stage of corona virus disease 2019 (COVID-19), the cases have only surged. A lot of research regarding the diagnosis of COVID through artificial intelligence using different cough samples has been accomplished [1]. The virus is deadly and causes severe health problems as its after effect. It is difficult to lessen the spread as the symptoms are unable to be tracked on time and report. Despite the testing and trials of vaccination, the count of cases to decrease to a single digit will take some time. Hence, for areas which fall under containment zone and where the infection is spreading at a faster rate, therefore monitoring the patients remotely is advisable. Going by the advancements in technology, the WSN based patient health monitoring system fits correctly in this scenario [2]. These health monitoring models are widely used in the healthcare sector [3]. Health monitoring systems with IoT provide remote monitoring and early diagnosis [4]. One of the benefit would be to secure the load of being quarantined in the hospital (Fig. 1). And the patient can save himself from the hassle of going to the doctor and wait in a queue [5].

Despite continuous efforts from the medical personnel, it gets difficult to keep a track as the number of patients keeps on increasing every day. Thus, the solution of remote patient monitoring can be used. Remote patient monitoring also comes with many benefits like the patient can stay at their homes, while the health line workers can keep a check from distant location [6]. In the situation, this system comes as a first-hand solution to control its spread [7]. Real-time wireless health monitoring finds its applications in monitoring various kinds of health issues and diseases such as measuring blood pressure, body temperature [8], and cardiovascular diseases [9].

The objective of this paper is to design and implement the patient health monitoring system for the people struggling with COVID-19. It has sensors that will keep

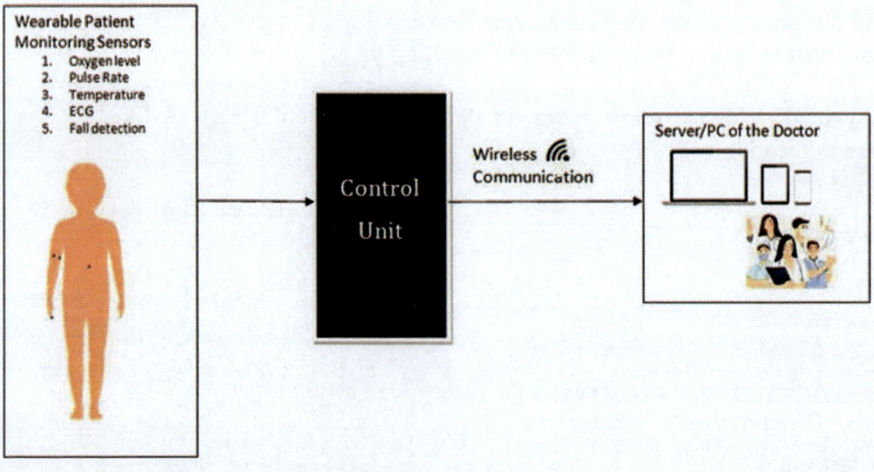

Fig. 1 Proposed system

track of the vital stats, thereby reducing the cost of visiting the doctor [10]. The nodes empower the network which is acquired over a wide area and process it which is further transmitted to ESP32. In case, the parameters fall out of the range described the buzzer rings. One main parameter to keep a check on the person's health is the heart rate of the patient [11, 12]. The common symptoms of COVID-19 include low oxygen level, high temperature, and high heart rate, and in some cases, the patient may lose balance. WSN (a self-configured) is wireless network responsible for gathering, processing, and distributing data to the sink where data is gathered in the database storage center. This database storage center acts as a medium among the network and the users [13, 14]

Recent literature survey and advancements in innovation have made it simpler to gather information anywhere, be it in the home, industry, and across urban communities [15, 16]. As this information is gathered and deciphered, the information would now be easily accessible. These steps are making what is known as the Internet of Things (IoT), the Internet of Everything, it is used to be known as Machine to Machine (M2M) correspondence [17]. Earlier GSM modules and Bluetooth devices were being incorporated to monitor the patient's health status. The current circumstance is advancing quickly with the making of low power WSNs [18]. Presently, the gathered information can be given to individuals who need it. Systems for health monitoring based on IOT are effectively put to use for various diseases [19–24].

2 Methodology

2.1 *Proposed System*

The main goal is to design and implement a wireless sensor network-based patient health tracking device for COVID-19 positive patients. Sensors are placed on the patient's body (arm/chest) suffering from COVID-19 or any other communicable disease to sense heart rate, oxygen level, and core body temperature of the virus contained patient and of the environment. Two sensors are placed on the arm to analyze heart rate and vibrations, and for fall detection. Along with four sensors, an emergency button is provided for notifying the health staff. The sensors are further interfaced to a control unit that calculates the values; the data is eventually then transmitted to the cloud server. The data can then be accessed by the medical staff or doctor at any other distant location. Therefore, based on the parameters (heart rate value, oxygen level, body and room temperature, the electrical activity of heart contraction and fall detection vibration), the doctor can analyze the virus-contained patient and therefore suitable measures could be taken.

2.2 Sensor

- Pulse oximeter measures the value of heart rate of a person along with oxygen level. The oxygen level is measured by sending the infrared light into capillaries in the finger, earlobe, or toe and detects the amount of light reflected off the gases. Pulses are digitally detected by the microcontroller to give the suitable outcome, explained with the formula:

$$\text{Beats per minute} = 60 * \text{f}, \ \text{where f is the pulse frequency}$$

- Temperature sensor is connected to the microcontroller via analog pin and through which the signal is transformed in digital value using ADC. This digital data gets converted into the actual temperature value in degree Fahrenheit using the equation:

$$\text{Temperature (F)} = [\text{temperature value} \ * \ 9/5 + 32]$$

- Electrocardiogram (ECG) sensor is used to determine the electrical waves of the heart to diagnose different heart conditions.
- Knock sensor measures the fall detection of any patient due to breathlessness. The sensor gives the value "0" when no fall is detected and gives the value "1" when the falling of a person is detected.
- Emergency Button allows the patient to notify the doctor or the medical staff incase he/she feels unwell.

2.3 Protocol Used

I2C communication inter-integrated circuit is a serial communication protocol, transmitting data bit by bit through a primary wire. As the data packets are to be transmitted after a particular duration, clock signal shared among the master as well as the slave is considered for synchronization of output of bits to sampling of bits.

Wi-Fi -the microcontroller implements Wi-Fi Direct specification and TCP/IP full 802.11 b/g/n/e/i WLAN MAC protocol. When used in station (client) mode, the processor can communicate with most Wi-Fi routers for easy access. Wi-Fi Direct is easier to setup, has high data transfer speed, and has advanced system interconnections.

Experimental Setup.

Temperature sensor, ECG, pulse oximeter sensors, knock sensor, and emergency button are monitored and displayed on the screen. The values are stored on cloud database. Range of heart rate is determined as in Table 1. The real-time value curve for heart rate in Fig. 2 is as given:

Table 1 Range for heart rate

Heart rate	State
60BPM–100BPM	Normal
<60BPM	Low
>100BPM	High

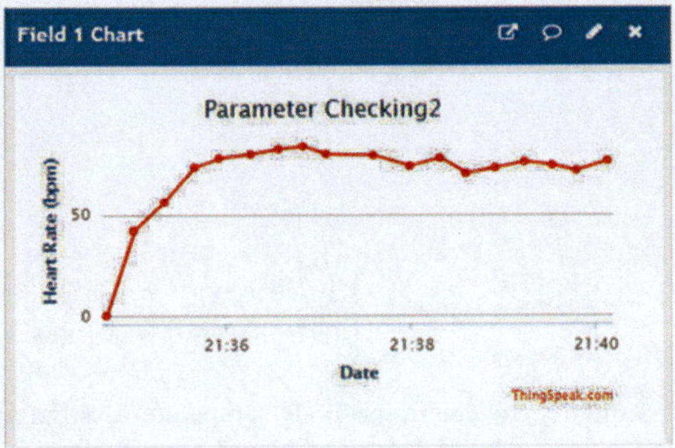

Fig. 2 Real-time curve for heart rate

$$\text{Normal} = \begin{cases} 1\ (\text{Healthy}),\ 60\text{BPM} <= x <= 100\text{BPM} \\ 0(\text{Unhealthy}),\ x > 100\text{BPM and } x < 60\text{BPM} \end{cases}$$

$$\text{Low} = \begin{cases} 1\ (\text{Healthy}),\ x > 60\text{BPM} \\ 0\ (\text{Unhealthy}),\ x < 60\text{BPM} \end{cases}$$

$$\text{High} = \begin{cases} 1\ (\text{Healthy}),\ x < 100\text{BPM} \\ 0\ (\text{Unhealthy}),\ x > 100\text{BPM} \end{cases}$$

For oxygen level of the patient, different range is considered and recorded as in Table 2. The real-time value curve for oxygen level in Fig. 3 is as given:

$$\text{Normal} = \begin{cases} 1\ (\text{Healthy}),\ 95\% <= x <= 100\% \\ 0(\text{Unhealthy}),\ x > 100\% \text{ and } x < 95\% \end{cases}$$

$$\text{Low} = \begin{cases} 1\ (\text{Healthy}),\ x > 95\% \\ 0\ (\text{Unhealthy}),\ x < 95\% \end{cases}$$

Table 2 Range for oxygen level

Oxygen level	State
95–100%	Normal
<95%	Low
>100%	High

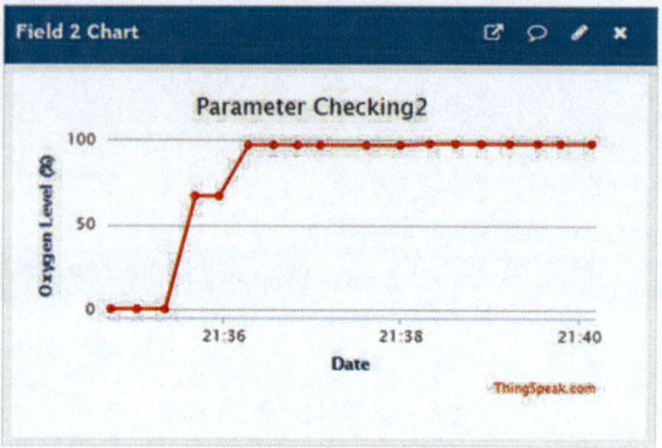

Fig. 3 Real-time curve for oxygen level

$$\text{High} = \begin{Bmatrix} 1\ (\text{Healthy}),\ x < 100\% \\ 0\ (\text{Unhealthy}),\ x > 100\% \end{Bmatrix}$$

Similarly, to determine body temperature, different range of body and room temperature values is also considered as in Table 3. The real-time value curve for body and room temperature in Figs. 4 and 5 is as given:

$$\text{Normal} = \begin{Bmatrix} 1\ (\text{Healthy}),\ 97^{\circ}\text{F} <= x <= 99^{\circ}\text{F} \\ 0(\text{Unhealthy}),\ x > 99^{\circ}\text{F and } x < 97^{\circ}\text{F} \end{Bmatrix}$$

Table 3 Range for body temperature

Body temperature	State
97–99°F	Normal
<97°F	Low
>99°F	High

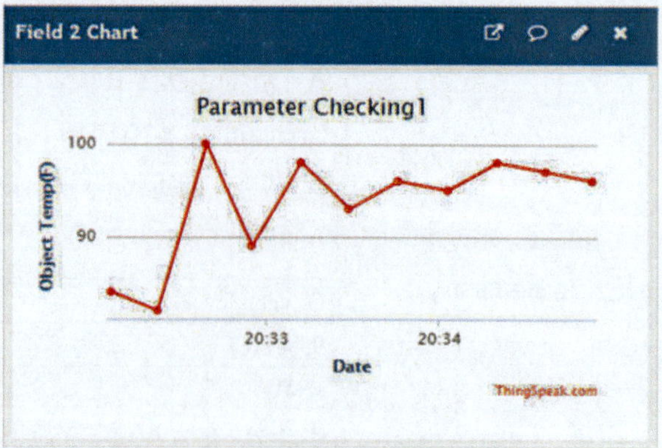

Fig. 4 Real-time curve for body temp

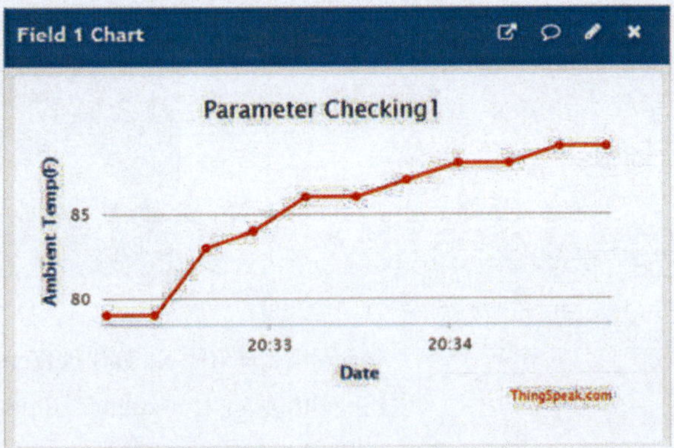

Fig. 5 Real-time curve for room temp

Table 4 Condition for fall detection

Fall detection	State
No fall detected	0
Patient fall detected	1

$$\text{Low} = \begin{Bmatrix} 1 \text{ (Healthy), x } > 97^{\circ}\text{F} \\ 0 \text{ (Unhealthy), x } < 97^{\circ}\text{F} \end{Bmatrix}$$

$$\text{High} = \begin{Bmatrix} 1 \text{ (Healthy), x } < 99^{\circ}\text{F} \\ 0 \text{ (Unhealthy), x } > 99^{\circ}\text{F} \end{Bmatrix}$$

For fall detection, the range lies between "0" and "1," which determines the falling of the patient. Value "0" states that no fall is detected and value "1" states that patient fall is detected as in Table 4. The real-time value curve for fall detection in Fig. 6 is as given:

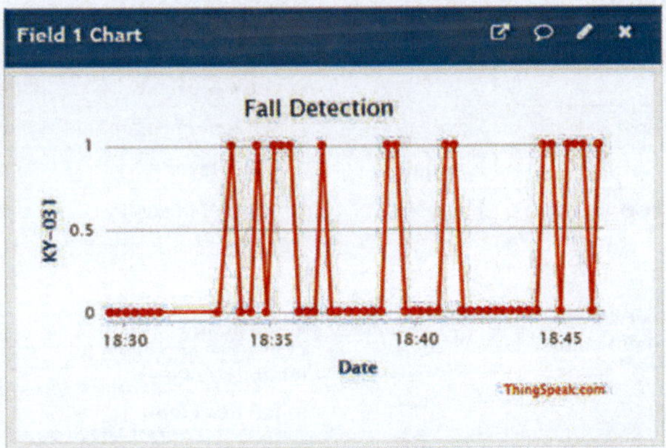

Fig. 6 Real-time curve for fall detection

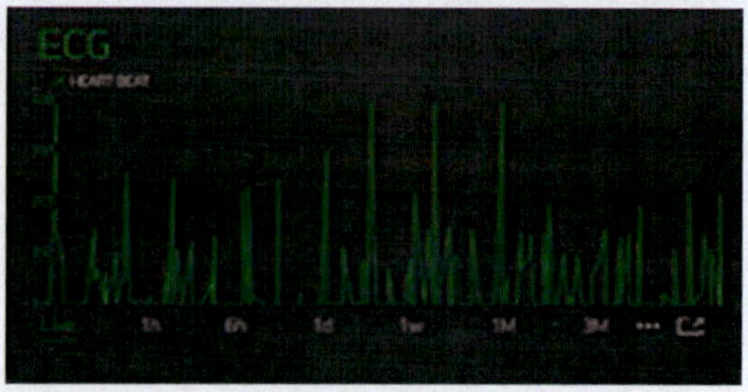

Fig. 7 Real-time curve for ECG-1

$$\text{Healthy} = \{0,\ \text{No fall detected}$$
$$\text{Unhealthy} = \{1,\ \text{Patient fall detected}$$

For electrocardiogram (ECG), values are determined by the electrical activity of the patient's heart at rest via electrical leads. Information like rhythm, heart rate, etc., are assessed, and P wave, QRS complex, and T waves are analyzed to detect any abnormality.

Analyzing the different range values for all parameters, the outcome for patient's health status is diagnosed in Figs. 7 and 8 which is as follows: Healthy, unwell, urgent checkup, low fever, and high fever as given in Tables 5 and 6.

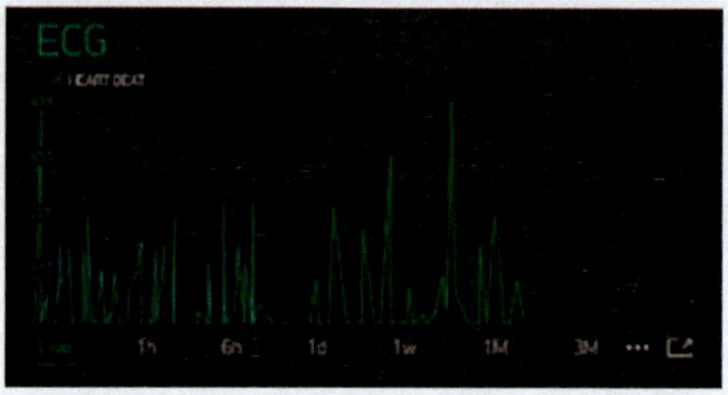

Fig. 8 Real-time curve for ECG-2

Table 5 Rules for analyzing health status

Heart rate	Oxygen level	Body and room temperature		
		Low	Normal	High
Low	Low	Urgent checkup	Unwell	Urgent checkup
Normal	Normal	Low fever	Healthy	High fever
High	High	Urgent checkup	Unwell	Urgent checkup

Table 6 Rules for analyzing health status

Fall detection (State)	Outcome
Patient fall detected	Urgent checkup
No fall detected	Healthy

The analysis of the COVID-19 positive patient's health status for all vital parameters can be summarized by considering the cases from Tables 5 and 6, and their health status can be determined by the doctor/medical staff. Cases are as follows:

1. If the output for heart rate/oxygen level along with patient temperature is (Low & Low) or (Low & High) or (High & Low) or (High & High), then the patient requires immediate medical attention.
2. If the output for heart rate/oxygen level along with patient temperature is (Low & Normal) or (High & Normal), then routine checkup is required.
3. If the output for heart rate/oxygen level and body temperature is (Normal & Low) or (Normal & High), then the patient is having low or high fever.
4. If the output for heart rate/oxygen level and body temperature is (Normal & Normal), then the patient is healthy.
5. If the patient fall is detected due to breathlessness, then an urgent medical checkup is required; otherwise, no fall is detected and the patient is healthy.

3 Result and Discussion

The pulse oximeter sensor, along with body temperature sensor, knock sensor (fall detection), ECG module, and emergency button is interfaced with the microcontroller. The complete prototype model can be seen in Figs. 9 and 10 where calculated data is displayed on the screen and visible to the doctor/medical staff observing the patient.

The readings measured are transferred to cloud center where the data is stored and accessed by the authorized user. The recorded data is displayed on the screen and the application as shown in Fig. 11.

The output from Fig. 11 signifies that there was some delay initially for the data received, but eventually it got stable just after few minutes, and an approximate real-time reading of **heart rate = 72.83 bpm** and **oxygen level = 98%** is observed for both parameters of sensor.

The output from Fig. 12 signifies that there was some delay initially, but eventually

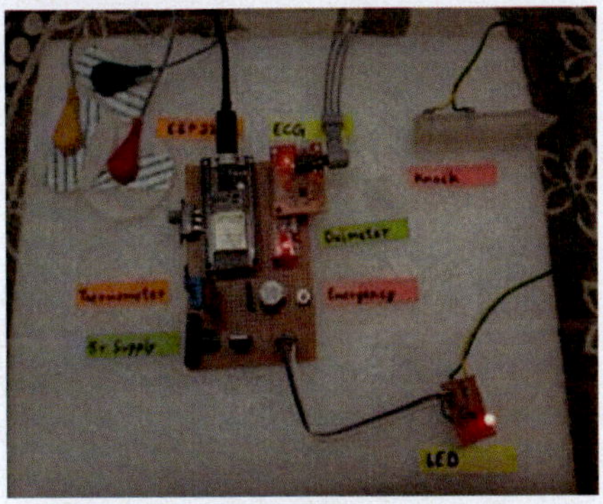

Fig. 9 System prototype—internal structure

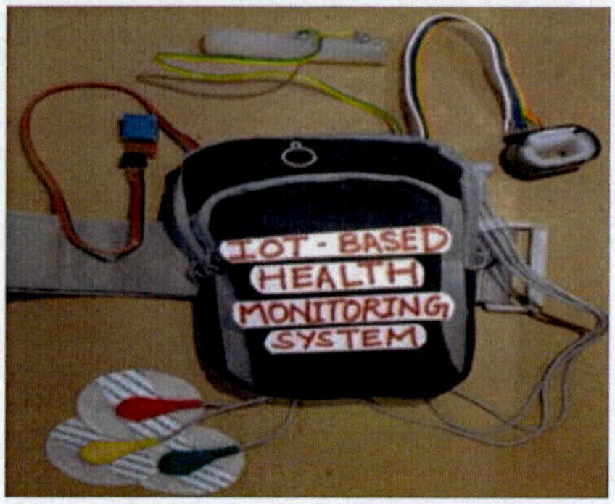

Fig. 10 System prototype

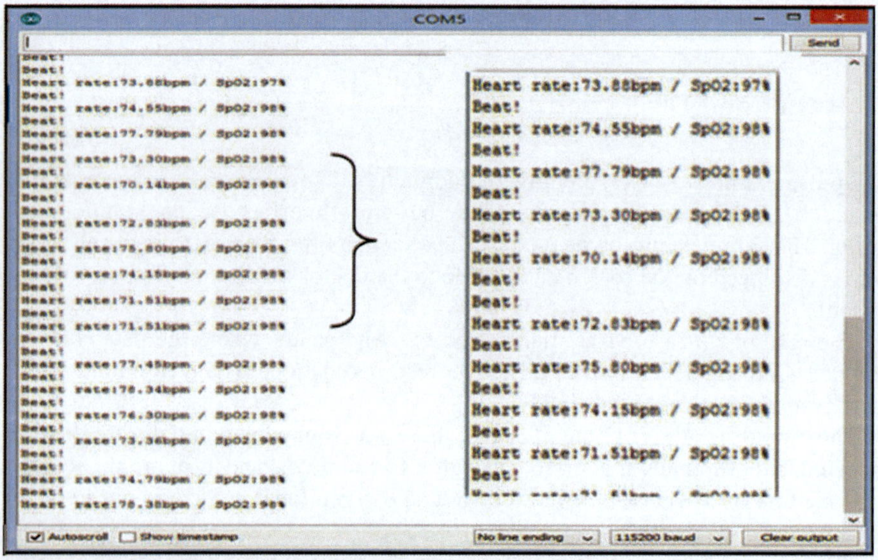

Fig. 11 Output on monitor for pulse oximeter

it got stable just after few minutes, and an approximate real-time reading of **ambient temperature = 89F** and **object temperature = 98F** is recorded for both parameters of the sensor.

From Fig. 13, reading was noted from the knock sensor which signifies the falling detection of any patient due to breathlessness. It is observed that the sensor gives the value **"0"** when no fall is detected and gives the value **"1"** when the falling of a person is detected. The vital parameters of the patient displayed on (Internet of Things) IoT application are shown below in Fig. 14.

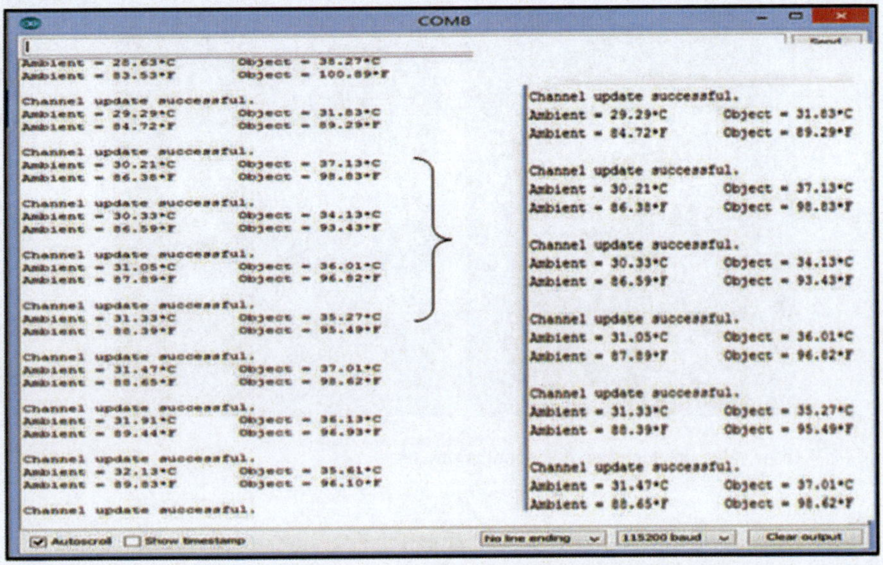

Fig. 12 Output on monitor for body and room temp

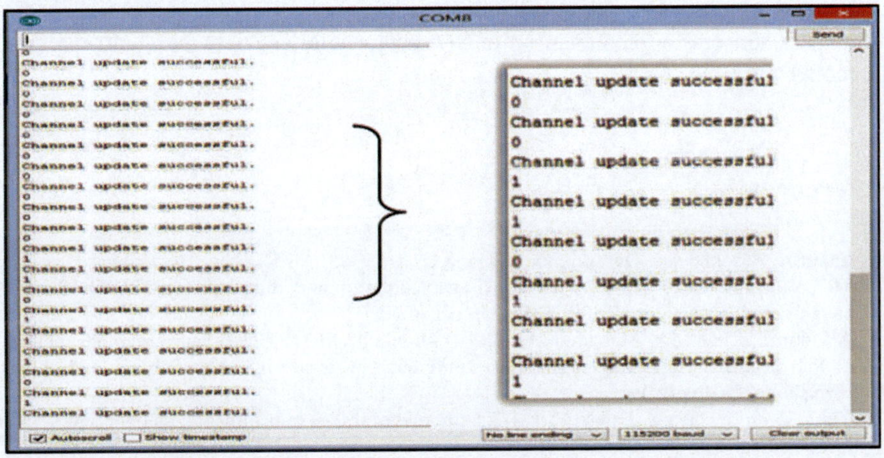

Fig. 13 Output on monitor for fall detection

4 Conclusion and Future Scope

To avoid coming directly in contact with the patients during the situation of the COVID-19 pandemic, a wireless sensor network (WSN)-based COVID-19 patient health monitoring system has been designed in this paper. Therefore, creating a health

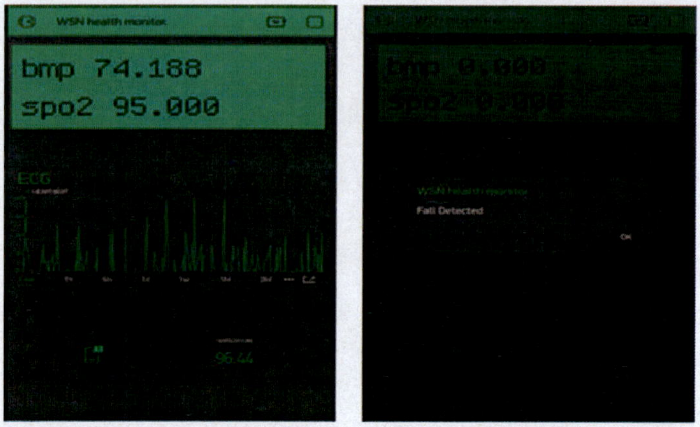

Fig. 14 Sensor value displayed on IoT application

monitoring system which transmits real-time data of the patients from a particular location to a targeted point contributes to the reduction in cases.

The existing WSN based health status monitoring systems majorly comprises of specific sensors which are required for a particular use. Some basic additional implementations has been done including reduction in the size of the hardware, addition of sensors, implementation of low power wireless networks, and making the model wearable.

References

1. Imran A, Posokhova I, Qureshi HN, Masood U, Riaz MS, Ali K, John CN, Iftikhar Hussain MD, Nabeel M (2020) AI4COVID-19: AI-enabled preliminary diagnosis for COVID-19 from cough samples via an app. Inform Med Unlocked 20
2. AlMotiri S, Khan MA, Alghamdi MA (2016) Mobile health (m-Health) system in the context of IoT. In: 2016 IEEE 4th international conference on future internet of things and cloud workshops (FiCloudW)
3. Yin Y, Zeng Y, Chen X, Fan Y (2016) The internet of things in healthcare: an overview. J Ind Inform Integr 1
4. Kotronis Cet al. (2017) Managing criticalities of e-Health IoT systems. In: 2017 IEEE 17th international conference on ubiquitous wireless broadband (ICUWB), Salamanca, Spain
5. Gupta N, Saeed H, Jha S, Chahande M, Pandey S (2017) IOT based health monitoring systems. In: 2017 International conference on innovations in information, embedded and communication systems (ICIIECS), Coimbatore, India
6. Rizwan P, Rajasekhara Babu M, Suresh K (2017) Design and development of low investment smart hospital using internet of things through innovative approaches. Biomed Res 28(11)
7. Malasinghe LP, Ramzan N, Dahal KP (2019) Remote patient monitoring: a comprehensive study. J Ambient Intell Human Comput
8. Lambat MM, Wagaj SC (2013) Review: health monitoring system. Int J Sci Res
9. Gogate U, Bakal J (2018) Healthcare monitoring system based on wireless sensor network for Cardiac patients. Biomed Pharmacol J

10. Patil S, Pardeshi S (2019) Health monitoring system using wireless body network sensor. Int Res J Eng Technol 05(04)
11. Lal Verma E, Bagga J (2015) Design and implementation of online heart rate monitoring system. Int J Sci Res 4(10)
12. Rathore DK, Upmanyu A, Lulla D (2013) Wireless patient health monitoring system. In: 2013 International conference on signal processing and communication, Noida, India
13. Piyare R, Lee SR (2013) Towards internet of things (IOTS): integration of wireless sensor network to cloud services for data collection and sharing. Int J Comput Netw Commun (IJCNC) 5(5)
14. Thwe HM, Tun HM (2015) Patient health monitoring using wireless body area network. Int Res J Eng Technol 04
15. Priyadharshini SG, Subramani C, Preetha Roselyn J (2019) An IOT based smart smetering development for energy management system. Int J Electr Comput Eng (IJECE) 9(4)
16. Al-Ali AR, Zualkernan IA, Rashid M, Gupta R, Alikarar M (2017) A smart home energy management system using IoT and big data analytics approach. IEEE Trans Consum Electron
17. Arshad A, Khan S, Alam AZ, Ahmad FI, Tasnim R (2014) A study on health monitoring system: recent advancements. IIUM Eng J 15(2)
18. Kirankumar CKR, Prabhakaran M (2017) Design and implementation of low cost web based human health monitoring system using Raspberry Pi 2. In: 2017 IEEE international conference on electrical instrumentation and communication engineering (ICEICE), pp 1–5
19. Sathya M, Madhan S, Jayanthi K (2018) Internet of things (IoT) based health monitoring system and challenges. Int J Eng Technol 7(1):175–178
20. Rahaman A, Islam M, Islam M, Sadi M, Nooruddin S (2019) Developing IoT based smart health monitoring systems: a review. Rev Intell Artif
21. Islam MM, Rahaman A, Islam MR (2020) Development of smart healthcare monitoring system. In: IoT environment in SN Comput. Sci, vol 1, 185p
22. Geetha Ramani J, Madhusudan S, Nila AL, Manibharathi S, Pradeep A (2020) IOT based employee health monitoring system. In: Conference: 2020 6th International conference on advanced computing and communication systems (ICACCS)
23. Valsalan P, Baomar TAB, Omar Baabood AH (2020) IOT based health monitoring system. J Crit Rev 7(4)
24. Larsen JR, Martin MR, Martin JD, Kuhn P, Hicks JB (2020) Modeling the onset of symptoms of COVID-19. Front Public Health 8:473. https://doi.org/10.3389/fpubh.2020.00473

Sentimental Analysis of Tweets During COVID-19 Pandemic: BERT Algorithm

Gurkirat Kaur, Munish Saini, and Amit Chhabra

Abstract As the coronavirus (COVID-19) grows its impact from China, expanding its catchment into surrounding regions and other countries, increased national and international measures are being taken to contain the outbreak. This perspective paper is written to capture and analyze the various mental state health issues being perceived via emotional analysis of Twitter data during the COVID-19 virus outbreak from a single nation further spread of to the whole world. A data-driven approach with higher accuracy as here can be very useful for a proactive response from the government and citizens. In the proposed work, tweets during the COVID situation have been collected and their sentiments are explored using BERT (Bidirectional Encoder Representation from Transformer) algorithm. BERT is the algorithm that takes text as input, and the trained basis on the epochs (number of passes performed). The performance parameters are computed such as accuracy, precision, recall, and F-measure. Further, the proposed approach is compared with other existing algorithms such as Naïve Bayes (NB), support vector machine (SVM), and logistic regression (LR). The performance measures indicate that the BERT algorithm outperforms all other existing algorithms with an accuracy of 86.7% as compared to 67.3%, 63.4%, and 61.2% with Naïve Bayes, support vector machine, and logistic regression, respectively. The government and other medical health agencies can use the outcomes of this paper for implementing and taking preventative measures to maintain the good mental and physical health of medical staff.

Keywords COVID · Twitter sentiment analysis · Novel coronavirus · BERT · Prediction algorithm · Metrics

G. Kaur (✉) · M. Saini · A. Chhabra
Guru Nanak Dev University, Amritsar, India

N. Marriwala et al. (eds.), *Emergent Converging Technologies and Biomedical Systems*, Lecture Notes in Electrical Engineering 841,
https://doi.org/10.1007/978-981-16-8774-7_11

1 Introduction

The health officials are the most prone to any devastating circumstance like a pandemic outbreak as a large number of patients are to be treated in a limited capacity with time constraints as well [7]. The effect of the pandemic not only causes physical pain and sufferings to the normal people of every society, but it has a huge mental impact on the persons who are held answerable for their cure and remedies during any highly evolving bad or even worse situations related to the health of *homo sapiens* [5]. The doctors, nurses, and even higher authority health officials, all have a huge responsibility on their shoulders to save people from the chaos and limit the worst outcomes of any pandemic like the COVID-19 virus. Every human is affected whether directly or indirectly during the sickness effective on a global level as shown in Fig. 1.

The state of mind of a normal person gets troubled and utterly disturbed when so much suffering is seen with their naked eyes. Such pain and remorse emotions are key factors in demotivating the person who is going to find a proper remedy to cure the suffering of their breed. The emotion of hope and faith gets lost somewhere during bad times that are affecting the whole world altogether [8]. Further, outcomes can be new ways of treatment and state-of-the-art new methods to be used to minimize the effects like localizing the spread as much as possible by quarantining affected citizens under proper surveillance.

People nowadays, express most of their emotions by sharing their views on social media Web sites like Facebook, Twitter, and other popular social media platforms by writing or even sharing images with captions along with them [15]. The popular trends are mentioned using a *hashtag,* through which the current hot topics can be tagged and further views are shared [11]. Tracking the emotions and sentiments of people during a pandemic will have mixed feelings of expressions due to widespread effects as in the whole world confirmed cases shown in Fig. 2.

In this paper, the focus is given on public opinion analysis via tweet data collected from tweepy API [2] in the English language to capture the various emotions and feelings expressed and then limiting the exploration toward the health-related text data.

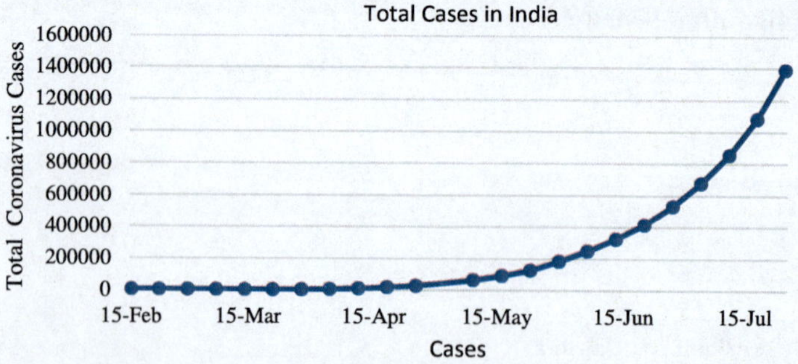

Fig. 1 Total cases in India during this pandemic [20]

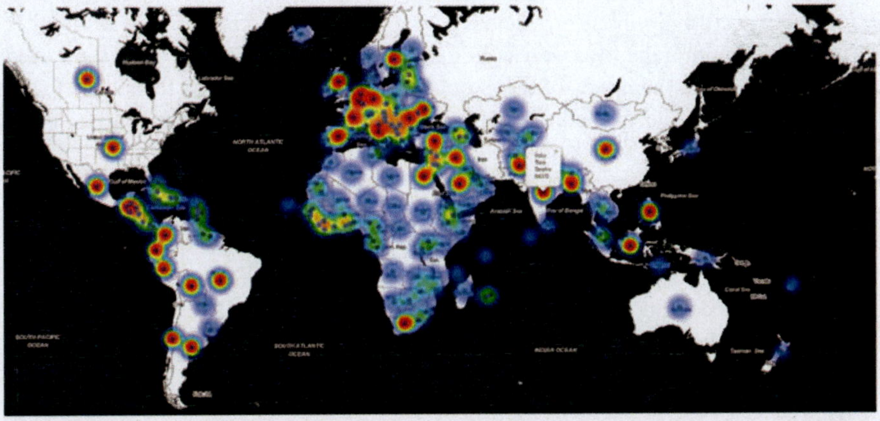

Fig. 2 Geospatial analysis of confirmed corona cases [3]

For performing this task, Twitter [9] is preferred because it is a famous social media platform having a plethora of information to be tapped and analyzed to preprocess as well as refine to gain the inside knowledge from the tweets. The tweets generally convey individual perspectives or feelings toward the subject referenced in the tweets. Sentimental analysis using natural language processing is one of the techniques that help to extract the feeling of the user in any situation [4]. Twitter provides an easier platform to retrieve user perspectives and feelings [18].

The objective of the research is to crawl through the various bundle of diverse sentiments articulated using Twitter, a social media platform. The crawled data is further refined and tokenized for accuracy in capturing the opinions and views of the people regarding health all over the world. Tweets with various health synonymous hashtags along with text data are used to analyze the psychological condition of various health officials.

Exploratory data analysis (EDA) is performed on tweets to check the performance of the model. It has achieved 82.3% accuracy. EDA is used to see the structure of the dataset collected. This step helps to expose patterns and relationships between the data. For further analyzing the data, natural language processing (NLP) and BERT methods are used, which brings out the resourceful information regarding peak levels of sentiments during the pandemic. Most of the authors have preferred machine learning methods to achieve high accuracy while analyzing the text data. Pang and Lee [17] have performed emotion classification using machine learning methods for the analysis of tweets. Besides applying machine learning strategies, natural language processing methods have been introduced. NLP helps to resolve uncertainty and add valuable information in the text. BERT is one of the best NLP techniques. BERT was designed by Google [19], which is a Fortune Five Hundred company. BERT is a trained model that works based on a transformer encoder. BERT set new state-of-the-art performance on various sentence classification and sentence–pair regression tasks. BERT uses cross-encoder [21].

This study will help the users, developers, researchers, academicians, and other stakeholders to comprehend as well as gain knowledge about the insights of the varied emotions running in the minds of the people around the globe. This further will help to get the state of mind of medical staff and other persons in any bad situation like pandemic, so that better measures can be taken beforehand.

In the rest of the paper, Sect. 2 places the work in the context of related work in this domain. Section 3 describes the research methodology. Section 3 discusses the methods, and a model for evaluating the popular tweets related to health are collected and used as part of the method process. Section 4 presents a discussion on the findings. We conclude the paper with some ideas for future work in Sect. 5.

2 Related Work

Much research interest has been directed toward sentiment analysis, particularly the challenges encountered in detecting word sentiment. The advent of technology has dramatically influenced human lives and their communities.

Sujatha et al. [21] have introduced a forecasting model to predict the COVID cases in India using the multilayer perceptron (MLP) method using the WEKA and Orange tools on COVID-19 Kaggle data and shown that their machine learning model is giving better results than their counterparts, that is, Linear Regression (LR) and vector auto-regression (VAR) methods. Mittal [13] researcher analyzes the current trend of COVID-19 based on certain criterion using "Exploratory Data Analysis." Exploratory Data Analysis (EDA) is the way to explore the data to extract useful and actionable information from it. EDA is the revelatory step in any kind of analysis.

Majid et al. presented a diagnosis model for the novel coronavirus infection detection. Based on Bayesian optimization and deep learning mechanisms, the model is using the convolution neural network (CNN) layered architecture approach to assist the field specialists, radiologists, and physicians to make better decisions in diagnosing the novel COVID-19 virus in the patients in a faster and reliable manner.

Mardani et al. [12] have published a new way of using fuzzy logistics called hesitant fuzzy sets used in designing a novel framework to address as well as assess the key challenges faced in the digital health during the pandemic outburst of coronavirus globally. By combining the unique fuzzy approach with Stepwise Weight Assessment Ratio Analysis (SWARA) and Weighted Aggregated Sum Product Assessment (WASPAS) methods, the work is done to rank the life-threatening challenges being faced by the current digital technologies while controlling the COVID-19 situation.

Tuli et al. [22] proposed a novel method called Deep Bayes-Squeeze Net-based COVIDiagnosis-Net to classify the COVID-19 cases as the COVID-19 or normal (healthy). The model ensures an end-to-end learning schema that can directly learn discriminative features from the input chest CT X-ray images and eliminate handcrafted feature engine.

Devlin et al. [6] developed Bidirectional Encoder Representations from Transformers (BERT) at Google AI Language. BERT is "*designed to pretrain deep bidirectional representations from the unlabeled text by jointly conditioning on both left and right context in all layers.*" The state-of-the-art BERT is pretrained on two unsupervised tasks—masked language modeling and next sentence prediction, thus making it an effective technique for eight sentiment classification. BERT is known to have achieved exceptional results in eleven natural language understanding (NLU) tasks.

Wang et al. [23] investigated the influence of air temperature and relative humidity on the transmission of COVID-19 by calculating the "effective reproductive number"(R), and under the "Linear Regression" framework, they found out that a one-degree Celsius rise in temperature and one percent increase in the relative humidity lower R by 0.0225 and 0.0158, respectively, and indicates that arrival of summer and rainy season in the northern hemisphere can effectively reduce the transmission of COVID-19.

Inferring from the latest trend nowadays as per the hashtags captured using Twitter data (tweets), it can be concluded that the people are having a rich amount of intensifying emotions. The state of the mindset especially of the people who are going to defend all of us from the outspread virus needs to be considered. The captured Twitter data is based on health-related tags to further narrow down our Web crawling and limiting the tweets, making it more relevant to this research.

3 Experimental Setup and Analysis Methodology

3.1 Experimental Setup

In this study, tweets are collected related to mental health during the COVID situation. The experiment is performed on Jupyter Notebook using Python 3.3.0. Dataset is taken in CSV format, with 20 columns such as TweetPostedTime, Tweet ID, TweetBody, TweetHashtags, UserID, UserName, etc. Firstly, Exploratory Data Analysis has been performed after that text has been classified using BERT algorithm.

3.2 Experimental Setup

This section discusses the steps performed for analysis (see Fig. 3).

Data Collection

The data was collected using the Tweepy API [2] for Python in which all the latest tweets related to the COVID pandemic were captured (refer to Table1). All the tweets have emotion and that was what needed for the research, and by applying sentiment

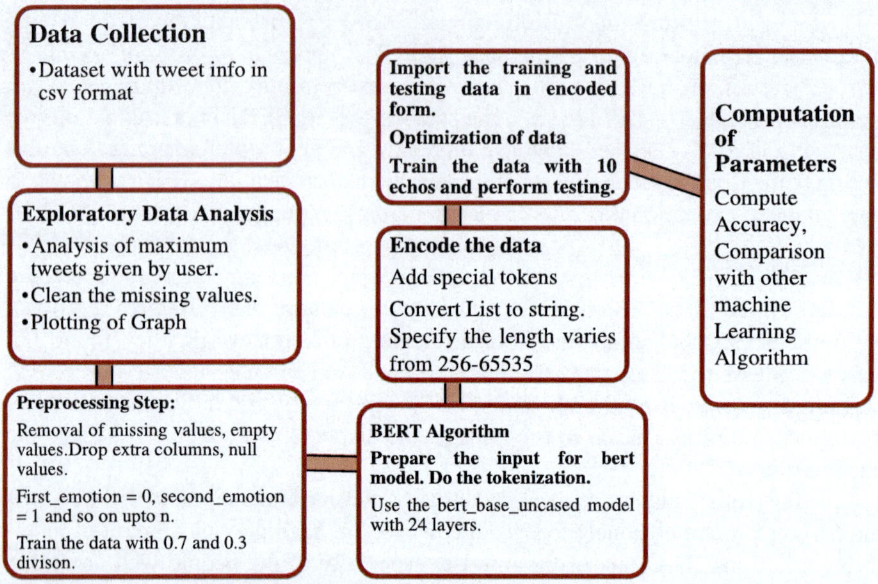

Fig. 3 Methodology of proposed work

Table 1 Attributes of the dataset

Attribute	Description
TweetPostedTime	It represents the timestamp of the collected tweet
TweetID	A Unique identifier associated with each tweet
TweetBody	It includes text mentioned in the tweet
TweetRetweetFlag	It is a flag for the indication of tweet retweet status. It is either true or false. The true flag represents the tweet is retweeted and false specifies it is not retweeted
TweetSource	It contains the location information for the tweet origin
TweetRetweetCount	It consists of the count of total retweets
TweetFavoriteCount	It stores the count of marked tweets
TweetHashtags	It represents the hashtags that are mentioned in the tweet
UserID	It specifies the unique user identifier
UserName	It represents the name of the user
UserLocation	The geographical location of the user
UserDescription	It contains the information related to the user
UserFollowersCount	It specifies the total number of followers

analysis, the captured tweets were grouped based on the emotions they possess. The usernames are kept anonymous focusing solely on the text in the tweet. The timestamp of the tweet is also considered to relate to the sentiments as time plays a vital role in understanding the mindset of the person, while they tweet [16]. The dataset that was considered, covered all the various other aspects of the tweet as well, such as time of the tweet, the description of the user, and the hashtags used in the tweet alongside description about the user posting the tweet. All these factors, when combined, provide more insight about the sentiments of the user while tweeting, and thus, we can further understand the state of mind of the user during the pandemic.

Exploratory Data Analysis

Exploratory Data Analysis (EDA) [1] is the first step while starting the analysis of the dataset. This process mainly focuses on efficiently understanding the dataset. The process of EDA is graphically presented in Fig. 4.

Figure 5 represents the top 10 trending hashtags that were exploited during the rise of the pandemic, having *#covid* as the most repeatedly used. It further depicts the mental state of the users who were more concerned about the disastrous outbreak rather than any other topic during that time.

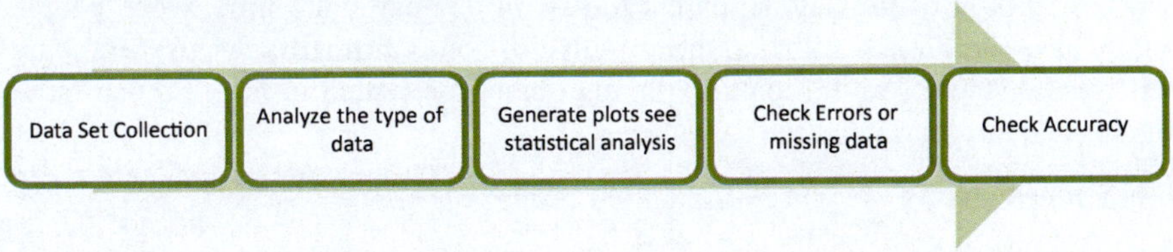

Fig. 4 General steps of exploratory data analysis

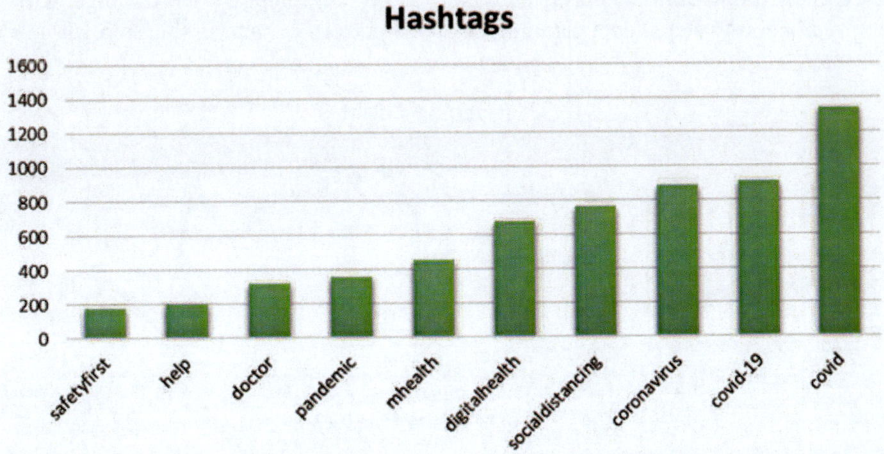

Fig. 5 Top 10 hashtags corresponding to their count

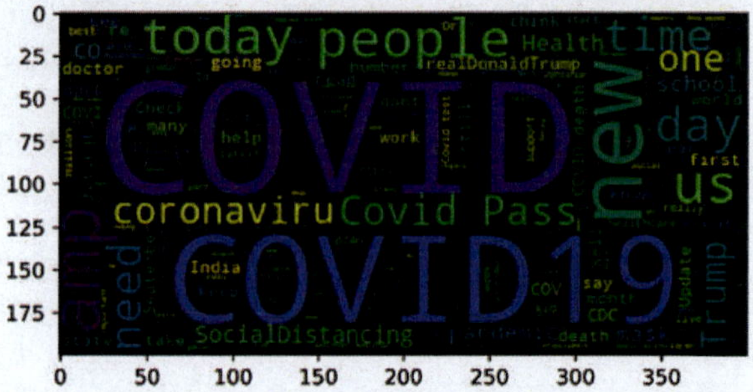

Fig. 6 Word cloud of tweet body

Moreover, analyzing the frequent hashtags is essential, but the Tweet_Body has much more rather than just hashtags. The text posted in the tweets is having as much significance as a hashtag. Figure 6 shows the wordcloud of most frequent phrases used in the Tweet_Body during the COVID outbreak, with the size of the text conveying the frequency of repetition of that word in the dataset.

This paper concentrates on the mental health analysis of a person, evident to reveal that the mood and emotions of a person get influenced by the time of the day as well. As shown in Fig. 7, the thoughts can be witnessed to be at their peak levels from 12:00 to 16:00 h of the day. Apparent to say, in this particular time, when people usually have their lunch, either alone or with close ones, primarily discuss and share their mental state of mind, making the data being presented in Fig. 7 much more obvious and appropriate at the same time.

Data Preprocessing

The tweet data has been extracted based on various hashtags such as #doctors, #socialdistancing, #coronaheros, #digitalhealth, #mhealth, #healthinnovations, and #medtech. Using these hashtags, 10,000 tweets are extracted. These all are labeled based on their emotions such as ['fear', 'surprise', 'sad', 'happy', 'trust', 'anger']. In the preprocessing steps, data cleaning has been performed, and in this step, all null

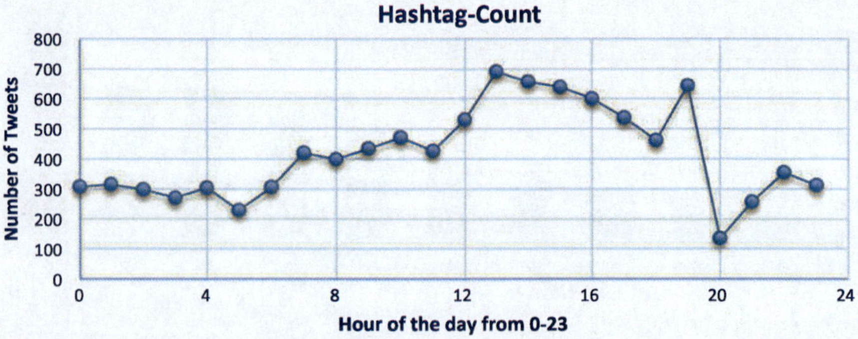

Fig. 7 Count of tweets corresponding to their hour

Table 2 Labels of sentiments

Sentiment	Label
Fear	0
Pride	1
Sad	3
Disgust	6
Sad	4
Surprise	5
Happy	2
Anger	3

has been extracted. Each emotion has been labeled using the enumeration function as given in Table 2.

Classification Using BERT Algorithm

BERT (Bidirectional Encoder Representations from Transformers) [24] model is used for unlabeled data to give bidirectional representation. This algorithm works from both the context, i.e., from left and right both. BERT is one of the efficient techniques to get high accuracy in natural language processing. The basic steps of the BERT algorithm are shown in Fig. 8.

To perform the text classification, we used a BERT model known as an advance supervised model. This component has used the emotion labeled data such as different emotions of doctors (sad, happy, and many more). These emotions are labeled further from 0 to n where n is the number of emotions. In our experiment, we have used the BERT of HuggingFace [24]. The following Fig. 9 shows the steps of the proposed algorithm.

Computation of Parameters

In this paper, the model is focused to compute the accuracy of positive emotions and negative emotions: positive emotions are considered happy and trust, and other emotions are considered in a negative impact [14]. The performance is measured on basis of true positive, true negative, false positive, and false negative. The following Fig. 10 shows the meaning of these terms.

Comparison of BERT with Traditional Machine Learning Algorithms

In this section, the BERT algorithm results are compared with support vector machine (SVM), Naïve Bayes (NB), and logistic regression (LR). These machine learning algorithms are used because of their effectiveness and performance.

Logistic regression (LR) [25] is the algorithm used to find the data which is dependent, and this helps to find the relation between the independent variable. Here, this model will help to predict the emotions are sad or anger based on other tweet emotions used for training. This model is useful for linear as well as nonlinear data. The LR model returns the 1 if true emotion and 0 if false emotion predicted. Here,

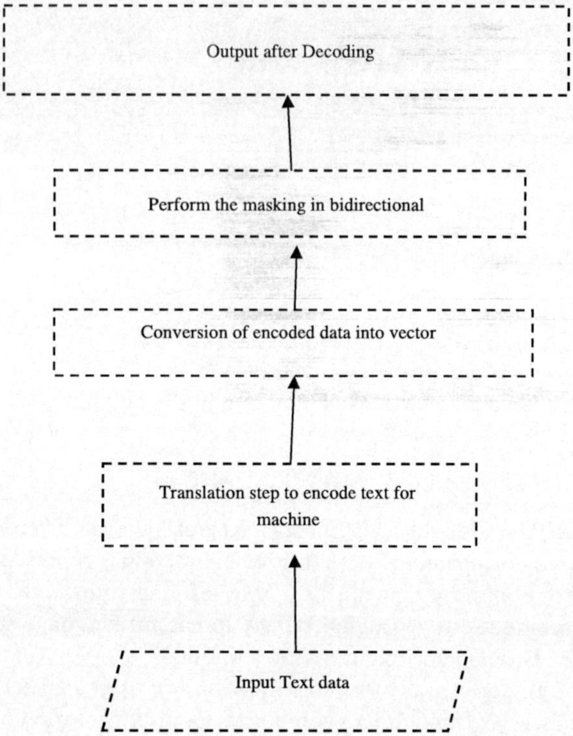

Fig. 8 Flow of BERT algorithm

the model is used for tweets, to find their probability of occurrence in this pandemic. Consider the tweets and their sentiments, the LR model will give the attributes of A(S|T) where S is the class of sentiments and T is tweets retrieved.

$$\text{A (class of sentiments | Tweets)} = \text{A(Tweets)} \tag{1}$$

It will return output in two values 1- for true predicted emotion values and 0 – for false predicted emotion values. In this, A(S|T) S are sentiments, and T is text so sentiment range various from 0 to n. Therefore, the equation will be used as an exponential function [10].

$$A(S|T) = \frac{1}{x} e^{w^T y} \tag{2}$$

where x is the normalizing factor. Naïve Bayes (NB) [9] is the algorithm that works on Bayes rule. This algorithm is used for text classification based on a supervised algorithm. In this paper, we computed the P(S) and P(T|S) using the equation.

$$P(S|T) = \frac{P(T|S)P(S)}{P(T)} \tag{3}$$

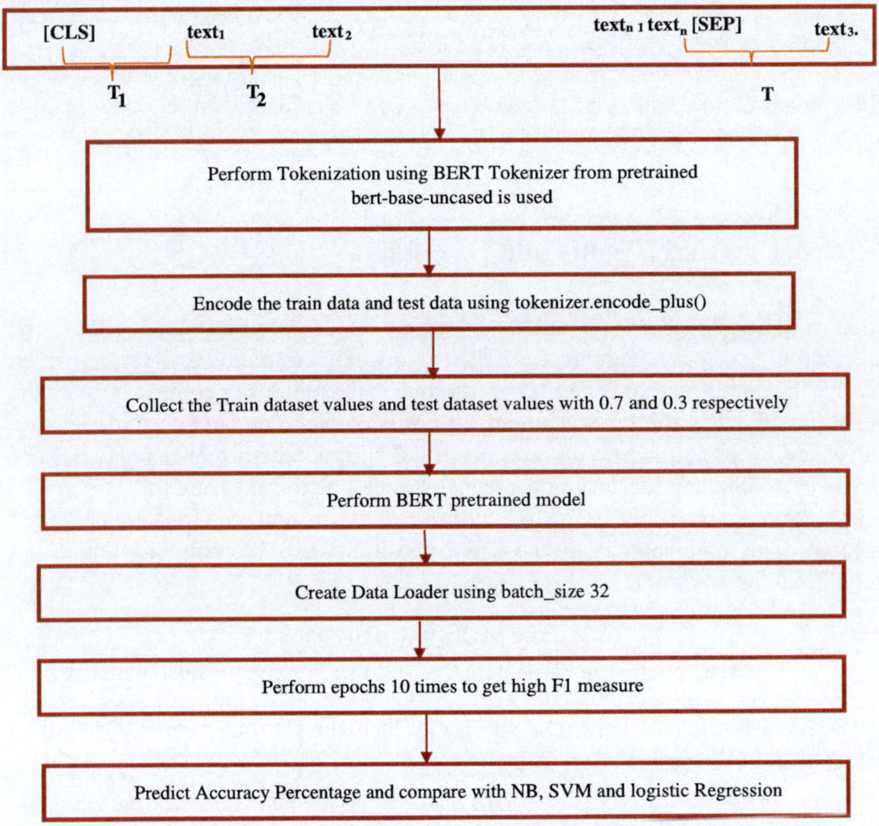

Fig. 9 Steps of proposed approach where T1, T2.... Tn is tweets

Predicted Emotion -ve	Predicted Emotion +ve	
False Negative	True Positive	Actual Emotion +ve
True Negative	False Positive	Actual Emotion -ve

Fig. 10 Confusion matrix

For estimating P(S), the relative frequency of each tweet has been targeted in trained data. Consider different tweets as $T_1, T_2, \ldots\ldots Tn$ are attributes and computed using

$$P(\mathrm{T1}, T2, \ldots\ldots Tn|S)P(S) = \prod_k P(Tk|S) \tag{4}$$

Support vector machine (SVM) is used for text classification. It focuses on more features, and estimate the discriminate function.

$$y(x) = w^T g(x) + b \tag{5}$$

where w is weight vector, g(x) is feature space, and b is biased. Here, due to a large number of tweets, the classification will be performed linearly separable.

4 Experimental Results and Discussion

After capturing the data and further assessing the acquired knowledge from the information gained by applying the BERT algorithm, we found these results which clearly explain the plethora of emotions running in the minds of people all around the world. To validate our proposed model, we have compared the proposed model with Naïve Bayes (NB), support vector machine (SVM), and logistic regression (LR). The parameters computed are accuracy, precision, recall, and F-measure.

The accuracy is defined as the total number of tweets and emotions are classified correctly. This parameter is to check the performance of a complete model that includes all the emotions.

$$\text{Accuracy} = \frac{\text{True positive} + \text{True negative}}{\text{True positive} + \text{True negative} + \text{false positive} + \text{false negative}} \tag{6}$$

The precision is also known as specificity. It is the ratio of correctly classified tweets to all of the correctly predicted tweets.

$$\text{Precision} = \frac{\text{True positive}}{\text{True positive} + \text{false positive}} \tag{7}$$

The recall is also known as sensitivity. Recall defines as the ratio of true positive and addition of true positive and false negative.

$$\text{Recall} = \frac{\text{True positive}}{\text{True positive} + \text{false negative}} \tag{8}$$

F-measure is also known as the F1-score. This term has a high predictive success rate. It can be calculated using the following formula:

$$F - \text{measure} = 2\left(\frac{\text{precision} * \text{recall}}{\text{precision} + \text{recall}}\right) \tag{9}$$

The tweets contain various emotions, the count of emotions is shown in Table 3, and Fig. 11 shows that fear emotion is more prominent during this COVID pandemic.

The data is divided into train and test data. After that, it has been compared with other algorithms and resulted in Table 4, and Fig. 12 shows the value of performance metrics.

Table 3 Dataset classification

Sentiment	Count	Count of test and train data
Happy	1419	Test-420
		Train-999
Sad	1448	Test-438
		Train-1010
Disgust	1442	Test-398
		Train-1044
Fear	1484	Test-439
		Train-1045
Anger	1417	Test-430
		Train-987
Surprise	1410	Test-450
		Train-960
Pride	1380	Test-425
		Train- 955
Total	10,000	

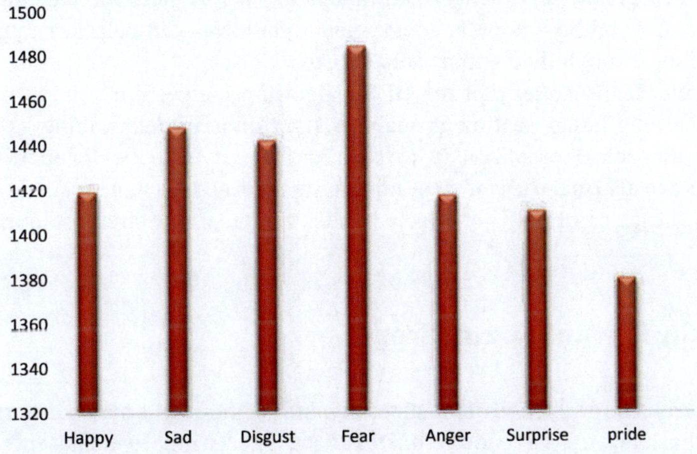

Fig. 11 Count of each emotion

Table 4 Comparison of the proposed algorithm with Naïve Bayes, SVM, and logistic regression

Algorithm	Accuracy (%)	Precision (%)	Recall (%)	F-measure (%)
Naïve Bayes	67.3	61.6	62.2	61.5
Support vector machine	63.4	63.0	62.3	60.3
Logistic regression	61.2	59.3	59.2	59.2
BERT (Proposed algorithm)	86.7	83.4	83.8	83.5

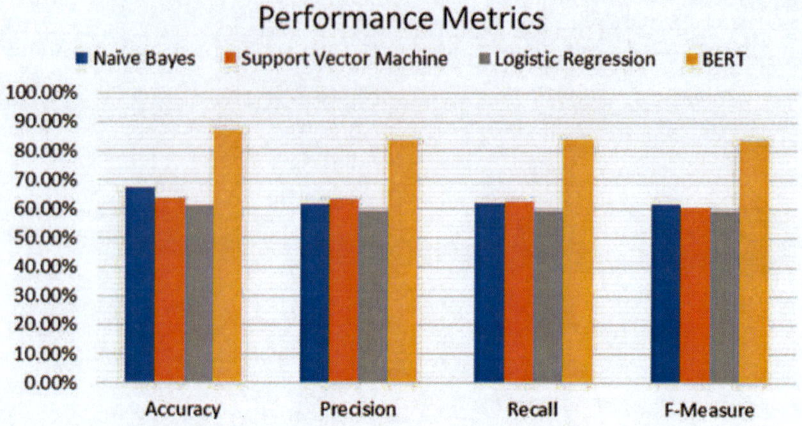

Fig. 12 Performance metrics computation of all the algorithm

The findings from this research clearly show how bad a pandemic can affect the intensity of the emotional mindset in the human beings, creating fear and sadness as the most powerful ones in comparison to additional primary sentiments. The research further explicates how sentiments of normal people get so much affected during the time of the day and how popular social media platforms can help in capturing all their emotions through their expressional posts.

The result clearly states that the BERT algorithm outperforms the other major machine learning-based sentiment analysis algorithms in determining as well as predicting the actual emotions in text-based data. It is to be noted that other researchers can also make use of these findings to learn about a more realistic mindset of persons, which can easily get affected under various major circumstances.

5 Conclusion and Future Scope

In this research, the prediction of the states of minds of the people has been normalized as per the hashtags used to capture the text data. The Twitter live dataset is used to justify as well as forecast the various sentimental challenges to be seen during the novel coronavirus widespread. BERT is used as a proficient model to understand as well as determine the rush of sentiments and deep emotions of the people facing the struggle during the COVID outbreak including the health officials and the other experts related to the field of medical sciences.

The proposed model can predict the sentiment residing in the tweets posted by tweet users, which makes the model much more accurate in analyzing the tweet data fed to the model. The results further articulate the accuracy in using the BERT algorithm for sentimental analysis of tweets used as test dataset. BERT algorithm performed well, and it can handle various emotions like sadness, anger, and disgust.

Further, in the future, we can work more on other machine learning algorithms to deal with emotions others that positive, negative, and neutral.

References

1. Alaparthi S, Mishra M (2020) Bidirectional encoder representations from transformers (BERT): a sentiment analysis odyssey. arXiv:2007.01127
2. Allen TT, Sui Z, Akbari K (2018) Exploratory text data analysis for quality hypothesis generation. Qual Eng 30(4):701–712
3. Belkacem S (2020) COVID-19 data analysis and forecasting: algeria and the world. arXiv: 2007.09755, RoessleinJoshua. "tweepy Documentation. http://tweepy.readthedocs.io/en/v3.5 (2009)
4. Cambria E, Poria S, Gelbukh A, Thelwall M (2017) Sentiment analysis is a big suitcase. IEEE Intell Syst 32(6):74–80
5. Ćosić K, Popović S, Šarlija M, Kesedžić I (2020) Impact of human disasters and Covid-19 pandemic on mental health: Potential of digital psychiatry. PsychiatriaDanubina 32(1):25–31
6. Devlin J, Chang MW, Lee K, Toutanova K (2018) Bert: Pre-training of deep bidirectional transformers for language understanding. arXiv:1810.04805
7. Galbraith N, Boyda D, McFeeters D, Hassan T (2020) The mental health of doctors during the Covid-19 pandemic. BJ Psych Bull:1–4
8. Huang L, Rong Liu H (2020) Emotional responses and coping strategies of nurses and nursing college students during COVID-19 outbreak
9. Hughes DJ, Rowe M, Batey M, Lee A (2012) A tale of two sites: Twitter vs. Facebook and the personality predictors of social media usage. Comput Hum Behav 28(2):561–569
10. Indra ST, Wikarsa L, Turang R (2016) Using logistic regression method to classify tweets into the selected topics. In: 2016 International conference on advanced computer science and information systems (ICACSIS). IEEE, pp 385–390
11. Kywe SM, Hoang TA, Lim EP, Zhu F (2012) On recommending hashtags in twitter networks. In: International conference on social informatics. Springer, Berlin, Heidelberg, pp 337–350
12. Mardani A, Saraji MK, Mishra AR, Rani P (2020) A novel extended approach under hesitant fuzzy sets to design a framework for assessing the key challenges of digital health interventions adoption during the COVID-19 outbreak. Appl Soft Comput:106613
13. Mittal S (2020) An exploratory data analysis of COVID-19 in India. Int J Eng Res Technol (IJERT). ISSN: 2278-0181
14. Mohammad SM, Kiritchenko S (2015) Using hashtags to capture fine emotion categories from tweets. Comput Intell 31(2):301–326
15. Nabity-Grover T, Cheung CM, Thatcher JB (2020) Inside out and outside in: How the COVID-19 pandemic affects self-disclosure on social media. Int J Inf Manag:102188
16. Naseem U, Razzak I, Musial K, Imran M (2020) Transformer based deep intelligent contextual embedding for twitter sentiment analysis. Futur Gener Comput Syst 113:58–69
17. Pang B, Lee L (2004) A sentimental education: sentiment analysis using subjectivity summarization based on minimum cuts. arXiv preprint cs/0409058
18. Parise S, Whelan E, Todd S (2015) How Twitter users can generate better ideas. MIT Sloan Manag Rev 56(4):21
19. Patel M (2019) TinySearch--semantics based search engine using bert embeddings. arXiv: 1908.02451
20. Sahoo S, Bharadwaj S, Parveen S, Singh AP, Tandup C, Mehra A, Grover S (2020) Self-harm and COVID-19 pandemic: an emerging concern–a report of 2 cases from India. Asian J Psychiatry
21. Sujath R, Chatterjee JM, Hassanien AE (2020) A machine learning forecasting model for COVID-19 pandemic in India. Stochast Environ Res Risk Assess:1

22. Tuli S, Tuli S, Tuli R, Gill SS (2020) Predicting the growth and trend of COVID-19 pandemic using machine learning and cloud computing. Internet Things:100222
23. Wang J, Tang K, Feng K, Lv W (2020) High temperature and high humidity reduce the transmission of COVID-19. SSRN 3551767
24. Wolf T, Debut L, Sanh V, Chaumond J, Delangue C, Moi A, Brew J (2019) HuggingFace's transformers: state-of-the-art natural language processing. Arxiv-1910
25. Zhang Z (2016) Model building strategy for logistic regression: purposeful selection. Annals Trans Med 4(6)

The Analysis of Plants Image Classification Based on Machine Learning Approaches

Sukanta Ghosh and Amar Singh

Abstract With the fast development in urbanization and populace, it has become a sincere errand to support and develop plants that are both significant in supporting the nature and the living creature's needs. Moreover, there is a requirement for saving the plants having worldwide significance both financially and naturally. Finding such species from the backwoods or bushes having human contribution is a tedious and expensive undertaking to perform. Classification and identification of plants-leaf are useful for individuals to viably comprehend and ensure plants. The leaves of plants are the main acknowledgment organs. With the advancement of artificial intelligence and computer vision innovation, plant-leaf recognition dependent on plant-leaf image investigation is utilized to improve the information on plant classification and insurance. Deep learning is the condensing of deep neural network learning technique and has a place with neural organization structure. It can naturally take in highlights from huge information and utilize artificial neural network dependent on back propagation methods to prepare and order plant-leaf tests. There are numerous machine learning approaches for identification and classification of plant-leaf image. Some of the famous and effective approaches are Random Forest, Support Vector Machines, ResNet50, CNN, VGG16, VGG19, PNN, KNN, etc. In this paper, we are going to apply 9 machine learning techniques on Flavia plant-leaf image dataset. Flavia plant-leaf image dataset consists of 32 different species of plant. The images are first preprocessed and then their shape, color and texture-based features are extracted from the processed image. Initial these images are in the size of 256*256 pixels. These images were preprocessed and taken up to the size of 64*64 for fast processing. ResNet50 has given the best results with an accuracy of 98%. Though SVM and S-Inception have also provided a good accuracy.

Keywords Image classification · CNN · SVM · Random forest · Thresholding · Multivariate data · Clustering

S. Ghosh (✉) · A. Singh
Lovely Professional University, Phagwara, India

N. Marriwala et al. (eds.), *Emergent Converging Technologies and Biomedical Systems*, Lecture Notes in Electrical Engineering 841,
https://doi.org/10.1007/978-981-16-8774-7_12

1 Introduction

Restorative plants are vital to humankind and creatures. In prior days, individuals were adequate to recognize the therapeutic parts of these plants in restoring different infections. The best technique to recognize plants effectively and effectively is a manual-put together strategy which depends much with respect to the intrinsic information on a specialist botanist [1]. Identification of legitimate restorative plants is very testing and it is an ideal opportunity to secure therapeutic plants since a few plant animal categories are getting wiped out.

It is assessed that there are around countless existing plants. They have various shapes, structures and ways of life. To comprehend and utilize plants, plants should be arranged. Plant scientific categorization has an assortment of classification techniques, for example, plant cell classification, plant hereditary classification, plant serum classification, and phytochemical classification. For by far most of non-research experts, it is hard to dominate some classification techniques, hard to work, and helpless common sense. The customary strategies for plant classification and acknowledgment require the recognizer to have an abundance of ordered information and long-haul common sense experience, and even to take the comparing key to finish the classification viably.

Recognizing plants utilizing flowers and fruits is an exceptionally tedious assignment and has been completed simply via prepared botanists. Nonetheless, notwithstanding this time concentrated undertaking, there are a few different disadvantages which are inaccessibility of required morphological data and utilization of natural terms that no one but specialists can comprehend. Leaves assume a significant part in plant ID since they can be handily found and gathered wherever at all seasons, while blossoms must be gotten at sprouting season. Plant leaves have two-dimensional nature and consequently they are generally reasonable for machine preparing, and the plants can be effortlessly arranged dependent on its different morphological highlights [1].

Programmed plant species acknowledgment with plant-leaf image handling has application in weeds identification, species revelation, plant scientific categorization, regular save park the board, etc. It is viewed as a fine-grained plant-leaf image acknowledgment issue and difficult to settle in light of the fact that [3]:

(a) The unpretentious contrasts between various species in a similar class. At some point, such fine contrasts can be in any event, testing to human specialists.

(b) Typically, this requires enormous preparing information; however, it isn't possible because of the quantity of species [2].

Computer vision strategies and deep learning (DL) approaches are used in the recognizable proof of plant species. The traditional computer vision strategy includes the pre-processing of plant images, extricating the handcrafted features, and classifying them utilizing machine learning (ML) calculations. DL technique requires the plant images to be preprocessed and it additionally plays out the cycle of both feature extraction and classification. A portion of the revealed exactness's for plant acknowledgment utilizing traditional computer vision approaches are 76.3% [5], 90% [6], and 91% [4]. The acknowledgment rate is additionally improved by DL draws near. Liu and Kan [7] detailed that the programmed distinguishing proof of plant species utilizing DL (precision of 93.9%) strategy performs in a way that is better than conventional classification strategies.

Convolutional neural network (CNN) is a supervised DL approach. It comprises of three main components that is convolution layers, pooling layers, and fully connected layers (FCLs). The presentation of AlexNet CNN approach opened the doorway to the improvement of new CNN models. A portion of the DL CNN models are VGG-16, VGG-19, Inception-v3, Inception-ResNet-v2, Xception, ResNet50, DenseNet-121, DenseNet-169, DenseNet-201, MobileNet and so forth [8–16].

In this article, we are going to apply 9 machine learning techniques namely Support Vector Machine, Random Forest, K-NN, S-Inception, PNN, VGG16, VGG19, ConvNet and ResNet50 on Flavia plant-leaf image dataset. Flavia plant-leaf image dataset consists of 32 different species of plant. The images are first preprocessed, and then their shape, color, and texture-based features are extracted from the processed image. Initially, these images are in the size of 256*256 pixels. These images were preprocessed and taken up to the size of 64*64 for fast processing. ResNet50 has given the best results with an accuracy of 98%. Though SVM and S-Inception have also provided a good accuracy.

The organization of this article goes like this. Section 2 will discuss the related work on plant-leaf image identification and classification. Section 3 describes the methodology for plant-leaf image identification and classification. Section 4 quotes the experimental analysis and the observation on plant-leaf image identification and classification. Section 5 summarizes the results.

2 Related Work

Wang et al. performed plant-leaf image classification by extracting the features using pulse-coupled neural network technique and classified using support SVM approach. The approach of Wang et al. is measured for three datasets, namely Flavia, Intelligent Computing Laboratory (ICL) and MEW2012. The reported accuracies for the above datasets are 96.67, 91.56, and 91.2% [17].

Liu et al. used the combined way using numerous texture and shape features to create a final feature vector. Texture features measured are local binary pattern, Gabor filters, and gray-level co-occurrence matrices. Hybrid deep belief networks with dropout are used for the plant-leaf image classification. This method was applied on ICL leaf dataset and provided an accuracy of 93.9% [7].

Tan et al. proposed a novel approach D-Leaf network which is a CNN-based method for feature extraction. Extracted features from this approach are then classified using various machine learning classifiers like SVM, ANN, KNN, NB, and CNN [18].

Ghazi et al. executed plant-leaf image classification using pre-trained DL model such as AlexNet, GoogleNet, and VGGNet on LifeCLEF 2015 plant dataset. The data augmentation is executed to diminish the overfitting issue. It was found that the performance of these pre-trained models was affected on the basis of the number of iterations and data augmentation [19].

Sun et al. developed a 26-layer ResNet model for plant-leaf image classification. This model is applied on a real-time dataset BJFU100 dataset. BJFU100 dataset is a collection of 100 classes of plant species. This method is further used to validate the Flavia dataset [20].

Lee et al. proposed a CNN-based DL model for plant-leaf image classification. It was able to find and analyze the feature of raw plant-leaf image. This approach produced better results on leaf venation as compared to leaf shape. Hybrid local global features were used to compare different approaches and comparison [21].

Liu et al. come up with a hybrid DL approach for feature extraction from a plant-leaf image. This approach is amalgam of two methods, AutoEncoder and CNN. These extracted features are then classified using SVM approach. This approach was tested on ICL leaf dataset and found that hybrid DL method with accuracy 93% performed better than SVM with accuracy 88%, AE with accuracy 90%, and CNN with accuracy 91%) [22].

Barré et al. come up with a DL based plant-leaf image classification approach known as LeafNet. It was found that CNN learns specific features better than hand-crafted features. LeafNet is a collection of many sets of convo layers with max pooling which is further, followed by three FCLs. This CNN approach was applied and evaluated on three datasets namely LeafSnap, Flavia, and Foliage [23].

Pawara et al. stress on comparison of the performance of the conventional method and DL method in plant-leaf image classification using AgrilPlant, LeafSnap, and Folio datasets. AgrilPlant is a custom dataset. It is having 10 classes. Each class contains 300 images of agri-plants. AlexNet and GoogleNet were trained from scratch and finely tuned for DL approach. The histogram of oriented gradient (HOG) with KNN classifier were used. In another approach bag of visual words (BOWs) with HOG as feature extraction and SVM, MLP as a classifier was used. AgrilPlant dataset produces an accuracy of 79.43 and 98.33% was obtained for HOG–BOW with SVM and fine-tuned GoogleNet [24].

Hu et al. came up with a multi-scale fusion CNN (MSF-CNN) for plant-leaf image classification. Images were reduced to 256×256, 128×128, 64×64, and 32×32 using bilinear interpolation operations method. Concatenation operation is performed for feature fusion between two different scales. Two datasets, namely Malayakew dataset and LeafSnap dataset are used for evaluation of MSF-CNN method [25].

For plant-leaf image classification researches have used numerous dataset such as Flavia Dataset [29], Leafsnap Dataset [30], UCI Plant-Leaf Dataset, UCI One-Hundred Plant Species Dataset, Herbarium Dataset. These are the standard datasets for implementing and testing machine learning or deep learning model. There are many datasets available for plant classification task.

Flavia Dataset [6]: Flavia dataset was used for training the algorithm and was obtained from: A Leaf Recognition Algorithm for Plant classification Using Probabilistic Neural Network, by Stephen Gang Wu, Forrest Sheng Bao, Eric You Xu,

Yu-Xuan Wang, Yi-Fan Chang and Qiao-Liang Xiang, published at IEEE 7th International Symposium on Signal Processing and Information Technology, Dec. 2007. The dataset provides extremely controlled plant-leaf images on white background and no stem is present. This dataset covers 32 species with only a single-training image.

UCI Plant-Leaf Dataset [34]: This dataset was created by Pedro F. B. Silva of Porto University. It is a multivariate plant-leaf dataset. It contains 40 distinct species with 340 illustrations.

UCI One-Hundred Plant Species Dataset [32]: James Cope of Royal Botanic Gardens has collected and created this database. It contains almost hundred plant species with 16 images from each species covering more than 1600 plant-leaf images.

Herbarium Dataset [31]: This dataset is created by the joint efforts of New York Botanical Garden (NY), Bishop Museum (BPBM), Naturalis Biodiversity Center (NL), Queensland Herbarium (BRI), and Auckland War Memorial Museum (AK). This dataset covers 65,000 species of plants. The data set includes more than 2.5 million leaf images. The split of data for training and testing is approximately 80% and 20%. All images are in JPEG format but irregular in dimensions.

LeafSnap Dataset [30]: This dataset is created using two different sources: Lab images (23,147) and Field images (7719). This dataset contains 185 different plant/tree species. Lab images are of high quality and taken of pressed leaves in lab conditions, whereas field images are taken using mobile devices in outdoor environment, hence, contains a lot of noise. Images in the dataset are segmented.

UCI Folio Data Set [33]: This dataset was created in the farm of the University of Mauritius and nearby locations. It consists of 32 different species with 20 images from each species. The leaves were taken on a white background. The pictures were photographed in daylight to ensure optimal light intensity.

3 Proposed Methodology

Basically, there are two approaches which is used for plant-leaf image classification namely traditional approach and deep learning approach. The same has been depicted in Fig. 1. In this paper, we have applied and tested both the approaches and find out the comparative differences among both the approaches.

3.1 About the Dataset

Flavia dataset was used for training the algorithm and was obtained from: A Leaf Recognition Algorithm for Plant classification Using Probabilistic Neural Network, by Stephen Gang Wu, Forrest Sheng Bao, Eric You Xu, Yu-Xuan Wang, Yi-Fan Chang and Qiao-Liang Xiang, published at IEEE 7th International Symposium on Signal Processing and Information Technology, Dec. 2007. The dataset provides

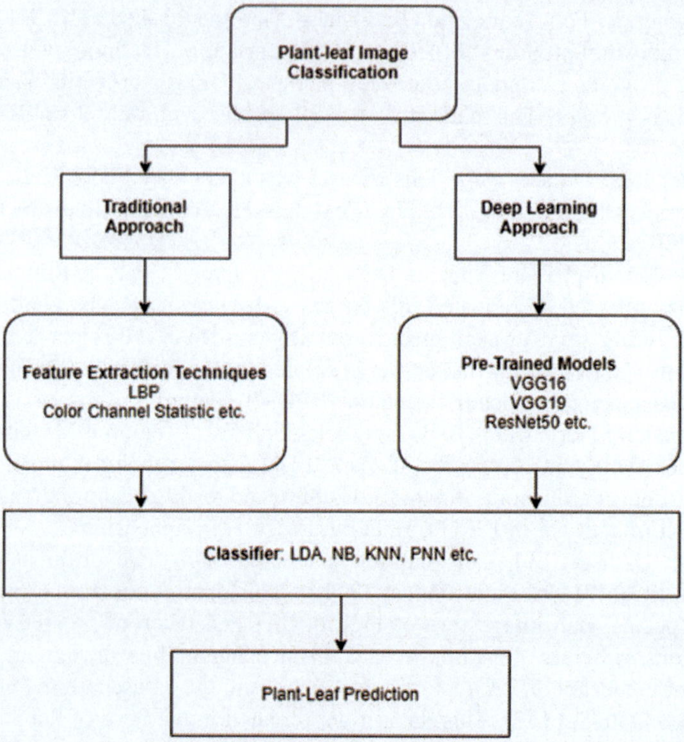

Fig. 1 Plant-leaf image classification approach

extremely controlled plant-leaf images on white background and no stem is present. This dataset covers 32 species with only a single-training image (Figs. 2, 3, 4 and 5).

Step 1: Load Original Image: There are multiple images from 32 classes of plants. Images are originally clicked on a white background and having a size of 256*256.

Step 2: Conversion of image from RGB to BGR: Open CV (python library for Image Processing), acknowledges pictures in RGB shading design so it should be changed over to the first configuration that is BGR design.

Step 3: Conversion of image from BGR to HSV: The basic answer is that not normal for RGB, HSV isolates luma, or the picture power, from chroma or the shading data. This is helpful in numerous applications. For instance, on the off chance that you need to do histogram balance of a shading picture, you presumably need to do that just on the power segment, and disregard the shading segments. Else you will get extremely peculiar tones. In computer vision, you regularly need to isolate shading parts from power for different reasons, for example, vigor to lighting changes, or eliminating shadows. Note, notwithstanding that HSV is one of many shading spaces that different tone from power (See YCbCr, Lab, and so on) HSV is

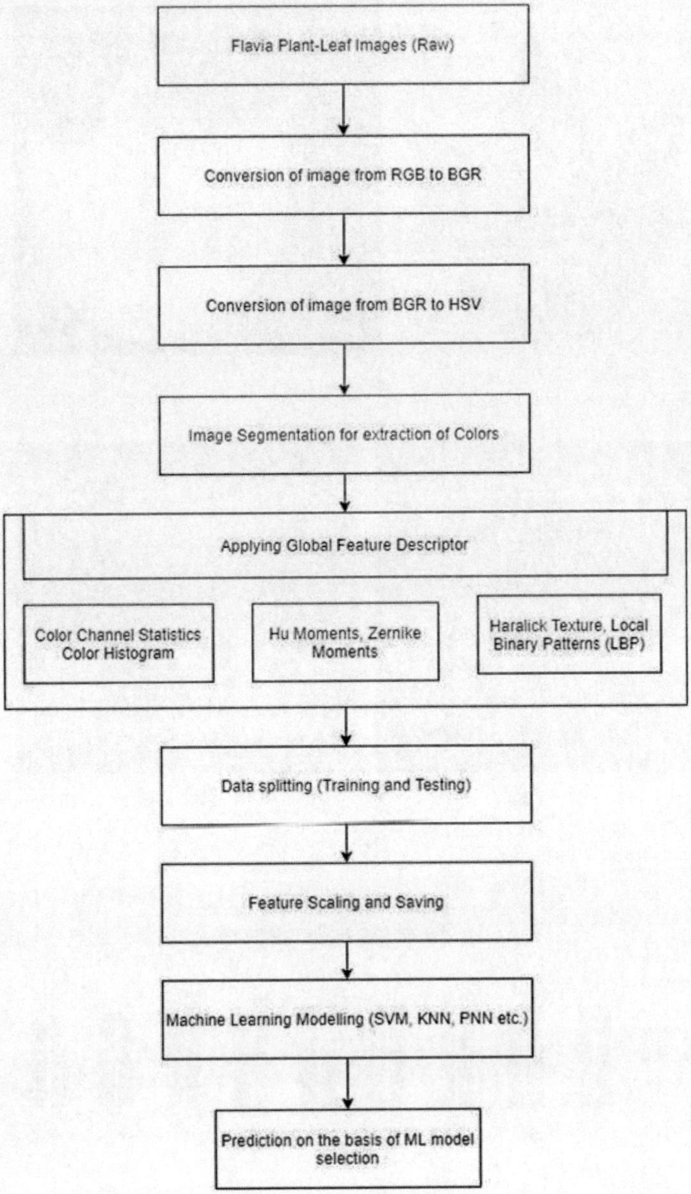

Fig. 2 Detail workflow for Plant-Leaf Image Classification

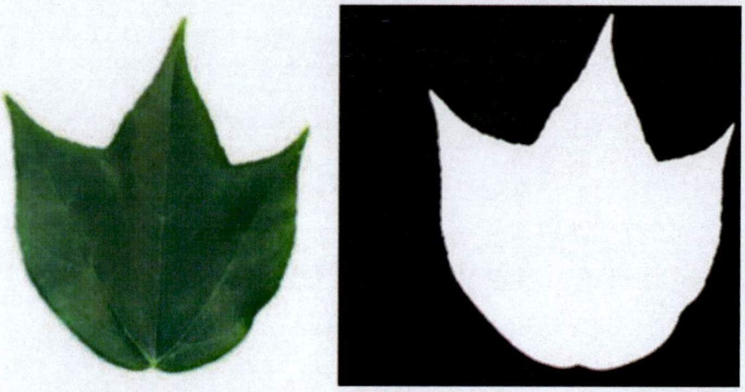

Fig. 3 Image pre-processing

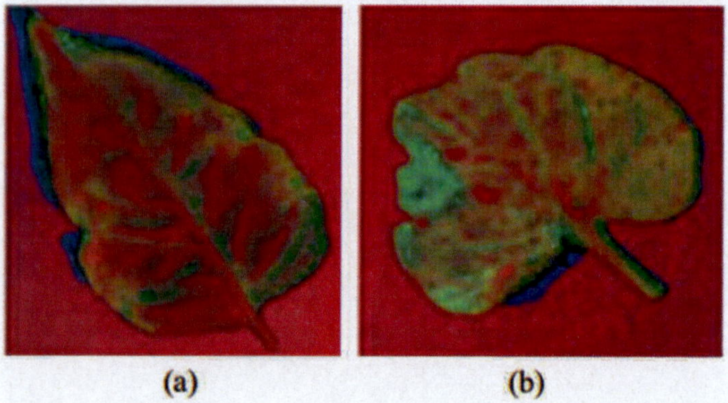

Fig. 4 Images converted to HSV

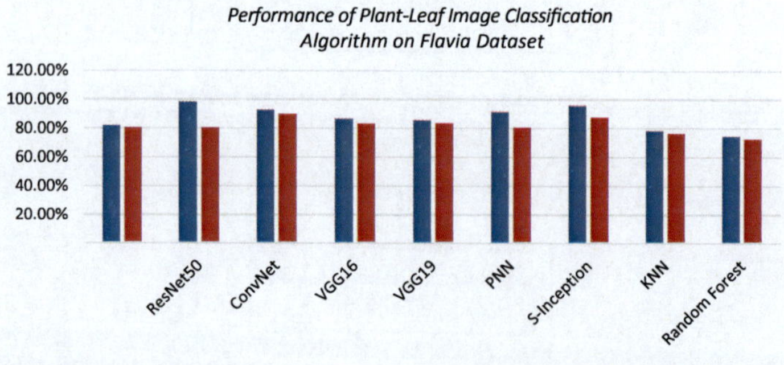

Fig. 5 Performance of Plant-Leaf Image Classification Algorithm on Flavia Dataset

regularly utilized essentially in light of the fact that the code for changing over among RGB and HSV is broadly accessible and can likewise be effectively actualized [27].

[45] RGB values are divided by max value that is 255 to get the new values of RGB. That is:

$$\begin{aligned}
R_{New} &= R/255 \\
G_{New} &= G/255 \\
B_{New} &= B/255 \\
C_{max} &= \max\left(R_{New}, G_{New}, B_{New}\right) \\
C_{min} &= \min\left(R_{New}, G_{New}, B_{New}\right) \\
dy &= C_{max} - C_{min}
\end{aligned}$$

Hue is calculated as:

$$H = \begin{cases} 60 * \frac{G_{New} - B_{New}}{\Delta} * mod6 & \text{if, } C_{max} = R_{New} \\ 60 * \frac{B_{New} - R_{New}}{\Delta} + 2 & \text{if, } C_{max} = G_{New} \\ 60 * \frac{R_{New} - G_{New}}{\Delta} + 4 & \text{if, } C_{max} = B_{New} \end{cases}$$

Saturation is calculated as:

$$S = \begin{cases} 0 & \text{if, } C_{max} = 0 \\ \frac{\Delta}{C_{max}} & \text{if, } C_{max} \neq 0 \end{cases}$$

Value is calculated as:

$$V = C_{max}$$

Step 4: Image Segmentation for extraction of Colors: The way toward parceling a plant-leaf image into different sections is characterized as image segmentation. Segmentation intends to separate a plant-leaf image into areas that can be more delegate and simpler to break down. Color image segmentation that depends on the color highlight of plant-leaf image pixels accepts that homogeneous colors in the image compare to isolate bunches and thus important items in the image. As such, each bunch characterizes a class of pixels that share comparable color properties. As the segmentation results rely upon the pre-owned color space, there is no single-color space that can give satisfactory outcomes to a wide range of plant-leaf images. [26]

Step 5: Applying Global Feature Descriptor: Local and global features are two methodologies for object acknowledgment. Global image features depict image as entire while local component speaks to as image patches. Global element sums up the entire image with single vector and likewise with local processes with various focuses on the image in this way making it stronger. In spite of strength in local component, global element is as yet helpful for applications where unpleasant segmentation of the article is accessible. Global features incorporate form portrayals, shape descriptors, and surface features. Global surface features and local features give distinctive data about the image on the grounds that the help over which surface is figured differs [28].

In computer vision, surface measurements are concocted to depict the perceptual ascribes of surface by utilizing discrete techniques. For example, surface has been depicted perceptually with a few properties, including: Contrast, Color, Coarseness, Directionality, Line-similarity, Roughness, Constancy, Grouping, Segmentation [28].

More spotlight was put on measurements that recognize little local features encompassing interest focuses in images. Feature descriptors added more subtleties from a window or fix encompassing each element, and acknowledgment depended on looking for sets of descriptors and coordinating descriptors with more unpredictable classifiers. Descriptor spectra included slopes, edges, and colors [28].

Step 6: Feature Scaling and Saving: Scaling is a method to standardize the autonomous features present in the information in a fixed reach. It is performed during the information pre-preparing to handle exceptionally fluctuating extents or qualities or units. In the event that element scaling isn't done, at that point, a machine learning calculation will in general weigh more noteworthy qualities, higher and consider more modest qualities as the lower esteems, paying little mind to the unit of the qualities.

Machine learning algorithms like linear regression, logistic regression, NN, and so on that utilization gradient descent as an optimization strategy expect information to be scaled. Investigate the equation for gradient descent underneath:

$$\theta_j := \theta_j - \alpha \frac{1}{m} \sum_{i=1}^{m} \left(h_\theta\left(x^{(i)}\right) - y^{(i)} \right) x_j^{(i)}$$

The presence of highlight esteem X in the recipe will influence the progression size of the gradient descent. The distinction in scopes of features will cause diverse advance sizes for each element. To guarantee that the gradient descent moves easily toward the minima and that the means for gradient descent are refreshed at similar rate for all the features, we scale the information prior to taking care of it to the model. Having features on a comparable scale can help the gradient descent unite all the more rapidly toward the minima.

Step 7: Model Training: The way toward preparing a ML model includes giving a ML calculation preparing information to gain from. The term ML model alludes to the model antiquity that is made by the preparation cycle. The preparation information should contain the right answer, which is known as an objective or target property. The learning calculation discovers designs in the preparation information that map the info information ascribes to the objective, and it yields a ML model that catches these examples. You can utilize the ML model to get expectations on new information for which you don't have the foggiest idea about the objective. For instance, suppose that you need to prepare a ML model to foresee if an email is spam or not spam. You would furnish custom ML calculation with preparing information that contains messages for which you know the objective (that is, a name that tells if an email is spam).

Custom ML calculation would prepare a ML model by utilizing this information, bringing about a model that endeavors to foresee if new email will be spam.

In this article, we are going to apply 9 machine learning techniques on Flavia plant-leaf image dataset. The algorithm is Support Vector Machine, PNN, KNN, Random Forest, S-Inception, VGG16, VGG19, ResNet50 and ConvNet.

Step 8: Plant Image Prediction: The models with best performance is them trained with whole of the dataset and score for testing set is predicted using Predict function. ResNet50 has performed well and achieved an accuracy of 98%.

4 Experimental Analysis and Result Discussion

The hardware environment of this experiment is Intel Core I3 CPU, the main frequency is 2.45 GHz, the memory is 12 GB; the operating system is 64-bit Windows 10 version, and the software environment used is Python using Anaconda IDE (Table 1).

We have taken a ratio of 70:30 for training and testing data. Accuracy has been taken for both Training Data and Testing Data. To improve the amount and nature of preparing information and lessen overfitting cases in preparing models, some generally utilized information upgrade strategies, for example, translation transformation

Table 1 A brief summary of applied classification techniques

Article Title	Classification Technique	Dataset	Accuracy	Conclusion
Identification of the Plants Based on Leaf Shape Descriptors [35]	Euclidean minimum Distance classifier	VISLeaf database	84.66 & 92.67 accuracy for ZM and HOG	High Accuracy and Speed but not good for Multidimensional and sparse data
Leaf Classification Using Shape, Color, and Texture Features [36]	Probabilistic Neural network (PNN) classifier	Flavia dataset	93.75	High Accuracy, Efficiency and multiple descriptors but uses high memory and Computation
Automatic Agricultural Leaves Recognition System [37]	SVM-PCA	200 images dataset of 4 plant species	77.96	High accuracy but having application in small dataset only
Automatic classification of plants based on their leaves [38]	Artificial Neural Network	Flavia dataset, ICL Dataset	96	Having high accuracy but need to be retrained if new leaf has been introduced

(continued)

Table 1 (continued)

Article Title	Classification Technique	Dataset	Accuracy	Conclusion
Leaf Recognition using Contour based Edge Detection and SIFT Algorithm [39]	SIFT, CSS	Flavia dataset	87.5%	Very robust algorithm but with average accuracy
Recognition of Leaf Based on Its Tip and Base using Centroid Contour Gradient [40]	Feedforward Backpropagation	Universiti Teknologi Malaysia custom dataset	99.47%	Provide a better accuracy than the previous methods but only work with one feature and on small dataset
SVM-BDT PNN and Fourier moment technique for classification of leaf shape [41]	SVM-BDT, PNN-PCA, Fourier Moments	Flavia dataset	69%	Provide high accuracy with hybrid approach but only work on shape and morphological features
Diagnosis of Diseases on Cotton Leaves Using Principal Component Analysis Classifier [42]	Principle Component Analysis and K Neighborhood classifier	Dataset of 110 Samples of cotton leaves	95%	Accurate and efficient but based on one feature (color) hence work for cotton plants only
Identification and Classification of Fungal disease Affected on Agriculture/Horticulture Crops using Image Processing Techniques [43]	ANN, PCA KNN, Neuro-KNN, PNN and SVM classifier	Plant pathology department of UAS, and UHS INDIA	91.54%	Provides high accuracy with pre-detection but uses different methods for different crops and also effected with outdoor conditions
Comparative Study of Leaf Image Recognition with a Novel Learning based Approach [44]	Dictionary based and bag-of words-based classification using SVM	Flavia dataset	95.47%	It provides high accuracy but work on limited features only

and rotation transformation, are embraced in the exploration article. The prediction has been taken for both DL based algorithms and non-DL based algorithm. The Table 2 is depicting the DL and non-DL based algorithm.

Table 3 depicts the performance of various plant-leaf image classification algorithm on Flavia dataset. The experiment was carried out in using python language and using various libraries like OpenCV, Keras, etc. The accuracy obtained by DL based methods is far better than non-DL based algorithm. ResNet50 has performed the best out of all with an accuracy of 98% on training data. SVM has also performed

Table 2 Classification of DL and Non-DL based plant image classification algorithm

Algorithm Name	Deep Learning Based	Non-Deep Learning Based
Support Vector Machine	No	Yes
ResNet50	Yes	No
ConvNet	Yes	No
VGG16	Yes	No
VGG19	Yes	No
PNN	No	Yes
S-Inception	Yes	No
KNN	No	Yes
Random Forest	No	Yes

Table 3 Performance of plant-leaf image classification algorithm on flavia dataset

Algorithm name	Accuracy (Training data) (%)	Accuracy (Testing data) (%)
Support Vector Machine	81.56	80.02
ResNet50	98	80.03
ConvNet	92.30	89.26
VGG16	86.20	82.65
VGG19	85.4	83.04
PNN	91.25	79.85
S-Inception	95.32	87
KNN	78	76
Random Forest	74	72

well in the table of non-DL based algorithm with an accuracy of 81.56% on training data. PNN and S-inception has also performed well with an accuracy of 91% and 95%, respectively.

5 Conclusion

Plant-leaf image classification is carried out using two approaches, traditional methods (Non-DL based) and deep learning-based method. Flavia datasets were considered for this experiment. It is observed from the experiment that the deep learning-based model performs better than traditional methods with a higher accuracy as compared to that of traditional methods. We have applied 9 machine learning techniques on Flavia plant-leaf image dataset. ResNet50 has given the best results with an accuracy of 98%. Though SVM and S-Inception have also provided a good accuracy. These accuracies can be further improved by increasing the number of images using data augmentation methods.

References

1. Cho S, Lee D, Jeong J (2002) Automation and emerging technologies: weedplant discrimination by machine vision and artificial neural network. Biosyst Eng 83(3):275280
2. Mallah C, Cope J, Orwell J (2013) Plant leaf classification using probabilistic integration of shape, texture and margin features. Signal Process Pattern Recogn Appl
3. Silva PFB, Marcal ARS, da Silva RMA (2013) Evaluation of features for leaf discrimination. Springer Lecture Notes in Computer Science, vol 7950, 197–204
4. Du JX, Wang XF, Zhang GJ (2007) Leaf shape based plant species recognition. Appl Math Comput 185(2):883–893
5. Jin T, Hou X, Li P et al (2015) A novel method of automatic plant species identification using sparse representation of leaf tooth features. PLoS One 10(10):e0139482
6. Wu SG, Bao FS, Xu EY et al (2007) A leaf recognition algorithm for plant classification using probabilistic neural network. In: IEEE International symposium signal processing and information technology. Cairo, Egypt, pp 11–16
7. Liu N, Kan JM (2016) Improved deep belief networks and multi-feature fusion for leaf identification. Neurocomputing 216:460–467
8. Goodfellow I, Bengio Y, Courville A et al (2016) Deep learning, vol 1. MIT Press, Cambridge, pp 322–366
9. Simonyan K, Zisserman A (2014) Very deep convolutional networks for largescale image recognition. arXiv:1409.1556
10. Szegedy C, Vanhoucke V, Ioffe S et al (2016) Rethinking the inception architecture for computer vision. In: Proceedings of the IEEE conference computer vision and pattern recognition, Las Vegas, USA, pp.2818–2826
11. Szegedy C, Ioffe S, Vanhoucke V et al (2017) Inception-v4, inception-ResNet and the impact of residual connections on learning. In: Proceedings of the 31st AAAI Conference artificial intelligence, San Francisco, USA
12. Chollet F (2017) Xception: deep learning with depthwise separable convolutions. 1610-02357
13. He K, Zhang X, Ren S et al (2016) Deep residual learning for image recognition. In: Proceedings of the IEEE conference computer vision and pattern recognition, Las Vegas, USA, pp 770–778
14. Huang G, Liu Z, Van Der Maaten L et al (2017) Densely connected convolutional networks. In: Proceedings of the IEEE conference computer vision and pattern recognition, Honolulu, USA, pp 4700–4708
15. Howard AG, Zhu M, Chen B et al (2017) MobileNets: efficient convolutiona neural networks for mobile vision applications. arXiv:1704.04861
16. Krizhevsky A, Sutskever I, Hinton GE (2012) ImageNet classification with deep convolutional neural networks. In: NIPS'12 Proceedings of the 25th International conference on neural information processing systems, vol 1, Lake Tahoe, Nevada, pp 1097–1105
17. Wang Z, Sun X, Zhang Y et al (2016) Leaf recognition based on PCNN. Neural Comput Appl 27(4):899–908
18. Tan JW, Chang SW, Kareem SBA et al (2018) Deep learning for plant species classification using leaf vein morphometric', IEEE/ACM Trans Comput Biol Bioinf :1. https://ieeexplore.ieee.org/abstract/document/8388220
19. Ghazi MM, Yanikoglu B, Aptoula E (2017) Plant identification using deep neural networks via optimization of transfer learning parameters. Neurocomputing 235:228–235
20. Sun Y, Liu Y, Wang G et al (2017) Deep learning for plant identification in natural environment. Comput Intell Neurosci 2017:6

21. Lee SH, Chan CS, Mayo SJ et al (2017) How deep learning extracts and learns leaf features for plant classification. Pattern Recognit 71:1–13
22. Liu Z, Zhu L, Zhang XP et al (2015) Hybrid deep learning for plant leaves classification. In: International conference intelligent computing, Cham, August 2015, pp 115–123
23. Barré P, Stöver BC, Müller KF et al (2017) LeafNet: a computer vision system for automatic plant species identification. Ecol Inf 40:50–56
24. Pawara P, Okafor E, Surinta O et al (2017) Comparing local descriptors and bags of visual words to deep convolutional neural networks for plant recognition. In: ICPRAM, Porto, Portugal, pp 479–486
25. Hu J, Chen Z, Yang M et al (2018) A multiscale fusion convolutional neural network for plant leaf recognition. IEEE Signal Process Lett 25(6):853–857
26. Lalitha M, Kiruthiga M, Loganathan C (2013) A survey on image segmentation through clustering algorithm. Int J Sci Res 2(2):348–358
27. PatilBharti JK (2011) Advances in image processing for detection of plant diseases. J Adv Bioinforma Appl Res 2(2):135–141
28. Krig S (2014) Computer vision metrics: survey, taxonomy, and analysis. Apress:85–129
29. Forrest Sheng Bao EYX (2009) Flavia leaf database. http://flavia.sourceforge.net/
30. Kumar N, Belhumeur P, Biswas A, Jacobs D, Kress W, Lopez I, Soares J (2012) Leafsnap: a computer vision system for automatic plant species identification, Computer Vision–ECCV. Lecture Notes in Computer Science. Springer, Berlin Heidelberg, pp 502–516
31. Tan KC, Liu Y, Ambrose B, Tulig M, Belongie S (2019) The herbarium challenge 2019 dataset. Comput Vision Pattern Recogn
32. Mallah C, Cope J, Orwell J (2013) Plant leaf classification using probabilistic integration of shape, texture and margin features. Pattern Recognit Appl
33. Munisami T, Ramsurn M, Kishnah S, Pudaruth S (2015) Plant leaf recognition using shape features and color histogram with k-nearest neighbor classifiers. Proc Comput Sci (Elsevier) J 58:740–747
34. Imah EM, Rahayu YS, Wintarti A (2018) Plant leaf recognition using competitive based learning algorithm, In Proceedings of the 2nd annual applied science and engineering conference (AASEC 2017), IOP Confernce. Series: Materials Science and Engineering, 288
35. Salve P, Sardesai M, Manza R, Yannawar P (2016) Identification of the plants based on leaf shape descriptors. In: Satapathy S, Raju K, Mandal J, Bhateja V (Eds) Proceedings of the second international conference on computer and communication technologies. Advances in Intelligent Systems and Computing, vol 379. Springer, New Delhi
36. Kadir A, Nugroho L, Susanto A, Santosa PI (2014) Leaf classification using shape, color, and texture features. abs/1401.4447
37. Puja D, Saraswat M, Arya K (2013) Automatic agricultural leaves recognition system. In: Bansal J, Singh P, Deep K, Pant M, Nagar A (Eds) Proceedings of seventh international conference on bio-inspired computing: theories and applications (BIC-TA 2012). Advances in Intelligent Systems and Computing, vol 201. Springer, India
38. Aakif A, Khan MF (2015) Automatic classification of plants based on their leaves. Biosyst Eng
39. Lavania S, Matey PS (2014) Leaf recognition using contour based edge detection and SIFT algorithm. In: IEEE international conference on computational intelligence and computing research, IEEE ICCIC 2014
40. Fern BM, Sulong GB, Rahim MSM (2014) Leaf recognition based on leaf tip and leaf base using centroid contour gradient. Adv Sci Lett
41. Singh K, Gupta I, Gupta S (2010) SVM-BDT PNN and fourier moment technique for classification of leaf shape. Int J Signal Process Image Process Pattern Recogn 3:67–78
42. Gulhane VA, Kolekar MH (2014) Diagnosis of diseases on cotton leaves using principal component analysis classifier. In: Annual IEEE India conference (INDICON). Pune, India, pp 1–5
43. Pujari JD, Yakkundimath R, Byadgi AS (2014) Identification and classification of fungal disease affected on agriculture/horticulture crops using image processing techniques. In: 2014 IEEE international conference on computational intelligence and computing research, Coimbatore, India, pp 1–4

44. Hsiao J, Kang L, Chang C, Lin C (2014) Comparative study of leaf image recognition with a novel learning-based approach. In: Science and information conference. London, UK, pp 389–393
45. Conversion from RGB to HSV color space at https://math.stackexchange.com/questions/556341/rgb-to-hsv-colorconversion-algorithm

Implementation of Blockchain in IoT

Rasmeet Kaur and Aleem Ali

Abstract The concept of the Internet of Things is arising and developing quickly. IoT addresses another innovation that empowers both virtual and actual items to be associated and interact with one another and gives rise to new digitized services that enhance our satisfaction. The IoT framework gives a few benefits; notwithstanding, the current incorporated design presents various issues including, security, protection, straightforwardness, and data integrity. The quick advancement and usage of IoT innovations have raised security concerns and made a sensation of vulnerability among IoT adopters. These difficulties impede the method of things to come improvements of IoT implementations. Shifting the IoT toward distributed ledger technology might be the right decision to determine such problems. Among the normal and well-known kinds of such innovation is the Blockchain. Coordinating the IoT with Blockchain innovation may induce incalculable advantages. The motivation behind this paper is to analyze the latest research patterns identified with security worries of the IoT idea and give an itemized comprehension of the point. Subsequently, this paper gives a thorough conversation of incorporating the IoT framework with Blockchain innovation. The study is elaborated into four segments. Segment 1 introduces the description of IoT. The next segment will present the fundamentals and working of Blockchain. Segment 3 portrays a few instances of utilization for Blockchain to give security and protection at IoT. In segment 4, various platforms for Blockchain are presented. Segment 5 presents the last contemplations.

Keywords IoT · Blockchain (BC) · Distributed ledger technology (DLT) · Security · Privacy

---

R. Kaur (✉) · A. Ali
Department of CSE, Global University Saharanpur, Saharanpur, U.P, India

N. Marriwala et al. (eds.), *Emergent Converging Technologies and Biomedical Systems*, Lecture Notes in Electrical Engineering 841,
https://doi.org/10.1007/978-981-16-8774-7_13

1 Introduction to IoT

The IoT is an extensive term alluding to progressing endeavors to associate a wide assortment of physical things to communication networks as shown in Fig. 1. IoT has a framework of organization that is worldwide where any article that is associated with the web has an identity and can speak with different gadgets on the web [1]. The gadgets contain microchips that interconnect every one of the gadgets. These computer chips track the surroundings and report in the network as well as to the humans.

Started during the 1990s, the idea of IoT is to expand over the Internet as well as to broaden the Internet. The most awesome aspect of IoT is that every single-actual substance can be imparted and is accessible. Currently, the Internet has connected

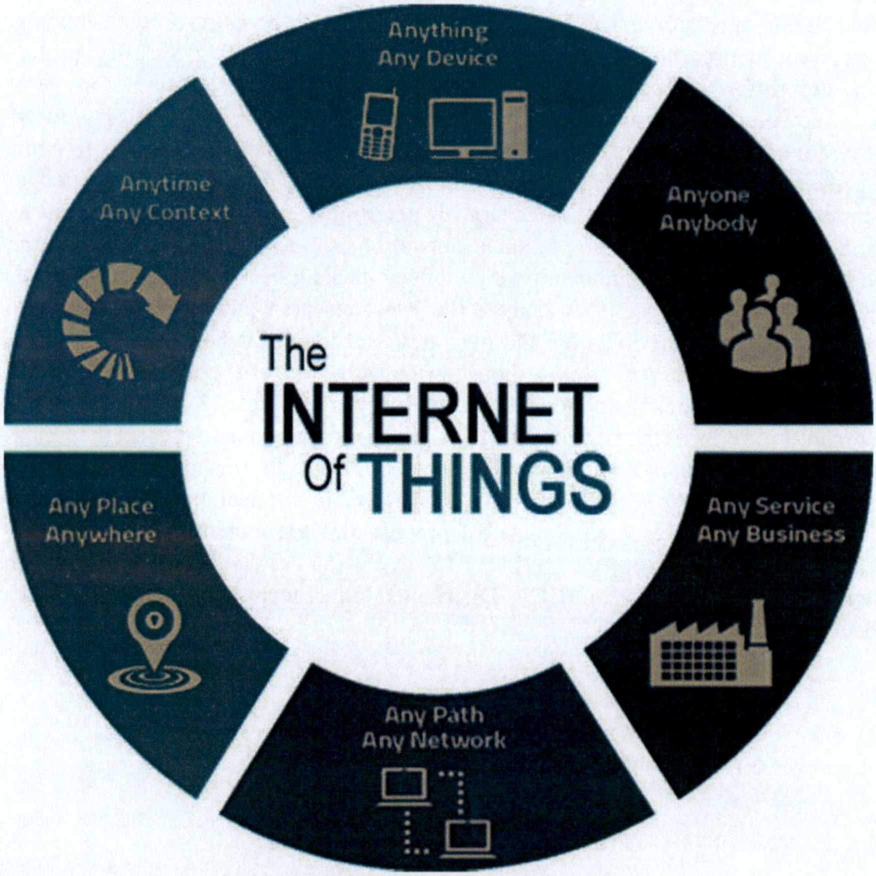

Fig. 1 Introduction to IoT

computers along with a wide heterogeneity of devices like TVs, workstations, refrigerators, ovens, electrical appliances, vehicles, and cell phones. In this new situation, projections show that the Internet will have more than 50 billion gadgets associated until 2020 [2].

The IoT framework offers various applications including, Smart homes, Smart cities, and Smart healthcare, etc. The essential component of this framework is the astute detecting assortment of information, which is then safely sent to the server [3]. The IoT domain has encountered fast advancement for over twenty years, and the quantity of IoT gadgets has developed dramatically, a pattern that enormously enhances social profitability and proficiency just as makes individuals' lives more helpful and astute.

There are remarkable benefits of IoT, still, it expanding the threat of openness to various privacy and security intrusions, and; a portion of such threats are new. Ahead of the concept of IoT, data leakage and denial of service were the most announced security concerns. Security and privacy alternatives need to be executed by attributes of heterogeneous IoT devices [4].

For these scenarios, BC plays a vital role, since one can use this technique to confirm, approve, and review the data given by the devices. Along with it, because of its decentralized nature, it disposes of the condition to trust in the outsider and doesn't have a single point of failure. BC is an idea that leads to decentralization as a safety effort, can make a worldwide file for all exchanges that happen in a given organization, and makes them permanent. It fills in as a public, shared, and general record.

Another main worry in the IoT domain is the secure storage of the data. Right now, numerous IoT data storage options preserve data on conventional centralized servers. Although, this strategy has some issues. First and foremost, all information is put away on a central server; hence, the performance needs, environment necessities, and upkeep expense for the central server are huge. The server must be equipped with a huge storage ability to preserve numerous data produces by IoT devices. When the server falls flat, the whole data storage framework won't work as expected.

Furthermore, as all IoT gadgets are associated with the central server, this will result in network blockage, high network delay, and non-sufficient space for data. At long last, when the main server is harmed by attackers, the data security will be incredibly compromised. Being a service of DLT, the Blockchain can take care of the issues that effectively happen in a centralized server [5].

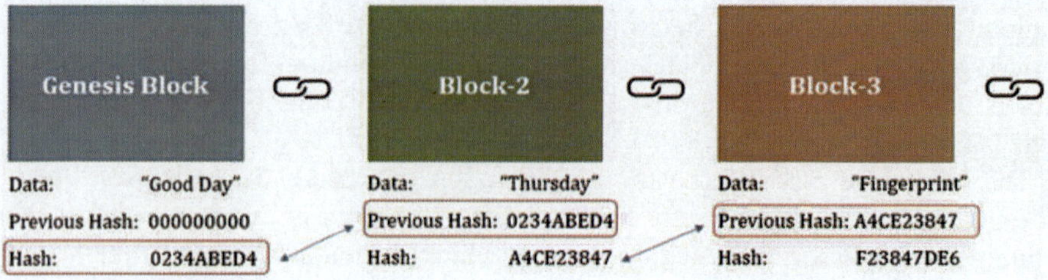

Fig. 2 Structure of blockchain

2 Blockchain

2.1 *Introduction*

Started in 2008, the embodiment of BC is to halfway keep a trustworthy data set arrangement through decentralization and distrust. The world kept using the centralized setup, where the main server is expected to manage the working until Szabo made decentralized computerized money toward the finish of 1990. After ten years, Bitcoin cryptographic money was advertised. BC turned out to be for the most part broad in 2009 after a study presented by Satoshi Nakamoto.

In a Blockchain, data is separated into a progression of blocks [6]. Every block of data can check the legitimacy of the data and create the succeeding block, which is associated in a sequential request into a chain-like arrangement as depicted in Fig. 2. BC is a non-centralized, distributed, and changeless log in which the data of the different exchanges that consistently occurred in a specific P2P network is kept. The process of storing an exchange/transaction in the distributed log demands a consensus mechanism.

A collection of exchanges are gathered and allocated a block in the ledger. To join a block to the preceding block, a hash function and timestamp of those blocks are used. In this way, numerous blocks are grouped as a chain and termed a Blockchain. The hash estimation approves the data integrity. The BC innovation advances sharing of information in which every taking part client/device in the structure maintains a duplicate of the actual ledger, hence every node is refreshed with recently added exchanges or blocks [7].

2.2 *Components of Blockchain*

The primary elements of the BC incorporate ledger, block, hash, transaction, minor, and consensus mechanisms shown in Fig. 3 [8].

A ledger can be defined as a data structure that is used to reserve different kinds of data.

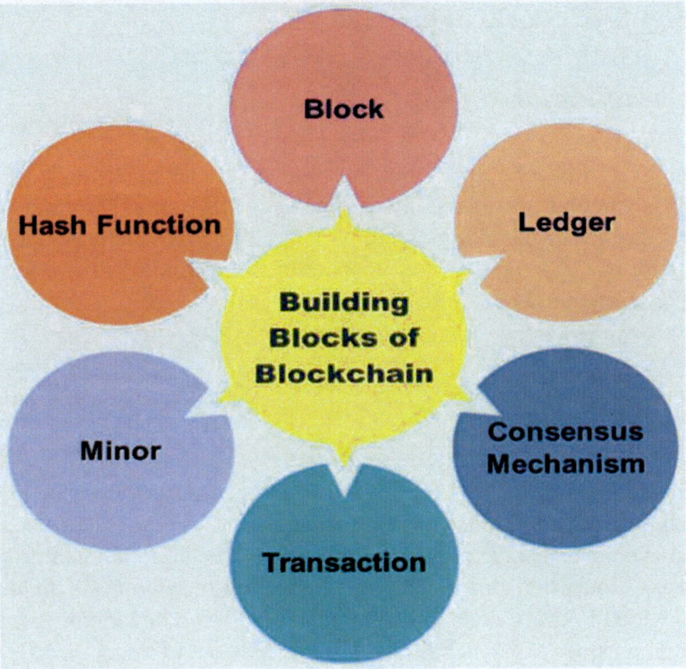

Fig. 3 Components of blockchain

A block is an essential part of the BC. Every block involves a bunch of exchanges. The blocks were linked to one another by putting away a hash estimation of the preceding block in the recent block. These linked blocks create a BC.

The hash estimation is utilized to authenticate the data integrity. Fundamentally, it is a mathematical issue that minors must break to discover a block. The motivation to utilize this estimation is it's free from collision nature in due to which it is exceptionally difficult to make two indistinguishable hashes for two diverse computerized data. In this way, allocating hash estimation for every block can fill in as an approach to distinguish the block and validate the data inside it.

The transaction is the littlest unit of an activity or process wherein a bunch of transactions is joined and reserved in a block. It is not easy to add a certain transaction in the block except if most of the co-operating nodes in the BC network mark their assent. The transaction size is significant for minors because the compact transactions consume limited energy and are simpler to approve.

Minors are PCs/specialists that endeavor to tackle a tough numerical issue to investigate another block. Finding another block is begun by communicating fresh transactions to every node, and afterward, every node consolidates a bunch of transactions into a block and starts finding the POW of the block.

3 Highlights of Blockchain

3.1 Decentralization

BC is commonly a decentralized and distributed setup that depends on the P2P correspondence among distributed nodes. The decentralization empowers using the handling force of every partaking client, which diminishes inactivity and abolishes the single point of failure issue. This attribute of BC technology helps in resolving the issue of a single point of failure [9–13].

3.2 Transparency

Rather than the centralized system, in which the central server is taking care of the whole control and admittance to all information, BC provides a decent degree of transparency wherein all nodes approach every one of the subtleties of the transactions that consistently occurred in the network. Furthermore, a copy of the distributed ledger is provided to every node to keep updated with modifications. Likewise, the shortfall of an outsider expands business agreeableness and trust [14, 15].

3.3 Immutability

The most vital attribute of BC is the capacity of ensuring the transactions' integrity by delivering unchanging records. In the case of the centralized model, the integrity of data is just overseen and safeguarded by the central authority, and this leads to a threat. On the other hand, the Blockchain utilizes collision-free hash estimations to connect every block to the preceding block which keeps up the respectability of the content of the block. Furthermore, blocks stored in the ledger are changeless, just if the greater part of the clients affirms that change.

3.4 High Security

Contrast to the existing solutions, BC innovation gives better security. Using the public key, BC gives a safe environment contrary to different sorts of attacks. Additionally, the consensus mechanism gives a reliable strategy that upgrades the security of the BC. Moreover, the shortfall of the single point of failure in the BC innovation gives higher security as compared to the centralized architecture [16, 17].

3.5 Anonymity

Regardless of BC using a record that is dispersed among all clients, BC gives an anonymous identity to secure the privacy of a node. This attribute can be used to give a protected and private democratic framework [18, 19].

3.6 Cost Decrease

As compared to a centralized model wherein the high level and complete equipment and programming framework is needed to assemble the centralized server, the BC innovation diminishes the costs identified with fitting and supporting enormous centralized servers as it uses the processing power of imparting gadgets [20].

3.7 Autonomy

The capacity to settle on self-ruling choices is amidst the highlights that Blockchain innovation can give. It permits the assembling of new gadgets that can make intelligent and self-sufficient choices [21]. For example, BC highlights including carefully designed and better security can be utilized to assemble better and secure independent vehicles.

4 Integration of IoT & Blockchain

Blockchain was initially utilized for monetary exchanges and digital currency where exchanges are executed and put away by every in the BC network. At that point, Blockchain is incorporated in different spaces because of the colossal advantages it gives [9, 22]. IoT framework is among these spaces. Joining Blockchain with IoT can give innumerable advantages to different IoT applications as shown in Fig. 4 [11–13, 23].

Here is the layered architecture, at the perception layer all the gadgets like sensors, actuators collect the data from the surroundings and pass it to the network layer. The network layer performs routing due to which all the devices that are joined together can interact across the internet. The third layer enables all the features associated with Blockchain. At last, the application layer which is the topmost layer provides the users with the features of data visualization and helps them to make appropriate decisions based on the gathered data.

Additionally, in this segment, we present a study on some use cases in which Blockchain is deployed with the IoT ecosystem.

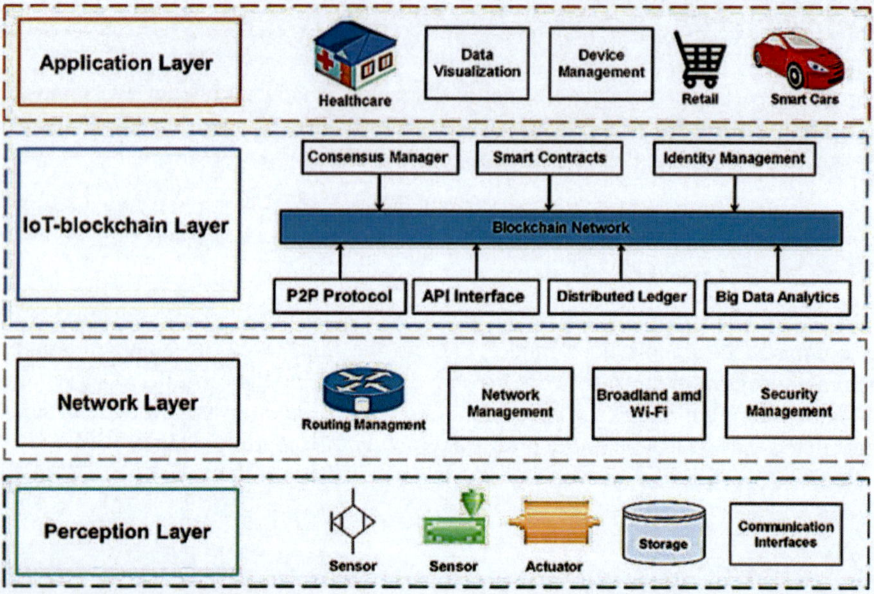

Fig. 4 Working of IoT with blockchain [21]

Oscar Novo addresses the scalability issue of overseeing access to a wide number of obliged gadgets in the IoT. Centralized frameworks come up short on the capacity to manage the increased load efficiently. The study presents another access management framework that resolves the problems related to dealing with various obliged IoT gadgets. The alternate is completely decentralized and dependent on BC innovation. Since most IoT gadgets are generally compelled to help BC innovation straightforwardly, the IoT gadgets in the proposed plan don't have a place with the BC network that makes the joining of the current IoT gadgets simpler to adjust to the proposed framework. The study gives a conventional, adaptable, and easily managed access control framework for IoT and implements a proof of concept (POC) model. All in all, the presented solution can adjust to different IoT situations affirming that Blockchain innovation can accept IoT innovation at its fullest [24].

Ali Dorri et al., design a lightweight BC-driven setup for IoT. This innovation essentially takes out the concerns of traditional BC, while keeping up the majority of its security and privacy advantages. IoT gadgets get an advantage from a private changeless log that acts like Blockchain yet is overseen centrally, to enhance energy utilization. The authors present a system that utilizes distributed trust to diminish the processing time of block validation. The methodology was investigated in a smart home [25].

Lei Hang and Do-Hyeun Kim proposed an incorporated IoT platform utilizing BC innovation to ensure observing data integrity. This designed framework aims to manage the cost of the gadget proprietor a useful application that gives an extensive, changeless record and permits easy access to their gadgets conveyed in various spaces. It likewise gives qualities of general IoT frameworks takes into account continuous checking, and control among the end client and gadget. The presented system is upheld by proof of idea execution in practical IoT situations, using Raspberry Pi gadgets and Hyperledger Fabric. The examination outcomes demonstrate that the fabricated setup is well-suited for the resource-constrained IoT setup and is versatile to be stretched out in different IoT situations [26].

Aafaf Ouaddah et al. demonstrate how BC can be appealing to confront various emerging difficulties. The authors present FairAccess that utilize the consistency of BC innovation to oversee access control for the benefit of obliged gadgets. In this study, the authors introduced another applicability space of BC that is access control through the FairAccess system. The proposed system uses the consistency provided by BC-based cryptocurrencies to tackle the issue of centralized and decentralized access control in IoT. In FairAccess, a straightforward and strong access control tool are provided [27].

Yunfa Li et al. consolidate the IoT with the BC, utilizing the benefits of BC decentralization, high dependability, and minimal cost to move and reserve image information of the users safely. Taking into account the security concerns, a secure transfer and stockpile option are proposed for detecting the image. First and foremost, this option brilliantly senses user image information, and partitions the detected information into intelligent blocks. Also, various blocks are encrypted and conveyed safely using encryption algorithms [28].

Jaspreet Kaur et al. created decentralized architecture utilized from Blockchain innovation combined with a centralized cloud setup which is client/servers setup with a basic BC at back end uphold with smart contract application. This architecture is implemented by the authors, and it was shown that how this design forestalls data misuse by utilizing the working of BC without any need to run a BC node by the IoT gadgets. For an end client experience, it will have all the earmarks of being the same as an ordinary web application and from the developer's point of view, the smart contract service will have equivalent software design to recent web applications along these lines permitting a simple change for both of centralized and decentralized techniques, while as yet holding the trust of decentralization [29].

5 Deployment of Blockchain with IoT

The implementation of BC in the IoT framework is certainly not a simple assignment. The initial and significant step is to pick the BC platform that will be embraced to blend the IoT with BC innovation [16]. Some well-recognized platforms can be used to implement the BC with IoT [10]. Table 1 shows the comparison of such platforms.

Table 1 Various platforms for blockchain

Platform	Type of blockchain	Smart contract	Consensus
Ethereum	Public and Permissioned	Yes	PoS
Hyperledger	Permissioned	Yes	PBTF
IOTA	-	Yes	-
Multichain	Permissioned	Yes	PBTF
Litecoin	Public	No	Scrypt
Lisk	Public and Permissioned	Yes	DPoS
HDAC	Permissioned	Yes	ePOW
Quorum	Permissioned	Yes	Multiple

5.1 Ethereum

This platform is used for BC, and it was reported in 2013. It creates an all-inclusive platform for different BC-driven applications. It was chiefly founded to implement smart contracts, preserved on the BC forever, and empower executing clients' requests. Even though Ethereum depends on smart contracts, the exchanges can keep various sorts of information.

This amplifies the probability for audibility and permits powerful extensions for different IoT services. The downside of this platform is that it requires somewhere in the range of 10 and 20 s to transfer a block. A few investigations used Ethereum to coordinate Blockchain with IoT [30].

5.2 Hyperledger

This platform is open-source, and it was intended to assist cross-industry BC innovations. It is overall open-source cooperation including pioneers from various ventures. It is a permission BC. However, most of the distributed records license opens deployment; this platform elevates and upgrades security to stay away from different kinds of attacks.

Before the usage of smart contracts in this platform is chiefly founded on chain-code usage, it gives quicker execution between peers in a few milliseconds. Along these lines, receiving chain-code smart contracts gives a powerful strategy to deploy BC in IoT services. Hyperledger fabric is among the most well-known and generally used structures.

5.3 IOTA

IOTA isn't treated as a BC platform as it principally relies upon Tangle, which is also a distributed ledger innovation. One can characterize this as a decentralized platform that encourages and measures different exchanges among interacting gadgets across the Internet. Essentially, IOTA executes an organized non-cyclic outline of transactions rather than chained blocks of various transactions. This gives a few advantages, for example, it gives a lightweight arrangement as the agreement doesn't need most interacting nodes to favor distinctive raised exchanges, instead, and two transactions can be checked by one node presenting an exchange themselves. This diminishes the exchange time and burden [21].

A few highlights of IOTA just as the utilization of facilitated non-cyclic graphs make the most versatile executions of a distributed log, forming it a productive alternative and platform for IoT services. Numerous scientists used IOTA to give a proficient platform to IoT services.

5.4 Multichain

Multichain permits the formation and implementation of private Blockchains. It utilizes an API, which scale-up the core of the actual Bitcoin API with new working, permitting the management of permissions, transactions, etc. Additionally, it gives a command-line tool to communicate with the network and various users that can communicate via JSON-RPC with the network such as Node.js, Java, C #, and Ruby.

5.5 Litecoin

This platform is technically similar to Bitcoin, yet provides quicker transaction confirmation times and enhanced storage capacity. It also provides the reduced generation time of a block and PoW. Moreover, the computational needs of Litecoin nodes are fewer, hence it is well-suited for IoT.

5.6 Lisk

It gives a platform that supports the concept of sub-blockchains that can be described with decentralized BC services and an option of cryptocurrencies to utilize. This platform also provides support to fabricate and implement decentralized services inside the platform used by the end clients directly. The services developed may utilize LSK currency or may produce custom tokens. This platform makes use of delegated proof of stake consensus.

5.7 *Quorum*

Quorum is fabricated to give the financial services industry permission implementation of Ethereum with support for transaction and contract privacy. It permits more than one consensus mechanism and attains data privacy via cryptography and segmentation. Quorum was being used by chronicled to build secure connections among physical assets and BC.

5.8 *HDAC*

This BC-based platform is an IoT contract and M2M transaction platform. The HDAC framework uses a mix of public and private Blockchains, and it assures security of these exchanges by using quantum random number generation. The HDAC cryptocurrency-enabled public BC can be proficiently utilized with multiple private Blockchains.

6 Conclusion

The study offers a remedy for IoT data security using Blockchain technology. Security challenges will continuously be increasing, so there is an urgent requirement for a decentralized and secure innovation to overcome these hurdles. Both IoT and Blockchain technology change ideas and make additional opportunities, each in their separate situations and it is possible to make applications that can possess the attributes of both. The BC innovation promises the security of data, and the intruder is not able to control or feed false data without breaking the chain. This paper also discusses the implementation of Blockchain with IoT. The study presented some use cases where both the technologies were integrated to preserve data integrity and privacy, and also discuss various platforms that provide a solution for various security breaches.

References

1. Husamuddin MD, Qayyum M (2017) Internet of things: a study on security and privacy threats. In: IEEE conference paper
2. Vignesh R, Samydurai A (2017) Security on the internet of things (IoT) with challenges and countermeasures. Int J Eng Develop Res 5(1):417–423
3. Lo'ai Tawalbeh et al (2020) IoT privacy and security: challenges and solutions. MDPI Appl Sci 10:4102
4. Jari Porras et al (2018) Security in the internet of things–a systematic mapping study. In: Proceedings of the 51st Hawaii international conference on system sciences, pp 3750–3759

5. Chandra U et al (2020) Internet of things (IoT) in agriculture. Inf Stud 7(2):32–36
6. Kaur R et al (2020) Internet of things: architecture, applications, and security concerns. J Comput Theor Nanosci 17:2469–2475
7. Kaur R (2020) Blockchain based technique for improving data security on IOT server platform. J Interdiscip Cycle Res XII(IV):334–344
8. Fernández-Caramés TM, Fraga-lamas P (2018) A review on the use of blockchain for the internet of things. IEEE Access 6:32979–33001
9. Kshetri N (2017) Can blockchain strengthen the internet of things? IEEE IT Prof (19)4:68–72,
10. Kumar M, Kumar P (2018) Blockchain technology for security issues and challenges in IoT. In: International conference on computational intelligence and data science, pp 1815–1823
11. Zheng Z et al (2017) An overview of blockchain technology: architecture, consensus, and future trends. In: IEEE 6th international congress on big data 2017, pp 558–564
12. Panarello A et al (2018) Blockchain, and IoT integration: a systematic survey. MDPI
13. Banerjee M et al (2018) A blockchain future for the internet of things security: a position paper. Digital CommunNetw 4:149–160
14. Reyna A et al (2018) On blockchain and its integration with IoT. Challenges and opportunities C. Future Gener Comput Syst 88:173–190 (Elsevier)
15. Sharma D et al (2020) Securing IOT communication using blockchain technology. Int J Adv Sci Technol 29(8):767–773
16. Pavithran D et al (2020) Towards building a blockchain framework for IoT, cluster computing. Springer Science+Business Media, LLC, part of Springer Nature 2020
17. Ahmad M et al (2018) IoT security: review, blockchain solutions, and open challenges. Elsevier Future Gener Comput Syst 82:395–411
18. WHunter G, Xu JC, Biaggi-Labiosa AM, Laskowski D, Dutta PK, Mondal SP, Ward BJ, Makel DB, Liu CC, Chang CW, Dweik RA (2011) Smart sensor systems for human health breath monitoring applications. J Breath Res 5:037111 (11pp)
19. Research article blockchain technology: is it a good candidate for securing IoT sensitive medical data? Article ID 9763937, Wiley Hindawi. Wireless Commun Mobile Comput 2018
20. Samaniego M et al (2016) Blockchain as a service for IoT cloud versus fog, In: IEEE international conference on internet of things and ieee green computing and communications and IEEE cyber, physical and social computing and IEEE smart data, pp 433–436
21. Atlam HF et al (2020) A review of blockchain in internet of things and AI, MDPI. Big Data Cogn Comput 4:28
22. Nguyen DC et al (2020) Integration of blockchain and cloud of things: architecture, applications, and challenges. IEEE Commun Surveys Tutor
23. Yaga D, Mell P, Roby N, Scrfone K (2018) Blockchain technology overview. National Institute of Standards and Technology Internal Report 8202
24. Novo O (2018) Blockchain meets IoT: an architecture for scalable access management in IoT. J Internet Things Class Files 14(8)
25. Dorri A et al (2017) Towards an optimized blockchain for IoT. In: IoTDI 2017, Pittsburgh, PA USA
26. Hang L, Kim D-H (2019) Design and implementation of an integrated IoT blockchain platform for sensing data integrity. MDPI Sensors 19:2228
27. Ouaddah A (2017) Towards a novel privacy-preserving access control model based on blockchain technology in IoT. Springer International Publishing, pp 523–533
28. Li Y et al (2020) A security transmission and storage solution about sensing image for blockchain in the internet of things. MDPI Sensors 20:916
29. Kaur J et al (2020) A blockchain-based solution for securing data of IoT devices. In: Yangui S et al (eds) ICSOC 2019 Workshops, LNCS 12019. Springer Nature Switzerland AG, pp 122–129
30. Xiang W, Atkinson I (2017) Internet of things for smart healthcare: technologies, challenges, and opportunities. IEEE Access

Advanced Approach Using Deep Learning for Healthcare Data Analysis in IOT System

Shaweta Sachdeva and Aleem Ali

Abstract A massive number of IOT devices creates a difficult volume of details. Cloud-based IOT computing approaches suffer from high and unpredictable network latency, leading to minimal expertise with real-time IOT deployment, such as healthcare. The data inference in edge computing starts from the data source to fix this issue (i.e., the IOT devices). Limited computational capabilities of the IOT device and power-hungry data transmission include an on-board processing-offload balance. The inference of IOT information, therefore calls for effective, lightweight techniques suited to this compromise and to confirm with limited resources in IOT devices such as wearables. A lightweight classifier performs directly on the IOT system in the first layer and determines whether to download or conduct the computer to the gateway. The second layer contains a lightweight IOT interface classifier (can identify a subset of groups only) and a complex gateway classifier (to distinguish the remaining classes). We introduced an advanced approach to utilizing deep knowledge for IOT Environmental Healthcare Data Review. The experimental findings (by utilizing a real-world data collection for the monitoring of human behaviors on a wearable IOT device) indicate greater precision (98% on average) or (90% on average).

Keywords Deep learning · CNN · Healthcare

1 Introduction

The rapid growth of wearable and smart phone apps has facilitated the use of IOT (Internet of Things) medical services. Monitoring human activities in real-time, in particular in activities of daily living, i.e., ADL, is a significant smart health challenge that facilitates patient healing and cares by the use of wearable or mobile sensors. As a result, the identification of personal interactions in human activity recognition (HAR) has become a problem to examine such that daily behaviors and relationships

S. Sachdeva (✉) · A. Ali
Department of CSE, Glocal University, Saharanpur, U.P, India

N. Marriwala et al. (eds.), *Emergent Converging Technologies and Biomedical Systems*, Lecture Notes in Electrical Engineering 841,
https://doi.org/10.1007/978-981-16-8774-7_14

between individuals, and their living environments are properly known and widely examined for the IOHT [1]. Various types of wearable sensors can be placed at different positions (e.g., head, forehead, upper arm, forearm, shine, etc.) to collect and relay real-time posture data (e.g., accelerometers and gyroscopes) using WSN [2].

Sensor technology provides possibilities for increasing multimodal information sensing and HAR fusion, which will allow the development of shuman-centered applications and services in cyber-physical-social networks in real-time Big Data [3, 4]. Since mobility data can easily be collected from wearable and mobile inertial sensors based on the physical movement of individuals, smart devices are widely used to identify, perceive and recognize the location of a person in several applications and systems [5, 6]. In HAR, however, the sensor data still poses many difficulties. For example, conventional machine learning approaches rely primarily on the availability of training data, which implies the extraction of features depends largely on a sufficiently labeled and well-determined data set [7, 8].

However, ADL data is continuously produced by the integrated sensor of intelligent devices, irrespective of whether people take sensitive action which results in an intensive laboratory phase in which well-labeled data are annotated and registered. Such wearable sensor data, namely a large number of unlisted data are combined a limited portion of classified data can be identified as motion data [9, 10] which are weakly labeled. A modern semi-monitored learning or weakly controlled learning system is required to cope effectively with such scenarios. To cope effectively with such a situation, it is necessary to create a new semi-supervised learning method or a weakly regulated learning system.

The signal from the on-body sensors is up to their position. Even for the same person, various positions of body sensors may create different patterns of motion. Exists can discern coarse-grain patterns by repetitive actions static activities (e.g., standing and standing) or simple transformations (e.g., standing and sitting) that are relatively consistent but face difficulties in identifying certain complex patterns with single-sensor data.

Sensor data obtained from multiple wearable devices, such as accelerometer, GPS, lighting, camera, etc., can be synchronized and optimized to capture more nuanced human behavior patterns from a multimodal and multi-positional point of view via a consolidated data fusion strategy. Besides, several subjects can create distinct motion patterns for the same form of action utilizing the same on-body sensors. For example, an elderly person and a child's falling trend can be entirely different. By contrast, traditional techniques for the extraction of HAR can only discern low-level features that could be necessary to identify fundamental physical or postural behaviors. However, without taking into consideration certain context-conscious or localizing challenges, it will be a struggle to grasp more relevant activities with semantic awareness, such as jogging, cooking, etc. It is also important to find an appropriate way to exploit high-level characteristics in a given context; this may help to distinguish patterns in human actions, gestures and representations of fine grain as shown in Fig. 1.

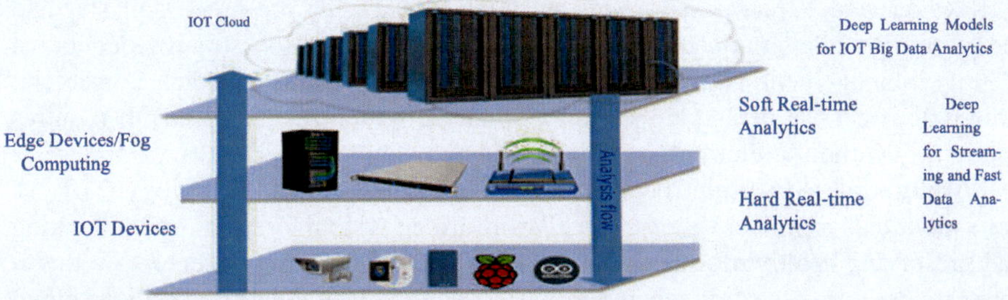

Fig.1 IOT data generation at different levels and deep learning models to address their knowledge abstraction

2 Related Works

Djenna et al. [1] proposed IOT-based healthcare has several security problems which, due to the dynamics of the environment and the nature of its goods, vary in methodologies, motivations and consequences. This paper outlines the latest IOT-based safety concerns. In summary, we discuss the likely threats and vulnerabilities and include a new description of cyber assaults that could have an effect on their protection at work.

Suguna et al. [2], proposed research contains surveys of cloud and IOT classification methods and diagnostic approaches to health data obtained by any register or sensor that collects and preserves real-time data in tablets to reflect the nature of the disease by any expert.

Subasi et al. [3], proposed the model that utilizes a data collection comprising body function records and vital signs with 10 subjects with different profiles while performing 12 functional activities to classify human behavior. The results show that the approach is extremely efficient, reliable and consistent in delivering m-Health-Services with 99.89 percent precision across different actions.

Panda et al. [4] proposed the results suggest that the Random forest, Decision Tree and Naive Bayes are appropriately classified. However, the model ranks for the deployment duration are Naive Bayes, Decision Tree and Random Woodland. The classifier concerned must be selected to be used in industrial environments based on IOT, depending on the parameters.

Bhoi et al. [5] concluded that the KNN senses are falling more consistently and that this is part of the classification process. When a fall happens, an alert message will be sent to the registered phone number via the Python module.

Ganesan et al. [6] define actual patient identification knowledge is used in the testing method to assess the nature of a disease. To be experimental, a reference data collection is analyzed using a number of classifiers, i.e., J48: Logistic Regression (LR) and (SVM). Simulation results have ensured superior performance for different parameters in the J48 classifiers, such as precision, reminder, F-score and kappa scores.

Ilavarasi et al. [7] proposed the results of the SMOTE-TL pre-processing step and the learning models indicate strong synergy. A decomposition strategy-dependent identity management algorithm is suggested for the class imbalance problem. This will affect the healthcare industry, where a written record of health requires anonymity without compromising the results of machine learning.

Miškuf et al. [8] define Cooperation between Operational Technology (OT), IT and individuals promotes the creation of an informed system for monitoring, tracking and preserving health information for patients in the ongoing care sector. We therefore propose our case study where we have captured hospital data and utilized cloud technologies for data processing and machine learning. We then designed a web application at the top of this concept and checked the project in the modern environment of the hospital.

Shinde et al. [9] proposed Random Forest (RF) and Latent Dirichlet Allocation (LDA) a few algorithms are introduced in the R module for more tangible results. The author conducted case studies to illustrate the realistic demonstration of the idea by assessing the fertility-related big data and constructing a mathematical model to better estimate these possibilities.

Yang et al. [10] proposed a rigorous safety analysis and detailed simulations of various main lengths and number of features and levels suggest that our scheme would significantly minimize overhead on IOT devices in the application of computer classifications.

3 Proposed Methodology

The introduction of Internet of Things (IOT) technology has modified conventional healthcare systems and many different applications are used for tracking. In comparison, the personalized wellness and disease reduction programs, the information obtained from the lifestyle component and behaviors research is largely based on the technique. Using smart data recovery and classification models, infections can be examined or abnormal health conditions can also be predicted. The Convolutionary Neural Network (CNN) model is used to replicate such abnormalities and may accurately diagnose disease prediction knowledge from record of medical is unstructured [11]. However, since CNN uses a fully connected network system, a lot of memory is used. In addition, the rise in the amount of layers would increase the difficulty analysis of the model. Consequently, in order to address these CNN model shortcomings, coefficient of Pearson correlation and normal behavior Model focused [12, 13] on the CNN-regular form of object detection and identification, in which the word "regular" denotes artifacts that are commonly seen and low-heterogeneity structures. In this context, we are developing a regular CNN data classification model for pattern discovery [14].

The primary health variables are selected in the first hidden layer and the study of related correlation coefficient is conducted in the second layer in order to differentiate between favorable and negative health influences [15]. In addition, repeated

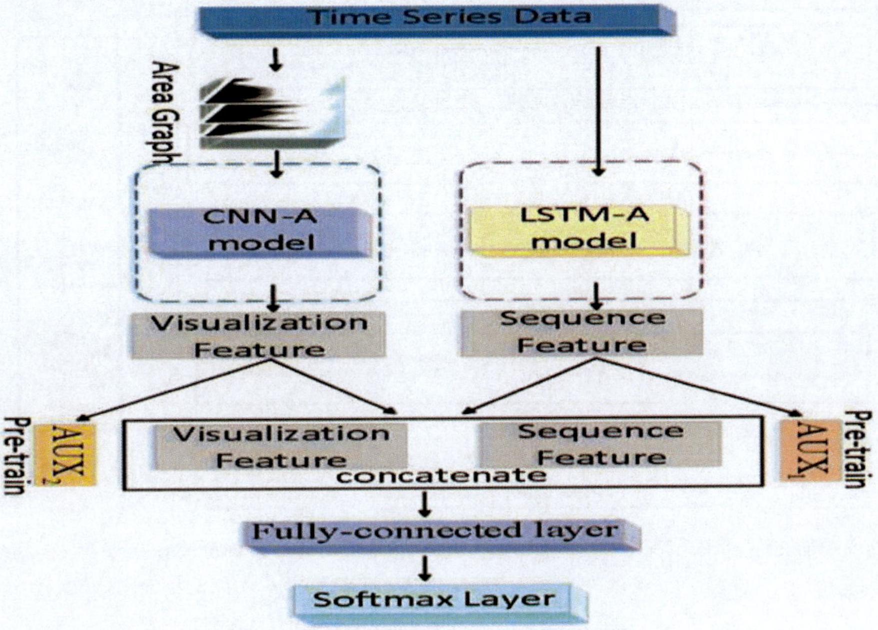

Fig. 2 Training and testing approach using deep learning based on CNN

behavioral patterns are defined by disrupting the daily pattern of classified health variables. Two different data sets are applied to address the implications of CNN's Model conventional exploration of information as shown in Fig. 2. Experimental data suggest that the model proposed in comparison with the three different learning models is more reliable and has a low computational load, which demonstrate the fundamental workflow of multiple organizations in a fog-dependent smart home environment. In the Intelligent Communication Mechanism [16, 17], the fog layer can collect the necessary data from the cloud layer on patient health information.

In conventional communication, fog-related warnings are conveyed to the cloud along with the information of patient for further potential action [18]. The platform used is a sensor network with the abilities of recording patient-oriented events effectively by combining numerous IOT devices, sensors and other internet-based hardware [19]. The aim of presented model is to observe the patients in need of intensive remote care through the fog-centric IOT technology as shown in Fig. 3 [20]. The fog layer contains nebulae at the edge of the network. In addition, fog features such as virtual services, accessibility support and scalability are ideal in an IOT-based health surveillance environment [21].

CNN based model various characteristics that affect diabetes and high pressure are studied for model efficacy studies. The set of health parameters are based on an attributes combination and correspondence coefficients are calculated of each attribute and achieve a coefficient of correspondence of 0.5 or higher. As a consequence, key characteristics are chosen for obesity, and the prediction of high blood

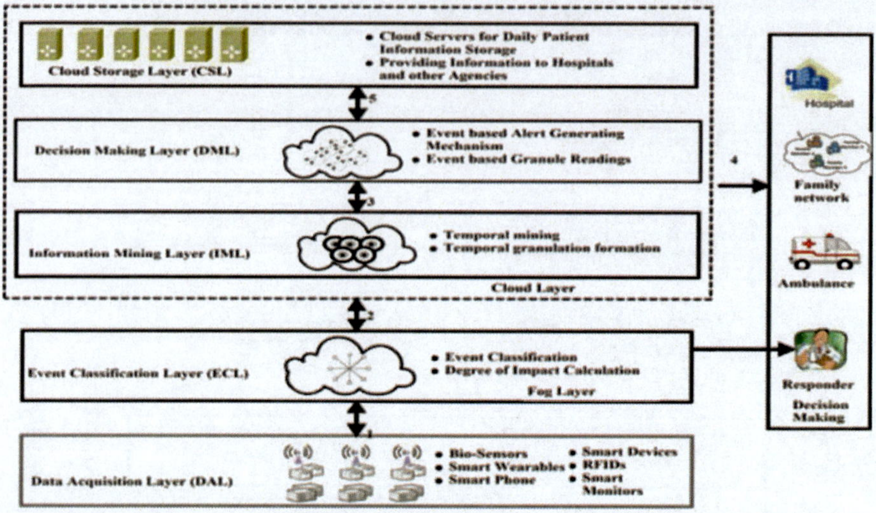

Fig. 3 Working of deep learning for healthcare data analysis in IOT environment

pressure. In addition, the relations between the selected characteristics are calculated and result differentiates in positive and negative relations. Correlated variables can help to better observe daily life these effects Regulation of the values of the negative related parameters may also predict an abnormality. CNN is used to separate them.

The experiment was performed on a 64-bit Core i5 processor with Windows 10 pro and 12 GB free RAM, SPSS [22]. The data presented to the Inspection Survey are used to research the proposed approach [23]. Context data include fitness metrics and some basic features. They give the results of 10,806 real-time health checks carried out by residents. Multivariate regression in SPSS is used to derive health-relevant variables that help to decrease numerical complexity [24] and efficiently diminish the number of characteristics without affecting the important values. Various characteristics that affect model obesity, elevated blood pressure and diabetes were investigated [25] efficiency studies.

The group of parameters related to health is based on the combination of characteristics and the calculated coefficient of correspondence of each characteristic and achieves a coefficient of correspondence of 0.5 or higher. As a consequence, the main traits for obesity, increased blood pressure and diabetes estimates are first selected [26]. In addition, the association between the chosen characteristics is determined and observed in positive and negative links. Identifying positively correlated variables can help for better daily life by monitoring these important positive effects. The monitoring of negative parameter values will also detect some anomalies [27, 28]. CNN technique is used to separate them easily. Regular factor activity is also evaluated to classify any external variables within the related factors that are chosen. The features of the parameter are measured as obesity, increased blood pressure and diabetes. This suggests which features are of a normal or irregular relationship

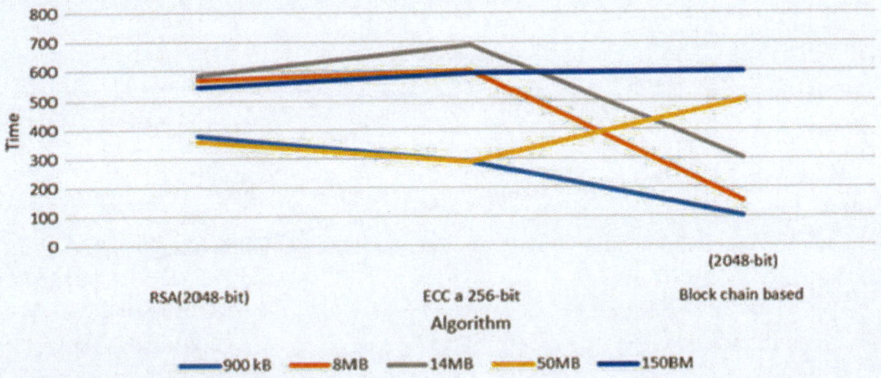

Fig. 4 Encryption time evaluation

[29]. It would dramatically improve wellness by increasing consciousness of obesity, elevated blood pressure and diabetes conditions and their origins when they emerge.

This study provides an algorithm for CNN based on the identification, reference and regular behavior of related health care parameters for three different diseases. Our model demonstrated its comparative research utility in 4,759,777 medical papers by using some of the knowledge from regular correlated algorithms. It also provides a comparison of the model's performance. Diagnosis precision and reference of our model are 80.43 percent; 80.85 percent; 91.49 percent; 82.61 percent; 95.60 percent with results from testing, respectively, based on LSTM model [30].To perform the simulation using python (compare the different algorithm, RSA, ECC, Blockchain).

This demonstrated that the data obtained after pre-processing is beneficial and removing only irrelevant data. The model often represents the potential precision of other traditional learning systems. Data mining and interpretation of medical evidence are also important for researching and diagnosing medical diseases and conditions [31]. The model we proposed would take advantage of the data obtained to demonstrate easy, reliable results for obesity, hypertension and diabetes as measured in form of Encryption time evaluation graph as shown in Fig. 4 and Decryption time evaluation graph as shown in Fig. 5.

4 Conclusion

Significant treatment options in the world of large medical data are supposed to help people retain their health status. This paper offers a CNN-based paradigm for daily exploration of health knowledge. The status of health research approach uses the wellbeing and behavioral patterns of chronic diseases introduced by IOT applications. A double-layer entirely connected in CNN architecture is used to pick and to identify the data which is collected for the process. Multivariate analysis continues with the recognition of core health variables. The description of these variables is then

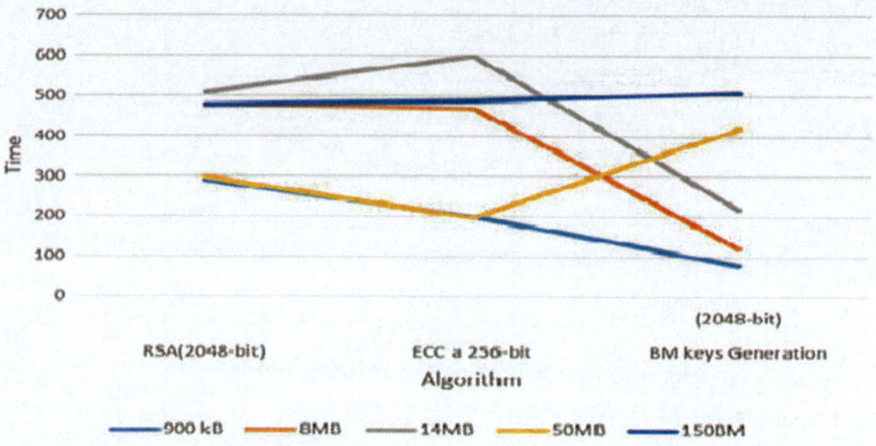

Fig. 5 Decryption time evaluation

performed in the second document. The main variable of the classified is assessed, and the main regular health items are picked. The model should recognize either the typical positive correlated factors that can be maintained in health care or negative factor as the usual factor that offer evidence to alter unhealthy lifestyles and activities in daily life. With respect to the effectiveness of the suggested model, this provides details relating to routinely correlated to the obesity and high pressure and diabetes wellbeing criteria. There are many type of illness will need further research and further vital proof of data gathered for future work. Thus, a variety of raw data are used for pre-processing methods to maintain the accuracy and reliability of the CNN learning model.

References

1. Djenna A, Saïdouni DE (2018) Cyber attacks classification in IOT-Based-healthcare infrastructure. In: 2nd cyber security in networking conference (CSNet). Paris, pp 1–4. https://doi.org/10.1109/CSNET.2018.8602974
2. Suguna M, Ramalakshmi MG, Cynthia J, Prakash D (2018) A survey on cloud and internet of things based healthcare diagnosis. In: 2018 4th international conference on computing communication and automation (ICCCA), Greater Noida, India, pp 1–4. https://doi.org/10.1109/CCAA.2018.8777606
3. Subasi A, Radhwan M, Kurdi R, Khateeb K (2018) IOT based mobile healthcare system for human activity recognition. In: 15th learning and technology conference (L&T). Jeddah, pp 29–34. https://doi.org/10.1109/LT.2018.8368507
4. Panda S, Panda G (2020) Intelligent classification of IOT traffic in healthcare using machine learning techniques. In: 2020 6th international conference on control, automation and robotics (ICCAR), Singapore, pp 581–585. https://doi.org/10.1109/ICCAR49639.2020.9107979
5. Bhoi SK et al (2018) FallDS-IOT: a fall detection system for elderly healthcare based on IOT data analytics. In: 2018 International conference on information technology (ICIT), Bhubaneswar, India, pp 155–160. https://doi.org/10.1109/ICIT.2018.00041

6. Ganesan M, Sivakumar N (2019) IOT based heart disease prediction and diagnosis model for healthcare using machine learning models. In: 2019 IEEE international conference on system, computation, automation and networking (ICSCAN), Pondicherry, India, pp 1–5. https://doi.org/10.1109/ICSCAN.2019.8878850
7. Ilavarasi AK (2020) Class imbalance learning for Identity Management in Healthcare. In: 2020 Fourth international conference on I-SMAC (IOT in Social, Mobile, Analytics and Cloud) (I-SMAC), Palladam, India, pp 995–1000, doi: https://doi.org/10.1109/I-SMAC49090.2020.9243420
8. Miškuf M, Zolotová I, Mocnej J (2018) Healthcare data classification—Cloud-based architecture concept, cybernetics & Informatics (K&I). Lazy pod Makytou:1–6. https://doi.org/10.1109/CYBERI.2018.8337557
9. Shinde PP, Oza KS, Kamat RK (2017) Big data predictive analysis: using R analytical tool. In: 2017 international conference on I-SMAC (IOT in Social, Mobile, Analytics and Cloud) (I-SMAC), Palladam, pp 839–842. https://doi.org/10.1109/I-SMAC.2017.8058297
10. Yang L, Li F (2018) Cloud-assisted privacy-preserving classification for IOT applications. In: 2018 IEEE conference on communications and network security (CNS), Beijing, pp 1–9. https://doi.org/10.1109/CNS.2018.8433157
11. Singh Rajawat A, Jain S (2020) Fusion deep learning based on back propagation neural network for personalization. In: 2nd international conference on data, engineering and applications (IDEA), Bhopal, India, pp 1–7. https://doi.org/10.1109/IDEA49133.2020.9170693
12. Biswas R, Pal S, Sarkar B, Chakrabarty A (2020) Health-care paradigm and classification in IOT ecosystem using big data analytics: an analytical survey. In: Solanki V, Hoang M, Lu Z, Pattnaik P (Eds) Intelligent computing in engineering. Advances in Intelligent Systems and Computing, vol 1125. Springer, Singapore. https://doi.org/10.1007/978-981-15-2780-7_30
13. Amin M, Shehwar D, Ullah A et al (2020) A deep learning system for health care IOT and smartphone malware detection. Neural Comput Appli. https://doi.org/10.1007/s00521-020-05429-x
14. Rajawat AS, Upadhyay AR (2020) Web personalization model using modified S3VM algorithm for developing recommendation process. In: 2nd international conference on data, engineering and applications (IDEA), Bhopal, India, pp 1–6. https://doi.org/10.1109/IDEA49133.2020.9170701
15. Philip JM, Durga S, Esther D (2021) Deep learning application in IOT health care: a survey. In: Peter J, Fernandes S, Alavi A (Eds) Intelligence in big data technologies—beyond the hype. Advances in Intelligent Systems and Computing, vol 1167. Springer, Singapore. https://doi.org/10.1007/978-981-15-5285-4_19
16. Zamanifar A (2021) Remote patient monitoring: health status detection and prediction in IOT-based health care. In: Marques G, Bhoi AK, Albuquerque VHC, KSH (eds) IOT in healthcare and ambient assisted living. Studies in Computational Intelligence, vol 933. Springer, Singapore. https://doi.org/10.1007/978-981-15-9897-5_5
17. Ahmadi H, Arji G, Shahmoradi L et al (2019) The application of internet of things in healthcare: a systematic literature review and classification. Univ Access Inf Soc 18:837–869. https://doi.org/10.1007/s10209-018-0618-4
18. Vyas T, Desai S, Ruparelia A (2020) Fog data processing and analytics for health care-based IOT applications. In: Tanwar S (eds) Fog data analytics for IOT applications. Studies in Big Data, vol 76. Springer, Singapore. https://doi.org/10.1007/978-981-15-6044-6_18
19. Mukherjee D, Paulson A, Varghese S, Nivelkar M (2020) SNAP N' COOK—IOT-based recipe suggestion and health care application. In: Pant M, Kumar Sharma T, Arya R, Sahana B, Zolfagharinia H (eds) Soft computing: theories and applications. Advances in Intelligent Systems and Computing, vol 1154. Springer, Singapore. https://doi.org/10.1007/978-981-15-4032-5_65
20. Chatterjee J, Das MK, Ghosh S, Das A, Bag R (2021) A review on security and privacy concern in IOT health care. In: Chakraborty C, Banerjee A, Kolekar M, Garg L, Chakraborty B (eds) Internet of things for healthcare technologies. Studies in Big Data, vol 73. Springer, Singapore. https://doi.org/10.1007/978-981-15-4112-4_12

21. Vaishnavi S, Sethukarasi T (2020) SybilWatch: a novel approach to detect Sybil attack in IOT based smart health care. J Ambient Intell Human Comput. https://doi.org/10.1007/s12652-020-02189-3
22. Mani JJS, Rani Kasireddy S (2019) Population classification upon dietary data using machine learning techniques with IOT and big data. In: Social network forensics, cyber security, and machine learning. SpringerBriefs in Applied Sciences and Technology. Springer, Singapore. https://doi.org/10.1007/978-981-13-1456-8_2
23. Rastogi R, Singhal P, Chaturvedi DK, Gupta M (2021) Investigating correlation of tension-type headache and diabetes: IOT perspective in health care. In: Chakraborty C, Banerjee A, Kolekar M, Garg L, Chakraborty B (eds) Internet of things for healthcare technologies. Studies in Big Data, vol 73. Springer, Singapore. https://doi.org/10.1007/978-981-15-4112-4_4
24. Puthal D, Ranjan R, Chen J (2019) Big data stream security classification for IOT applications. In: Sakr S, Zomaya AY (eds) Encyclopedia of big data technologies. Springer, Cham. https://doi.org/10.1007/978-3-319-77525-8_236
25. Puthal D, Ranjan R, Chen J (2018) Big data stream security classification for IOT applications. In: Sakr S, Zomaya A (eds) Encyclopedia of big data technologies. Springer, Cham. https://doi.org/10.1007/978-3-319-63962-8_236-1
26. Pandey P, Pandey SC, Kumar U (2020) Security issues of internet of things in health-care sector: an analytical approach. In: Verma O, Roy S, Pandey S, Mittal M (eds) Advancement of machine intelligence in interactive medical image analysis. Algorithms for Intelligent Systems. Springer, Singapore. https://doi.org/10.1007/978-981-15-1100-4_15
27. Sharma D, Jinwala D (2015) Functional encryption in IOT E-health care system. In: Jajoda S, Mazumdar C (eds) Information systems Security (ICISS 2015). Lecture Notes in Computer Science, vol 9478. Springer, Cham. https://doi.org/10.1007/978-3-319-26961-0_21
28. Hsueh PYS, Hu X, Cheung YK, Wolff D, Marschollek M, Rogers J (2020) Smart learning using big and small data for mobile and IOT e-Health. In: Firouzi F, Chakrabarty K, Nassif S (eds) Intelligent internet of things. Springer, Cham. https://doi.org/10.1007/978-3-030-30367-9_13
29. Syed L, Jabeen S, Manimala S, Elsayed HA (2019) Data science algorithms and techniques for smart healthcare using IOT and big data analytics. In: Mishra M, Mishra B, Patel Y, Misra R (eds) Smart techniques for a smarter planet. Studies in Fuzziness and Soft Computing, vol 374. Springer, Cham. https://doi.org/10.1007/978-3-030-03131-2_11
30. Onasanya A, Elshakankiri M (2019) Smart integrated IOT healthcare system for cancer care. Wireless Netw. https://doi.org/10.1007/s11276-018-01932-1
31. Sujatha R, Nathiya S, Chatterjee JM (2020) Clinical data analysis using IOT data analytics platforms. In: Raj P, Chatterjee J, Kumar A, Balamurugan B (eds) Internet of things use cases for the healthcare industry. Springer, Cham. https://doi.org/10.1007/978-3-030-37526-3_12

An Integration of AI, Blockchain and IoT Technologies for Combating Covid-19

K. Ashok Kumar, Vanga Karunakar Reddy, and A. Narmada

Abstract An entire world is facing epidemic from past one year due to Covid-19. With effect this, lot of countries and lot of states are collapsed their economic and also mainly common man suffers during lockdown. One of main reasons to get vaccination and drug delayed is variable characteristics of Covid-19 from individual to individual hence, it difficult to finalize characteristics and symptoms. Recently, there are huge research going on Covid-19 and presenting various directions to prepare vaccine and drug. This paper presents novel platform such as integrated IoT based AI with Blockchain technology to combat Covid-19. AI discusses with required ML and DL algorithms for prediction and analyzes data of Covid-19. This paper also directs new direction to prepare vaccine and drug based on AI hence updating and storing data of infected individuals automatically.

Keywords Covid-19 · AI · IoT · Blockchain · Vaccine · Integrated technology

1 Introduction

Corona virus disease-2019 (Covid-19) is spreading rapidly to entire globe from infected human beings. According to World Health Organization (WHO), total number of confirmed cases is 6,194,533 effected to 216 countries throughout the world by June 02, 2020 hence total number of deaths is 376,320 which is approximately 6.07%. The Covid-19 is mainly caused by Severe Acute Respiratory Syndrome (SARS) virus and rapid spreading results the global pandemic approximately four months. Main characteristics Covid-19 are identified from huge cases that are fever, pneumonia, respiratory problems, reduced count of lymphocyte and also decreased white blood cells (WBC) count in human body. In the absence of a vaccination, social distance is only solution which is widely adopted throughout world to suppress the spreading of virus as it is confirmed that the virus transmitted through human–human. An early detection is another acceptable solution to avoid spreading

K. Ashok Kumar (✉) · V. Karunakar Reddy · A. Narmada
Matrusri Engineering College, Saidabad, Hyderabad, Telangana, India

N. Marriwala et al. (eds.), *Emergent Converging Technologies and Biomedical Systems*, Lecture Notes in Electrical Engineering 841,
https://doi.org/10.1007/978-981-16-8774-7_15

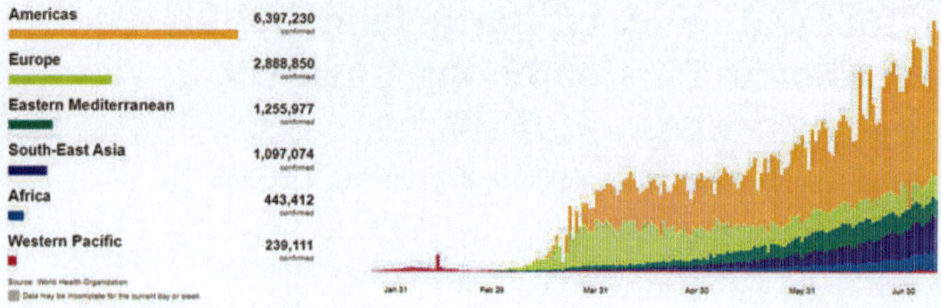

Fig. 1 The statistics of Corona virus region-wise (*source* WHO)

because of the virus is contagious nature. A reverse transcription polymerase chain reaction (RT-PCR) used golden standard for the diagnosis of Covid-19. However, RT-PCR has adequate, very limited supply and great delay in requirements of laboratory thereby posing unprecedented overheads for preventing the spread of virus especially at center of epidemic places. This is because of many factors like sample collection and its quality control whereas image accessing is easy in clinical practices such X-ray, Computed Tomography (CT) scan to clinicians in terms of assistance.

An exact source of virus is unknown and scientists are mapped genome of sequence of corona virus thereby identifying bats are the main source for Covid-19. The first human affected and reported from Wuhan city of china in December 2019, and then it is spreading massively throughout the world. As per WHO, approximately 213 countries and union territories are affected by Corona virus. Figure 1 shows statistics of Corona virus effected regions as per the WHO. Americans are the most effected region among all the regions and the maximum confirmed positive cases are reached to 6,397,230 till June 30.

The rapid increase in number of Corona cases throughout the world indicates that an immediate requirement of the vaccine or safety which leads to Covid-19 outbreak. The outbreak was linked to seafood and other animals in wholesale market of Wuhan. A β-Corona virus, SARS-CoV-2 is deemed responsible for outbreak of Covid-19. The characteristics of Corona virus is extremely contagious nature and proportionally long in period (1–14). A person may be infected in this period but it will not show any symptoms hence infected people spread carriers of virus unknowingly. The Covid-19 exhibits symptoms majorly fever, dry cough, sputum production and fatigue. In addition to this, headache, sore throat, breathlessness and myalgia are also shoed rarely in some infected humans. Table 1 shows symptoms of Covid-19 from much infected patients.

The remaining part of paper is as follows: Section-II presents related work and section-III propounded novel methodology to predict of Corona virus. Section-IV presents approximated results, and section-V concludes paper.

Table 1 List of basic symptoms (*source* WHO)

Most common symptoms	
Fever	88%
Dry Cough	67%
Fatigue	38%
Sputum Production	34%
Less Symptoms	
Shortness breath	19%
myalgia	15%
sore throat	14%
Headache	13.5%
Chills	11%

2 Related Work

An outbreak of Covid-19 prompted different researchers, scientists, scientists and organizations throughout the world to do research for developing vaccination and also treatment for Corona virus. As per WHO, the cause of most of the viral diseases is different viruses such as Corona virus and then severe effect on public health. In most recent, the Corona virus indicates danger bells to mankind because of change in symptoms periodically. As spherical range of corona virus is approximately 600 Å to 1400 Å, the best way of avoid Covid-19 is to wear mask and wash hands frequently. The various form SARS-COV and Middle East Respiratory Syndrome Corona virus (MERS-COV) witnessed for past two decades [1]. The first case of MARS-COV is found in Saudi Arabia and then spread large scale thereby resulting outbreak in Middle Eastern countries [2]. To identify characteristics of Corona virus, Wang et al. [3] analyzed and presented approximately 140 patients from Wuhan city, China. They considered medical history such as symptoms, signs, and demographics to determine clinical characteristics and effect on different organs of the patient body. Chen et al. [4] reviewed data of 100 patients and among 50 infected people are had direct effect from seafood market, Wuhan. They have investigated radiological, epidemiological and clinical characteristics and then reported 17% of patients developed acute respiratory distress syndrome (ARDS). They found approximately 11% of infected patients are died with multiple organ dysfunction syndrome (MODS). Jiang et al. [5] studied 6 published manuscripts on primary characteristics of Corona virus and also summarized findings overview of corona virus features and probable treatment for Covid-19. They have reviewed on CT scan features on Covid-19. Patel [6] focused on antimicrobial paper for combating bacteria and viruses which is very effective to arrest spread and dead novel corona virus. The difference of SARS-COV1 and SARS-COV2 is identified initially there after discussed survival period of SARS-COV2. There are two types of categories of paper production that are first category is antimicrobial paper with long lasting function and antimicrobial paper with short period. Another category of paper is ag- ion based microbial paper. Patel

Table 2 Simulated results [7] of deep learning model

S.No	Parameters	Specification
1	Accuracy	0.982
2	Sensitivity	0.976
3	Specificity	0.988

also proposed antibacterial nano particles which are integrated with minerals such as montmorillonite or pigments used as coating. Antimicrobial papers are effective to stop spreading corona virus on different surfaces (Table 2).

With reference of above literature, identification and restricting of spreading novel corona are prime concern of outbreak. Most of the literature is concentrating on techniques for identification of corona. Still, no one presents standard method to identify and treatment. Hence, this paper tries to direct unique technology for experimenting and producing standard medicine of novel corona virus.

3 Novel Methodology

Human being is the most intelligent creatures in the universe. The intelligence is integrated to any machine artificially known as artificial intelligence (AI). The intelligence is embedded into machine through computer programming hence it activates the senses like learn, think and applying intelligence similar to human beings. If the machine programmed properly, AI system produces incredible results in terms of accuracy and precision after experimenting at different conditions. AI primarily needed computational power to obtain intelligence from basic information. Initially, AI is broad area which is combined with machine learning later on it is combined with deep learning.

i. **Integration of AI with IoT**

In the modern age, there are lots of sources to generate massive data such as social media, search engines and e-commerce, etc. This generated data from sources is in the form of unstructured or raw data in the primary stage, and it requires huge time to sort this massive data. To solve this complex work, deep learning algorithms are used in AI. The word deep learning is known driving number of hidden layers in the processing of a problem. The deep learning utilizes supervised data through parallel processing mechanism. Machine learning algorithms are used to collect data thereafter trained from gathered data, and hence correctly predicted. Most of the algorithms are based on different approaches such as cluster learning, tree learning and Bayesian networks and so on. Computer vision is the best area for machine learning algorithm to obtain the objectives of AI. This technique targets to involve computer to interface real world and also able to understand time dependent conditions. The computer vision is mainly working based on digital image processing, signal processing and deep learning algorithms thereby identifying and classifying

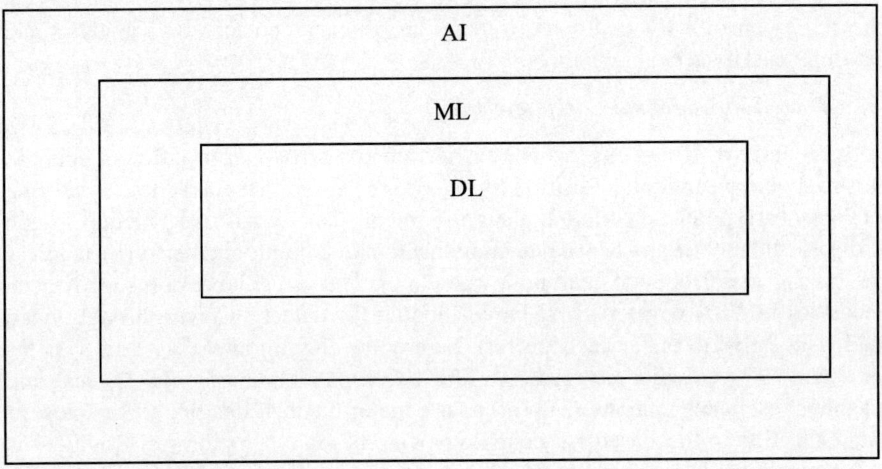

Fig. 2 Concept of AI, ML and DL technologies

of the objects to react accurately as similar as human. It is primarily requires certain algorithms of edge detection and filter circuit to detect shape and movement of object. Figure 2 depicts an idea for concepts of AI, ML and DL technologies.

The broad term of AI includes combination of machine learning (ML) and deep learning (DL) technologies and also fundamental requirement to adopt real-time conditions. There is a huge research going on this domain to analyze data and predict accurately. There are many complex attributes to predict accurately such as black-box strategy. IoT is another new strategy using in AI to process attributes and provide accurate results. AI-IoT based devices are interacted and communicated each other full duplex manner. The integrated technology of AI-IoT is structured transmitter, receiver and wireless sensor networks to explore high performance for future applications. Hence, integrated IoT based AI technology is the leading when compared to traditional techniques. Still, this technology needs huge amount of data to predict accurately.

ii. AI used in Covid-19

As IoT based AI technology is major technology in the present situation such as Alexa, Cortana, Siri and Google-Assistant from the companies of Amazon, Microsoft, Apple and Google, respectively. This pandemic situation occurred Covid-19 leads to outbreak in entire world. The IoT based AI technology plays major role in contagious disease such as treatment and prediction. Hence, contribution of this technology is begun in terms of combating Covid-19 disease. To reduce spreading of Corona virus, lockdown is used as one of best options entire worldwide. IoT based AI is the alternative method for Lockdown as face recognition through thermal cameras, cameras and also thermal screening at crowded places. Various steps are involved for combating covid-19 with AI technology that are data collection and early detection, observing behavior for treatment, tracing out primary contacts, data analysis and development of vaccine and drugs.

(a) *Data Collection and Early detection*

In the country of Hongkong, whenever new person arrives from different country, person should wear Global Position System (GPS) based bracelet hence monitoring movement at quarantine period. India is also tracing Corona positive patients through ArogyaSethu mobile app hence detecting location of patients and performs action as per Law in case disobey of quarantine guidelines. The surveillance company Athena Securities in USA developed AI based module for detecting fever through video feed. This helps to make decision fast thereby developing new diagnosis systems for Covid-19 by utilizing required algorithms. Computed tomography (CT) scan and magnetic resonance imaging (MRI) scan are major medical imaging techniques for data collection in IoT based AI technology. One of main symptoms of Covid-19 is high temperature fever hence encouraging symptomatic persons to be quarantined to reduce the spread of Corona Virus. It also proved in china at early detection period, and temperature detection is primary key for combating Covid-19. These methods are used to data collection of protection and privacy individuals. Passive mode of data collection is not suitable for privacy and also need to be updated automatically. Many of European Countries are utilizing AI based data automation to combat epidemic.

(b) *Observing behavior for treatment*

Most of the corona patients are curing by themselves without consulting any doctor. This type of virus called as mild Covid-19 and recommended patients to be home quarantine to avoid additional health issues. Another type of virus is called severe and critical Covid-19, and these types of patients are recommended to visit hospital. These types of category patients are mostly experiencing hypoxemia which needs external set up for oxygen either through ventilator or face mask. AI based technique is an intelligent platform for prediction and monitor automatically of Corona virus. A neural network develops for AI based technique to extract features of virus thereby monitoring and providing exact treatment for affected ones. This technique is also update itself to record patient's data which helps to develop vaccine for Covid-19.

(c) *Tracing out primary contacts*

Contact tracing is the method of identifying people based on history of Covid-19 affected ones. This also helps not to test large set community. However, tracing out primary contacts are quite challenge through conventional methods as data of affected patients is not updated automatically. AI based methods identify primary contacts through bracelets which are composed with GPS navigation and ArogyaSethu application from affected ones. It is recommended to affected persons to be home quarantined to avoid spray to community. According to the WHO, the identification of primary contacts composed with three steps.

i. The individuals who are direct contact with infected individuals
ii. Maintaining record the details of infected ones

iii. Get details of individuals to be tested soon

The process of tracing primary contacts is highly useful to avoid community spread at first and second stages. AI based technique helps to analyze the levels of spreading thereby identifying "hot spots" and clusters successfully.

Blockchain

Blockchain technology is used mainly to track primary contacts and preserving details of patient. It is also enabling methods of encryption, distribution and security of digital medical field. It simplifies the tracking of drug trails and also record activities of trails. Blockchain technology has capability of summarize continuous varying data such as Covid-19. Hence, Blockchain technology plays an important role at combating of Covid-19 such as tracking primary contacts, protecting of privacy information and managing supply chain at medical domain. There are two types of Blockchain methods to analyze data of Covid-19 that are CIVITAS and MiPasa.

CIVITAS

An application (app) developed based on Blockchain technology in Canada to provide security to Covid-19 patients and also assists various aspects to different nations. This app indicates whether the candidate come out from home through official ID given while registration in app. This app also provides ideal time and busy for patient to reduce risk individual and also others by carrying required items. In addition to this, CIVITAS app offers telemedicine such as consultation of doctor and record of patient details.

MiPasa

MiPasa is a platform of data streaming composed on Hyperledger Fabric which is built from IBM Company by integrating Blockchain and cloud. This platform mainly used to share patient details and record health information among doctors, authorities and also cluster of hospitals. The WHO also approved and acknowledged this application to share information among doctors efficiently to develop vaccination for Covid-19.

d. *Data Analysis*

AI based technology forecasts and tracks the characteristics of Corona virus for recorded data from different platforms such as social media and media platforms thereby measuring risk of infection. The data analysis of AI based technology predicts the number of infected individuals and number death cases at particular region. This helps to measure the most affected regions, countries and community of people thereby providing safety measures, respectively. Before data analysis, data of corona patients initially processed three steps that are pre-processing for normalization, segmentation and classification. Different methods are used for above mentioned steps for data collection and analysis efficiently. AI based technique provides the latest information of vaccination for Covid-19 with help of data analysis. It predicts and refers probable infection level by virus, requirement of beds and required equipment for treatment during epidemic. AI based technology is highly helpful in future such as second wave of Covid-19 as well as other epidemics. Pelaez and Loayza [7] analyzed different simulation parameters such as accuracy, sensitivity and specify by applying deep learning models for Covid-19.

e. *Development of Vaccine and Drugs*

AI based technology plays a vital role at development of vaccine and drugs for Covid-19 as it is adopt different conditions and update it. It is mainly using in drug research because vaccine needs huge amount of data from the different regions of patients. This technology accelerates the development of vaccine and also provides status of vaccine and drug. Because of adopt real-time conditions, AI based technology becomes a set of powerful tool for combating Covid-19 epidemic. This also recommends the positive case need to hospitalized or not based on severity of infection level by virus.

iii. Different algorithms involved in ML/DL

Algorithms of machine learning are broadly divided into two categories that are supervised and unsupervised algorithms. Figure 3 depicts broad classification of algorithms used in both ML and DL. The supervised learning is composed with classification and regression methods, and classification is implemented with Image classification and machine translation. The regression is implemented with stock prediction and image masking methods. The unsupervised learning is used in both machine learning and deep learning. The ML algorithm is composed with dimension reduction and clustering methods, whereas DL is composed with representation learning model and generative model. Principle Component Analysis (PCA) and t-SNE methods are utilized for dimension reduction and K-means, GMMs, HMMs are used for clustering technique. Mutual information, disentanglement and information bottleneck are techniques used in representation learning whereas GAN and VAE are used for generative model.

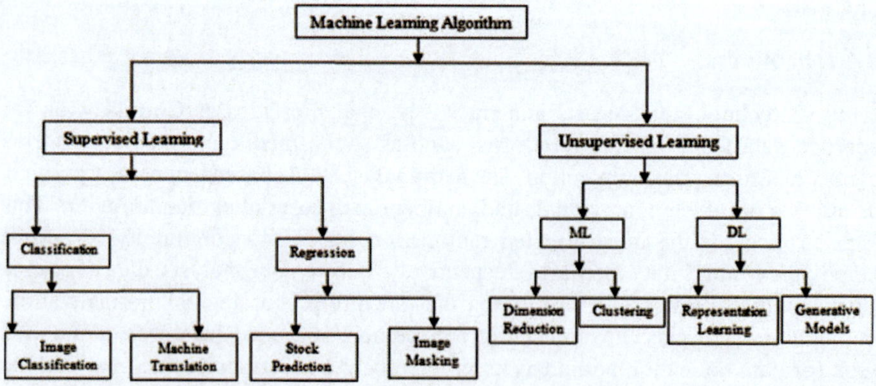

Fig. 3 Classification of algorithms of ML/DL

4 Conclusion

This paper presented novel platform by integrated different technologies such as AI, IoT and Blockchain for combating corona virus. Initially, this paper discussed corona effected countries by the region-wise which taken from WHO thereafter presented characteristics and required equipment to confirm Corona effected individuals. This paper is propounded IoT based AI technique with Blockchain for analysis of Corona characteristics and developing vaccine and drug. The novel platform IoT based AI with Blockchain discussed how it is suitable to combating Covid-19 with ML/DL algorithms. Finally, this paper tries to give the new direction for avoiding Covid-19.

References

1. Chan-Yeung M, Xu R (2003) SARS: Epidemiology. Respirology 8:S9–S14
2. World Health Organization (2020) Middle east respiratory syndrome coronavirus (MERS-CoV). Accessed 20 Apr 2020. https://www.who.int/emergencies/mers-cov/en/
3. Wang D, Hu B, Hu C, Zhu F, Liu X, Zhang J, Wang B, Xiang H, Cheng Z, Xiong Y, Zhao Y, Li Y, Wang X, Peng Z (2020) Clinical characteristics of 138 hospitalized patients with 2019 novel coronavirus–infected pneumonia in Wuhan, China. J Amer Med Assoc 323(11):1061
4. Chen N, Zhou M, Dong X, Qu J, Gong F, Han Y, Qiu Y, Wang J, Liu Y, Wei Y, Xia J, Yu T, Zhang X, Zhang L (2020) Epidemiological and clinical characteristics of 99 cases of 2019 novel coronavirus pneumonia in Wuhan, China: a descriptive study. Lancet 395(10223):507–513
5. Jiang F, Deng L, Zhang L, Cai Y, Cheung CW, Xia Z (2020) Review of the clinical characteristics of coronavirus disease 2019 (COVID- 19). J Gen Internal Med 35:1545–1549
6. Patel M (2020) Antimicrobial paper embedded with nanoparticles as spread-breaker for corona virus. Virus 3(1):001–012
7. Pelaez E, Loayza F (2020) A deep learning model to screen for Corona Virus Disease (COVID-19) from X-ray chest images. In: 2020 IEEE Andescon. IEEE, pp 1–6

Automated Parkinson's Disease Diagnosis System Using Transfer Learning Techniques

Rohit Lamba, Tarun Gulati, and Anurag Jain

Abstract Parkinson's disease is a neurodegenerative disorder that develops in an individual when the required amount of dopamine is not produced by respective neurons. The most common symptoms of this disease are tremors or shaking in hand/arms, changes in handwriting, muscle stiffness, slowness during walking, and change in speech. It is an incurable disease, but managing its symptoms can delay its progression, which is possible only if it is diagnosed at an early stage. Prior research work had proved that variation in handwriting can be considered as a quantitative marker for Parkinson's disease diagnosis. The authors present an automated Parkinson's diagnosis system using transfer learning techniques. The performance of the presented system is analyzed by using Parkinson's spiral drawing dataset. Four transfer learning architectures ResNet 34, DensNet 121, VGG 16, and AlexNet are used to classify spiral images of Parkinson's patients and healthy individuals. The performance of these architectures was examined in terms of accuracy, sensitivity, specificity, and ROC-AUC. After fine-tuning, it was noted that the performance of all architectures improved and the AlexNet architecture outperformed with 93.33% accuracy and 0.96 AUC.

Keywords Parkinson's disease · Spiral images · Transfer learning · AlexNet · VGG16 · ResNet34 · DenseNet121

R. Lamba (✉) · T. Gulati
Department of Electronics & Communication Engineering, Maharishi Markandeshwar Engineering College, Maharishi Markandeshwar (Deemed to be University), Mullana, Ambala, Haryana, India
e-mail: rohitlamba14@mmumullana.org

T. Gulati
e-mail: gulati_tarun@mmumullana.org

A. Jain
School of Computer Sciences, University of Petroleum & Energy Studies, Dehradun, Uttarakhand, India
e-mail: anurag.jain@ddn.upes.ac.in

N. Marriwala et al. (eds.), *Emergent Converging Technologies and Biomedical Systems*, Lecture Notes in Electrical Engineering 841,
https://doi.org/10.1007/978-981-16-8774-7_16

1 Introduction

Parkinson's disease (PD) is a neurodegenerative disorder that badly affects the patient's life and usually develops after the age of 60. The core cause of the disease is a deficiency of dopamine, a brain chemical produced by neurons. When these dopamine-producing neurons start dying, results in less dopamine production and starts of Parkinson's disease [1]. The cause of these neurons dying is still to be seen. PD is incurable, so early diagnosis is the only way to improve the patient's life. Symptoms of the disease can be restrained by using a balanced diet, proper medication, and regular exercise [2]. Medications such as levodopa are used for PD treatment, as these medications aggravate left dopamine-producing neurons to produce more dopamine [3].

The symptoms of PD are divided into two types, motor, and non-motor symptoms. The slowness, tremor, instability in posture, and rigidity are some of the motor symptoms [4]. Sleep problems, depression, constipation, and anxiety are some of the non-motor symptoms. Symptoms developed in PD patients vary from patient to patient. Symptoms are mild and sometimes not noticeable at the starting of the disease, but the symptoms go severe as the disease progresses. The life of PD patients is badly affected by this disease, in some of the cases patient is not easily able to do some of the daily need works like writing or typing, eating food, walking up from the bed and washing dishes, etc. [5].

Neurologists and movement order specialists can diagnose this disease by doing an in-depth review of the patient's medical history and performing some radiological scans, for which patients have to visit the doctors repeatedly [6, 7]. As this disease mostly develops in the later stage of life around the age of 60, visiting hospitals is not easy for PD patients, so there is a scope of developing a tool for PD diagnosis which can help the health care professionals during PD diagnosis. This is the major motivation behind this research work because, in developing countries like India, health care professionals and services are limitedly available [8, 9]. Recently for disease diagnosis, deep learning techniques are widely used because of the promising results provided through data augmentation and transfer learning techniques [10, 11].

The researchers had proposed various Parkinson's detection tools by applying and utilizing different data science techniques. They have used handwritten drawings [6], speech signals [12], freezing of gait (FoG) [13], MRI images [14], SPECT images, EEG Signals [15], and EMG signals [16]. They have applied various data science techniques to the above-said numerous signals. A tremor on one side of the arm or body is one of the earliest symptoms of PD, which adversely affects the patient's handwriting or typing ability.

Parkinson's diagnosis using a handwritten drawing is been taken as an objective of this research work. To formulate the above-said objective, authors have applied transfer learning techniques to classify the spiral images of PD patients and healthy individuals. The Parkinson's spiral drawing dataset used in this work has been taken from the Kaggle repository. The substantial contributions of this research work are:

1. Initially, the authors present an automated Parkinson's disease diagnosis system using spiral drawn by PD patients and healthy individuals.
2. Furthermore, the results of four transfer learning architectures namely ResNet34, DenseNet121, VGG16, and AlexNet were compared in terms of accuracy, sensitivity, specificity, and ROC-AUC.
3. Finally, the authors have achieved an accuracy of 93.33% and an AUC of 0.96 by fine-tuning AlexNet model.

The remaining sections of this paper are organized as follows: the earlier research work is presented in Sect. 2 followed by materials and methods in Sect. 3. The results are outlined and discussed in Sect. 4. The conclusion and future scope are presented in Sect. 5.

2 Related Works

Researchers have recently used different techniques and methods for Parkinson's diagnosis using handwritten drawings. Some of the recent research work is related to automating Parkinson's diagnosis is summarized here.

Pereira et al. [17] proposed an automatic Parkinson diagnosis system and made HandPD dataset publicly available. The dataset was composed using a smartpen by Sketching Spiral and Menders by Parkinson's patients and healthy controls. Images were generated from the data collected by the sensors of the smartpen. Three transfer learning architectures such as ImageNet, LeNet, and CIFAR-10 were employed for image classification. Experiments were done by dividing the dataset into 75:25 and 50:50 train and test ratios. Results show that the CIFAR-10 gives the best classification accuracy. Pereira et al. [18] proposed CNN-based architecture to learn features derived from handwritten dynamics. The authors also made the NewHnadPD dataset publicly available. Images generated from the time-series signals collected by smartpen sensors were fed into the CNN networks. Six CNN networks each were employed for the various exams and finally, majority voting was used. Two CNN architectures namely CIFAR-10 and ImageNet were also employed. Khatamino et al. [19] proposed a CNN-based method for Parkinson's diagnosis in which the features were learned from handwritten drawing samples drawn by Parkinson's patients. The authors also introduced a new dynamic spiral test as well as a static spiral test. The data was collected from 57 PD patients and 15 healthy controls. The data was collected in two ways first, the spirals images were collected and in the second five features X, Y, Z, Pressure, and grip angle were extracted. Results suggested that the dynamic test is more discriminative than the static test. The dataset is divided into 75:25 train and test ratios and the authors achieve an accuracy of 88%.

Moetesum et al. [20] presented a study of how visual attributes can be used from handwriting datasets for the diagnosis of PD. The PaHaW dataset was used in this study which does not contain any image. Eight different handwriting tasks were performed by individuals during the data collection process. Images were generated for every task from time-series signals by plotting x, y coordinates. Features from generated images were extracted and grouped into a combined feature vector by CNN architecture pre-trained with AlexNet. These combined feature vectors were fed into eight SVM classifiers one for each task and by majority voting and classification between healthy and Parkinson's patients was done. The results show an accuracy of 83% by ten-fold cross-validation method. Diaz et al. [21] presented how handwritten task images constructed from time-series signals of PaHaW dataset could be utilized to detect PD. 3-layer CNN architecture was used to classify the images generated from the eight different handwritten tasks. Transfer learning was also employed for performance enhancement and finally, majority voting was done at the classification stage. The authors achieved an accuracy of 86.67%. Razzak et al. [22] have analyzed different drawing tasks for Parkinson's diagnosis using deep learning techniques. PaHaW, HandPD, New HandPD, and Parkinson's drawing datasets were used to find the best drawing task that contributed more to classifying the drawing drawn by Parkinson's patients and healthy individuals. Four transfer learning architectures VGGNet, AlexNet, ResNet, and GoogleNet were employed for image classification. Experiments were performed by combining images of different datasets. The highest 96.08% accuracy was achieved by VGG16 architecture by combining the images of Parkinson's drawing, New HandPD, and HandPD datasets. Naseer et al. [23] proposed a CNN-based Parkinson's detection system using handwritten images. The study used the PaHaW dataset in which samples were collected from 75 subjects by performing eight different tasks. AlexNet, ImageNet, MNIST transfer learning techniques were employed on the dataset. The results were improved by data augmentation and fine-tuning techniques. Accuracy, precision, sensitivity, and specificity were the performance matrices used. The authors achieved 98.28% accuracy on spiral images using a trained fine-tuned network. Shaban, M. et al. [24] have proposed a PD diagnosis approach based on deep learning techniques. This study uses spiral and wave handwriting datasets downloaded from the Kaggle repository. The dataset consists of 102 wave and spiral images. The CNN fine-tuned VGG-19 architecture is used for classifying the images. Images were resized and augmented because the dataset is small in size. The proposed model achieved 89% and 88% accuracy for spiral and wave datasets respectively.

Chakraborty et al. [25] proposed a convolutional neural network approach to analyze the spiral and wave drawing patterns to detect Parkinson's disease. Dataset images were first resized and then contrast enhancement was performed using histogram equalization. Because the dataset consists of 102 spiral and wave images, hence data augmentation was applied to generate synthetic samples. Two classifiers logistic regression and random forest were used to form a Meta classifier. The proposed system achieved 93.3% accuracy with fivefold cross-validation technique. Kamran et al. [26] presented a Parkinson's diagnosis system using handwriting samples of PD patients. Images from various datasets HnadPD, NewHandPD, PaHaW, and Parkinson's spiral and wave were used in this study. Data augmentation techniques like threshold, flipping, contrast, illumination, and flipping were applied on datasets images. AlexNet, VGG16, GoogleNet, ResNet50, VGG19, and Resnet101 transfer learning techniques were used in this study.

3 Materials and Methods

3.1 Parkinson's Drawing Dataset

The Parkinson's drawing dataset used in this study is publicly available at Kaggle repository [27]. The dataset was collected by drawing spirals and waves from Parkinson's patients and healthy controls. Only spiral images are used in this study because most of the researchers have used spiral images for the diagnosis of this disease. Training and testing were two subsets in which the spiral image dataset was already segmented. The training subset and the test subset constitute 72 and 30 spiral images, respectively. Half of the images in both sub-categories are from patients with PD while the rest are from healthy individuals. The sample of images drawn by PD patients and healthy individuals is shown in Fig. 1.

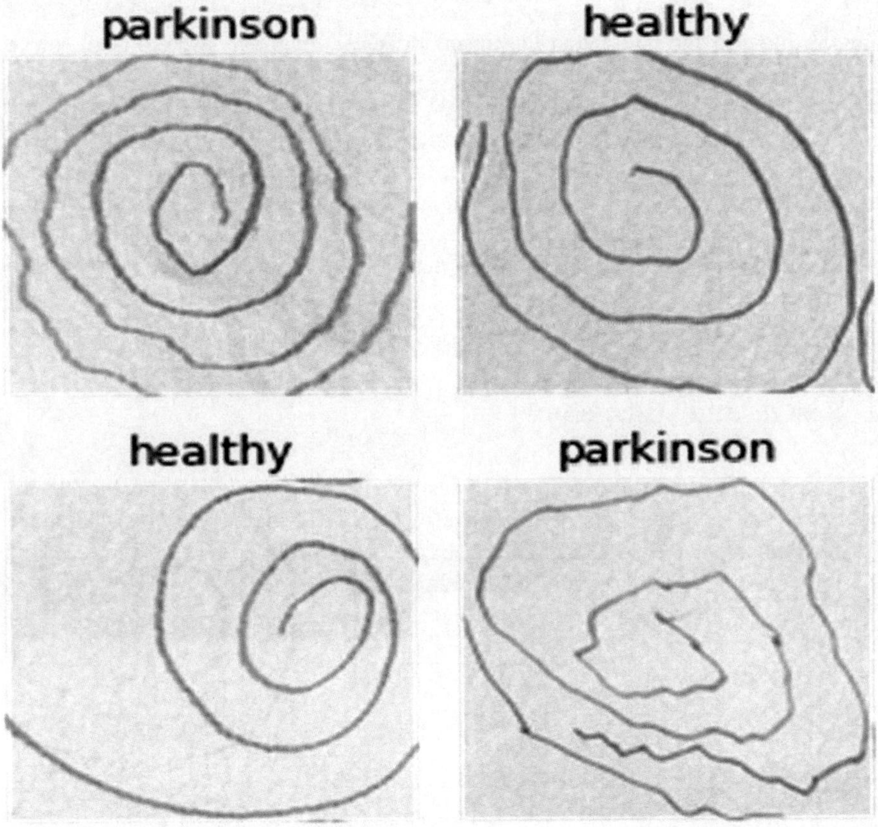

Fig. 1 Sample images from the dataset

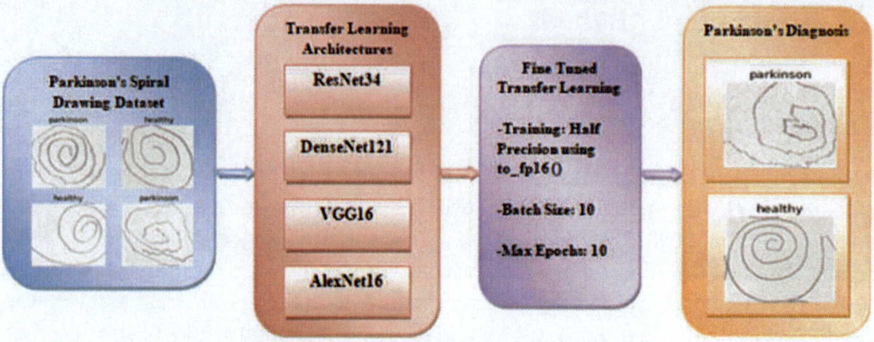

Fig. 2 Workflow of automated Parkinson's disease diagnosis system

3.2 Methodology

The workflow of the automated Parkinson's disease diagnosis system is shown in Fig. 2. The publically available Parkinson's spiral images dataset has been used in this study. This is a balanced dataset with 51 spiral images from PD patients and the remaining 51 images from healthy individuals. ResNet 34, DenseNet 121, VGG16 and AlexNet transfer learning architectures have been used to classify spiral images. Accuracy, sensitivity, specificity, and ROC-AUC parameters are taken to analyze the performance of transfer learning architectures. All the transfer learning architectures were then fine-tuned and AlexNet outperforms with the best results in all performance measures.

4 Results and Discussions

The paramount goal of this research is to design a PD diagnosis system using a spiral drawing of PD patients. The performance of the four transfer learning techniques namely ResNet34, DenseNet121, VGG16, and AlexNet are measured in terms of accuracy, specificity, and sensitivity as defined below.

$$\text{Accuracy} = \left(\frac{\text{TP} + \text{TN}}{\text{TP} + \text{FP} + \text{TN} + \text{FN}}\right) * 100$$

$$\text{Specificity} = \left(\frac{\text{TN}}{\text{TN} + \text{FP}}\right) * 100$$

$$\text{Sensitivity} = \left(\frac{\text{TP}}{\text{TP} + \text{FN}}\right) * 100$$

Here.

TP (True Positive): The individual is Parkinson's patient and the model has also detected it as Parkinson's patient.

TN (True Negative): The individual is healthy and the model has also detected it as healthy.

FP (False Positive): The individual is healthy and the model has detected it as Parkinson's patient.

FN (False Negative): The individual is suffering from Parkinson's and the model has detected it as healthy.

In all the transfer learning models used, CNN networks were used as a backbone with a fully connected head and a single hidden layer as a classifier. In the starting initial layers were frozen and weights are learned on the last fully connected layers means only the classification layer was trained. Then by running and experimenting with different epochs, architectures were saved when the best results were achieved. Finding the correct learning rate plays an important role in transfer learning architectures. Then the best learning rate was obtained by a function called lr_find. After that, all the layers were unfreezing and architectures were trained with the best learning rate. The batch size is taken as 10 during the training phase.

It was seen that as the number of batches escalated, the training and validation loss plummeted. The training and validation loss versus batch process for the ResNet34, DenseNet121, VGG16, and AlexNet are shown in Figs. 3, 4, 5 and 6 respectively. The performance of any classification model can be evaluated by confusion matrix. It is an M by M matrix in which M is the output class number. This matrix is drawn between the actual value and predicted value. The Confusion matrix for ResNet34, DenseNet121, VGG16, and AlexNet are shown in Figs. 7, 8, 9 and 10 respectively.

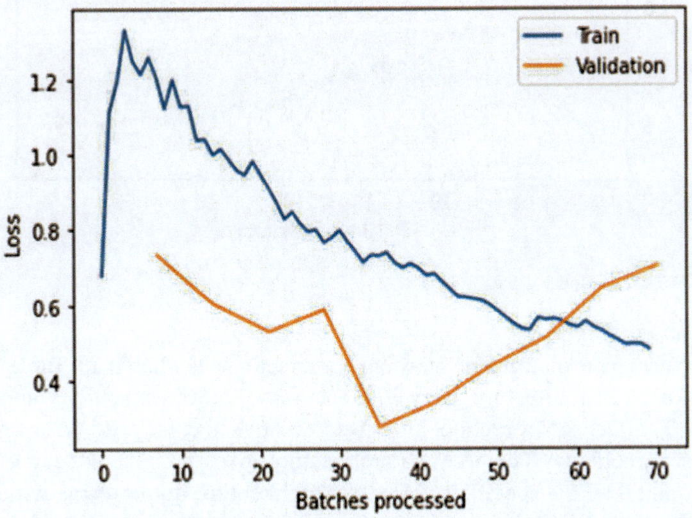

Fig. 3 ResNet34-Train and validation loss

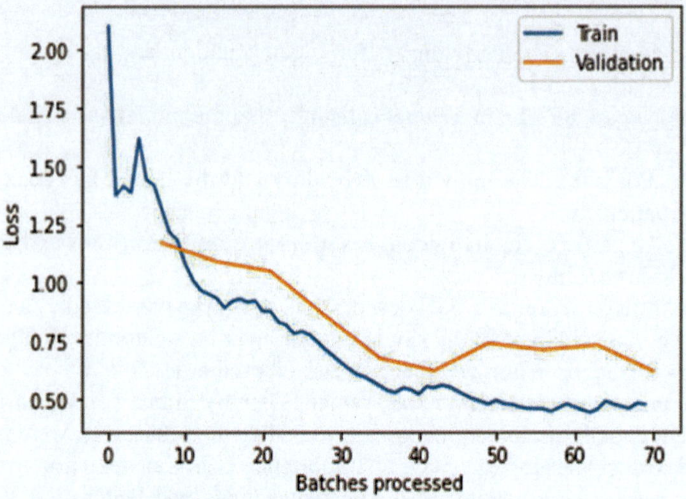

Fig. 4 DenseNet121-Train and validation loss

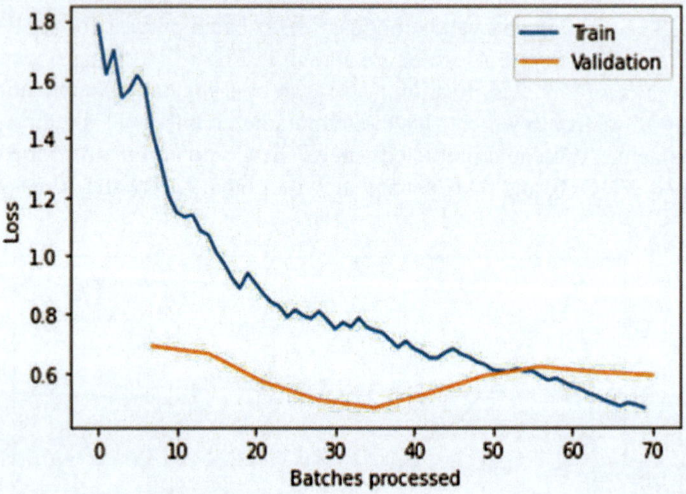

Fig. 5 VGG16- Train and validation loss

The performance of transfer learning architectures is shown in Table 1. After fine-tune, ResNet Architecture gives 90% accuracy, 86.66% specificity and 93.33% sensitivity. The DenseNet architecture gives 86.66% accuracy, 86.66% sensitivity, and 86.66% specificity. The VGG16 architecture gives 83.33% accuracy, 73.33% sensitivity, and 93.33% specificity. AlexNet architecture outperforms with 93.33% accuracy, 93.33% sensitivity, and 93.33% specificity as shown in Fig. 11.

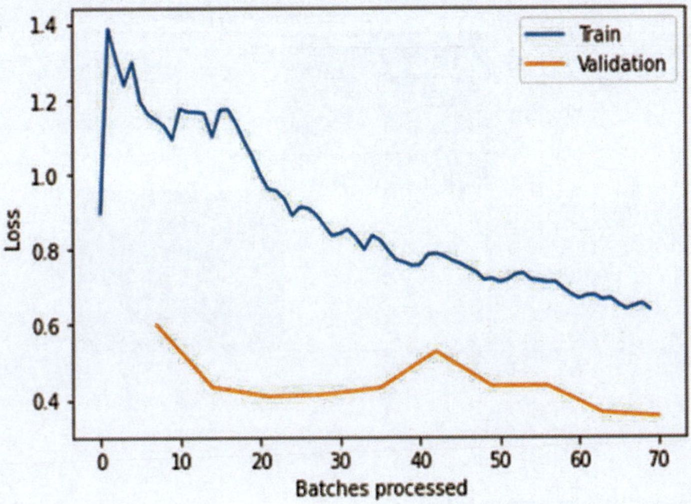

Fig. 6 AlexNet-Train and validation loss

Fig. 7 ResNet34-Confusion matrix

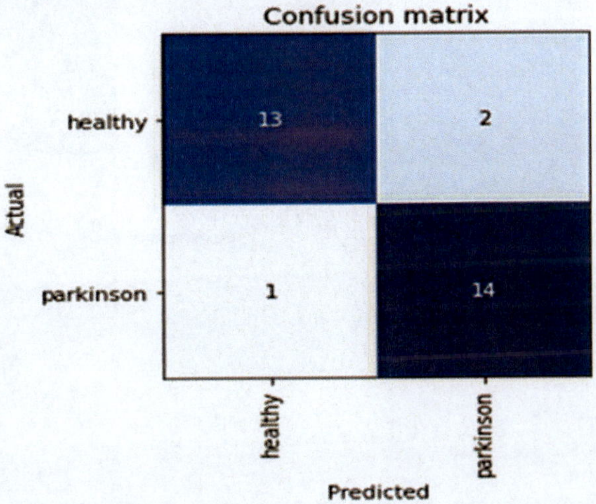

ROC is a graphical 2-D plot drawn between the true-positive rate and false-positive rate. Under this performance metric, the area under the curve (AUC) is calculated which lies between zero to one. AUC of the transfer learning architectures is been measured and shown with this graph. The higher the AUC means the model is more efficient to classify the spiral images drowned by PD patients and healthy individuals. ROC curve of transfer learning architecture is shown in Fig. 12.

Due to technological enhancement, computer-assisted medical diagnosis systems are gaining momentum as medical resources are limitedly available in developing

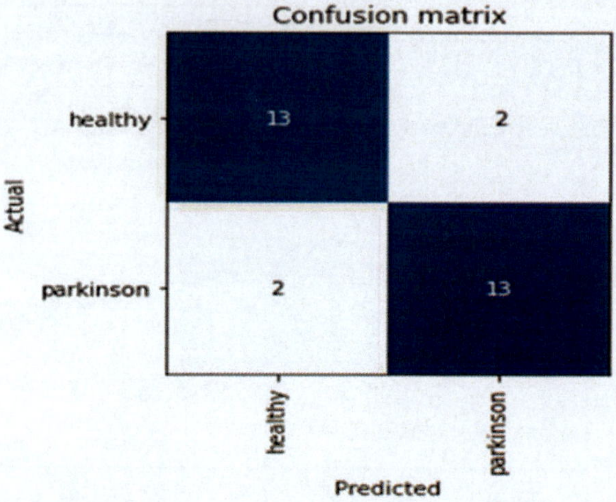

Fig. 8 DenseNet121-Confusion matrix

Fig. 9 VGG16-Confusion matrix

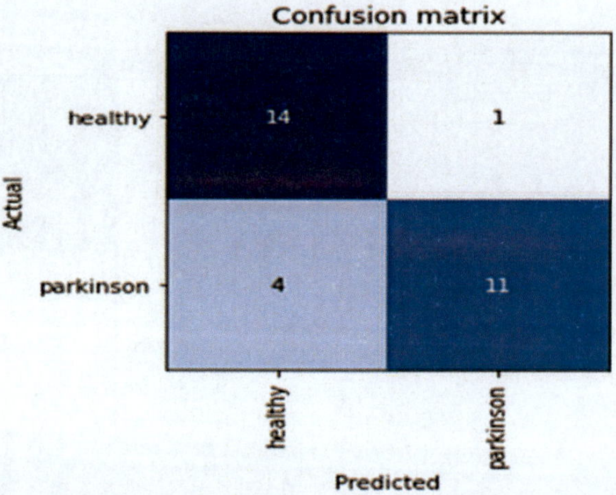

countries like India. The results are propitious and advocate that the proposed automated system can be used for PD diagnosis but it has some limitations.

The presented automated system is not able to find the severity of Parkinson's disease; it can only classify spirals drown by PD patients and healthy individuals.

There is a need to test this automated system on other Parkinson's drawing datasets for a reliable diagnosis.

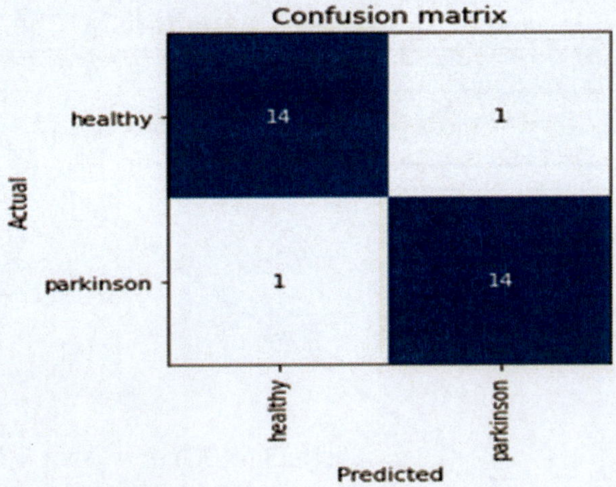

Fig. 10 AlexNet16-Confusion matrix

Table 1 Performance comparison of fine-tuned transfer learning architectures

Model	Accuracy %	Sensitivity %	Specificity %
ResNet34	90.00	93.33	86.66
DenseNet121	86.66	86.66	86.66
VGG16	83.33	73.33	93.33
AlexNet	**93.33**	**93.33**	**93.33**

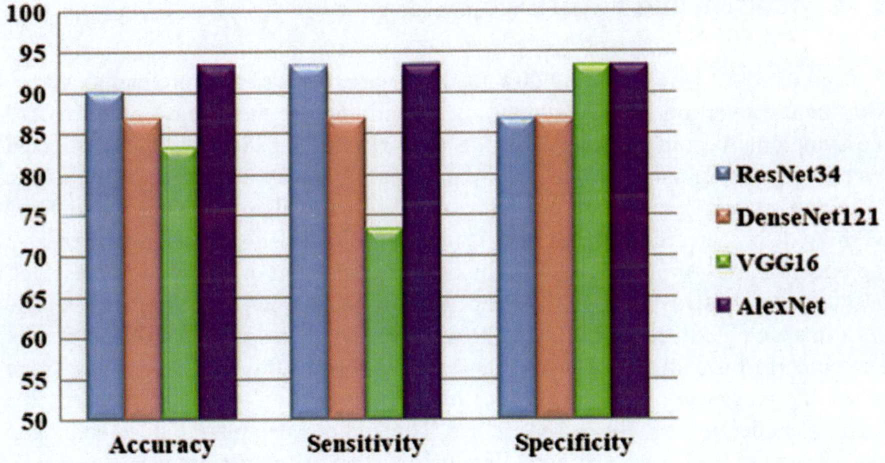

Fig. 11 Performance comparison of transfer learning architectures

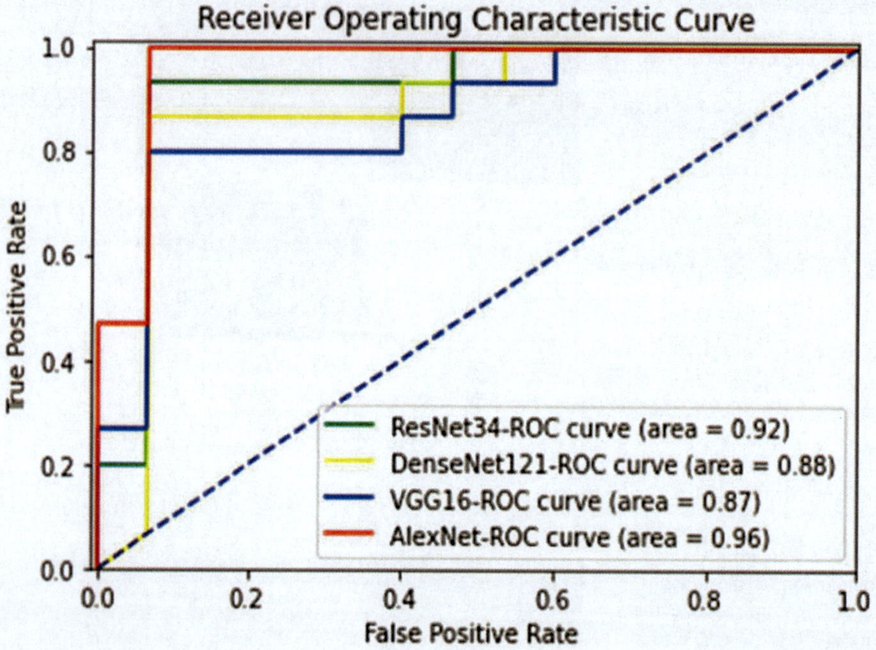

Fig. 12 ROC curve

5 Conclusion and Future scope

Parkinson's disease is a chronic disease that is progressive in nature and its symptoms appear over time. Initial symptoms are mild and as the disease goes forward the symptoms become critical. The life of Parkinson's patients is badly affected by this disease, in some of the cases patient is not easily able to do some of the daily needs works like writing or typing, eating food, walking up from the bed and washing dishes, etc. Since the disease is incurable, its timely diagnosis can improve the patient's life. An automated Parkinson's disease diagnosis system is presented in this research work by applying deep learning techniques on spiral images. The performance of four transfer learning architectures was analyzed. AlexNet architecture outperforms with the highest 93.33% accuracy and 0.96 AUC. The authors plan to test the presented automated system on other Parkinson's drawing datasets like wave, meander, and circles in near future. The authors also plan to develop a deep learning-based Parkinson's disease diagnosis system using MRI images.

References

1. Kotsavasiloglou C, Kostikis N, Hristu-Varsakelis D, Arnaoutoglou M (2017) Machine learning-based classification of simple drawing movements in Parkinson's disease. Biomed Signal Process Control 31:174–180. https://doi.org/10.1016/j.bspc.2016.08.003
2. Lamba R, Gulati T, Jain A (2020) Comparative analysis of Parkinson's disease diagnosis system. Adv Math Sci J 9(6):3399–3406. https://doi.org/10.37418/amsj.9.6.20
3. Ma A, Lau KK, Thyagarajan D (2020) Voice changes in Parkinson's disease: What are they telling us? J Clin Neurosci 72:1–7. https://doi.org/10.1016/j.jocn.2019.12.029
4. Ascherio A, Schwarzschild MA (2016) The epidemiology of Parkinson's disease: risk factors and prevention. Lancet Neurol 15(12):1257–1272. https://doi.org/10.1016/S1474-4422(16)30230-7
5. Bhat S, Acharya UR, Hagiwara Y, Dadmehr N, Adeli H (2018) Parkinson's disease: cause factors, measurable indicators, and early diagnosis. Comput Biol Med 102:234–241. https://doi.org/10.1016/j.compbiomed.2018.09.008
6. Lamba R, Gulati T, Al-Dhlan KA, Jain A (2021) A systematic approach to diagnose Parkinson's disease through kinematic features extracted from handwritten drawings. J Reliable Intell Environ:1–10. https://doi.org/10.1007/s40860-021-00130-9
7. Lamba R, Gulati T, Alharbi HF, Jain A (2021) A hybrid system for Parkinson's disease diagnosis using machine learning techniques. Int J Speech Technol:1–11. https://doi.org/10.1007/s10772-021-09837-9
8. Rani P, Kumar R, Ahmed NMOS, Jain A (2021) A decision support system for heart disease prediction based upon machine learning. J Reliab Intell Environ:1–13. https://doi.org/10.1007/s40860-021-00133-6
9. Jain A, Tiwari S, Sapra V (2019) Two-phase heart disease diagnosis system using deep learning. Int J Control Autom 12(5):558–573
10. Tiwari S, Jain A (in press)Convolutional capsule network for COVID-19 detection using radiography images. Int J Imaging Syst Technol. https://doi.org/10.1002/ima.22566
11. Rani P, Kumar R, Jain A, Chawla SK (2021) A hybrid approach for feature selection based on genetic algorithm and recursive feature elimination. Int J Inf Syst Model Design (IJISMD) 12(2):17–38. https://doi.org/10.4018/IJISMD.2021040102
12. Behroozi M, Sami A (2016) A multiple-classifier framework for Parkinson's disease detection based on various vocal tests. Int J Telemed Appl. https://doi.org/10.1155/2016/6837498
13. Ertuğrul ÖF, Kaya Y, Tekin R, Almalı MN (2016) Detection of Parkinson's disease by shifted one dimensional local binary patterns from gait. Expert Syst Appl 56:156–163. https://doi.org/10.1016/j.eswa.2016.03.018
14. Sivaranjini S, Sujatha CM (2019) Deep learning based diagnosis of Parkinson's disease using convolutional neural network. Multimed Tools Appl:1–13. https://doi.org/10.1007/s11042-019-7469-8
15. Oh SL, Hagiwara Y, Raghavendra U, Yuvaraj R, Arunkumar N, Murugappan M, Acharya UR (2018) A deep learning approach for Parkinson's disease diagnosis from EEG signals. Neural Comput Appl:1–7. https://doi.org/10.1007/s00521-018-3689-5
16. Loconsole C, Cascarano GD, Brunetti A, Trotta GF, Losavio G, Bevilacqua V, Di Sciascio E (2019) A model-free technique based on computer vision and sEMG for classification in Parkinson's disease by using computer-assisted handwriting analysis. Pattern Recogn Lett 121:28–36. https://doi.org/10.1016/j.patrec.2018.04.006
17. Pereira CR, Weber SA, Hook C, Rosa GH, Papa JP (2016) Deep learning-aided Parkinson's disease diagnosis from handwritten dynamics. In: 2016 29th SIBGRAPI conference on graphics, patterns and images SIBGRAPI. IEEE, pp 340–346. https://doi.org/10.1109/SIBGRAPI.2016.054
18. Pereira CR, Pereira DR, Rosa GH, Albuquerque VH, Weber SA, Hook C, Papa JP (2018) Handwritten dynamics assessment through convolutional neural networks: An application to Parkinson's disease identification. Artif Intell Med 87:67–77. https://doi.org/10.1016/j.artmed.2018.04.001

19. Khatamino P, Cantürk İA, Özyılmaz L (2018) A deep learning-CNN based system for medical diagnosis: an application on Parkinson's disease handwriting drawings. In: 2018 6th international conference on control engineering & information technology CEIT. IEEE, pp 1–6. https://doi.org/10.1109/CEIT.2018.8751879
20. Moetesum M, Siddiqi I, Vincent N, Cloppet F (2019) Assessing visual attributes of handwriting for prediction of neurological disorders—a case study on Parkinson's disease. Pattern Recogn Lett 121:19–27. https://doi.org/10.1016/j.patrec.2018.04.008
21. Diaz M, Ferrer MA, Impedovo D, Pirlo G, Vessio G (2019) Dynamically enhanced static handwriting representation for Parkinson's disease detection. Pattern Recogn Lett 128:204–210. https://doi.org/10.1016/j.patrec.2019.08.018
22. Razzak I, Kamran I, Naz S (2020) Deep analysis of handwritten notes for early diagnosis of neurological disorders. In: 2020 International joint conference on neural networks (IJCNN). IEEE, pp 1–6. https://doi.org/10.1109/IJCNN48605.2020.9207087
23. Naseer A, Rani M, Naz S, Razzak MI, Imran M, Xu G (2020) Refining Parkinson's neurological disorder identification through deep transfer learning. Neural Comput Appl 32(3):839–854. https://doi.org/10.1007/s00521-019-04069-0
24. Shaban M (2020) Deep convolutional neural network for parkinson's disease based handwriting screening. In: 2020 IEEE 17th international symposium on biomedical imaging workshops, ISBI Workshops. IEEE, pp 1–4. https://doi.org/10.1109/ISBIWorkshops50223.2020.9153407
25. Chakraborty S, Aich S, Han E, Park J, Kim HC (2020) Parkinson's disease detection from spiral and wave drawings using convolutional neural networks: a multistage classifier approach. In: 2020 22nd International conference on advanced communication technology, ICACT. IEEE, pp 298–303. https://doi.org/10.23919/ICACT48636.2020.9061497
26. Kamran I, Naz S, Razzak I, Imran M (2021) Handwriting dynamics assessment using deep neural network for early identification of Parkinson's disease. Futur Gener Comput Syst 117:234–244. https://doi.org/10.1016/j.future.2020.11.020
27. Parkinson's Drawings Dataset (2021) https://www.kaggle.com/kmader/parkinsons-drawings Accessed 10 Jan 2021

Manual and Automatic Control of Appliances Based on Integration of WSN and IOT Technology

S. Karthikeyan, Adusumalli Nishanth, Annaa Praveen, Vijayabaskar, and T. Ravi

Abstract As indicated by the Internet of Things, the future home the purported Smart Home, will be a consistent mix of actual savvy objects, interfacing, among them and with the general climate. Furthermore, since handsets are often used to manage certain aspects of people's lives, the capability to power and monitor Smart Households from they will become a requirement. The justification for the Home Automation System is to monitor the limits such as voltage, current and temperature using remote network architecture that operate on a screen. The main aim is to reduce a smart condo's excessive energy consumption. It aids with an improvement of controlling organisation introduction. The aim of its project is to design a well-thought-out intra smart home system that allows the consumer to monitor all of their electric and electronic devices from every other mobile. This project's use includes features such as screen surveillance, light and fan power, fire warning and greenhouse service. The detectors are linked to the Pic microcontroller, which sends the sensor' position to the email address. The Arduino is used to interfere with device and Wlan is also connected to the Arduino to have a Domain name from either an adapter. With the use of WSN, this research framework provides a solution for providing extremely accurate monitoring and scheduling position of current state of gear.

Keywords Home automation · Arduino · Bluetooth · WSN · Smartphone

1 Introduction

A Wireless Sensor Network (WSN) is a centralised organisation made up of dispersed and automatic modules that monitor material or chemical concentrations using sensors. The WSN arrangement is created by combining hubs or self-administering with a gateway and toggle. Household computerisation or flat designs, according to some reports, may use resources more effectively than conventional systems. As a result, a few researchers have advocated for the use of remote monitoring to reduce

S. Karthikeyan (✉) · A. Nishanth · A. Praveen · Vijayabaskar · T. Ravi
Department of ECE, Sathyabama Institute of Science and Technology, Chennai, India

N. Marriwala et al. (eds.), *Emergent Converging Technologies and Biomedical Systems*, Lecture Notes in Electrical Engineering 841,
https://doi.org/10.1007/978-981-16-8774-7_17

energy consumption. In the drafting, also suggested clear housing assemblages get the WSN (Wireless Sensor Network) [1] as a manifestation of ineffable creation because of its flexibility and long battery life, the WSN has indeed been widely seen in controller and inspecting implementations that instead Wi-Fi. Humans differ from most other animals in that they have special supervisory powers, which necessitate proper details and knowledge of history or rather its general situation. Monitoring systems are used to obtain data through structures and their average soil characteristics in a motorised or dynamic device to reduce the energy acquiring [2]. The sensor is a sensor that can augment or replace a person's Sight, hearing, taste, smell and interaction are the five students. For use of a master device network is shown to be versatile and effective inside a variety of situations. Even a variety of settings, including domestic digitalisation, manufacturing engineer and control threats, among others. A far-flung mobile device [3] uses spatiotemporal confiscated free devices to measure and regulate body temperature, voltage and budget constraints. Because of the abundance of high straightforwardness and ease by laptop connectivity and internet, the remained of domestic digitalisation has been rising amazingly since later last year. A mobile electric drivetrains system connects electronic components in a residence. The methods used in household distributed computing are similar to those used in housing industrialization and urbanisation and management of local tasks such as smart tv setup, pot plant including yard planting and pet care, among other things. Devices can be connected by a personal organiser and licenced for web connection from web to experiences related from a PC. The use of technology advancements and management structures to reduce human labour is referred to as a product advancement method. The rapid advancement in technology encourages one to use cells to power home equipment in an indirect manner. Computerised devices have the potential to operate with agility, dedication and a low rate of errors.

Home scientists and home computer partnerships, the bolster method is a huge problem. If the client lies and outside the house, a consumer pneumatic tires culture is built on automation operating intelligent home gadgets. Home computer technology allows a person to monitor various aspects of their home usually. A personal computer is a system or tool designed to perform a particular function, usually a mechanical unit for home use, such as with a refrigerator. House digitization combines the monitoring of lighting, temperature, equipment and different models to provide offers with a feature, functionality, efficiency and protection. Household mechanisation may be a replacement for formal thinking for hampered and elderly people. Household digitalisation or construction urbanisation, combined with the fuel concept, makes living in today's world incredibly easy. It includes personalised control of overall electrical and electronic devices in the household, as well as disorders that can lead via long-distance messaging. This arrangement allows for unified monitoring of lighting, water heating, sound/video facilities, surveillance mechanisms, kitchen machinery and all other remaining devices used in homes frameworks. Canny home can be defined as a "propelled bedroom" because it combines power of devices with vision.

Home People with advancement deficiency, the elderly, having poor vision, sensory people who are blind and mentally impaired human beings all need an electronic device. A large number of individuals one of its primary goals of sharper households is to reduce energy consumption. Smart systems can be used in a controller to accomplish this impartiality. Furthermore, led lighting management systems should take signature light into account (daylight). As a result, a few studies have shown that in industry or administrative structures, daytime will stand in for mainly lighting control. Scanners and fast controls use light to reduce the amount of energy used to operate external light [4], ensuring that a room is adequately illuminated. Despite numerous suggestions for intelligent street lights for fuel savings in beautiful houses, a precise electric lighting framework of strong fearlessness and assist in ensuring is yet to be uncovered. The current arrangement's main goals are to broaden the scope of automatic monitoring considerations and reduce the effect of a remote barrier for connected home structures [5] on the WSN collecting data interface. A large number of narrow reach peer far away sensor line segments make up a dispersed sensor. By merging two different forms of advancement, such as converter and long-distance connectivity. Before submitting results to the device, WSN [6] notices, receives and manages paper material in its concealing region. The WSN is commonly used in manager and tracking apps due to its flexibility and lightweight. WSN in a genius home cooperative [3] consists of confiscated free gadgets with extensive applications, such as surveillance, military tracks and intelligent motorised vehicles. Every unit within organisation in WSN for connected homes [7] is freed from various places; they are power energised, small in scale and have good indicators. Via a visual functional tissue, a brilliant home current controller that used a far-off network system was already developed for healthy products in this article. It will, in turn, be realised without the involvement of customers in the future. As a result, it is simple to securely monitor and manage the insightful household using web-based technologies.

2 Related Work

Pawar et al. [1] have designed a Home Automation System concept that includes the Arduino ATmega328 microchip, a Wi-Fi device and motion sensors. The CPU is the core computer, which communicates the with Wi-Fi unit and takes requests to view monitor computers. The steelworker manages the communication between the programme and the chip, as well as the buyers and the creations. The platform for the items conversation system is an Android device that establishes a connection for the client to communicate only with a processor. The proposed setup involves a staff, a client, several contact networks, that are all managed by connection tools.

Choudhary et al. [2] have suggested a flexible wireless home mechanisation device that utilises Wi-Fi technology to link its dispersed instruments to a homes framework labourer. In this article, an Arduino Uno R3 microcontroller and a connecting wires Voltage regulator are being used to power a variety of equipment and programming and other devices with a large amount of energy. PIR meter, when PIR-based technology locators are used to the discerning enhancement of humans, pets, or different posts, thermocouple, etc. for testing heat and moisture content, design identifiable evidence, video seeing, etc. are among the different sensors used during device structure [5].

Sagar et al. [3] Assign probabilities to build a ringed home coordination device using an Arduino Microcontroller pic microcontroller with a simple Wi-Fi card slot, in addition to the serial communication sensors (sensors) that are used. As a result, the Galileo serious progress functions as a network specialist, allowing the development layout to be passed from web programmes on any main Computer in a comparable LAN using journeyman carpenter IP and from any PC or network globally using Network IP Wi-Fi technology is the organisation used in this article. Thermocouple and moisture, construction transparency, fire and smoke field, light scale and on/off function for multiple devices are all included in the proposal components. [8]

Pooja et al. [4] The aim of the External Keyword Powered Consumer Products Monitor Progress Program was to analyse data from the Microcontroller, initialise the Hdtv and Arduino show and display the circumstance with physical pressures on the LCD. The machine is familiar with the divider's wiring clicks. And using direct current devices, the danger of dangerous electrocution may be held to a minimum. The design employs two user interfaces, one for the PC the other for the Device. This GUI may be used to determine the status of the creations, such as whether they are on or off. Any time the story with the hardware shifts, a quick suggestion appears here on GUI. Only after Device's Wireless is connected to the PC's HDMI, the screen GUI will most likely act like a professional to advance or transfer any info to both the mobile and the main power pad. If the network card between both the PC or PC and the power fence fails, connection may be s right by connecting via USB. The person can control and operate the devices using IOT of any mobile location on the network.

Dhakad Kunal et al. [5]. A system's components are divided into three types: PCB, toughness processor and Microcontrollers controller. On the PCB, the LPT port, transistors and diode shunt resistor are all connected. They connected two gadgets to the PCB, such as a machine and a lamp. The Arduino and the dampness transmitter are connected. It can also tell the difference between temperature and moisture. PC is connected to Arduino and the PCB Arduino and PCB can connect along others through the Window. They measured the mass and also the amount of dust in the atmosphere. They have just a fixed time when temperatures but moisture are accurately resourced. It consistently services temperature and tensed muscles at regular intervals throughout the screengrab. Predilections (a) Increases safety by controlling appliances (b) Obtains the home by using web access Increment usability by regulating the temperature (c) loses time (d) reduces costs and adds relaxation (e) allows computers to be regulated while the user is away [8].

Santhi et al. [6] capture how the innovations and correspondence production are used to achieve a company's home medicine expenses or information technology. Rate focused on strewn data registration assist in connecting with matters encompassing all because one can know that it is simple to get to something at any moment and in any location in a simplistic manner with beautifully portrayed line stuff. As a result, cloud will most likely serve as a gateway to IoT. The inspiring opportunities for constructing the organisation and connection of mobile gadgets for homes advancement reasons to the internet that are still accessible.

Jain. Stevan Maineka et al. [7] depicts The Internet of Things (IoT) as a case inside which objects, species, entities were granted specific identity as well as the ability to send data over the network without the need for a person link. The term ‘Web of Things’ refers to a variety of capabilities and investigative tools that allow the Net to delve into the current reality of actual items. Summary the furthest contacts, RFID, unreferenced and far smart cities (WSNs), are all a component of the Internet of Things (IoT). The use of IoT technology and then a large network to digitalise the writing activities greatly integrates basic digital units to it and the devices are operated sufficiently indirect via the site. This report covers the potential of WSN, IoT and connected home architecture.

Existing System

The Bluetooth, ZigBee and Snapdragon software are currently used for home automation. The system necessitates a time-consuming and expensive powered installation as well as the use of an end PC. Gestures are used to organise a home control system. The controller transmits hand gestures to the system using a glove. A cell phone remote controller for office automation. The system differs now that all communications are conducted over a specific phone system rather than over the network. Any mobile that supports double tone different reoccurrence can be used to access the system (DTMF). Our project’s current setup does not access the internet of Things concept to power home appliances. This is fitting for modern technologies that allow you to monitor devices anywhere on the globe. As a result, we’ve decided to use IoT engineering as a basis for our connected home project (Fig. 1).

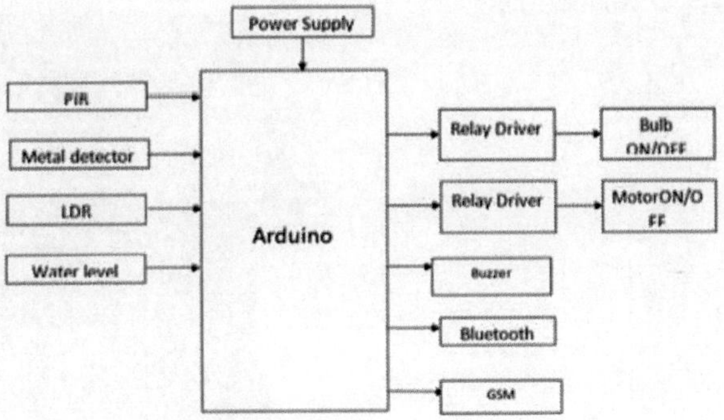

Fig. 1 Overview of the proposed system

3 Proposed System

The suggested plan inside this paper is not identical to one of the regular WSN-based superb residences [9], that are using WSNs to pass controlling orders for home working frameworks. The main motivations for the designed antenna are to raise awareness of a clear home remote controller and to reduce the effect of far-off resistance on the WSN [10] innovation for a sharp layout and data collection device. The proposed platform, which is intended for protection and to screen, consists primarily of Arduino software and a meter. To monitor the hardware, the Micro-controller board is connected to the internet through the Modulated signal Killing (MODEM) GUI. When an individual enters the house and the PIR sensor detects them, it sends out a different task to regulate, such as turning on the light and fan. We may use Wearable technology to control domestic electrical equipment such as light bulbs, fans and engines (IOT). For identifying metal for identifies cheat, the product tracking device is used. If some unknown party comes into another phone app zone, it would be personal to the property owners. Following that, a water reservoir is used to assess the total available in the drain pipe. LDR is used to naturally switch on the lighting in the evenings and turn off lights all through the day.

The A PIR sensor can also be placed above the hospital's head so that when he wakes up, the switch in the police station turns on, alerting the hospital personnel. The LDR sensors measure illumination from inside the hospital and control the lighting in the corridors and other areas. The metal detector sensor can be placed in the doctor's office so that if someone approaches the room playing metal ions, the bomb sounds off and the doctors and nurses are notified (Fig. 2).

Hardware Implementation

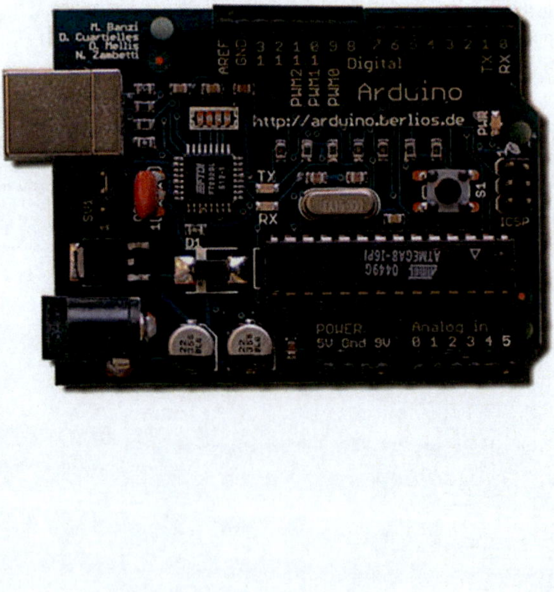

Fig. 2 Aurdino UNO

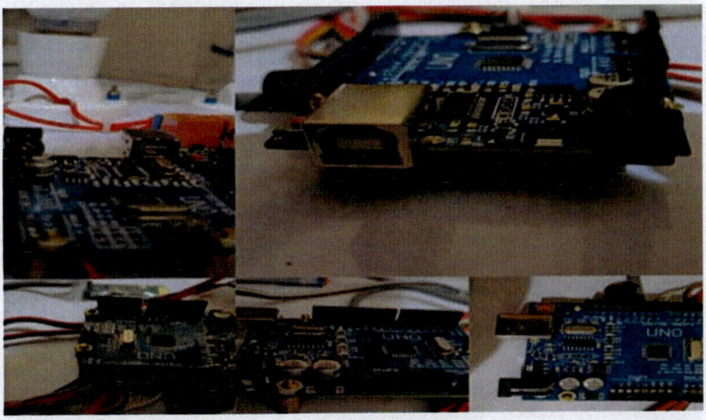

Fig. 3 Hardware Aurdino UNO

3.1 Aurdino UNO

Arduino Uno Arduino is a device that allows you to appear well-intentioned when controlling a larger portion of the adult situation beyond your computer. It's an active real-time computing platform based on a simple microcontroller module, as well as a development environment for writing programs for the system. The ATmega328 is used in the Arduino, which is a microcontroller. A USB connection, a force jack, an Honest view and a 16 MHz clay transformer light switch are among the 14 computerised feedback pins (of which six can be used as PWM returns). It includes anything needed to assist the processor; basically, attach it to a PC through USB or compel that with an Ond cable or battery to get started."Arduino is a real-time recording level that is open-source. The Buying framework is built on a basis so I also row and an enrichment layout. The microcontroller can be used to make self-contained connected devices. Otherwise, it could be linked to the computer's coding." A real Input/Output (I/O) board with such a configurable Embedded System (IC) (Fig. 3).

3.2 Bluetooth

Bluetooth HC-05 module The HC-05 The Bluetooth module is also used to connect between Arduino Ide and a device over a distance. The HC-05 is a slaves device that runs on 3.6 to 6 V of fuel. State, RXD, TXD, GND, VCC and EN are the six pins. Assign the TXD pin of the Bluetooth enabled device HC-06 to RX (pin 0) of the Arduino Board and the RXD pin to TX (pin 1) of the Arduino Uno for equipment. Adriano's connection with the Bluetooth (BT) unit is sketched forth (Fig. 4).

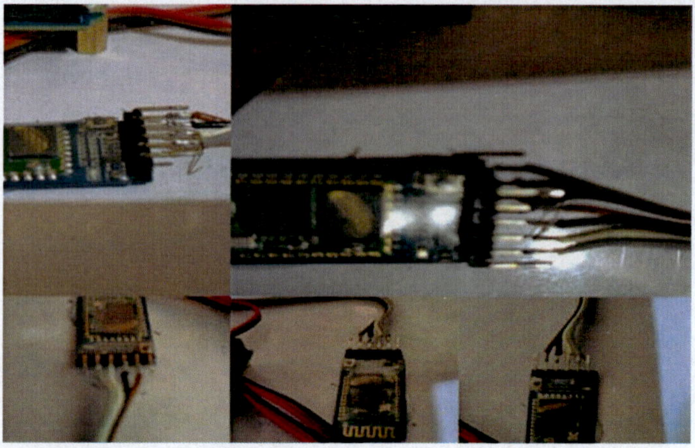

Fig. 4 Bluetooth hardware

3.3 Pir

A PIR tracker senses activity by detecting the heating emitted by a living body. These are often mounted on security cameras so that they can switch on as soon as an individual approaches. They are incredibly convincing when it comes to upgrading home surveillance systems. The sensor is turned off because, but instead of sending lighting or metastasis, it really should be obstructed by a passing individual to "sense" The person, the PIR, is sensitive to the cosmic rays emitted by all living things (Fig. 5).

At an intruder walks into the field of view of the monitor, the tracker "sees" a sudden increase in thermal energy. A PIR sensor light is expected to turn on as someone approaches, but it won't react to someone passing. The lighting is set up in this manner.

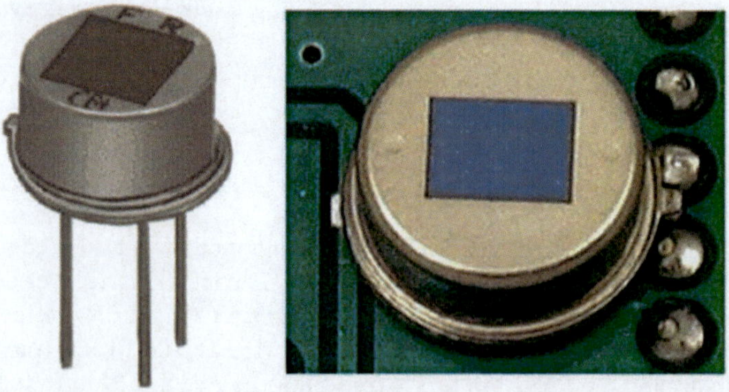

Fig. 5 PIR

The spatial production of the PIR sensor is obtained in Fig. 7 and also the operational amplifier of the PIR sensor is obtained in Fig. 7. The PIR sensor is primarily used only for action track and to reduce power usage. When an individual walks into the room, the colour will change on and the transfer function will be produced and in PC, as seen in Fig. 6.

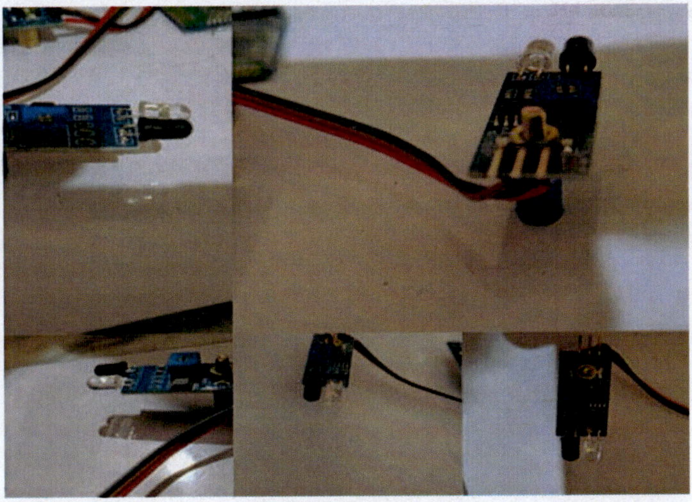

Fig. 6 Hardware PIR

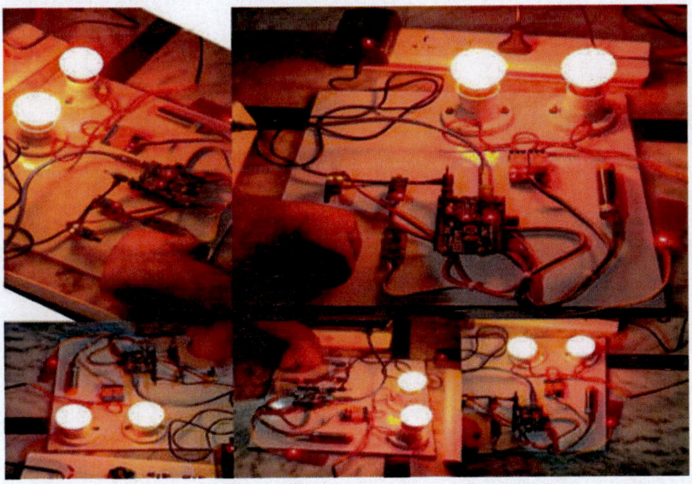

Fig. 7 PIR sensor output

3.4 Metal Detector

Metal A locator is an automated visual depiction of metal in the immediate vicinity. Metal detectors are useful for locating metal speculations hidden inside objects or metallic articles deep underground. They routinely involve a handheld unit with a sensor. This is a test that can then be run on the land or on different posts. A shifting sound in earbuds or a needle proceeding forward a pointer appear if the indicator steers against a hunk of iron. The device frequently provides a sign of location; the closest the metal is to the headphones, the louder the sound or the further the device goes. Set "walk around" iron reminders used for security bugs at ways in confinement workplaces, civic centres and airports to detect rotating steel arms on a part of the body are also another basic kind. As the LC circuit, which really is L1 and C1, receives a dissonant repeat on any material nearby, an electromagnetic field is generated and causes a stream to flow up and down and alters the sign direction through twist. In comparison to the circuit, a reference voltage is often used to adjust the togetherness indicator. It is far smarter to verify the distance as there is a circle and no strategy for dealing with the material (Fig. 8).

Right LC circuit may have altered sign as the metallic is seen. The modified sign is sent to the proximity indicator (TDA 0161), which will detect the shift in the flag and react accordingly. The attract system yields 1 mA when no object is observed and around 10 mA once the circle is near to the earth. Once the express trigger is high, the resistor R3 can give a reference voltage to silicon Q1. Q1 will indeed be switched on and the drive will shine, as well as the doorbell. The regulator r2 limits the current channel (Fig. 9).

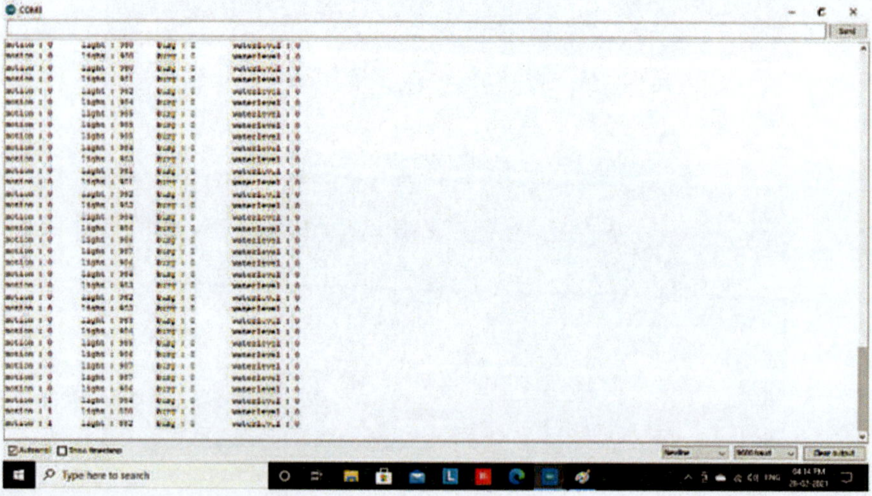

Fig. 8 Digital sensor PIR output

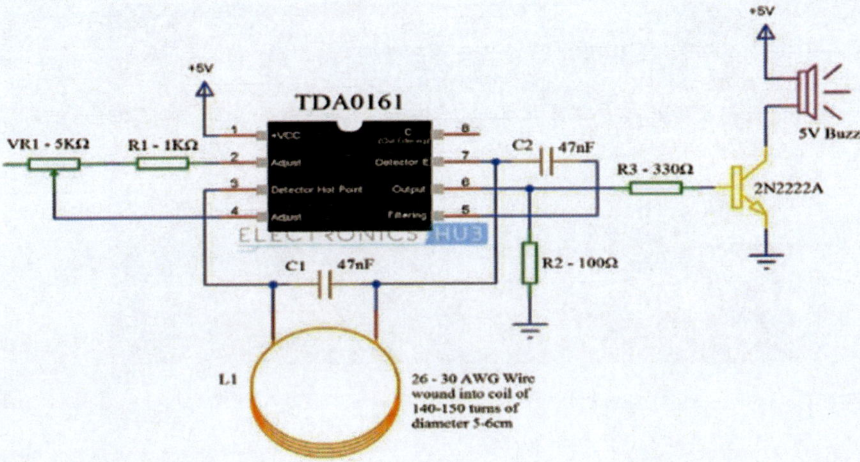

Fig. 9 Digital sensor PIR

The real out of the metal detector sensor is seen in Fig. 11 above, while the voltage signal of the metal detector sensor is shown in Fig. 11. The metal detector is mostly used to locate metal and for safety purposes. When an object is detected and also an alarm sounds, the display can be seen in Fig. 10 and also the sensor signal received in a PC is seen in Fig. 12.

LDR Sensor

A heat variable, also known as a photographic diode, colour resistor (LDR), or photoconductor. A picture resistor's opposing decreases as the event illumination

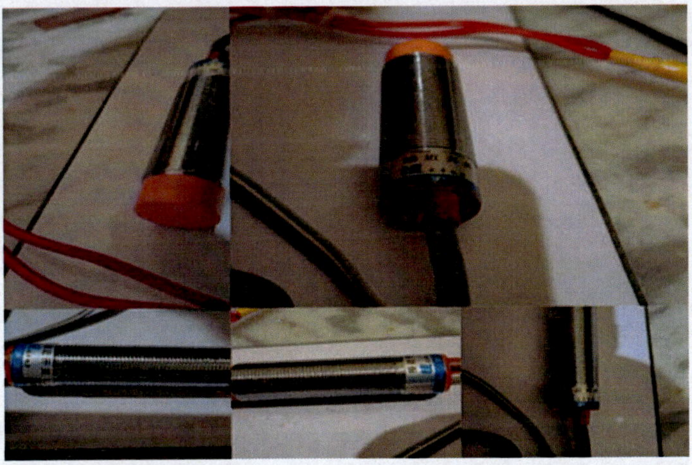

Fig. 10 Hardware of metal detector

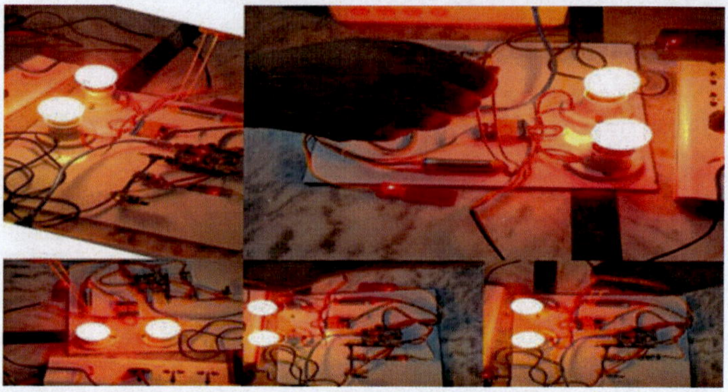

Fig. 11 Output of metal detector

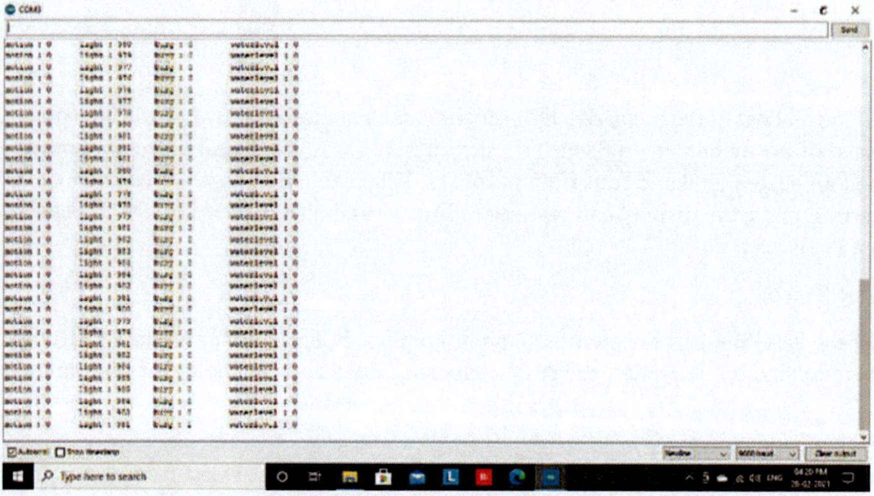

Fig. 12 Digital output of metal detector

voltage increase, indicating photoelectric effect. In light-sensitive identifier circuitry and glow dim activated sharing protocols, an image regulator may be used. An image resistor is produced of a transistor with high resistance. An image resistor can get an obstruction as high as a few mega ohm (M) in the dark, in the sun, it can have distortion as low as very few hundred ohms. If the incidence light on a photosensor exceeds a predetermined occurrence, photons consumed by the semiconductor provide enough energy for bound electrodes to jump into the conduction band following that, the charge carriers (and their opening companions) guide force, lowering conflict. The distortion scope and assorted variety of a picture blocker can vary greatly between different devices. In fact, fascinating photo transformers can react differently to photons within particular frequency categories (Fig. 13).

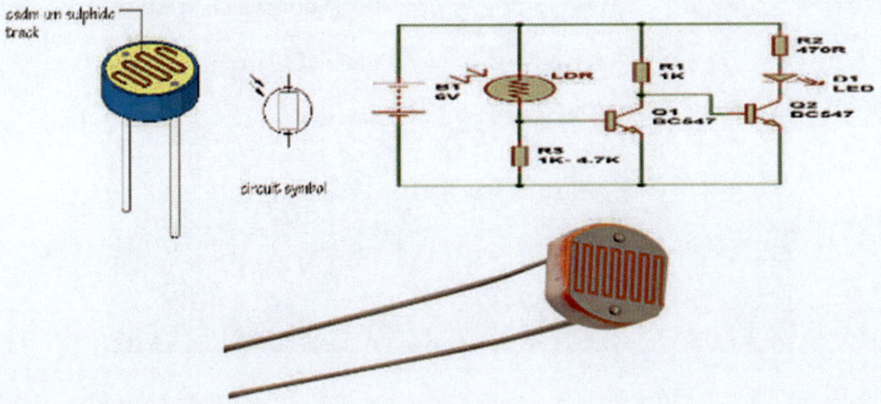

Fig. 13 LDR sensor

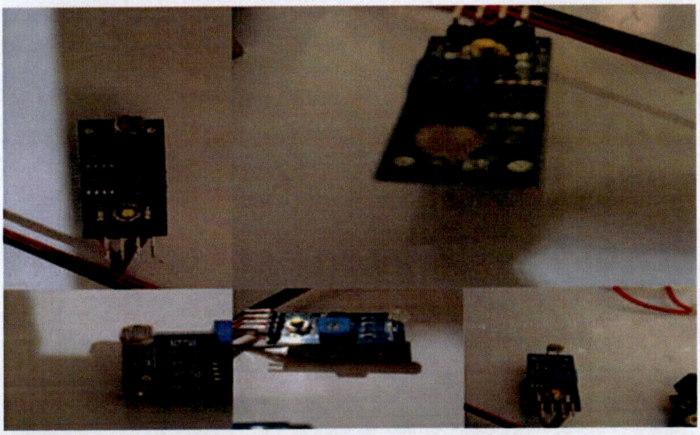

Fig. 14 Hardware of LDR sensor

The visible out of the LDR sensor is shown in Fig. 15, or the operational amplifier of the LDR sensor is shown in Fig. 16. The LDR sensor senses light output and turns on the lighting so when intensity of light in it is extremely low, as seen in Fig. 15, which is great for students who could really toggle on the lights at a certain time. Figure 16 depicts the display screen achieved in a Device (Fig. 14).

3.5 *Water Level Sensor*

Level Neurotransmitters discern various oils and fluidised bed particles such as blends, ridged materials and powders with a higher solid body. Level sensors can

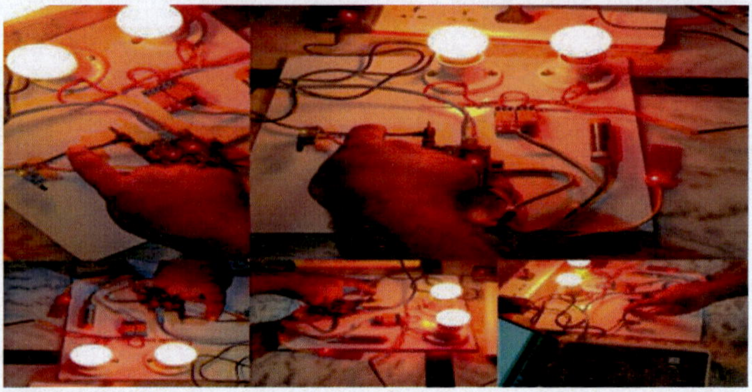

Fig. 15 Output of LDR sensor

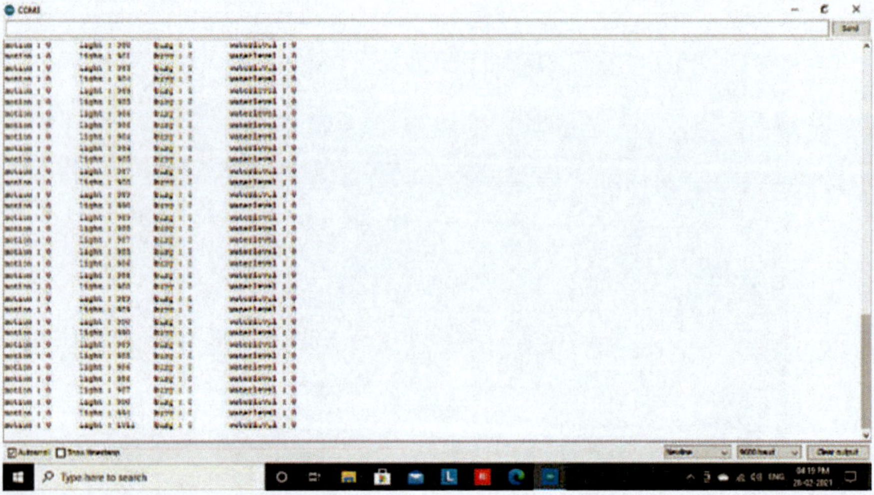

Fig. 16 Digital output of LDR sensor

detect the level of free-flowing liquids, as their name suggests. Fluids include water, grease, mixtures and other emulsions, as well as solid particles of cement matrix, which are included in those materials (solids which can stream). These compounds can, in general, because of the force, become at balance or in storage facilities, maintaining their amount in closed condition. The level of a sensor is measured against a standard index (Figs. 17 and 18).

The visible output of the water level sensor is obtained in Fig. 19 and the voltage signal of the water level sensor is obtained in Fig. 20. A water level sensor is primarily used for detecting water level and motor switch, as seen in Fig. 19 and indeed the voltage signal obtained is observed in Fig. 20.

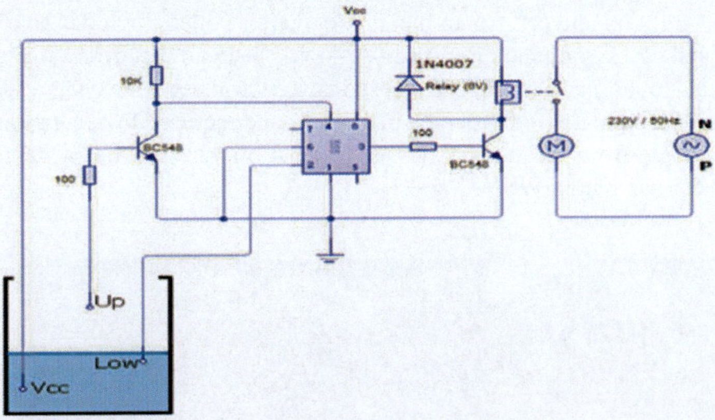

Fig. 17 Water level sensor

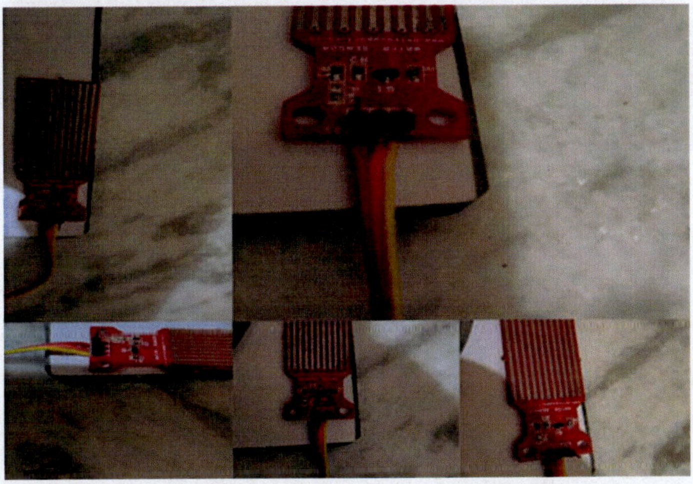

Fig. 18 Hardware of water level sensor

Relay Module

A leg is an electrically driven mechanism that could be turned down the brightness. This device is used in the field of force coverage. This is applicable to all AC and DC systems. This device is small, consistent and secure. It regulates an input torque. The turn component is depicted in Fig. 22. The first section is the genius transfer apparatus, which is connected to the existing wiring of machine tools in the home, such as a roof cooler and lights to obtain electricity. This unit will significant contributions from the lifestyles and unrelated home stocks that are linked to the action module. With a 5 V amplifier style Dc power Wi-Fi connection, it is 240 VAC to turn from (AC) to (DC). The hand-off component's potential as a usual switch "ON" and "OFF" will toggle a light on and off. An ambient recognizing system includes an ultrasonic camera as well as a switch module and an Arduino Wi-Fi connection. Wi-Fi is an RF module with a lot of features that can be used on a central network system. The IEEE 802.15.4 standard greatly reduces the amount of code required to ensure knowledge exchanges. Aside from its data warehousing capabilities, Wi-Fi has a slew of other advantages for use with a WSN (Fig. 21).

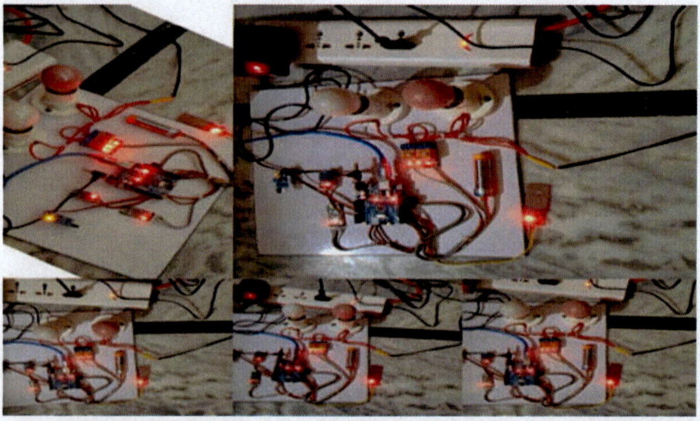

Fig. 19 Water level sensor output

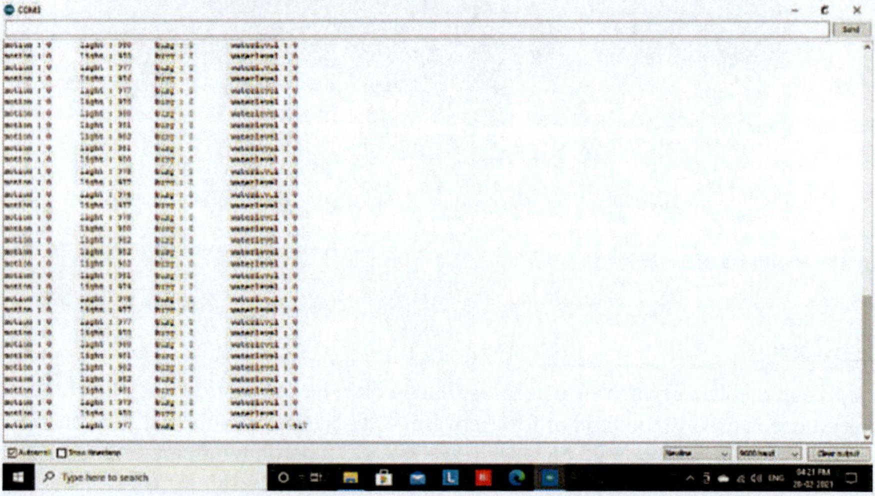

Fig. 20 Digital output of water level sensor

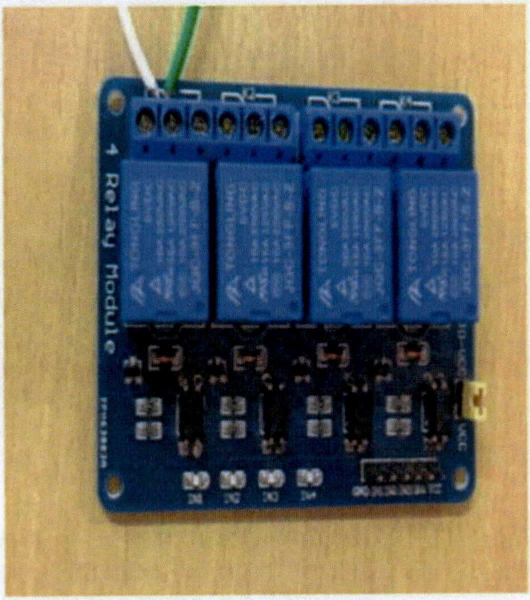

Fig. 21 Relay module

3.6 GSM

The GSM protection platform sends immediate messages based on the sensors used in this module. If the PIR sensor detects something out of the norm, the server will be notified immediately. This indicates that there is someone close to the house who is not the customer. With the aid of fire detection, the GSM also plays an important role in the fire alarm system. When smoke is detected, the guide dog an SMS alert via GSM.

4 Conclusion

The proposed kit is a practical method for partnering with your house. It also has a management structure that is used for interaction. It improves the intelligence and efficiency of household partnerships. A structure and production concept for a fantastic home advancement device based on the Arduino microcontroller board is published in this research scheme. The microcontroller board is connected to the sensing. Due to any signals received from similar sensors, the residential mechanically installations can be tested, managed and accessed normally. The device is reliant on electricity. The partnership will be terminated and SMS ready restrictions will be lifted if the power source falls short of expectations. For defence productivity, every power centrepiece energises the security mechanism. It is not able to achieve

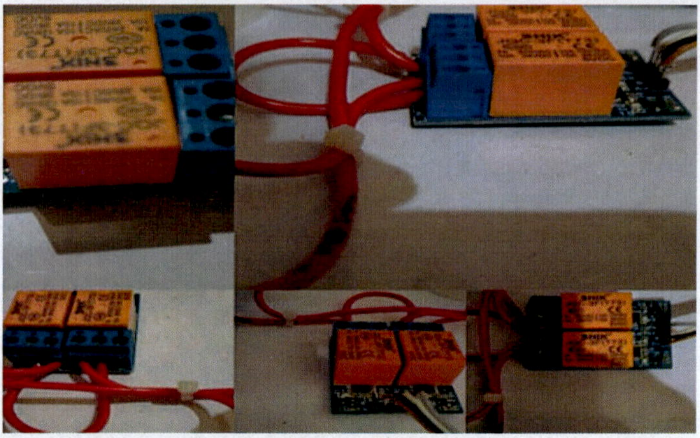

Fig. 22 Relay driver hardware

the framework without a security framework. Any base cost may even be induced in the conceptual proposal for dream homes or buildings. It alters the problem of establishing trading centres in WSNs and expands the effect of far-flung blocks. The suggested system was said to be a foundational, monetarily informative and adaptable system.

References

1. Pawar NPS (2016) A home automation system using Internet of Things. Int J Innov Res Comput Commun Eng 4(4)
2. Choudhary V, Parab A, Bhapkar S, Jha N, Medha Kulkarni Ms (2016) Design and implementation of Wi-Fi based smart home system. Int J Eng Comput Sci 5(2)
3. Vinay Sagar KN, Kusuma SM (2015) Home automation using internet of things. Int Res J Eng Technol (IRJET) 2(3)
4. Pawar PN, Shruti Ramachandran P, Varsha V Wagh4 (2016) A survey on internet of things based home automation system. Int J Innov Res Comput Commun Eng 4(1)
5. Kunal D, Tushar D, Pooja U, Vaibhav Z, Lodha V (2016) Smart home automation using IOT. Int J Adv Res Comput Commun Eng 5(2)
6. Santhi H, Gayathri P (2016) A review of home automation using IoT applications. Int J Comput Sci & Eng Technol ISSN : 2229-3345 7(07)
7. Jain SA, Maineka S, Nimgade P (2017) Application of IoT-WSN in home automation system: a literature survey. Multidiscip J Res Eng Technol 3(1):916–922
8. Gwang JK, Jang CS, Yoon CH, Jin Janz S, Woo Lee J (2013) The implementation of smart home system based on 3G and zigbee in wireless network system. Int J Smart Home 7(3):311–320
9. Bangali J, Shaligram A (2013) Design and implementation of security systems for smart home based on GSM technology. Int J Smart Home 7(6):201–208
10. Anuja P, Murugeswari T (2013) A novel approach towards building automation through DALI-WSN integration. Int J Sci & Res Publ 3(4):1–5
11. Goldsmith A (2017) "Wireless sensor networks technology for smart buildings" for Funded project final survey report in precourt energy efficiency center, pp 1–5

Eye Controlled Wheel Chair System for Physically Challenged People

S. Karthikeyan, M. Maheshwar Reddy, Md. Dhariq Refai, R. Narmadha, and S. Jayanthi

Abstract As per another report mutually set up by the World Bank and the WHO, on the planet there are 15% handicapped are incapacitated. Utilizing an amazing wheelchair to drive paddling is one of the principal steps to coordinate individuals with extreme physical and scholarly inabilities into society. For seriously incapacitated individuals, driving a wheelchair is a troublesome assignment except if the tongue is utilized to control the toy stick. Simultaneously, the visually impaired and the handicapped deal with two issues, which establish an unforgiving climate for them, which imply haughtiness and limitation. Different projects have been intended to conquer the previously mentioned issues lastly permit clients to perform safe activities and perform significant day-by-day life undertakings. The mechanical wheelchair utilizes eye development and head development to control the wheelchair. Moreover, we can speak with room gear, for example, fans, by utilizing a similar head development to give more autonomy to the incapacitated. Use RF transmitter and collector to finish this correspondence. Utilizing this capacity, you can undoubtedly control different gadgets.

Keywords Wheel chair · RF transmitter · Visually impaired

1 Introduction

Wheelchairs are intended to assist individuals with inabilities to move around and perform day-by-day exercises, yet consider the possibility that the debilitated have serious incapacities. There are many savvy wheelchairs being produced. With the headway of innovation, new and more brilliant wheelchairs entering the market will help the seriously impaired. Our wheelchair is the exertion of beginning, standing, and moving the wheelchair through the simple developments of the eyes and head.

S. Karthikeyan (✉) · M. Maheshwar Reddy · Md. Dhariq Refai · R. Narmadha
Department of ECE, Sathyabama Institute of Science and Technology, Chennai, India

S. Jayanthi
Department of ECE, Sri Manakula Vinayagar Engineering College, Pondicherry, India

N. Marriwala et al. (eds.), *Emergent Converging Technologies and Biomedical Systems*, Lecture Notes in Electrical Engineering 841,
https://doi.org/10.1007/978-981-16-8774-7_18

Furthermore, we likewise associated different modes in the wheelchair room and associated them with the RF module. Hence it is more conscious of walking for elder people's neediness. Because the foveal vision is very important for old age people compared to younger ones. The significance of a focal or fringe sightsees misfortune on the vision procedure acclimated manage strolling adopt by mensuration strolling techniques for outwardly obstructed adherents. Companion in treatment vivid virtual setting was adapted separately the standard procedures for the optic-stream and egocentric-heading approaches by counteracting the walker's inspiration of reading from the precise course of strolling. Conditions comprised of an objective at spans a coppice, the detached alone, or the backwoods alone after a speedy show of the objective. Marginal vision is the main important procedure for ambulatory. It has to be stabilized and making the flexibility in an appropriate way. The mind requires data from the eyes until it can see objects in the atmosphere. When this evidence is available, the cerebrum will use it to build an emotional picture of the situation. In general, we have the imprint that we see the refinements of our environmental influences unmistakably, and our visual perception is smooth and consistent. The expansion of firmly fitting contact lenses has resulted in supplementary precise eye undertaking soundtracks, and ways like compelling search coils are the greatest effective choice for scientists working the dynamic and physiology underlying eye movement. This approach permits eye movements within the vertical, horizontal, and torsion directions.

2 Related Work

An enormous number [1] of individuals create spinal line wounds each year, and about a portion of them cause quadriplegia. Loss of human portability is one of the significant changes in life achieved by quadriplegia, and strolling has become a deep-rooted battle. Quadriplegics depend on electric wheelchairs to move, however without hands control frameworks are right now huge and costly. The point of the undertaking is to plan an electric wheelchair with another control framework, reasonable for quadriplegics with a face shape, and a brilliant camera and flicker sensor changed before the client's face. Face zone was discovered dependent on the Ada Boost learning calculation. At that point utilize the Flandmark Detector to distinguish milestones. In this paper [2] uplifted wheelchair constrained by eye-to-eye connection and squinting. The camera is set before the wheelchair client and is used to take photographs of subtleties. Successive pictures are deciphered as visual direction and flicker structure. The course of the view is addressed by the even review point, which can be found in the triangle framed by the focuses of the eyes and nose. The review and flickering aides are utilized to give directional guidelines and time, individually. The course order is identified with the development bearing of the electric wheelchair, and the time grouping is identified with the development season of the wheelchair.

In this paper [3], electric wheelchairs with high portability affectability are quite possibly the main strides for individuals with serious physical and mental inabilities to mingle. For individuals with extreme incapacities, wheelchair access is a drawn-out undertaking other than the control of toy twig using their patois. The visually impaired and the incapacitated need to manage two issues at a time, which can make them become diverted, which is the development and the standing position. To conquer the issues referenced above, different projects are being created to permit end clients to do more secure exercises and complete certain significant undertakings in everyday life. The venture [4] examined wheelchairs dependent on eye-to-eye connection and non-verbal communication. This task is helpful for individuals who can't do anything because of sickness, injury, or inability. They can move the wheelchair to one side and right by taking a gander along the edge you need, or they can use different eyes and body hands to begin and position the wheelchair.

3 Existing System

In this framework, we would now be able to utilize optical sensors to control the wheelchair dependent on the development of the eye cover. It can begin and balance the wheelchair in a matter of moments.

Regardless of whether you flicker or open your eyes, squint. With the assistance of lighting the appreciation, the optical sensor works, and in addition to that the palpebra in ultraviolet region and uses a phototransistor and a differential circuit to identify changes in mirrored light.

At the point when the eyes flicker, it implies that the wheelchair can push ahead. Multiple times implies turning left and multiple times implies turning right. Supplementing Communication Potentials [5] between People with Agility Losses and their Close Situation. With the help of eye blink sensors [6, 7] and software solutions (keil) [8, 13] solve the difficulties of ailment individuals. Solution also produces with the help of [6, 9, 10] special instruments. Existing systems have its own limitations solution given with [11, 12] image processing.

4 Proposed System

In this system, we used eye blink sensor to control the wheelchair. Firstly we map the house or any area and then we give the command to the wheelchair by eye blink sensor and the controller.

When the eye blink sensors detect two blinks means it goes to move first room and then it detects three blinks means it goes to move to next room, three times means goes to move fourth room and, etc.

The projected arrangement is very useful and no need to regulator the helm chair as per the direction.

5 Implementation of Prototype Model

5.1 Motor Driver

The 16 pin L293D is a popular IC used for driving the motor. It is used principally for driving the motor alone. This IC has the power to drive two motors of DC sort at the same time and it's additionally ready to management the direction of motors severally. This IC will be the correct high-quality if the engines with the power of less than 36 V, with the presence of 600 mA which can be measured by circuits of 555 timers, op-amp, Arduino, ARM, PIC, etc. The motorized heavy is made humble using this L293D IC.

Half H-bridge is the employed attitude of this integrated route. Here, using H-bridge set up the motorized innings together in anti-clockwise and clockwise courses. As supposed earlier, this integrated device can run the motor at a comparable time; the arrangement for this is shown in Fig. 1. In this we used 15v battery to function motors it is associated with motor motorist (Fig. 2).

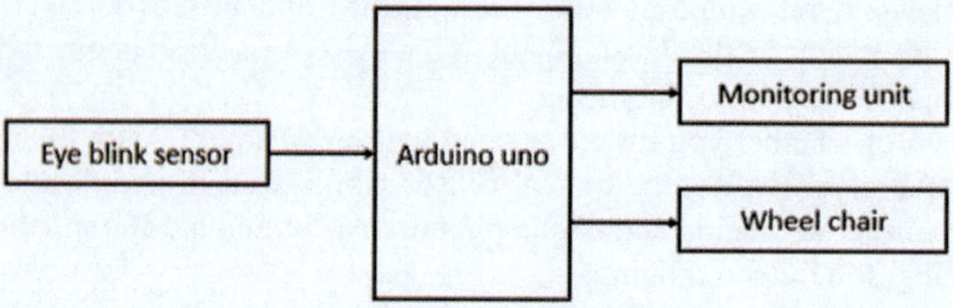

Fig. 1 Proposed system with sensors and software solutions

Fig. 2 Motor driver

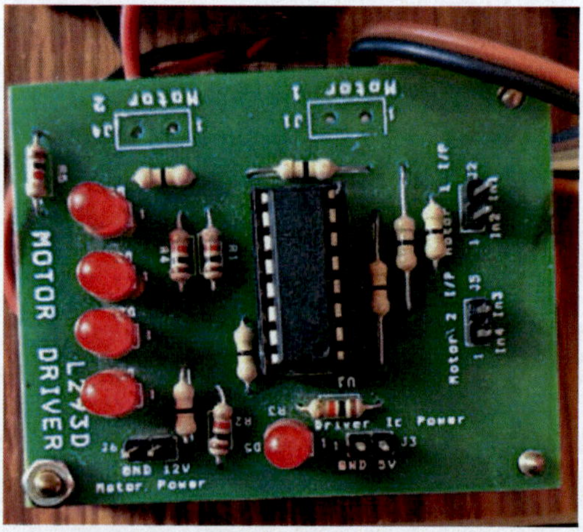

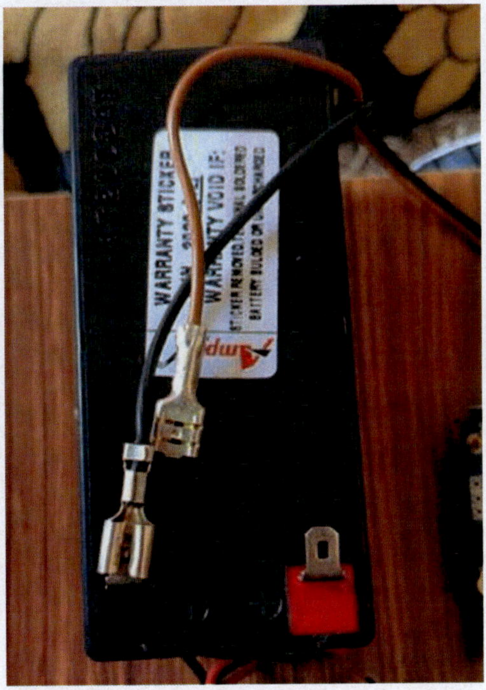

Fig. 3 Battery

5.2 *Eye Blink Sensor*

Figure 3 is used for emitting and detecting infrared radiation. In Fig. 4 there are two parts which are LED for light production and the handset. If the thing is adjacent to the device, the IR frivolous from connection rectifier can get reflected off to the thing and it'll be detected by the receiver appearance. The proximity sensors are used for detection of the obstacles. An Active Infrared sensor will be acting as proximity sensor here. The diversity outside the eyes will change with the blink of an eye. When the eyes are closed, the output is high and the output is low. This knows whether the eye is closed or open area. This output is equipped with a signal circuit to indicate an alarm. Since you don't understand the eyes, you can use it for projects including risk management.

5.3 *Arduino UNO*

Figure 5 is an Arduino board which are used for the supervisory of the definite world than the Individual Processer management. This dispensation period is an exposed foundation for the microcontroller boarding and it can be intelligent to do development software design on the boarding. This boarding is a microcontroller that

Fig. 4 IR sensors

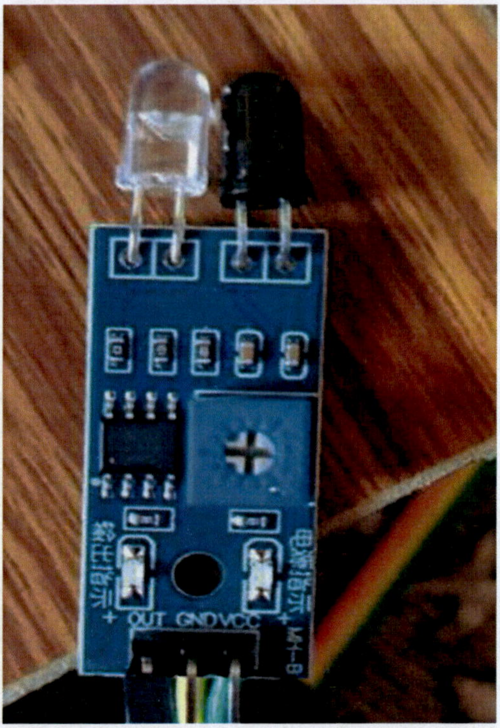

is contingent on ATmega328. It has electronic 14 input/produce pins, in which six pins are material sources which are of 16 MHz clay resonator, force jack, ICSP header, switch for rest, and USB connotation. It has all that can be help the microcontroller in interfacing to individual processer with a USB or with an AC current to DC current get-together or it necessitates a cordless to inaugurate. "Using the software solution must be an open-source genuine recordkeeping period."

5.4 Sensor Output

From Fig. 5 we know that it is in on state if give a command like two blinks then it will move to first room. Same if we give three blinks means it will move to second room.

From above figures, if the LED's are blinking as shown in Fig. 6 then it is moving in forward direction. If it is blinking like shown in Fig. 7 then it is moving backward direction. If it is blinking like Fig. 8 then it is turning left. If it is blinking like shown in Fig. 9 then it is turning towards the right.

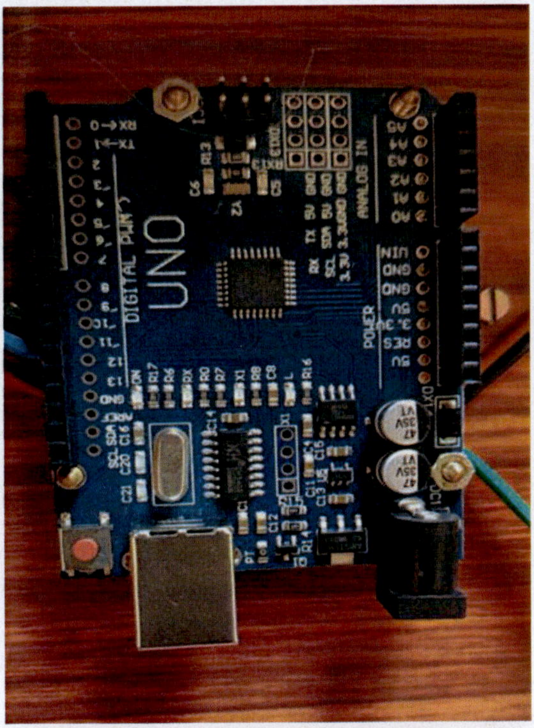

Fig. 5 Arduino

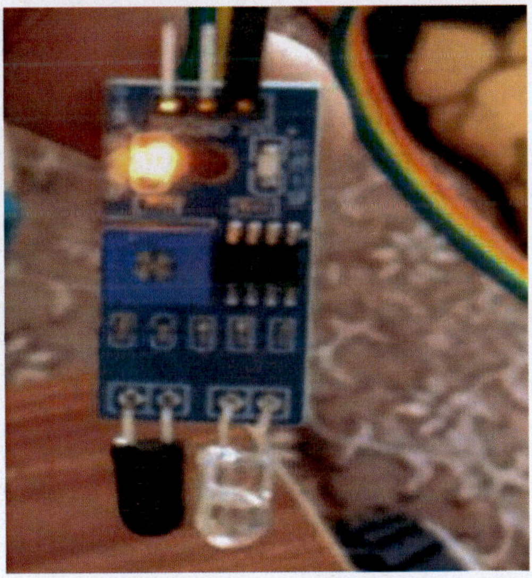

Fig. 6 IR sensor

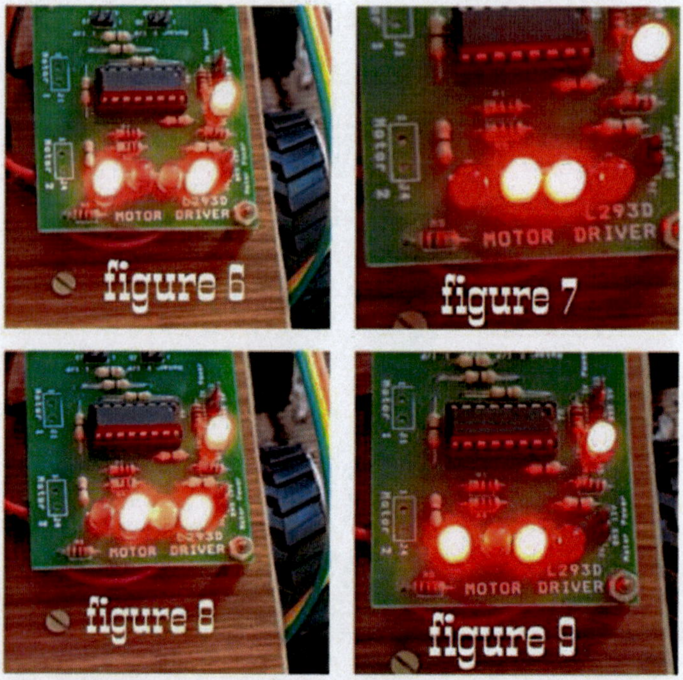

Fig. 7 Motor driver connections

Fig. 8 Output in off state

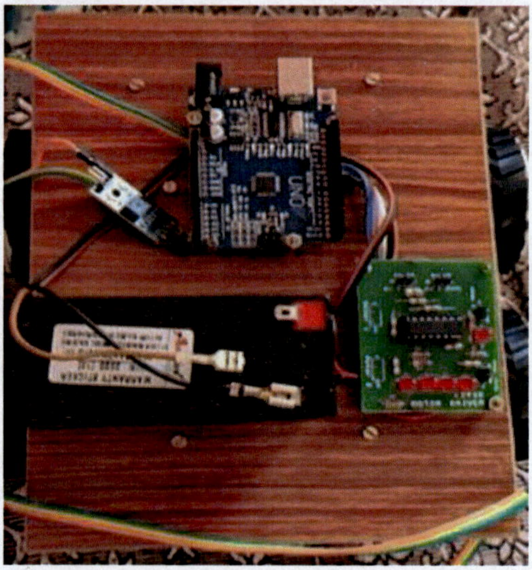

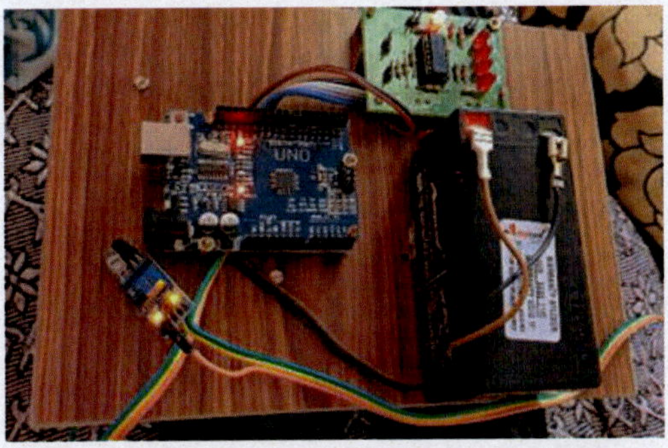

Fig. 9 Output in on state

5.5 *Vision Status and Mobility*

The wheelchair is in the off state after connecting to the battery and it is in on state, now it is ready to move.

For two blinks it will move upto	5000 ms
For three blinks it will move upto	10000 ms
For four blinks it will move upto	15000 ms
For five blinks it will move upto	20000 ms

Identification of substitute is done even on illumination except if the enhancing is covering the complete eye, this is on the estates that when the light hits the pupil and brightening banquets on the student casing complete replacement which indifferences those pixels so as we treat the bright spots it will permission behind most life-threatening modification edges that can't be strong-minded and the administrator will believe another situation to be an iris area. This communication works notwithstanding of whether depiction taken in negligible dim temperature.

References

1. Teodiano FB-F, Auat Cheein F, Member, IEEE, Müller SMT, Celeste WC, de la Cruz C, Cavalieri DC, Sarcinelli Filho M, Amaral PFS, Perez E, Soria C, Ricardo Carelli, Senior Member, IEEE (2013) Towards a new modalityIndependent interface for a robotic wheelchair. In: XXIV CongrEsso BrasIlEIro Em EngEnharIa BIomédICa, 2014
2. Gajwani PS, Chhabria SA (2010) Eye motion tracking for wheelchair control. Int J Inf Technol Knowl Manag 2(2):185–187
3. Perez E, López N, Orosco E, Soria C, Mut V, Teodiano F-B (2013) Robust human machine based on head movements applied to assistive robots. Sci World J 2013
4. Mazo M, Rodriguez FJ, Zaro JlL, Ureia J, Garcia JC (1995) Wheelchair for physically disabled people with voice, ultrasonic and infrared sensor control. Auton Robot 2(3):203–224

5. Caon M, Carrino S, Ruffieux S, Abou Khaled O, Mugellini E (2012) Augmenting interaction possibilities between people with mobility impairments and their surrounding environment. In: Communications in computer and information science, pp 1–11
6. https://learn.sparkfun.com/tutorials/accelerometer-basics/all
7. http://www.keil.com/c51/c51.asp
8. https://www.pantechsolutions.net/sensors/user-manual-for-eyeblinksensor#sthash.Rv5vb3yy.dpuf
9. http://www.engineersgarage.com/electroniccomponents/rf-module-transmitter-receiver
10. https://www.sparkfun.com/datasheets/Components/ADXL330_0.pdf
11. Koshy MM, Karthikeyan S (2017) A survey on advanced technology for communication between deaf/dumb people using eye blink sensor & flex sensor. In: Proceedings of international conference on innovations in information, embedded and communication systems (ICIIECS)
12. Balaji SR, Karthikeyan S (2017) A survey on moving object tracking system using Image Processing. In: Proceedings of 11th international conference on Intelligent systems and control, IEEE explorer conference, pp 11–16
13. Narmadha R, Rajkumar I, Sumithra R, Steffi R (2020) Continuous monitoring of electricity energy meter using IoT. Adv Intell Syst Comput 1057:731–738

Improved Sparse PLSR and Run-To-Run Algorithms for Traffic Matrix Prediction in Software-Defined Networks

Madhwaraj Kango Gopal, M. Amirthavalli, and B. Meenakshi Sundaram

Abstract Predicting the correct traffic matrix is crucial in addressing many network issues like routing, availability of networks, clear communication, etc.... In conventional networks, link load measurements are used for better traffic matrix prediction. The precision of a system, however, is small since this method does not evaluate the fundamental series of linear equations governing the problem of traffic prediction. Software-Defined Networks(SDN) offer statistics of certain forms of movements, thus providing different ways of solving issues with the traffic matrix. A network's performance and complexity can be measured using SDN. In this research work, a deep traffic matrix prediction model is proposed to evaluate the traffic in a better way. Further, the network traffic can be forecasted by using the traffic knowledge of a particular network. Gradient descent is considered to be an iterative machine learning modeling method that helps in reducing errors, optimizing weights, and thereby lowering the cost function. Evaluating the gradient of the negative likelihood equation in calculating the traffic matrix is a challenging part since all state models are composed of the gradient. In the traffic matrix, some methods deliver correct predictions, and some do not. In the proposed work, we have introduced two algorithms, the sparse PLSR and Run-2-Run algorithms for traffic prediction. A comparative study between the proposed algorithms and the already existing algorithms was done based on the training efficiency and performance in traffic prediction.

Keywords Traffic matrix · Software defined networks · Deep learning

M. K. Gopal (✉) · B. Meenakshi Sundaram
Department of Master of Computer Applications, New Horizon College of Engineering, Bengaluru, India
e-mail: dr.madhwaraj@newhorizonindia.edu

M. Amirthavalli
Department of Information Technology, SSN College of Engineering, Kalavakkam, India

N. Marriwala et al. (eds.), *Emergent Converging Technologies and Biomedical Systems*, Lecture Notes in Electrical Engineering 841,
https://doi.org/10.1007/978-981-16-8774-7_19

1 Introduction

SOFTWARE DEFINED NETWORK (SDN) is called a form of network engineering that enables the network to be operated with software applications intelligently as well as centrally or 'programmed'. This assists operators in managing the entire network continuously as well as holistically, regardless of the network innovation that underlies it. SDN is based on logically centralized network topologies for controlling and managing intelligent network resources. Present approaches to network management are distributed. With little knowledge of network status, computers usually run independently. For the type of unified control that an SDN-based network has, bandwidth management, maintenance, security, as well as regulation can be highly complex and automated, and an organization can reach a holistic point of the network. The generalization and centralization of the operation of company networks are done using SDN. Traffic programmability, flexibility as well as the opportunity to produce policy-driven network supervision and implementation of network automation are seen to be the most common benefits of SDN. Its greatest advantage is that a system for supporting more data-intensive technologies such as big data and virtualization can be developed. Machine learning techniques have been used across many disciplines too and have found to be more effective in delivering predictions [13–16].

Machine learning approaches are now being used with software-defined networks. The use of machine learning methods in SDN [1] is acceptable and effective for the reasons mentioned below. Initially, the new advances of computational technology such as the Graphics Processing Unit (GPU) and the Tensor Processing Unit (TPU) could offer a strong opportunity for promising techniques in machine learning (e.g., deep neural networks) to be applied in the network field. First, for machine learning techniques, knowledge is important for driving. The unified SDN controller has a greater knowledge of the system and could gather multiple network data for implementations of the machine learning methodology. Third, through data processing, network modeling, automatic network service delivery, machine learning algorithms focused on real-time as well as historical network data can add the intellectual capacity to the SDN controller. Finally, the programmability of SDN enables optimum network remedies (e.g., setup and allocation of resources) through machine learning techniques or deep learning architectures.

Nowadays, SDN's are used for large-scale networks too. Global network management can be comfortably done and also well-supported while using SDNs via their control plane, unified control provides large-scale network management. In wired networks, nodes are largely static but connected to high-speed links. Many reviews have recently been carried out to resolve the limitations of traditional wireless mesh networks (WMNs) in adapting the SDN architecture to WMN administration. A hybrid routing scheme was designed to enable and communicate with traditional as well as SDN-based wireless devices for existing side-by-side in the data plane.

Therefore, by using a methodology called traffic matrix prediction in a deep belief network, we deployed a traffic analysis framework for a large-scale network.

For traffic matrix estimation, we investigated a sparse partial least square regression (PLSR) and Run-2- Run PLSR algorithms.

1.1 Traffic Matrix Prediction

For network operators to incorporate heterogeneous network planning and control on a massive scale, traffic information is an important configuration input. A Traffic Matrix (TM) represents the amount of traffic that flows between all feasible nodes of origin–destination pairs (OD) in a network. Different network management operations are selected on the basis of particular types of network traffic. The problem that estimates the future traffic network from current and previous traffic network data is known as traffic matrix prediction. The advantages of prediction of the traffic matrix are as follows. Traffic flow adoption between nodes of origin and destination and two. Estimating potential network activity using known traffic data. In this work, a deep architecture for the calculation of TM has been proposed. Subsequently, by using the proposed deep architecture using known network traffic information, we predicted potential network traffic. The known TM, we assume, is X with x as its entry. First, we standardize the TM X here by splitting the X limit, such that all X entries become [0, 1]. For simplification, the TM is viewed as the standardized one without special comment during the remainder of this section.

2 Literature Survey

Two methodologies, Deep Convolution Neural Networks (DCNN) and Deep Belief Network (DBN) for large-scale networks, were suggested by Fadlullah et al. [2]. They obtained improved results depending on the rate of packet loss as well as throughput in the large-scale network. The computational complexity was significantly reduced in this work.

Nie et al. [3] recommended a deep framework for prediction and calculation of the traffic matrix. They investigated the time-varying network traffic properties in a data center network and introduced a new form of network traffic prediction focused on a deep conviction network and a logistic regression model.

Xie et al. [1] suggested node mobility to solve the traffic balancing problem. To decrease SDN controller response time, a two-layer supervised learning method was introduced in helping the controller forecast node mobility as well as connection probability of failure in adynamic network topology. They suggested an alternative selection method for the route, accomplished optimum traffic balance, and at the same time reduced the overhead control plane.

Gongming et al. [4] suggested PLSR-DBN for the recognition of a non-linear system. They removed over-fitting as well as a local minimum outcome from gradient-based learning, however in the unsupervised training process, a contrastive divergence algorithm was utilized. Utilizing PLSR- DBN, they achieved improved results on non-linear system recognition.

Tian [5] incorporated the use of SDN for the estimation of the traffic matrix. Traffic Control And Monitoring (TCAM) efficiency improved while calculating the traffic using SDN. They also achieved major productivity improvements over other strategies too.

Traffic steering methods used for the existing SDN-based SFC (Service Function Chaining) methods were applied by Hantouti et al. [6]. They used this methodology in real-life networks and found that they were performing better than the existing methods largely due to scalability and versatility.

A Gradient Boosting Decision Trees (GBDT), a community learning approach, was developed by Yang et al. [7] to predict short-term traffic based on traffic volume data collected from detectors of the freeway loop. The performance was described by integrating the data on the volume of traffic obtained as a reference by different upstream and downstream instruments, increasing prediction quality.

Camacho et al. [8] suggested a Partial Least Squares (PLS)-based gradient descent system. They also improved this approach with the usage of sparse variants of PLS. The latest published real case analysis showed the useful application of the method, revealing the relevant enhancement in detecting performance as well as the evaluation of network attacks.

A gradient fixing model was introduced by Fei et al. [9]. They designed a gradient fixing-based Gibbs sampling training algorithm (GFGS) and gradient fixing-based parallel tempering algorithm (GFPT) based on gradient fixing. They also performed a comparative analysis of novel methodologies and current methods too. They effectively resolved the gradient error issue and achieved greater training precision at low cost of computational time.

3 Traffic Matrix Estimation Framework Based on SDN—Methodology

Network problems are addressed by various traffic matrices such as congestion control, network, and traffic engineering. Calculating a precise traffic matrix of network is difficult to achieve. The reason for this is as follows. The network's traffic matrix is T = t(o,d) since t(o,d) d denotes the motion (o, d)-load of traffic from origin to destination d. The aim of the traffic matrix prediction is to find a load of each o–d flow provided each word in the matrix of traffic corresponds to one o–d.

T is defined in vector form as M = [m 1, m 2.......m J]^T, the entire traffic collection is p.

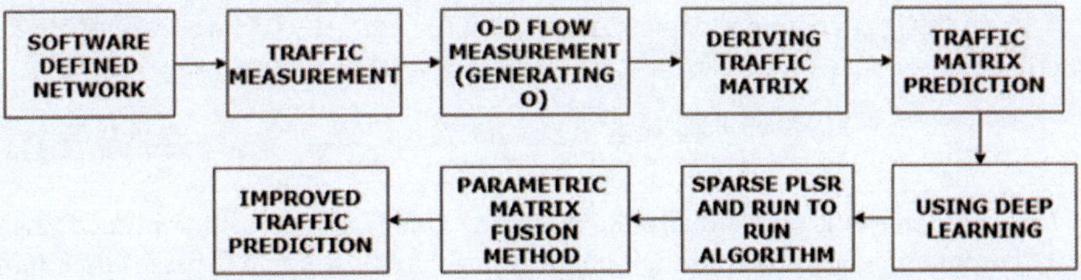

Fig. 1 Overview of the proposed work

3.1 *Traffic Measurement*

The overview of the proposed work is depicted in Fig. 1. In this work, three different types of traffic measurements [6] have been discussed:

1. Link loads: SNMP protocols are used to perform these calculations.
2. Destination-based flows: For routing, SDN flow table has a flow for each destination since this network uses shortest path routing.
3. Origin–destination (o–d) flows: SDN node flow table uses origin–destination flow for calculating traffic (as directed by the centralized controller).

The traffic matrix is calculated with the above three forms of measurements. The measurements of connection loads (type 1) and routing flows (type 2) in the network are unaltered. The measurements of Type 3 are self-selected, which is the purpose of our research. In the traffic matrix, each o–d flow resembles one variable. Ideally, as far as possible, certain flows have been used in an appropriate way for traffic calculation. For traffic estimation, we use a handful of these flows, and the focus of this paper is how to successfully carry out this process. Flow signifies o–d flow here and other flow forms may be indicated as destination-based flows.

3.2 *Underlying Linear Equations*

The network is supposed to be streamlined. There are routing nodes (conventional routers), node Band one SDN router on this network. As specified in Eq. (1), p, L, and other nodes mentioned below are added.

V: The set of nodes.
L: The set of links.
p: The set of all o–d flows. Note that $|P| = |V|(|V| - 1)$
I: The set of SDN nodes in the network, I $\subseteq$ V

A linear equation of m is defined for any flow measurement. Traffic prediction is done by considering the limitations of the linear equation.

The following equation depicts the measurements of first series(load link calculation):

$$R \cdot m = Q^R \tag{1}$$

It is noted that R is denoted as a binary matrix [L| | P| as well as link in each row, is R. Through connection J-through connection l, the flow 1 and 2 passes then the row is [1 1 0 . . . . . . .0] in R.The corresponding row will be [1 1 0 . . . . . . .0] in R.

Flow-based destination is computed from the following equation:

$$D \cdot m = Q^D \tag{2}$$

whereas $Q^D = [\, Q_1^D,\, Q_2^D \ldots\ldots\ldots\, Q_n^D]^T$ and the outcome of destination-based flow is represented as Q_i^D in the table of flow, the total number of flows based on destination is denoted as n_d, as well as D denotes a $n_d \times |P|$ binary matrix. The construction of flow based on destination is denoted by every other row in D. For example, the row in D becomes [1, 0, 0, 1, 0 . . . . . . 0] , if a flow-based destination contains o–d flow 1–4.

Measurement of o–d flow is done with the following equation:

$$O \cdot m = Q^O \tag{3}$$

whereas $Q^O = [\, Q_1^O,\, Q_2^O \ldots\ldots\ldots\, Q_n^O]^T$ as well as Q_i^O represents the measured outcome for o–d flow i.O is a $n_O \times |P|$ binary matrix. In O, each row denotes the creation of an O–d flow. Therefore, it consists of only one in each row.

By adding three pairs of equations that are linear, we get

$$A.m = Q \tag{4}$$

whereas $Q = \begin{pmatrix} Q^R \\ Q^D \\ Q^O \end{pmatrix}$ as well as $A = \begin{pmatrix} R \\ D \\ O \end{pmatrix}$.

If the network comprises multiple SDN nodes, D and O apply to multi-node measurements. Notice that certain D-rows from distinct SDN nodes can be the same because they denote the same movement depending on the destination, and the controller may delete those redundant rows. Since the controller does not install the same o–d flow for traffic measurement in separate SDN nodes (one calculation is very sufficient), all entries in O must be unique.

Before any debate, the two major characteristics of matrix A are underlined. Note that P tends to all o–d flows in the set numbers start from 1 to 1 as well as each flow the corresponding load of traffic is defined as $m = [m_1, m_2 \ldots\ldots .m_J]^T$. M is the traffic matrix–vector form, to put it another way.

- Each row in A belongs to a categorized flow type. Suppose in row A, for instance, is [1 1 0…….0], there are two o–d flows such as o–d 1st flow and o–d 2nd flow in the pooled flow.
- A flow of o–d applies to each column at A. In a column, the count of 1 s shows how many times the o–d flow occurs as other clustered flows are formed. For instance, if a column is [1, 0, 0, 1, 0…… 0], this implies that the grouped flows would contain this flow.

Rows 2 and 3 are related to A. There is one point that needs to be mentioned. Multi-path routing may be utilized along with the shortest path routing when multiple paths are of equal distance. For the traffic matrix, the only variation triggered through this multi-path routing would be that fractions, not only binary numbers, might be the value in the R as well as D matrices. And the whole system isn't evolving at all.

3.3 Generating O–d Flow

For traffic measurement selecting flow (O–d flow) relates to one row in the O matrix. The requirement for choosing an o–d flow for the traffic measurement are described in the below sections.

(i) **Prioritizing Flows**

Several tools are necessary to give a rough estimate of the flow rate. The gravity model uses the process below to predict $t_{o,d}$ (o–d load from origin o to destination d movement). Suppose.

$$m^g = [m_1^g, m_2^g \ldots\ldots m_{|J|}^g]^T,$$

whereas m_j^g denotes the flow estimated load j in J. Remember that, in the traffic matrix, m_j^g relates to one $t_{o,d}$. In that same way the resulting m_j^g is determined by the concept of gravity:

$$t_{o,d} = \frac{d_o a_d}{g}$$

whereas d_o denotes total traffic leaving its origin o, total traffic occurring at destination d is denoted as a, all of that is accessible from SNMP measurements, and constant of normalization is denoted as g which is equivalent to the inclusion of all actual traffic loads,

$$\text{i.e.,} \sum_o d_o \text{ or } \sum_d a_d \text{ or } \sum_{o,d} t_{o,d}$$

The tomgravity model is described to be improved and it is given as,

$$v^{tg} = \sqrt{m_1^g}, \sqrt{m_2^g} \ldots\ldots\ldots \sqrt{m_{|J|}^g}]^T \quad (5)$$

$$m^{tg} = [m_1^{tg}, m_2^{tg} \ldots\ldots\ldots m_{|J|}^{tg}]^T, \quad (6)$$

whereas m_j^{tg} denotes a revised value for m_j^g, m_j^{tg} derived using solved following quadratic Equation.

$$mini\left\|\frac{m^{tg} - m^g}{v^{tg}}\right\| s.t\, Q^R = R.m^{tg}, \quad (7)$$

whereas ||.|| denotes the L_2-Norm of a vector. Every MK denotes the refined predicted output from m_K^{tg}

We'll utilize m_K^{tg} throughout this section, the flow weight j in J. For the metric to be added to the flow chart, the weight is used as its initial value: the greater the weight, the greater the significance.m^{tg} is used as an original estimate of the traffic matrix. In this paper, an enhanced calculated matrix of traffic based on m^{tg} is obtained by the estimation process.

(ii) **Rank Increasing Selection Principle (RISP)**

No additional details on the traffic matrix can also be used with the inclusion of an o–d flow to the flow graph. Taking the example below into account. Tell that there will be two separate SDN nodes in the two destination-based flows, Q1 and Q2. It defines the formulations as follows:

$$Q_1 = m_1 + m_2 + m_3 \quad (8)$$

$$Q_2 = m_1 + m_3 \quad (9)$$

Next, y-1 and y-2 are calculated and then we can calculate the load of m-4. The traffic matrix will be given by the addition of o–d flow 4 to the traffic calculation flow graph with no additional information. The proposed traffic measurement method would guarantee that the load that is measured from this flow is not derived from the predominant flows of the flow tables when the centralized controller selects an o–d flow for calculation. This assures that the flow that is corresponding to the inserted flow in A is autonomous of other A rows. The added row should dramatically increase the rank of A to satisfy the requirement. In this case, the rank-increasing selection principle is followed for flow selection.

4 Deriving the Traffic Matrix

Calculating the initial traffic matrix,m^{tg}.Then enhance the estimate by measuring flows in Q. Along with Q, potential traffic matrix solutions have been situated on a hyper plane $Q = A \cdot m$. We'll pick the projected point m^{tg} on this hyperplane to render the final approximation. That is, we pick M to reduce $\left|\left|m - m^{tg}\right|\right|$.

$$\min\left|\left|m - m^{tg}\right|\right| s.t. Q = A.M$$

Traffic calculation is estimated from the above and obtained a matrix form of network traffic data. Lastly, using traffic measurement and o generation (o–d flow estimation), the traffic matrix is derived.

In our proposed work, estimation of the traffic matrix will approximate the deep learning process and Run-2-Run algorithm is used to enhance deep learning better than the current methodology. These techniques are useful in predicting the future traffic of the network. The techniques are discussed below.

4.1 Traffic Matrix Prediction Using Deep Learning

The traffic matrix forecast calculates the potential traffic of the network from previous traffic data over the network. For TM estimation, an SDN-based deep architecture has been proposed. Further, by training the proposed deep structures across established traffic data from the network, the potential network traffic was accurately predicted.

The challenging part of the deep learning-based estimation of the traffic matrix[3] is to measure the negative probability function gradient, even if the gradient consists of all state models. Since gradient descent is considered to be an iterative machine learning optimization technique that reduces cost function to a great extent, precise traffic matrix predictions are done through this model. In earlier works, they had used a contrastive divergence algorithm for estimating this gradient instead of directly computing it.

In the proposed work, we improve the gradient using deep learning instead of directly computing it. We also used the sparse PLSR variants and Run-2-Run algorithm for computing gradient. It improves optimization performance, learning ability, and computational efficiency. These techniques are useful to estimate gradients when compared with the existing contrastive divergence algorithm.

4.2 Partial Least Squares (PLS) Regression

To find the gradient, regression methods could be used for optimization. Regression methods are used to analyze high dimensional sets rather than high dimensional parameters such as scaling and gradient parameters. PLS is a regression technique, common in cases with large dimensions, and has been found to be useful in the presence of collinearity while generating the predictors.

The PLS algorithm defines H subspace that significantly increases its covariance with L, including a N ?? O solution matrix L and a N ?? M set H of predictor variables. It contains o–d flow (origin and d- destination) in traffic matrix M.

Model PLS shall be described as:

$$H = T \cdot I^T + B$$

$$L = T \cdot J^T + O$$

- Residual X and Y matrices. Where L and O are residual matrices, A is known to be a latent vector, T is N ?? A score matrix.
- The residual matrix used for the consistency model determination. The discrepancy between the observed variable and the estimated data value is used in regression analysis.
- I, J are o × d and m × d loading matrix for predictors.
- While T is defined as the matrix of the N/A score, the number of latent variables (LVs) is A, used to fit the formula. And O-A and M-A loading matrices for the predictors as well as the outcome are known as P and Q. Similarly, the residual matrices N'M and N'O are defined as E and F. A traffic predictor model was derived as follows:

$\boldsymbol{m_{n,t+1}}$ **and** $(\boldsymbol{m_{n,t}}, \boldsymbol{m_{n,t-1,\ldots.,}}, \boldsymbol{m_{n,t-w+1}})$

4.2.1 Sparse PLSR

Even though PLS can manage noisy predictor variables efficiently, the addition of variables that are not important for estimation of the response typically reduces the model's predictive efficiency.

This family of algorithms is termed as sparse partial least square regression. It is used for very high dimensionality data and also improves learning ability in the traffic matrix. In addition, the performance of the network is also improved while employing this technique.

By restricting (i.e., forcing 0) the loads that appear to be the PLS model's calculation of the relative value of each vector by solving the optimization problem, a sparse PLS solution can be obtained:

$$arg\ \mathrm{mini}||\mathrm{c} - \mathrm{p}q^t||^2{}_f + \lambda_1||p||_1 + \lambda_2||q||_2$$

4.2.2 Group-Wise PLSR

The recently suggested Group-wise PLS (GPLS) is another method for achieving sparse PLS solutions, whereby the result is derived by identifying classes of associated predictor variables instead of regularization. The GPLS algorithm will start shortly by describing a set of K (potentially overlapping) sets of associated variables derived from the M-M relationship map M calculated from the M-M relationship map M is $C = X^T Y$. The scores and weights of K PLS systems along with 1 LV are then calculated, each of which takes into account only the set of variables relevant to one of the classes. Among these, it preserves the one with the highest association with Y while the other ones are discarded. This is iterated in the case of several LVs.

For data discovery, GPLS analysis is particularly suitable. However, in terms of predictive goodness, the approach substantially outperformed PLS and SPLS once data is constrained in a GroupWise way, i.e., while there are classes of associated aspects linked to the response. To classify the variables group in M, the GPLS method fitting requires the formulation of a threshold, aiming to regulate both the size and number of the variables groups to be used simultaneously. Optimum values are graphically chosen for analyzing the correlation map M, by controlling as well as by exchanging between group size and dimension.

4.2.3 Run-To-Run Algorithm

The gradient is estimated in the previous section using PLSR Method. Let us define input as R (traffic matrix), needed to optimize network performance and predict the traffic in an SDN. W is considered as output (predicted values). The goal of this algorithm is to optimize the output W value using input R. The algorithm gave a very accurate traffic prediction.

The Run-to-Run optimization technique, used in PLS, SPLS as well as GPLS for a general optimization issue, can be described below:

Select an initial prediction parameter s and v_c (level of exploration).

1. Initialize the input R_i for i = 0.
2. Repeat initial predictor parameter from PLS method $s = \{1 \ldots\ldots\ldots S\}$
3. Generate the input R (traffic matrix)$R_i^k = R_i + v_c + v_i^k$, for v_i^k drawn from the multi-normal distribution.
4. Apply input R_i^k to the system and measure the output W_i^k
5. Setup a PLS model with k cases, then organize the input in R_i^k rows as well as the output in row R_i^k.

$$W_i = W \cdot B_i + F \tag{10}$$

6. Compute the next input $R_{i+1} = R_i + 3 \ldots B_i$
7. Check the solution for convergence and otherwise loop back to step 11

In our previous section, we discussed the process of improving the gradient using deep learning. We use PLSR, sparse PLSR, and GroupWise PLSR for improving the learning rate, and the performance of the network has also improved. A traffic predictor model as $m_{n,t+1}$ and $(m_{n,t}, m_{n,t-1,....}, m_{n,t-w+1})$ was obtained. After estimating traffic matrix prediction, the closeness, and period were calculated using the Spatio-temporal technique. After this process, these two were fused by using a parametric-based matrix. Therefore, it becomes possible to predict the traffic, maintain daily history, and also predict the traffic in SDN in an easy effective manner.

5 Spatio-Temporal Dependence

After calculating traffic matrix prediction in SDN, by treating output of predicted traffic data set as images, Spatio-temporal analysis [10] was done to find the closeness and period for predicted traffic. The output predicted traffic can be split into two-time slots, one is closeness and the other the periods. Assuming the target to be measured is the estimated amount of t slot traffic, the periods preceding t are split into two parts, i.e., the latest time and the daily history.

Let's define I as the duration of the dependency on closeness and the traffic of the current time fragment to design the dependency on temporal proximity could be defined as

$$Z_{tc} = Z_{t-i}, Z_{t-(i-1)}, \ldots\ldots\ldots\ldots Z_{t-1} \tag{11}$$

The above equation refers to closeness (recent times)of predicted traffic. The recent times come under the hour, minute, seconds. This temporal closeness dependence is called short-term traffic prediction.

In the same way, the duration of time dependency is expressed by j and the sampled traffic from everyday history can be represented as temporal dependence as follows:

$$Z'_{tp} = Z_{t-j*24}, Z_{t-(j-1)*24}, \ldots\ldots\ldots Z_{j-24} \tag{12}$$

$$Z''_{tp} = [Z_{t-j*24}, Z_{t-(j-1)*24}, \ldots\ldots\ldots Z_{j-24}] \times 7 \times Z'_{tp} \tag{13}$$

$$Z'''_{tp} = [Z_{t-j*24}, Z_{t-(j-1)*24}, \ldots\ldots\ldots Z_{j-24}] \times 4 \times Z''_{tp} \tag{14}$$

5.1 *Parametric Matrix-Based Fusion*

According to the above understanding, it is understood that the traffic of different cells is related to both proximity and time, but the significance varies from one to another.

To achieve this interaction, a parametric system based on a matrix is suggested to combine the closeness and time characteristics. Suppose that the output of the SDN is Z_C^{L+1} and Z_d^{L+1} respectively. After fusion, we have

$$Z_O = Z_C \odot Z_C^{L+1} + Z_d \odot Z_d^{L+1} \tag{15}$$

whereas $\odot$ is represented as a Hadamard product, Z_C and Z_d are the learnable parameters that demonstrate the relationship between the time of closeness and wireless traffic.

6 Results and Discussion

6.1 Performance Analysis of Traffic Prediction Ratio

The three different algorithms that were taken for performance comparison in traffic prediction are plotted in Fig. 2.

Figure 2 also depicts the traffic prediction of proposed sparse PLSR when compared with other existing methods to analyze its performance (Table 1).

In comparison, the gradient for the deep learning algorithm was determined by the contrastive divergence algorithm [3]. Traffic prediction learning rate can be increased by using this methodology. The only limitation of this method is that it is not adaptable for high-dimensional data.

The DBNSTCS algorithm [11] is used to predict the network traffic in two ways, i.e., long-range component and fluctuation dependence by low pass component and

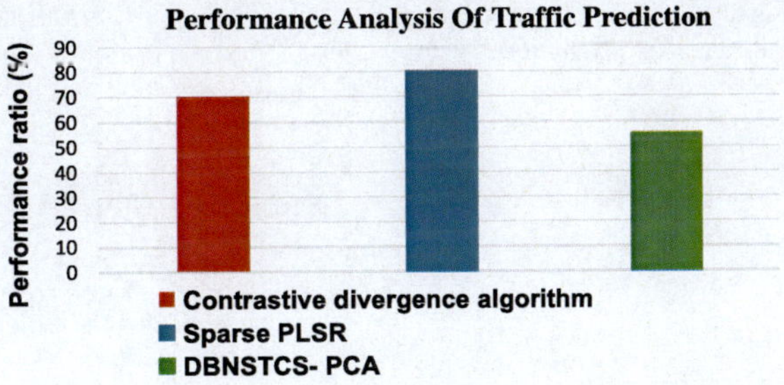

Fig. 2 Performance improvement ratio

Table 1 Comparison of performance of traffic prediction

Algorithm	Performance ratio (%)
Contrastive divergence algorithm	70
Sparse PLSR	80
DBNSTCS- PCA	55

high pass component. Owing to the lack of gradient improvement in deep learning, the efficiency study of traffic prediction was lagging to an extent.

In our proposed work, sparse PLSR is used for deep learning based on traffic matrix prediction. PLSR is used to compute the gradient of high dimensional and it is more robust. It increases learning ability and more reliably forecasts traffic. Compared to current approaches, the overall efficiency of traffic matrix estimation in large-scale networks is increased.

6.2 Training Efficiency

We equate the training efficacy of the proposed Run-to-Run algorithm with other existing approaches, as depicted in Fig. 3. It is obvious that the Run-to-Run algorithm performs better when compared with the Contrastive Divergence Algorithm and WSTNET (Table 2).

The contrastive divergence algorithm [3] is a learning algorithm that improves the training efficiency of traffic prediction based on deep learning. The only limitation is that it takes more average training time for large-scale networks. In WSTNET algorithm [12], the traffic gets predicted accurately, but there were issues while employing it on practical networks. Further, it also increased the training time, and the performance efficiency was also seen to lag while using it on a large-scale network.

Initially, in our proposed solution network-wide traffic data is processed on large scale by enabling SDN, derived from a technically centralized control system. The SDN control plane also tends to be programmable to enable the modular implementation of new network features, making it possible to incorporate the TM prediction method alongside controllers as an application. This can be used for practical

Fig. 3 Training efficiency of traffic matrix prediction

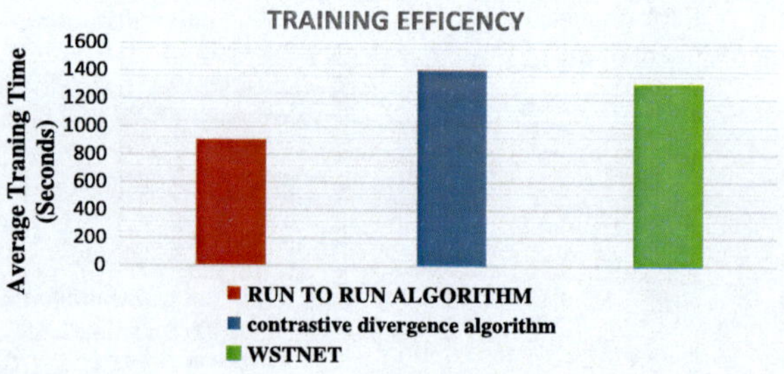

Table 2 Comparison of training efficiency

Algorithm	Average training (seconds)
Run-2-Run algorithm	600
DBN	780
WSTNET	1300

SDN implementations and mostly more reliably and efficiently follows methods of forecasting TM. Using a Run-to-Run algorithm, traffic data can be quickly trained into SDN. The training performance in deep learning-based traffic prediction gets increased and the total training time for traffic data in large-scale networks also gets decreased.

7 Conclusion

In this work, a heterogeneous framework for solving the traffic matrix prediction in a large-scale SDN has been developed. Firstly, SDN facilitates the processing of massive network-wide traffic data on a wide scale, taking advantage of the technically centralized control structure. The modular introduction of new network features is facilitated by the programmable control plane of SDN. Incorporating the TM model as an application has also become simple and looks effective. This is used for practical SDN implementations, is more reliable, and efficiently follows TM forecasting strategies. Different forms of flow were generated in SDN which gave additional opportunities to resolve the issue with the traffic matrix. A deep architecture has been suggested for traffic matrix prediction in this research work. Additionally, the proposed deep architecture was trained using known network traffic data and was found to reliably predict network traffic. The Sparse PLSR was used as the traffic matrix estimation algorithm. For high dimensional data, sparse PLSR was used and it was found to be more robust than PLSR. In this proposed work, instead of computing the traffic and gradient directly, the gradient was strengthened using deep learning. For computing gradient, we used sparse PLSR variants and the Run-2-Run algorithm. The output optimization, learning capacity, and computing efficiency were increased considerably. When compared with the existing algorithms, our approach was an effective one while calculating gradients.

References

1. Xie J, et al (2018) A survey of machine learning techniques applied to software defined networking (SDN): research issues and challenges. IEEE Commun Surv & Tutor 21(1):393–430
2. Fadlullah ZMd, et al (2018) On intelligent traffic control for large-scale heterogeneous networks: a value matrix-based deep learning approach. IEEE Commun Lett 22(12):2479–2482
3. Nie L, et al (2016) Traffic matrix prediction and estimation based on deep learning for data center networks. IEEE Globecom Workshops (GC Wkshps)
4. Gongming W, et al (2017) Nonlinear system identification using deep belief network based on PLSR. In: Proceedings of 36th Chinese control conference (CCC). IEEE
5. Tian Y, Chen W, Lea C-T (2018) An SDN-based traffic matrix estimation framework. IEEE Trans Netw Serv Manage 15(4):1435–1445
6. Hantouti H, et al (2018) Traffic steering for service function chaining. IEEE Commun Surv & Tutor 21(1):487–507

7. Yang, Senyan, et al. (2017) Ensemble learning for short-term traffic prediction based on gradient boosting machine. J SensS
8. Camacho J, et al (2019) Semi-supervised multivariate statistical network monitoring for learning security threats. IEEE Trans Inf Forensics Secur 14(8):2179–2189
9. Fei LI, Xiaoguang GAO, Kaifang WAN (2018) Training restricted boltzmann machine using gradient fixing based algorithm. Chin J Electron 27(4):694–703
10. Zhang C, et al (2018) Citywide cellular traffic prediction based on densely connected convolutional neural networks. IEEE Commun Lett 22(8):1656–1659
11. Nie L, et al (2018) Network traffic prediction based on deep belief network and spatiotemporal compressive sensing in wireless mesh backbone networks. Wirel Commun Mob Comput
12. Zhao J, et al (2019) Spatiotemporal traffic matrix prediction: a deep learning approach with wavelet multiscale analysis. Trans Emerg Telecommun Technol 30(12):e3640
13. Bellie V, Gopal MK, Venugopal G (2020) Using machine learning techniques towards predicting the number of dengue deaths in India—A case study. Int J Eng Trends Technol (Special Issue):130–135
14. Gopal MK, Bellie V, Venugopal G (2020) A novel machine learning technique towards predicting the sale of washing machines in a small organization. Int J Psychosoc Rehab 24(5):6969–6976
15. Gopal MK, Amirthavalli M (2019) Applying machine learning techniques to predict the maintainability of open source software. Int J Eng Adv Technol 8(5S3):192–195
16. Gopal MK, Venugopal G, Amirthavalli M, Meenaskhi Sundaram B (2021) A recommendation model for cultivating crops using machine learning. In: Proceedings of the Northeast Green Summit 2021, National Institute of Technology, Silchar, 16–18 November 2021

An Efficient Object and Railway Track Recognition in Thermal Images Using Deep Learning

Rohini Goel, Avinash Sharma, and Rajiv Kapoor

Abstract To avoid rail accidents, an efficient railway safety system is essential. The collision between the trains and obstacles on the railway track is one of the main reasons for accidents that result in terms reduced safety and higher financial burdens. Researchers are ceaselessly working to enhance railway safety for curtailing the accident rates. In this paper, a novel technique is discussed for recognizing the objects (obstacles) on the railway track in front of moving train. This methodology presents identification of the railway track along with deep network-based technique for recognition of obstacles on the railway track. The deep network gives the model understanding of real-world objects and enables obstacle recognition. The thermal image data is used for the training and validation of deep network. In this work, Faster R-CNN is utilized to effectively recognize obstacles on the railway tracks. This work can be an incredible assistance for railway to curtail mishaps and monetary burdens. The results demonstrate that the proposed work assists to boost railway safety with good accuracy.

Keywords Thermal imaging · Railway track detection · Hough transform · HSV color space segmentation · Faster R-CNN

1 Introduction

These days, because of the development of high-speed railways, the safety [1] prerequisites of the railways are additionally increasing continuously. As the high-speed railways straightforwardly lead to an increase in train mishaps. Numerous individuals lose their lives in train mishaps every year. The elements liable for the mishaps are, such as obstacles on the railway tracks, human mistakes, and unfavorable climate

R. Goel (✉) · A. Sharma
CSE Department, Maharishi Markandeshwar (Deemed to be University), Mullana, Ambala, Haryana, India

R. Kapoor
Department of ECE, Delhi Technological University Delhi, Delhi, India

N. Marriwala et al. (eds.), *Emergent Converging Technologies and Biomedical Systems*, Lecture Notes in Electrical Engineering 841,
https://doi.org/10.1007/978-981-16-8774-7_20

conditions. The obstruction due to obstacles is because of the carelessness of pedestrians and vehicles crossing the tracks, animals strolling on the tracks and any other heavy non-living item fallen on the track from the overpass. The human error can happen because of the laxity of driver/railway staff. The unfavorable natural conditions like low visibility because of haze and rain can cause issues. Many railways crossing in various countries need sufficient admonition devices like gates and lights. These issues cause troubles for the travelers as well as lead to monetary loss to railways as train cancellations and accidental compensations paid to infested individuals. These problems can be vanquished by utilizing an early admonition framework that not just tracks the obstacles and earlier cautions the driver yet also aids in unfavorable climate conditions. This framework can enormously mitigate the number of train mishaps occurred because of obstacles and troublesome climate conditions. The object on the railway track might be a moving body [2]. Several research has been done to distinguish and recognize moving object, such as M. Irani et al. [3] discussed a unified methodology dependent on the separation of the moving object detection in situations and relating techniques. R. Cucchiara et al. [4] introduced an HSV color space analysis-based shadow detection and suppression method for moving visual object identification and tracking. S. Mockel et al. [5] delineated a multisensory obstacle detection framework dependent on fusion of active and passive optical sensors. J. J. Garcia et al. [6] showed an intelligent framework dependent on optical emitter and codification technique to recognize obstacles in railway tracks. N. Hautiere et al. [7] introduced a strategy for estimating visibility distance under hazy climate utilizing vehicle-mounted camera and implementing Koschnieder's Law. S. Wu et al. [8] portrayed a novel strategy for crowd modeling and anomaly detection dependent on particle trajectories, chaotic dynamics, and probabilistic systems. J. J. Garcia et al. [9] proposed a multisensory framework comprised of infrared and ultrasonic that can inform about the presence of obstacles on railway tracks. X. Zhou et al. [10] combined object recognition and background learning by proposing a unified system named DECLOR for moving object identification. Y. Chen et al. [11] proposed a technique dependent on image matching and frame coupling to handle the object detection issue caused by moving camera and object motion. A. Berg et al. [12] proposed a technique for obstacle detection on the railway track utilizing monocular thermal camera and gained a novel data collection. H. Mukojima et al. [13] proposed a background subtraction based strategy to distinguish obstacles on the railway tracks utilizing images captured from train frontal view camera. D. Sinha et al. [14] introduced an object identification approach on railway tracks utilizing vibration sensors and filter out the sign from high-level acoustic noise utilizing a novel Monte Carlo based Bayesian analysis. V. Amaral et al. [15] portrayed obstacle detection systems in railway level crossing utilizing 3D point clouds gained with 2D laser scanner. Y. Wu et al. [16] introduced a coarse to fine thresholding plan on particle trajectories in video of moving objects captured by moving camera. M. Karaduman [17] presented the obstacle recognition framework utilizing laser distance meter and trained installed camera.

R. Manikandan et al. [18] introduced an obstacle identification approach utilizing thermal camera and ADA boost algorithm. G. M. Shafiullah et al. [19] built up a forecasting model to examine the vertical–acceleration behavior of railway wagons attached to moving trains utilizing regression algorithms. O. Rat et al. [20] proposed a hybrid way to combine CRBM and ESN for predicting time series of railway speed limitations. S. Mittal et al. [21] introduced a vision-based railway track observing methodology utilizing deep learning classifier for uncontrolled real-world data. G. Krummenacher et al. [22] introduced two machine learning techniques dependent on SVM and neural network [23] to identify rail wheels.

M. E. Garcia et al. [24] proposed a methodology for autonomous train stop activity utilizing monocular vision-based methodology and Deep Learning models. In this paper, a framework is intended to distinguish tracks through Hough transform first and afterward segment the moving objects from the image utilizing color HSV segmentation. At last, the Faster Region-Convolution Neural Network (Faster-RCNN) is utilized to identify the obstacles on the track region.

The paper is organized in different subsections as follows: segment II discusses the proposed technique in detail including data collection steps utilizing thermal imaging, detection of railway tracks, and deep network [25] (Faster R-CNN) for recognition of objects. The results and discussion are given in segment III. Finally, the paper is concluded in segment IV.

2 Proposed Method

The proposed technique is utilized to recognize the railway track along with the obstacle on it from the frames of thermal video sequence [26]. The essential block diagram of the proposed strategy is shown in Fig. 1. The frames are separated from the thermal video sequence for further processing. The different steps of the proposed approach for the identification of the railway track along with obstacles on the railway track are shown in Algorithm 1 and discussed in following subsections.

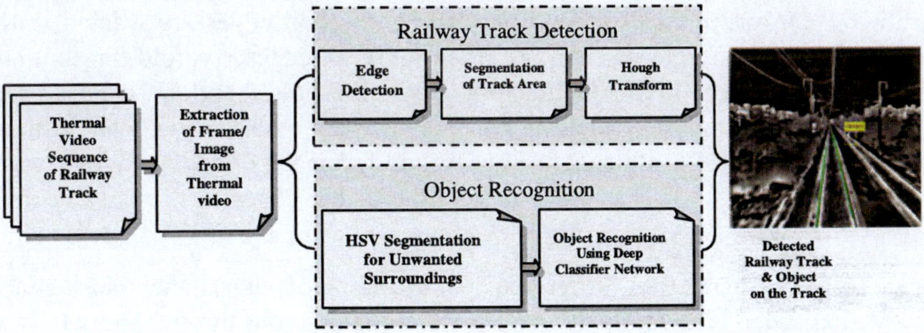

Fig. 1 Basic block diagram of the proposed method used to detect railway track and along with object on the track

2.1 Detection of Railway Track

The first and most significant element in the proposed work is the identification of railway tracks. The railway track recognition step includes edge detection utilizing canny edge detector [27], segmentation of track area utilizing handcrafted triangular mask and finally, the utilization of Hough transform [28] as line detector as the railway track appears as straight lines in the frames. The details of the steps followed for the detection of the railway track are given as follows:

Edge Detection. After the extraction of frames from the video successions the edge recognition is applied to the frame utilizing canny edge detector [27]. The frame is changed over into grayscale image as just luminance channels are needed for distinguishing the edges. The canny edge detector is computationally more affordable than other edge identification techniques. In canny edge detector, at first, the noise and undesirable subtleties in the video frame is decreased by utilizing Gaussian filtering [29] as

$$F(x, y) = h(x, y) * I(x, y) \tag{1}$$

$$\text{Where, } h(x, y) = \frac{1}{2\pi\sigma^2} e^{-\frac{i^2+j^2}{2\sigma^2}}$$

Where $I(x,y)$ is the input frame. At that point the gradients of the filtered frame $F(x,y)$ is determined utilizing the gradient operator as given below:

$$F_M(x, y) = \sqrt{F_i^2(x, y) + F_j^2(x, y)}$$

$$\text{And } \quad F_\theta(x, y) = \tan^{-1}\left[F_j(x, y)/F_i(x, y)\right] \tag{2}$$

After finding the gradients, the dispersing of the widened edges is performed by utilizing non-maximum suppression [30], as the thin edges are wanted in the final output image of edge detector. To filter out weak edges, twofold thresholding techniques are applied. In this methodology, two threshold l_t and h_t (where $l_t < h_t$) are utilized to acquire strong edges and suppress weak edges. The choice of these two values l_t and h_t will influence the general performance of canny edge detector. Fundamentally this stage is capable to find the actual edges in the railway track image.

Track Area Segmentation. After the identification of edges, the track area is segmented as video of the railway track containing numerous things nearby railway tracks. The removal of undesirable zones helps in efficient detection of railway tracks. It is seen that the area containing railway track looks like the geometry of the isosceles triangle as demonstrated in Fig. 2a. The track area is segmented [31] by utilizing a triangular mask on the desired zone. The height h and base b of the triangle are

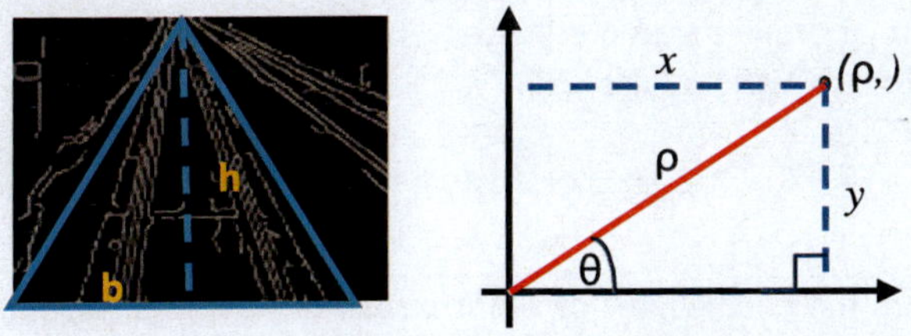

(a) (b)

Fig. 2 **a** Railway track area Mask dimensions (h & b) for segmentation of railway track area. **b** Transformation of a point from line space (x,y) to parameter space (ρ, θ) [28]

acclimated to find the optimum mask dimension. The bitwise AND operation is performed between the image and mask to segment track region is given as:

$$I_{Track}(x, y) = F_T(x, y) \&\& T_{mask} \tag{3}$$

where, $M_{triangle} = triangle[(0, 0), (0, b), (h, 0.5 * b)]$

$F(x, y)$ & $I_{\text{Track}}(x, y)$ are the input and output image respectively and T_{mask} is the triangular mask three vertices.

Algorithm 1: Detection of Railway Track & Object Recognition

Input:
Thermal Video Sequence of Railway Track
Output:
Detected Railway tracks and obstacles on the track
begin
1. Extract frames $\boldsymbol{I(x,y)}$ from the thermal railway track video sequence
Case 1: Detection of Railway Track
2. Apply Canny edge detection on each frame to extract edges $\boldsymbol{F_T(x,y)}$
3. Segment the Railway track region from $\boldsymbol{F_T(x,y)}$
4. Apply Hough transform to find the coordinates $\boldsymbol{(i,j)}$ of railway tracks
Case 2: Recognition of Object
5. Apply HSV color space segmentation on the input frame $\boldsymbol{I(x,y)}$ to remove noise from the frame
6. Identify the object from the HSV segmented frames using the Faster R-CNN
7. The coordinates of the railway track and object information are unified to generate the final output
8. Combine all the output frames as video sequence
End

Hough Transform. After the track region segmentation, a confined search space is found to distinguish the railway tracks. The Hough transform [28] approach is utilized as a line indicator to recognize the railway tracks. The Hough transform is an efficient strategy for recognizing lines in the images. In Hough transform, every straight line can be represented by a single point in the parametric space. A straight line is determined by the angle 'θ' of its typical and its algebraic distance 'ρ' from the origin utilizing normal parameterization as demonstrated in 2b. The identification of presence of line is depicted as:

$$\rho_i = x_i * \cos\theta_i + y_i * \sin\theta_i \tag{4}$$

where (x_i, y_i) are the coordinates of point in the x–y plane in the segmented track region. If the count in the given cell (θ_i, ρ_i) is 'C' then 'C' figure points lie along the line whose normal parameters are (θ_i, ρ_i).

2.2 *Object Recognition on the Railway Track*

When the railway tracks are distinguished, the next stage is to recognize objects (obstacles) on the railway tracks. At first, the noise (undesirable surroundings) is taken out from the image and afterward, objects are recognized utilizing Faster R-CNN [32] network.

HSV Segmentation for Noise (unwanted surrounding) Removal. The undesirable surroundings of the track like trees, poles, and buildings are considered as noise. Human and other living objects discharge more noteworthy infrared radiations than other non-living objects. Due to thermal imaging, the living objects seem brighter than others. Subsequently, HSV segmentation [33] is applied to eliminate the less bright objects. In the initial step of HSV segmentation [33], the image is changed over from RGB color space to HSV color space as given below:

$$H = \begin{cases} 1 + (G - B)/\Delta(\text{if } R = \max(R, G, B)) \\ 3 + (B - R)/\Delta(\text{if } G = \max(R, G, B)) \\ 5 + (R - G)/\Delta(\text{if } B = \max(R, G, B)) \end{cases}.$$

$$S = [\max(R, G, B) - \min(R, G, B)]/\max(R, G, B)$$

$$V = \max(R, G, B) \tag{5}$$

where $\Delta = [\max(\mathrm{R, G, B}) - \min(\mathrm{R, G, B})]$ and (R, G, B) is the RGB color space at pixel location (x,y) in the image. Consequently, the lower limit l_{T} and upper edge h_{T} threshold of the HSV color space is performed to separate the white color from the image that addresses living obstacles.

$$I_{\mathrm{Seg}}(x, y) = \begin{cases} 1 \ (\text{if } l_{\mathrm{T}} \le I_{\mathrm{HSV}}(x, y) \le h_{\mathrm{T}}) \\ 0 \qquad \text{else} \end{cases} \tag{6}$$

where '1' and '0' addresses white and black tones respectively, $I_{HSV}(x,y)$ input image in HSV color space and $I_{Seg}(x,y)$ is output image after noise removal. Finally, the obstacles are segmented from the image, and the surrounding is suppressed.

Object Recognition using Deep Network. Faster R-CNN [32] is utilized to recognize obstacles on the railway tracks. The Faster R-CNN comprises of two modules: initial, a deep fully convolutional network used to propose regions and second is the Fast R-CNN detector [32] that recognizes the objects utilizing region proposals. The Region Proposal Network utilizes 'attention' system to tell the Fast R-CNN detector network where to look. In this work, VGG-16 network model [34] is utilized in Faster R-CNN model [32]. The small network is slid over the convolutional feature maps that produce the set of rectangular object proposals. It is hard to portray objects of various shapes by going through a fixed-sized window hence distinct size anchors are utilized. By default, the anchors are at position of image having 3 scales and 3 ratios.

The Fast R-CNN network [35] is utilized for classification which has two fully connected layers. The one-layer classifies the proposals in $N + 1$ distinctive class. Another fully connected layer is utilized for better adjustment of bouncing box for 'N' classes utilizing regression prediction. For the Region Proposal Network (RPN) preparing, all the anchors are categorized in two distinct categories. The anchors that overlap the ground truth with an Intersection over Union (IOU) more than 0.7 are classified as foreground and the anchors that don't cover any ground truth object (IOU under 0.3) are classified as background. The loss function to be limited is given as:

$$F_{\text{Loss}}(\{m_v\}, \{n_v\}) = \frac{1}{C}\sum_{v} L_c(m_v, m_v^*) + \gamma\frac{1}{R}\sum_{v} m_v^* L_r(n_v, n_v^*) \quad (7)$$

where m_v is the predicted probability of anchor v being an object. Vector n_v signifies the parameterized coordinates of predicted bouncing box. L_c and L_r are the classification and regression loss respectively. For classification, Cross Entropy Loss is utilized and for Bounding Box Regression smooth L1 loss is utilized. The normalization parameters C and R are mini batch size (i.e., $C = 256$) and number of anchor locations (i.e., $R = 2400$). The term 'γ' is the weight balancing parameter set to 10 (default value).

3 Result and Discussion

This segment presents the experimental details of the methodology to assess its performance. The experimental results are illustrated as.

3.1 Experimental Setup

In this work, the thermal video of the railway track is utilized to figure out the performance of proposed approach. The 749 frames from the railway track video are separated for implementation of the proposed work. The implementation of Faster R-CNN is performed using a system with configuration Intel(R) Core(TM) i5-1035G1CPU @ 1.00 GHz, 1.19 GHz, 16 GB RAM, and NVIDIA MX230 GPU.

3.2 Detection of Railway Track

For the detection of the railway track, as a matter of first importance, the frames are extracted from the video sequence as demonstrated in Fig. 3a. At that point, the Canny edge detection approach is applied to the frame to visualize the edges that are the initial step of railway track detection. The performance of the canny edge detector relies upon the double threshold (low l_t and high h_t). Consequently, the values of these thresholds are picked so that only desired data is acquired in terms of edges. It is seen that the desired results of edge detection are acquired at $[l_t, h_t] = [150, 200]$ for this railways image data. Subsequently, the lower threshold 'l_t' is set at '150' and higher threshold 'h_t' at '200' for this proposed technique. The output of the Canny edge detector is at the optimized threshold value is shown in Fig. 3c.

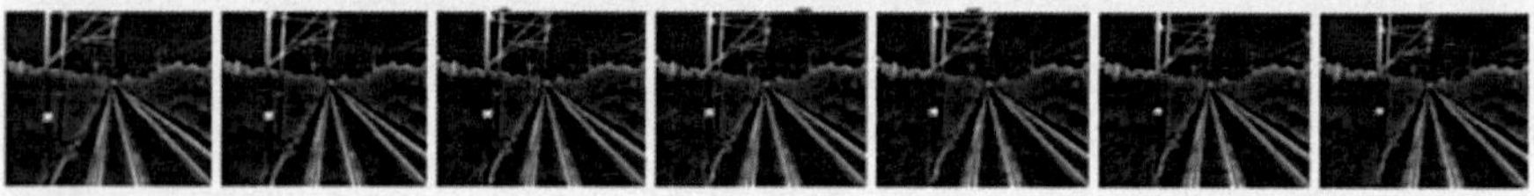

Fig. 3 **a** Extracted frames from the thermal video sequence. **b** Original frame. **c** Result of edge detection at threshold values $l_t = 150$ and h_t. **d** Railway track area segmentation at Mask dimensions ($h_M = 0.6 \times h$ & $b_M = 0.5 \times b$). **e** Input frame. **f** Detected railway track at $\Delta\rho = 1$ and $\Delta\theta = 1$

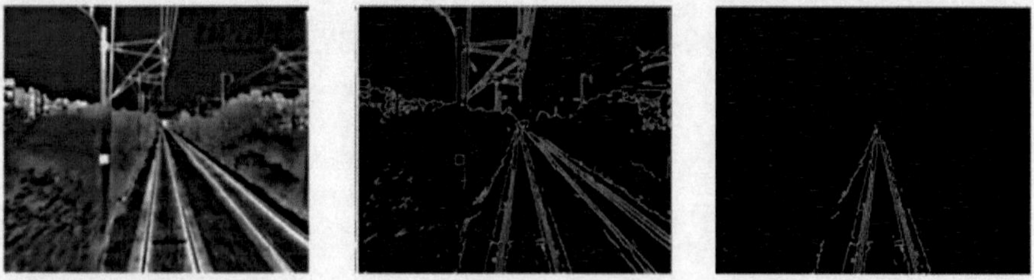

(b) (c) (d)

Fig. 3 (continued)

Fig. 3 (continued)

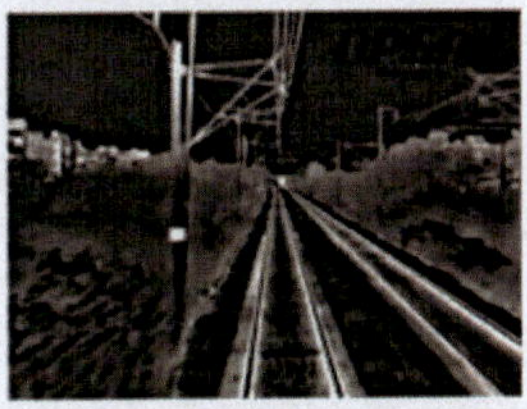

(e)

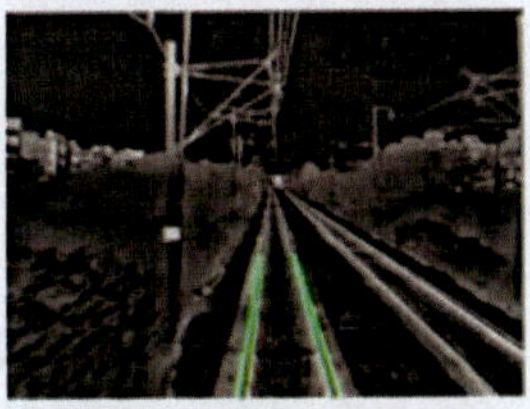

(f)

When the edge detection in all the frames is done, at that point the edges of the track region are extracted from the entire scene edges in the image. The segmentation of the track region edges is done by utilizing masking of the frames. It is seen that the contour of the railway track area looks like the isosceles triangle. The height h and width b of the frame is utilized to find the optimized size of the mask. It is seen that for smaller mask measurements the segmented area loses some desired railway track area and for higher values, the output contains some undesirable surrounding regions. It is analyzed that the mask measurements ($h_M = 0.6 \times$ h & $b_M = 0.5 \times b$) better portions the desired railway track region when contrasted with other mask measurements. The segmentation performed similarly well for all frames. The segmentation of the edge detector output with the mask dimensions ($h_M = 0.6 \times h$ & $b_M = 0.5 \times$ b) has appeared in Fig. 3d.

After the extraction of the railway track territory with some surroundings, the following stage is to recognize and visualize the railway track. As talked about in Sect. 2, the geometrical model of railway tracks look like straight lines so the Hough transform is utilized as a line identification strategy to distinguish the railway tracks. In Hough transform, the track identification accuracy is influenced by quantization parameters $\Delta\rho$ and $\Delta\theta$, so the values of the quantization parameters are to be chosen carefully. The values of $\Delta\rho$ and $\Delta\theta$ are varied from 0.1 to higher range. The Hough transform is applied to detect railway tracks at different combinations of $\Delta\rho$ (0.1–2.0) and $\Delta\theta$ (0.1–5.0). The results illustrate that the detected railway tracks efficiently fitted with the ground truth at $\Delta\rho = 1$ and $\Delta\theta = 1$. The experiment is carried out with different frames of the video sequence data and the optimized values of $\Delta\rho = 1$ and $\Delta\theta = 1$ performed well for distinct frames. The input image and the detected railway track output are shown in Fig. 3e, f.

3.3 Object Recognition

When the railway track is identified and visualized, the subsequent stage is to recognize an object (obstacles) on the rail line track. At first, HSV segmentation approach is utilized for the removal of undesirable surroundings. In the previous section, obstacles appear whiter than other objects when captured by the thermal camera So HSV segmentation performs well for noise removal. For masking, two thresholds (l_T &

h_{T}) are utilized for white color. As the obstacles seem whiter than all other objects in the scene, so the upper threshold h_{T} is set to '1'. In the experiment, the lower limit l_{T} value is varied between ranges (0–1) to get the optimum segmentation result. The optimum results are recorded at threshold values ($l_{\mathrm{T}} = 0.85$, $h_{\mathrm{T}} = 1$) for the frames containing obstacles. The consequences of the HSV segmentation at the optimum threshold values ($l_{\mathrm{T}} = 0.85$, $h_{\mathrm{T}} = 1$) are appeared in Fig. 4b.

At last, HSV segmented image is input to the Faster R-CNN Network which gives recognized obstacles at the output. The important parameter to optimize is Intersection over Union (IoU) threshold to assess the accuracy of the network. In general, the IoU value between 0.7 to 0.9 is considered an acceptable range for the accurate recognition utilizing Faster R-CNN Network. The initial results are obtained by detection network utilizing threshold value 0.7 as demonstrated in Fig. 4c yet the obstacle is recognized at a shorter distance from the train. The lower IoU values give better outcomes in terms of timely identification yet, in addition, confronted challenge of lower accuracy. To take care of this issue, an optimum IoU threshold value '0.5' is acquired which timely perceive the obstacles on the track with good accuracy as demonstrated in Fig. 4d. The final results of railway track and obstacle recognition of the proposed algorithm have appeared in Fig. 4e, f. The performance of the proposed strategy is assessed with the assistance of following parameters:

$$\text{Accuracy} = \frac{(\text{True Positive} + \text{True Negative})}{\text{Total Number of images}} \tag{8}$$

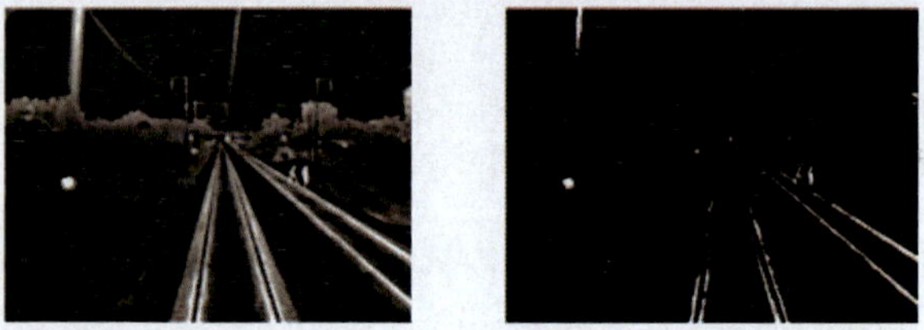

(a) (b)

Fig. 4 **a** Input frame **b** surrounding removal at threshold values $l_T = 0.85$ and $h_T = 1$. **c** Faster R-CNN result with at IoU = 0.7 **d** at IoU = 0.5. **e** The final results of railway track detection and obstacle recognition with Faster R-CNN at IoU = 0.7 **f** at IoU = 0.5

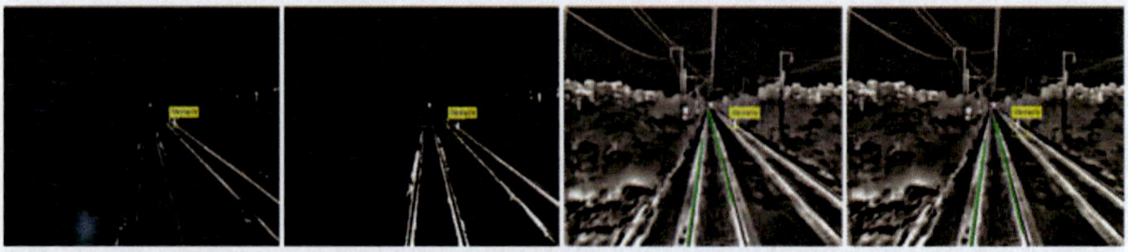

(c) (d) (e) (f)

Fig. 4 (continued)

Table 1 Performance of the proposed method for different IoU

IoU	Classification accuracy	Precision	Recall
0.5	0.8297	0.8312	0.8716
0.7	0.7627	0.7789	0.8106

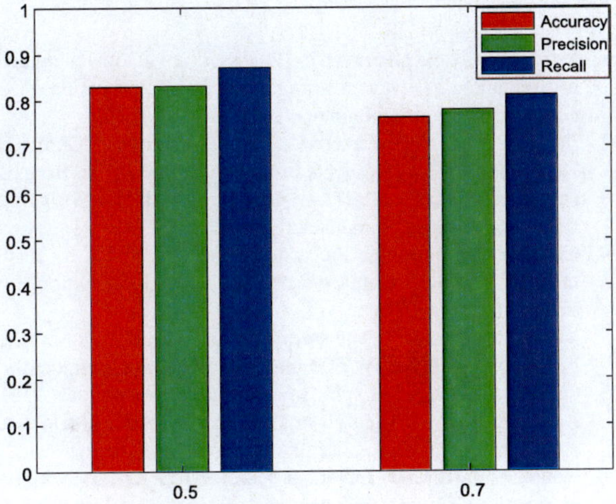

Fig. 5 The classification accuracy, precision, and recall for different values of IoU

$$\text{Precision} = \frac{\text{True Positive}}{\text{True Positive} + \text{False Positive}} \tag{9}$$

$$\text{Recall} = \frac{\text{True Positive}}{\text{Number of images having object class}} \tag{10}$$

These parameters are assessed for various values of the Intersection over Union (IoU) as demonstrated in Table 1. Figure 5 represents that the performance of the proposed strategy is better at IoU $= 0.5$ with an accuracy of around 83%.

4 Conclusion and Future Scope

The proposed technique performs satisfactorily for the detection of railway tracks and objects recognition on the track. This paper introduced a novel methodology dependent on deep learning network to distinguish the railway tracks as well as to recognize obstacles on the railway track in a thermal video sequence. Thus, this work can be a robust technique to build up an early warning framework to avoid railway mishaps for railway safety enhancement. This technique will be additional cost-effective as it doesn't need any critical change in the train's infrastructure as well as will diminish the monetary burden of railways regarding accidental compensation.

As future work, the framework will be extended to efficient recognition of other object classes close to the railway track to boost the adequacy of the framework.

References

1. Sabnis OV, Lokeshkumar R (2019) A novel object detection system for improving safety at unmanned railway crossings. In: Fifth international conference on science technology engineering and mathematics (ICONSTEM, IEEE)
2. Vazquez J, Mazo M, Lazaro JL, Luna CA, Urena J, Garcia JJ, Cabello J, Hierrezuelo L (2004) Detection of moving objects in railway using vision. In: IEEE intelligent vehicles symposium
3. Irani M, Anandan P (1998) A unified approach to moving object detection in 2D and 3D scenes. IEEE Trans Pattern Anal Mach Intell 20(6)
4. Cucchiara R, Crana C, Piccardi M, Prati A, Sirotti S (2001) Improving shadow suppression in moving object detection with HSV color information. In: Proceedings of IEEE intelligent transportation systems
5. Mockel S, Scherer F, Schuster PF (2003) Multi-sensor obstacle detection on railway tracks. In: Proceeding in IEEE IV2003 intelligent vehicles symposium
6. Garcia JJ, Losada C, Espinosa F, Urena JS, Hernandez A, Mazo M, Marziani CD, Jimenez A, Bueno E (2005) Dedicated smart IR barrier for obstacle detection in railways. In: 31st annual conference of IEEE industrial electronics society
7. Hautiere N, Tarel J, Lavenant J, Aubert D (2006) Automatic fog detection and estimation of visibility distance through use of an onboard camera. Machine Vision and Applications (Springer) 17:8–20
8. Wu S, Moore BE, Shah M (2010) Chaotic invariants of lagrangian particle trajectories for anomaly detection in crowded scenes. In: IEEE conference on computer vision and pattern recognition (CVPR), pp 2054–2060
9. Garcia JJ, Urena J, Hernandez A, Mazo M, Jimenez, Alvarez JA, Marziani FJ, Jimenez CDA, Diaz MJ, Losada C, Garcia E (2010) Efficient multisensory barrier for obstacle detection on railways. IEEE Trans Intell Transp Syst 11(3)
10. Zhou X, Yang C, Yu W (2013) Moving object detection by detecting contiguous outliers in the low-rank representation. IEEE Trans Pattern Anal Mach Intell 35(3):597–610
11. Chen Y, Zhang RH, Shang L (2014) A novel method of object detection from a moving camera based on image matching and frame coupling. J PLOS ONE 9(10)
12. Berg A, Ofjall K, Ahlberg J, Felsberg M (2015) Detecting rails and obstacles using a train-mounted thermal camera. image analysis, scandinavian conference on image analysis (SCIA), vol 9127. Springer, pp 492–503
13. Mukojima H, Deguchi D, Kawanishi Y, Ide I, Murase Ukai HM, Nagamine N, Nakasone R (2016) Moving camera background-subtraction for obstacle detection on railway tracks. In: Proceeding in IEEE international conference on image processing (ICIP)
14. Sinha D, Feroz F (2016) Obstacle detection on railway tracks using vibration sensors and signal filtering using bayesian analysis. IEEE Sens J 16(3)
15. Amaral V, Marques F, Lourenco A, Barata J, Santana P (2016) Laser-Based Obstacle Detection at Railway Level Crossings. Hindawi Pub. Corp. J Sens
16. Wu Y, He X, Nguyen TQ (2017) Moving Object Detection with a Freely Moving Camera via Background Motion Subtraction. IEEE Trans Circuits Syst Video Technol 27(2):236–248
17. Karaduman M (2017) Image processing based obstacle detection with laser measurement in railways. In: 10th international conf. on electrical and electronics engineering
18. Manikandan R, Balasubramanian M, Palanivel S (2017) Vision Based Obstacle Detection on Railway Track. Int J Pure Appl Math 116(24)
19. Shafiullah GM, Ali ABMS, Thompson A, Wolfs PJ (2010) Predicting vertical acceleration of railway wagons using regression algorithms. IEEE Trans Intell Transp Syst 11(2):290–299

20. Fink O, Zio E, Weidmann U (2013) Predicting time series of railway speed restrictions with time-dependent machine learning techniques. Expert Syst Appl (Elsevier) 40(15):6033–6040
21. Mittal S, Rao D (2017) Vision based railway track monitoring using deep learning. Comput Sci, ArXiv
22. Krummenacher G, Ong CS, Koller S, Kobayashi S, Buhmann JM (2018) Wheel defect detection with machine learning. IEEE Trans Intell Transp Syst 19(4):1176–1187
23. Goel R, Sharma A, Kapoor R (2019) Object recognition using deep learning. J Comput Theor Nanosci 16:4044–4052
24. Garcia ME, Labayen M, Zamalloa M, Arexolaleiba NA (2020) Application of computer vision and deep learning in the railway domain for autonomous train stop operation. IEEE/SICE Int Symp Syst Integr (SII)
25. Goel R, Sharma A, Kapoor R (2020) State-of-the-art object recognition techniques: a comparative study. In: Soft computing: theories and applications. Advances in Intelligent Systems and Computing (Springer)
26. Singh S, Khosla A, Kapoor R (2019) Object tracking with a novel visual- thermal sensor fusion method in template matching. Int J Image, Graph Signal Process (IJIGSP) 7, 39–47
27. Vishwakarma DK, Kapoor R, Dhiman A (2016) Unified framework for human activity recognition: an approach using spatial edge distribution and R-transform. Int J Electron Commun (Elsevier) 70(3):341–353
28. Niblack W, Petkovic D (1990) On improving the accuracy of the Hough transform. Mach Vis Appl (Springer) 3:87–106
29. Flusser J, Farokhi S, Hoschl C, Suk T, Zitova B, Pedone M (2016) Recognition of images degraded by Gaussian Blur. IEEE Trans Image Process 25(2)
30. Rothe R, Guillaumin M, Gool LV (2014) Non-maximum suppression for object detection by passing messages between windows. In: Asian conference on computer vision. Springer, pp 290–306
31. Kapoor R, Rohilla R (2014) Modified Foreground Segmentation for Object Tracking Using Wavelets in a Tensor Framework. Int J Electron (Taylor and Francis) 102(9):1560–1582
32. Ren S, He K, Girshick R, Sun J (2017) Faster R-CNN: towards real-time object detection with region proposal networks. IEEE Trans Pattern Anal Mach Intell 39(6):1137–1149
33. Burdescu DD, Brezovan M, Ganea E, Stanescu L (2009) A new method for segmentation of images represented in a HSV color space. In: Proceedings of international conference on advanced concepts for intelligent vision systems
34. Tammina S (2019) Transfer learning using VGG-16 with deep convolutional neural network for classifying images. Inter. l. J Sci Res Publ
35. Girshick R (2015) Fast R-CNN. In: Proceedings of IEEE international conference on computer vision (ICCV)

Employee Health Monitoring System for Industry 4.0

Devansh Atray and Rajeshwar Dass

Abstract With the advent of Industry 4.0, degree of automation in the industrial sector has been rising exponentially over the past decade. Though this trend is that of a rapid increase, it hasn't yet manifested as complete independence from the human workforce. This paper aims to facilitate health monitoring of human workforce in large industrial setups. This is achieved using the principles of Internet of Things (IoT). By collecting daily data points of employee health on three metrics: Blood Pressure, Body Mass Index, and Temperature, it aims to prevent deterioration in their health and seeks to help diagnose of clinical conditions, which may not otherwise be identified early. Collected data are sent to a cloud server where these are stored and made available for remote visualization using Grafana. The system also provides alerts in case of serious deviations from accepted value ranges.

Keywords Industry 4.0 · Internet of Things · Grafana · Healthcare · Remote visualization · Remote monitoring

1 Introduction

Industry 4.0 consists of the overall transformation of an industrial setup using principles of digitization and intelligent engineering. Digitized products and services are a necessity for any industrial system under Industry 4.0. Increased productivity and reduced costs are achieved in modern industries with the help of intelligent communication, internet of things, remote sensing, monitoring and control, big data, and artificial intelligence [1, 2].

Although their nature of roles and responsibilities have been changed due to the fourth industrial revolution, people are still key players in the overall process and functioning of the industry. Thus, it becomes essential that health and safety of Human resources are ensured in such environments.

D. Atray (✉) · R. Dass
DCRUST, ECED, Murthal, Haryana, India

N. Marriwala et al. (eds.), *Emergent Converging Technologies and Biomedical Systems*, Lecture Notes in Electrical Engineering 841,
https://doi.org/10.1007/978-981-16-8774-7_21

It has been shown that good employee wellbeing and health have salutary influence at societal level and also contributes to overall business success in the long term. By placing an increased focus on improving workplace health, organizations have the potential to reduce operational costs and thus increase cost savings. To enhance strategic success, it is essential that both employees and organizations recognize the importance of workforce health [3].

The waste of human potential due to ill-health represents a significant economic and societal cost and impedes the prospects of many individuals in their field of work [4].

Estimated percentage of sickness absenteeism in the Indian Industry is 66.9%. Overall 16.5 and 16.2 days are lost by male and female workers, respectively, in a single year because of sickness absence. Blue-collar workers approximately lose 21 days while white-collar workers lose 11 days per year. The prevalence of ailments relating to the musculoskeletal system is highest at 31.4% among workers followed by that of the gastrointestinal system at 25.8%. Hypertension affects 24.4% of the workers and illnesses related to respiratory system affect 18.1%. 7.4% workers are hospitalized at least once in 12 months due to sickness and 81% experience at least one health event in 12 months [5].

This contribution aims to provide a scalable and cost-effective approach to monitor workforce health across the industry. Unlike the Body Sensor Network (BSN) approach, the infrastructure available for such measurements is shared among a specific number of people [6]. This ensures low upfront cost of this method. Also, the problem of asset management, due to non-zero attrition rate in an organization, when employing separate devices for each individual of the workforce is eliminated. By establishing a regular measurement routine, consistent and reliable individual health data may be obtained.

Here, measurement of three main body parameters is considered, i.e., Body Mass Index (BMI), Body Temperature, and Blood Pressure (BP).

At present, among the world's population, 11 and 15% of men and women, respectively, are suffering from obesity. The percentage of population suffering from obesity has been consistently rising and has nearly tripled in the last five decades [7, 8]. As adult population forms the backbone of industrial workforce, it is important that such condition is identified early from evidence-based data and preventive action may be taken. Another prevalent non-communicable disease is elevated blood pressure, also called Hypertension. It is known to cause an increased risk of other medical conditions related to heart, brain, and kidney. An estimated 15% of the world's population suffers from hypertension, most of whom live in middle and low-income countries. Hypertension is a major cause of premature deaths worldwide [9, 10]. Due to the homeothermic nature of human body, a certain temperature is maintained to direct and coordinate its metabolic activities [11]. Significant deviations from this normal level always occur due to abnormalities within the body and should never be overlooked [12].

Thus, by measurement of the above parameters, comprehensive data is obtained which corresponds directly to the overall health of an individual. This data is sent to medical officers inside the factory for remote viewing and analysis, ensuring occupational health and safety of employees.

The paper is divided into five sections. In Sect. 1, introduction was covered. Section 2 consists of a system overview while methodology used is provided under Sect. 3. Results obtained from the system are discussed in Sect. 4 followed by Sect. 5 that covers the conclusion and future work.

2 System Overview

Figure 1 denotes the overall block diagram of the system. Each component is labeled and is detailed in the following sub-sections separately.

2.1 *Microcontroller*

Arduino is an open-source electronic prototyping platform that uses different AVR microcontrollers, each having its own unique features and functions. Arduino platform consists of a physical board for hardware and an Integrated Development Environment (IDE) which uses language identical to C++ for board programming. The presence of a USB port that handles both power and communication ensures Arduino's ease of use [13]. In this paper, Arduino Mega with ATmega 2560 microcontroller (MCU) is used because of the presence of four hardware serial ports on the board.

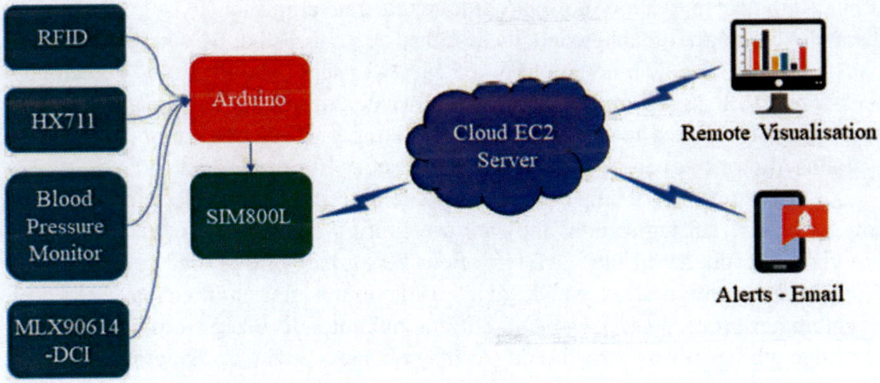

Fig. 1 Basic block diagram of the system

2.2 Blood Pressure Measurement

Sunrom 1437 Blood Pressure sensor is a digital sensor with serial output at 9600 baud. Each reading consists of 15 bytes and reading packet's last byte is always an enter key character. Serial output consists of 8 data bits along with 1 stop bit but no parity bit. All the output parameters are in ASCII format. Its output consists of systolic, diastolic, and pulse readings. It operates on a regulated 5 V power supply [14]. The single output wire from the sensor is connected to Arduino's UART at RX pin. The incoming ASCII data has to be converted into Integer format before any further processing can be done.

2.3 Body Mass Index Measurement

Body Mass Index (BMI) is measured indirectly using the body weight of an individual. As the height of an individual is fixed from start of adulthood, from the below equation BMI is obtained.

$$\text{BMI} = \frac{\text{Weight (kg)}}{[\text{Height (m)}]^2} \quad (1)$$

For purposes of body weight measurement, HX711 is employed which is characterized by a selectable dual channel analog-to-digital converter (ADC). It has a 24-bit output precision that provides a resolution of 4 milli-grams. The output data bits are denoted in 2's complement format and in case of overflow output saturates at value of 800000 h. Internally, the two channels are selected via a multiplexer whose output is connected to a low-noise programmable gain amplifier (PGA). The gain of Channel A is programmable where it can either be set to 128 or 64 whereas Channel B has a gain of 32 which is fixed. For a 5 V power supply, at a gain of 128 and 64 on Channel A, $\pm$ 20 mV and $\pm$ 40 mV of full-scale differential voltage are obtained respectively. It features an internal crystal oscillator for clock generation. At internal crystal oscillator frequency, output data rate is set at 10 samples per second.

HX711 is controlled using external hardware pins and does not require programming of its internal registers as they are pre-configured. MCU is interfaced to the chip via a two-pin serial interface [15]. Four 50-kg half-bridge load cells are used in full-bridge configuration which yields a maximum measurement of 200 kg of weight, under proper load placement. Differential output is taken from both arms of the bridge which corresponds directly to the unbalance in the bridge circuit.

2.4 Temperature Measurement

MLX90614-DCI is used for non-contact high precision temperature measurements with a 5° Field-Of-View (FoV). It comes in TO-39 sized package which integrates the infrared sensor and the signal conditioning circuitry in a single package. The MLX90614 comes factory calibrated for temperature ranges of −40 to 125 °C for ambient and −70 to 380 °C for object temperature. Output temperature value is obtained by averaging all temperatures of all the objects present in FoV. DCI variant used in this paper provides an accuracy of ± 0.2 °C at human body temperature range and ± 0.5 °C at room temperature range [16]. Measured values are accessed by 2 wire serial I2C interface with MCU which provides a resolution of 0.02 °C. Also, thermal gradients, which can lead to inaccurate measurements, are measured internally and the measured temperature is compensated for them. The sensor is operated via a 3.3 V supply from MCU.

2.5 SIM800L

SIM800L is a miniature cellular module that uses General Packet Radio Service (GPRS) to connect with the internet. It features an inbuilt TCP/IP stack that can be accessed with the help of AT commands. Due to these reasons, SIM800L is used in applications of data logging where low bandwidth is available on the network. The recommended supply voltage is in the range of 3.4–4.4 V [17]. Several modules are available based on SIM800L with inbuilt level shifting for interfacing with TTL-based MCUs. The module used here is one such variant. Serial Interface is used to communicate with the module using AT commands. Message Queuing Telemetry Transport (MQTT) is implemented on the application layer using MCU.

2.6 MFRC522

It is a highly integrated Radio Frequency Identification and Detection (RFID) reader-cum-writer IC for contactless data exchange at 13.56 MHz ISM band. The reader supports ISO/IEC 14,443 A/MIFARE and NTAG cards and labels. Data framing and error detection is done in accordance with ISO/IEC 14,443 A which includes both CRC and parity functionality. RFID module is powered by a 3.3 V supply from MCU and uses SPI to transmit data serially to MCU at 10 Mbit/s [18]. Unique compatible passive tags are used for employee identification before the measurement of data.

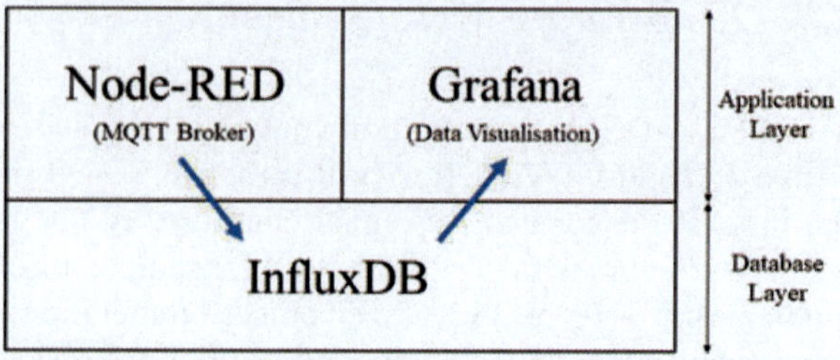

Fig. 2 Two-layered deployment on EC2 instance

2.7 *Cloud EC2 Server*

Amazon AWS provides infrastructure as a service platform known as EC2. For purpose of this system, a Windows EC2 instance was created to serve as a cloud server.

Two layers of deployment on this instance are shown in Fig. 2. InfluxDB serves on the database layer where data sent from sensor nodes are stored. As this application inherently generates time-series data, use of a time-series database is preferred over other relational databases. With the use of INSERT statement, available data are stored inside the database, and using SELECT statements are retrieved from the database [19]. On the application layer, we have two applications, namely, Node-RED and Grafana.

Node-RED is an open-source flow-based development tool for visual programming in event-driven applications [20]. MQTT broker is deployed in this environment as a Node using which relevant topics are subscribed, where sensor node publishes employee data. Received data are processed and written to in InfluxDB [21].

Grafana is an open-source web application, used for data visualization and data analytics, developed by Grafana Labs. It features different types of charts, graphs, and tables that can be used for visualization of data from supported sources [22]. Here, Grafana is configured with InfluxDB as a data source. Grafana also features alerts where if the alert rule is satisfied, a notification is pushed onto the configured notification channel.

3 Methodology Used

Figure 3 denotes the process flow of the implemented system. Before measurement of any kind of data from the sensors, employee is identified using a unique RFID tag. This approach uses event-driven data transmission, where data is sent to the cloud server only when an employee is available for measurement. After successful identification, BMI measurement takes place where the data from load cells is communicated serially to Arduino. Similarly, blood pressure and temperature values are acquired by Arduino. After acquiring the three parameters, they are collectively sent to the cloud server using SIM800L. The advantage of using GSM rather than other network

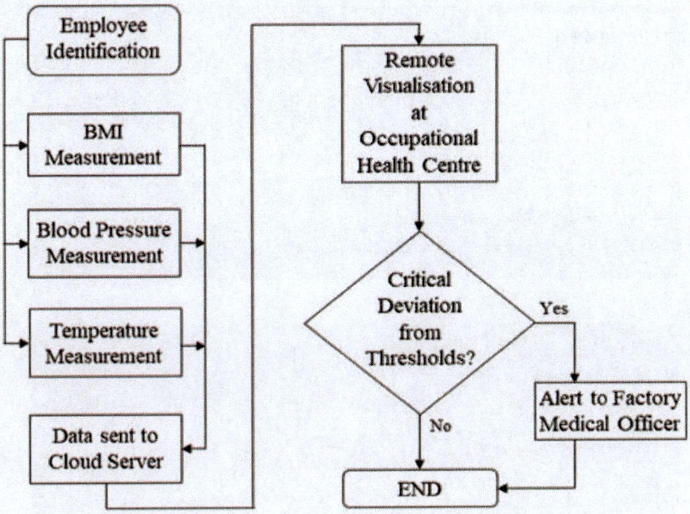

Fig. 3 Process flow diagram

technologies like Wi-Fi is that functioning of such a system is independent of the condition of organization's network. Also, multiple such devices may be used in geographies where organization's network is either unavailable or not of appropriate strength.

For data transfer through MQTT, three separate topics are created, each for a different metric. MQTT broker in the cloud server listens to these topics and thus receives data sent from the sensor node. Apache web-server running on the EC2 instance redirects all the incoming HTTP traffic to the Grafana port so that remote visualization may be obtained.

At Occupational Health Centre (OHC) of the factory, employee-wise data is visualized where the staff reviews the trends. If a metric value deviates from the specified band, Grafana issues an alert on the defined notification channel via Simple Mail Transfer Protocol (SMTP) so that the factory medical officer is notified of the event and corrective action is taken.

4 Results

After successful implementation, it is observed that the acquired parameters from employees are viewed on the Grafana dashboard. Figure 4 represents the screenshots from one such dashboard which is allocated for a single employee. Here, Fig. 4a denotes the most recent measured values of the employee using simple tiles of data. Here, unique color is used for each individual metric and it does not correspond to any other information. Figure 4b–d shows the line chart visualization of measured

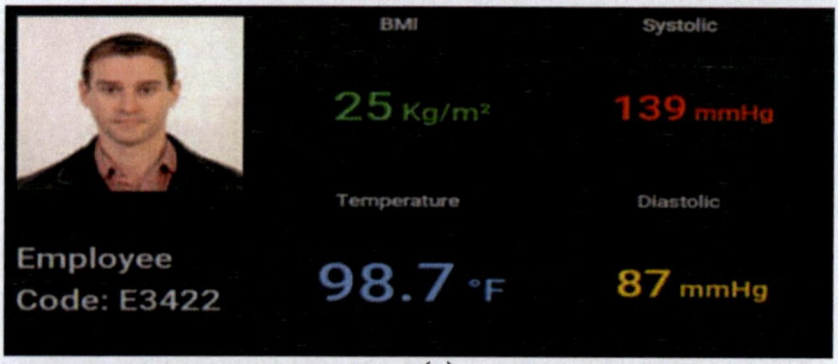

(a)

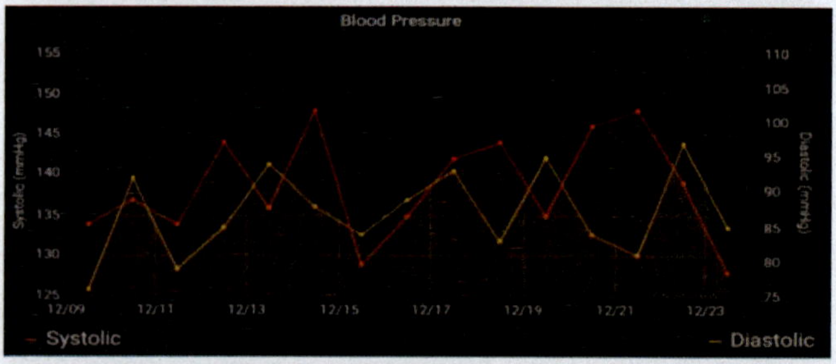

(b)

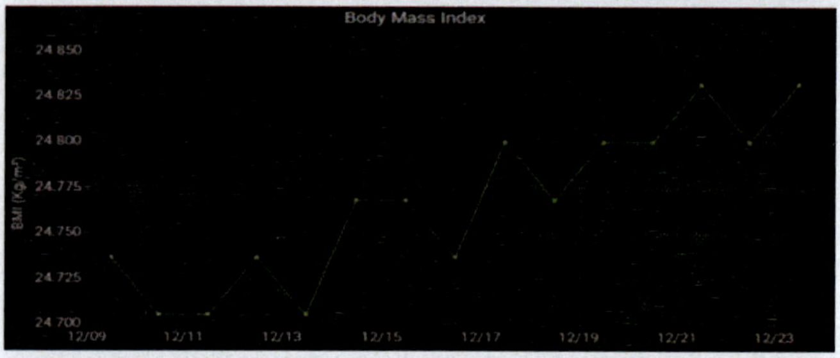

(c)

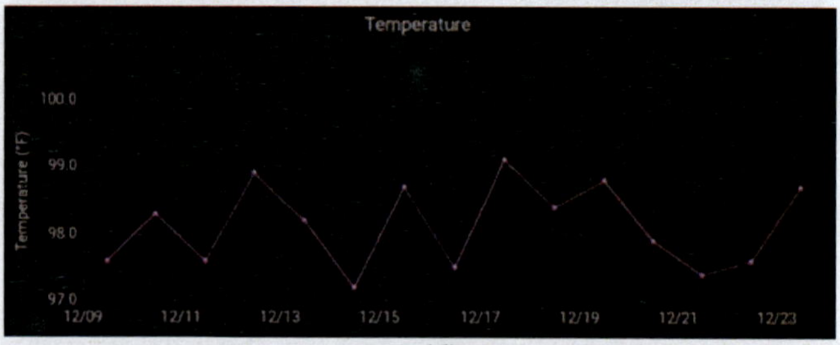

(d)

Fig. 4 Representation of measured metrics in Grafana for Remote Visualization (**a**) Latest metric values in tile format (**b**) Blood Pressure metric's line chart (**c**) Body Mass Index metric's line chart (**d**) Temperature metric's line chart

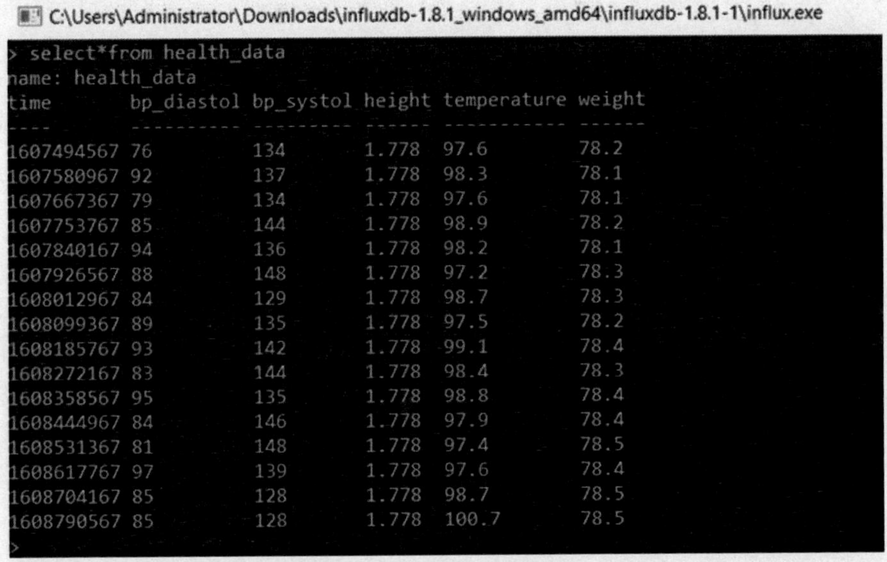

```
C:\Users\Administrator\Downloads\influxdb-1.8.1_windows_amd64\influxdb-1.8.1-1\influx.exe
> select*from health_data
name: health_data
time       bp_diastol bp_systol height temperature weight
----       ---------- --------- ------ ----------- ------
1607494567 76         134       1.778  97.6        78.2
1607580967 92         137       1.778  98.3        78.1
1607667367 79         134       1.778  97.6        78.1
1607753767 85         144       1.778  98.9        78.2
1607840167 94         136       1.778  98.2        78.1
1607926567 88         148       1.778  97.2        78.3
1608012967 84         129       1.778  98.7        78.3
1608099367 89         135       1.778  97.5        78.2
1608185767 93         142       1.778  99.1        78.4
1608272167 83         144       1.778  98.4        78.3
1608358567 95         135       1.778  98.8        78.4
1608444967 84         146       1.778  97.9        78.4
1608531367 81         148       1.778  97.4        78.5
1608617767 97         139       1.778  97.6        78.4
1608704167 85         128       1.778  98.7        78.5
1608790567 85         128       1.778  100.7       78.5
>
```

Fig. 5 Database created in InfluxDB

data where a measurement on the three parameters was taken from a single employee each day at a specific time for sixteen days.

Figure 5 shows a measurement created inside an InfluxDB database where the received values from the controller are stored in a time-series format. The height of the employee is assumed to be already available and a node-red flow appends the incoming data with the height value each time it is written into the database. Height is thus assumed to remain constant throughout the testing.

Figure 6 is that of an alert mail sent to factory medical officer when the temperature of employee was more than 100 °F and less than 96°F during measurement. Critical thresholds for BMI were taken at 25 kg/m^2 whereas for systolic and diastolic at 150 mmHg and 100 mmHg respectively.

5 Conclusion and Future Work

A scalable system was developed which is capable of monitoring employee health based on three parameters—Blood Pressure, BMI, and Temperature—and providing real-time alerts for Industry 4.0 environments. Measured data are sent to cloud via MQTT protocol where it is stored and made available for purposes of remote visualization. Future work includes implementation of deep learning algorithms on acquired data for long-term health predictions and integration of these data with organization's Human Resource Management System (HRMS). This may open up

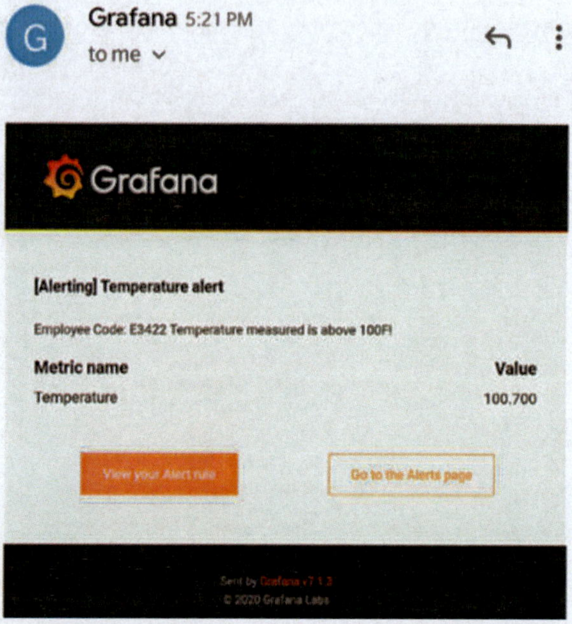

Fig. 6 Email received after critical deviation

the possibility of existence of long-term employee health records and allocation of work to employees on the basis of their health.

References

1. Muhuria PK, Shuklaa AK, Abraham A (2019) Industry 4.0: A bibliometric analysis and detailed overview. Eng Appl Artif Intell 78(2):218–35.
2. Wollschlaeger M, Sauter T, Jasperneite J (2017) The future of industrial communication: Automation networks in the era of the internet of things and industry 4.0. IEEE Ind Electron Mag 11(1):17–27.
3. Black C (2008) Working for a healthier tomorrow. The stationery office, London.
4. Hulshof CTJ (2009) Working for a healthier tomorrow. Occup Environ Med 66(1):1–2.
5. Manjunatha R, Kiran D, Thankappan KR (2011) Sickness absenteeism, morbidity and workplace injuries among iron and steel workers—a cross sectional study from Karnataka, Southern India. Australas Med J 4(3):144–7.
6. Poon CC, Lo BP, Yuce MR, Alomainy A and Hao Y (2015) Body sensor networks: In the era of big data and beyond. IEEE Rev Biomed Eng 8:4–16.
7. Obesity and overweight WHO Media Centre, https://www.who.int/news-room/fact-sheets/detail/obesity-and-overweight. Accessed 01 Dec 2020
8. Csige I et al. (2018) The impact of obesity on the cardiovascular system. J Diabetes Res 2018.
9. Chobanian AV (2003) The seventh report of the Joint National Committee on Prevention Detection Evaluation and Treatment of High Blood Pressure. JAMA 289(19):2560–72.
10. World Health Organisation, https://www.who.int/health-topics/hypertension. Accessed 01 Dec 2020

11. Chen W (2019) Thermometry and interpretation of body temperature. Biomed Eng Lett 9(1):3–17.
12. Wunderlich CA (1871) On the temperature in diseases: a manual of medical thermometry. The New Sydenham Society, London.
13. Arduino guide, https://www.arduino.cc/en/guide/introduction. Accessed 02 Dec 2021
14. Sunrom Blood Pressure Sensor 1437, https://www.sunrom.com/p/blood-pressure-sensor-serial-output. Accessed 04 Dec 2020
15. HX711 sensor, https://blog.csdn.net/hudoudoudechuntain/article/details/7883231. Accessed 04 Dec 2020
16. MLX90614 Datasheet, https://www.melexis.com/media/files/documents/datasheets/mlx90614-datasheet-melexis.pdf. Accessed 04 Dec 2020
17. SIM800 Hardware Design V1.08, https://pdf.direnc.net/upload/sim800-gsm-module.pdf. Accessed 04 Dec 2020
18. MFRC522 Datasheet, https://www.nxp.com/docs/en/data-sheet/MFRC522.pdf. Accessed 04 Dec 2020
19. InfluxDB homepage, https://www.influxdata.com/. Accessed 02 Dec 2020
20. Node-RED, https://nodered.org/about/. Accessed 05 Dec 2020
21. Gulati U et al. (2019) Intelligent car with voice assistance and obstacle detector to aid the disabled. In: international conference on computational intelligence and data science 2019. Procedia Comput Sci 167:1732–38.
22. Grafana—The open platform for analytics and monitoring, https://grafana.com/. Accessed 02 Dec 2020

Intelligent Tutoring System for Preschooler Enhancement

P. Raja, Rajesh Sigh, and Anita Gehlot

Abstract The Preschooler is children aged from 2 to 6 years old. The Intelligent Tutoring System (ITS) review is done to learn various existing solutions and future scope in the field of ITS. The need for a robot to exponentially benefit the preschooler with the knowledge and IQ is a demanding need and making children learn basics is a normal schedule. Making it controlled by a robot that is trained to serve the purpose will help the nation for the betterment. The system proposed has modules that can be accessed remotely by the robots to educate a Preschooler. A wide range of literature work is done to precisely state the different existing technologies to ensure the novelty of developing an innovative solution to serve better. The implementation part of the system is discussed and the module attachment on clouds and Machine learning in the domain model is to be carried out in further research.

Keywords ITS · ICT · Preschooler · Tutoring Robot

1 Introduction

Children, the backbone of the nation are affected mentally due to social problems at an age of 2–6. The betterment of the future is in the hands of the children. The way they are grown up decides the mentality and health of the future. The need to ensure good growth forces us to focus on the preschooler age where the child changes from toddler to a world explorer. The Preschooler children are intended to learn new things and the age where they love exploring things and learn basics. Verbalizing one thought loud gives a persistent gain in a week [1–3]. The things learned at this

P. Raja (✉) · R. Sigh · A. Gehlot
Lovely Professional University, Phagwara, Punjab, India
e-mail: raja.21019@lpu.co.in

R. Sigh
e-mail: rajesh.23402@lpu.co.in

A. Gehlot
e-mail: anita.23401@lpu.co.in

N. Marriwala et al. (eds.), *Emergent Converging Technologies and Biomedical Systems*, Lecture Notes in Electrical Engineering 841,
https://doi.org/10.1007/978-981-16-8774-7_22

age are the basics which are going to serve as the basics for the future. Alphabets, grammar, colors, social behavior, public actions are some basics that are learned at this age. The children at this age have a strong grasping power and could think of situations in a multidimensional manner. The lack of time that the parents spend with their children pushes them into stress and emotional disorder. The children are curious to explore but the resources they get in pre-kinder garden or in home is not sufficient to calm down the hunger for knowledge acquisition. The children get addicted deep into the mobile gadgets. They see gadgets as advanced tools, where they could find better resources. But the resource they often go through isn't relevant to the mental development of children. They land up affected with radiation from gadgets neither with the knowledge. This affects mentally and which leads to some dangerous diseases like Autism. The medication could help get rid of the built-up problems, but the technology could help, not getting into the problem.

The world is running behind technology which has both a boon and bane. The use of technology is a good way would help fight the issues caused due to the bad way of the technology or by emotional and physical disorders. There are lots of solutions proposed to make a kid interactive and to act as an unlimited knowledge source. The Intelligent Tutoring System (ITS) has been evolved to provide multi-disciplinary solutions to raise up an intelligent kid. The system to tutor kids is a social problem these days that require attention and proper research work which could serve better.

Autism Spectrum Disorder (ASD) is especially seen in the age of 2–5. ASD is specially defined as the mental stress and disorder of children who lack mental growth. This usually happens due to the workload of the parents or not taking care of the children. The parents don't have enough time to spend with children and mostly appoint a caretaker, the work of the caretakers isn't immense and that leads to various disorders. To encounter the problems of ASD and to bring good health of children in future, this problem is stated, and a literature work is done. The radiation from electronic gadgets is the second thing that is being focused on for the research work. An eco-friendly green environment is intended to be built by the end to serve children with sufficient and efficient resources. The paper would help us identify the flaws in the existing system and would help us recommend a change in the society for the betterment. The previous work stated, is focused on children from age 6 to 12 years old. 12 children with ASD are selected and undergo a one-month training with a robot and positive results are seen in their social activities [4]. The use of a similar system in the younger ages would help in avoiding the children getting ASD. The previous research work is not focused on the 2–5 age group which is focused to ensure the health and emotions of the children. In this paper, author has planned to implement the system to enhance the learning skill of children using the proposed system. The paper includes the various related work under significance of Intelligent Tutoring System and the relationship model to the teaching–learning process and algorithm and enabling of features in Smart Tutoring system is detailed.

2 Significance of Intelligent Tutoring System

Robots are classified based on the different domains. Industrial, domestic, military, medical, education, Security robots are the major domains available in the field of robotics. The same is shown in Fig. 1. The proposed framework lies in the education sector. The various robots in the education domain are taken into consideration, the Intelligent Training System (ITS) based robots serves the purpose efficiently.

Intelligent Training System (ITS) is a System that holds a set of rules and principles where a system is trained beforehand to train humans later. The system may be ML enabled, Big data-enabled, the purpose of the system is to reduce human intervention. There are several types of ITS. ITS is applied in the field of healthcare, education, social effects, companionship, and social definition [5]. The most seen and used method is social robots [6]. The social robots have the ability to read and learn from the user in an easy manner and train humans in the same way again. ICT by teachers, personal and contextual factor is seen [7]. Let's consider an example to make it clear. Let's have a tutor, she has a lot many students to take care. She could focus only on one student to give a better knowledge. So, an ITS-based robot could serve by learning from a tutor and replicate the same like the tutor to the children [8]. The tutor teaches the robot to play three-note harmonies and the robot further teaches the children. The training in design and manufacturing of the gears is also done through ITS using ML algorithms and which is some application of the ITS [9]. One more application for elders in the field of ITS would be the social development of a student meeting his faculty and moving on to a manager in a company. The needs of a manager and the knowledge that a teacher gives in a college are trained to make

Fig. 1 Classification of Robots based on different domains

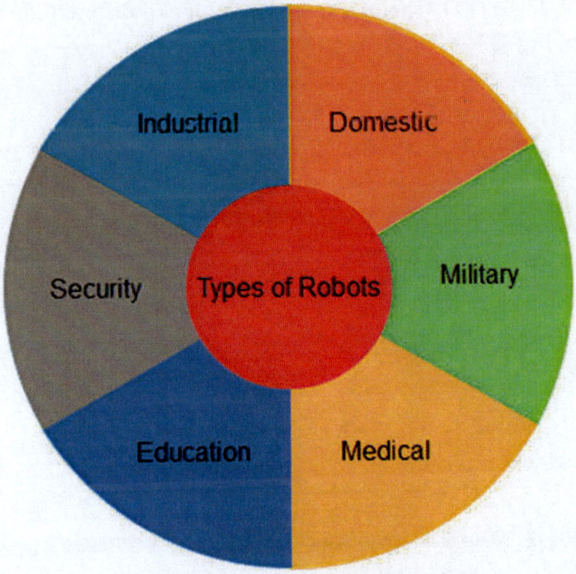

students learn the things and standards that a manager expects [10]. ITS is a subpart of Machine Learning (ML), but not compulsory that ML is the only solution to take care of the model efficiency [11]. ITS consists of four major models or nodes which makes it an efficient full-fledged system.

Domain model: The behavior and knowledge are located in this model.

Student model: Gaining the students' knowledge and AI functioning essentiality is defined.

Teaching model: Lessons and activities are completed in this node.

Learning Environment: The student interaction interface.

Various technologies are used based on the application and problem statement. The personalized learning time in robots is proposed in the paper and the efficient positive results in the mental growth of the children are seen. The interface is given with four kinds of activities, which a child is initiated to do, based on the mood and thinking of the child. The four operations are a game (tic-tac), physical exercise (standup, raise your hands, clap your hands), refocusing (Find a number), relaxing (breathe In and Out). The timing management within a continuous session would help better in learning things [12]. Curriculum gap identification based on the student test assessment, attendance, and syllabus covered helps in training the module to frame curriculum [13]. Some technologies even claim to calculate age, emotion, and gender based on the children's speech [14]. Images-based lessons are the other new way to easily teach the students with basic flowers, fruits, vegetables, animals and, etc. [15].

Tutoring robots are classified into various types based on the applications. The different learning techniques such as formulas, calculations, simple mathematical problems, and problem-solving basics are discussed in the paper [16]. Robots are again classified based on the positive and negative impacts. Focusing on the positive part is the best thing that a person should peruse for the betterment in the case of children [17]. The research percentage of different countries based on ITS is shown in Fig. 2.

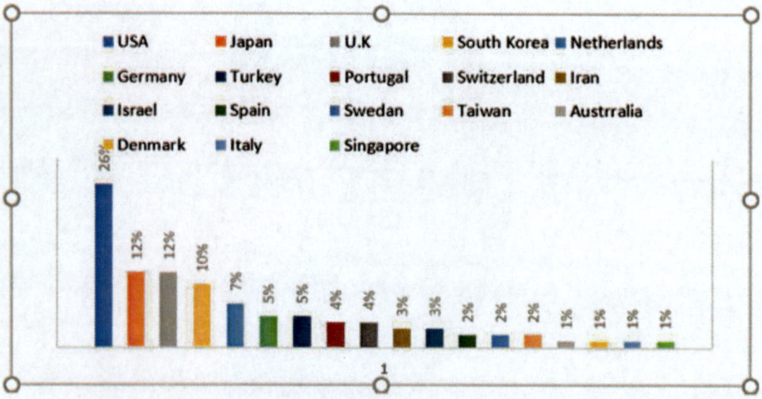

Fig. 2 Nations where the research studies were carried out

The language is a barrier between the machine and a child. Considering an English-speaking nation, it is fine that a child is fluent enough in English to communicate and learn with the machine. The system should be capable enough to communicate in the mother tongue which would provide better experience with the robot. One such is a storytelling session. The story is narrated by a robot in Spanish and the child is asked to translate it into English, On the successful translation to English, the story is continued. This is a two-week course with five sessions and each session would have 30–40 sentences and could go up to 20 min [18]. Building a system with multiple languages would make it unique and useful. Some negative vibes are produced by robots in the field of education for preschoolers which would ruin the child to the core. The possible ways are mentioned over here which one has to stay away from [19]. There are three different ways proposed in managing the affective state of the children like engagement, disengagement, negative engagement [20]. The technology could take in any way, that depends on the study purpose. In some places, even learning programming was done easily using ITS [21]. The factors that may affect the influence of adaptation are real survey, attitude towards ICT, teacher level, technological, lack of time, and resistance to change [22].

3 The Teaching–Learning Process and Algorithm

Towards the behavioral intervention, learning outcomes, and Internal motivation the system is developed to tutor the child in a better way. Every child has their own way to learn things. Knowing they started and giving customized teaching would help in bringing up a brighter student. A solution with NAO with a mobile application is proposed to serve the problem statement [23]. NAO, Robo vie R3, TIRO, Pepper, Maggie, Mio Amico are robots that are used as social robots in the language learning class [24]. The percentage of application of several robots in the field of ITC is shown below in Fig. 3. Applications proposed with NAO [12, 18, 23–29]. Sometimes a

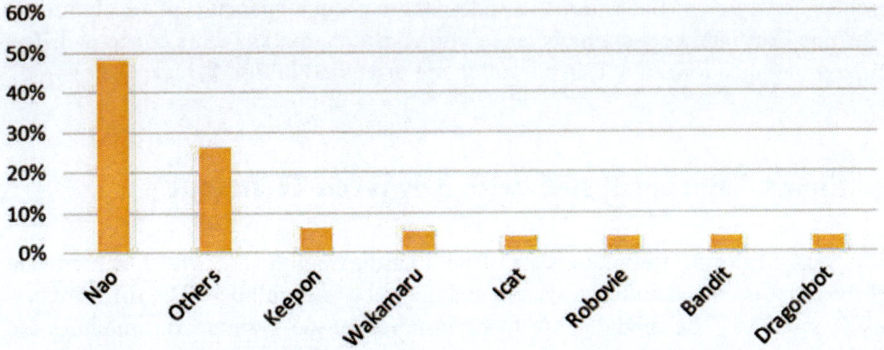

Fig. 3 Types of robots used in the studies

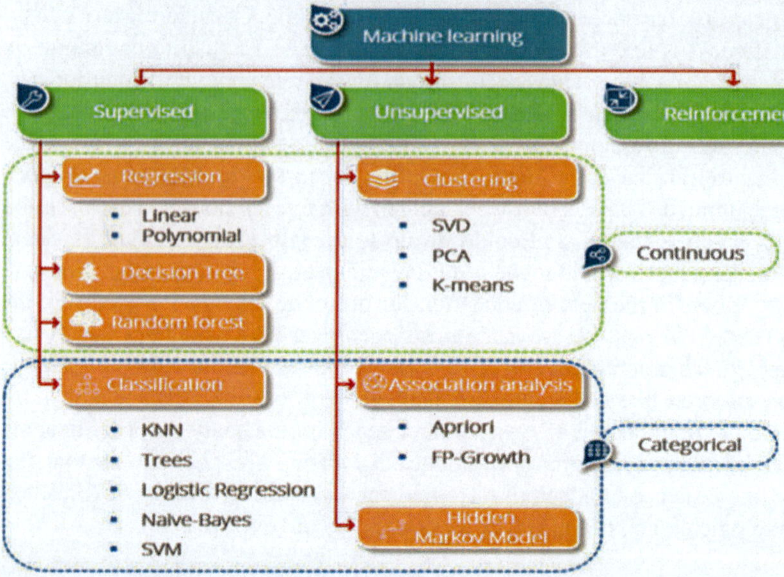

Fig. 4 Types of machine learning algorithms

robot is forced to learn from children to train the children for future. The perceptual, language, and social development is observed in the baby and trained [25]. Affect and learning is another relationship model that helps in social interaction enhancement [30].

The research articles are based on different Machine learning Algorithms. The classification of algorithms is done based on the efficiency of input data and the type of data. The different types of supervised, unsupervised, and reinforcement learning algorithms are discussed and the continuous or categorial data-based classifiers are separated and shown in a better way in Fig. 4.

Machine learning has a wide range of applications. The applications serve different problem statements. Each problem statement expects a special type of algorithm. Machine learning in education is taken into consideration as ITS is concerned. The different applications of ML in education are discussed in Fig. 5.

4 Smart Tutoring System with Advanced Techniques

The Smart Tutoring Robot consists of both hardware and software. The hardware of the robot is considered as a system and the same is developed. The software part is the modules. The modules are to be installed in the system. The modules are different activities or games that are intended to provide knowledge to the children. The system encloses a display that is programmed with a Microprocessor (Raspberry

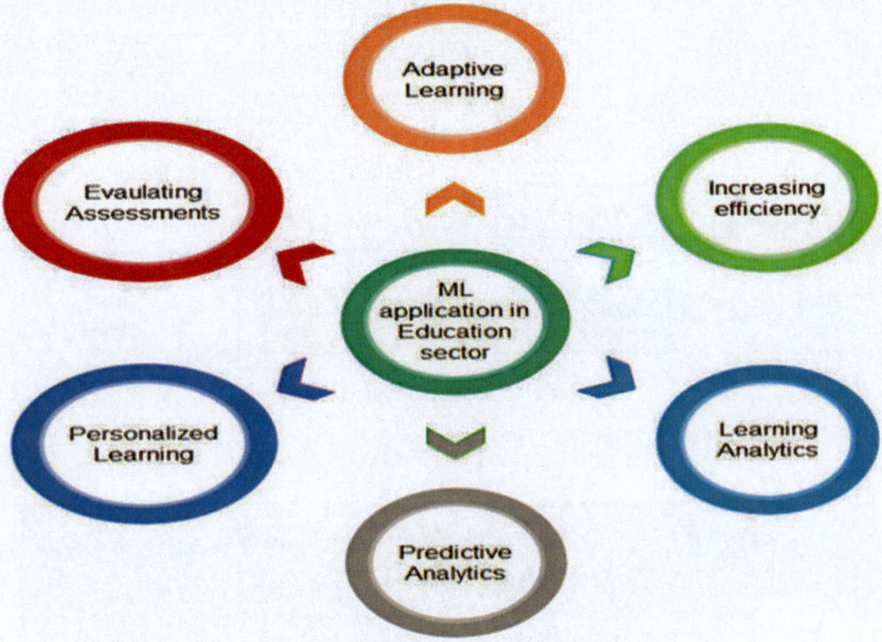

Fig. 5 ML application in education sector

Pi) which is enabled with Google API for voice commands. The system consists of a Microphone and Speaker which helps in communication part and the vision sensor is used to monitor the child. The system enclosed an Encoded DC motor to drive the motor. The system is enabled with a basic structure of ITS which comprises a set of sensors to monitor the children and an actuator to respond and communicate with children to make the system user friendly. The block diagram of the proposed work is stated in Fig. 6.

The proposed system includes a microphone (Respeaker 4 Mic Array V2), image sensor, speaker, and microprocessor. The indication circuit is added to show the user interaction by glowing LED. The system is implemented and working. The implementation of the proposed work is shown in Fig. 7. Different modules are to be installed which will be discussed further. The modules include alphabets detection, numbering, shapes, etc. The system teaches the child if he/she is wrong and appreciates the correct move. The system is featured to display a set of alphabets, shapes, or numbers. The character is selected randomly through the Raspberry Pi and displayed. The child must touch the character as said. The training of the kid in an interactive way, such as voice assistant and visual guidance helps the child better way. The complete implementation including the modules in cloud and validation of the system with the children is to be done further.

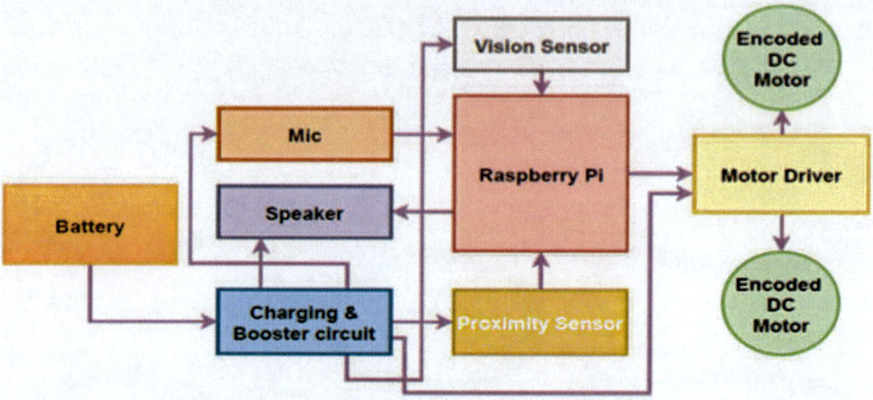

Fig. 6 Block diagram of the system

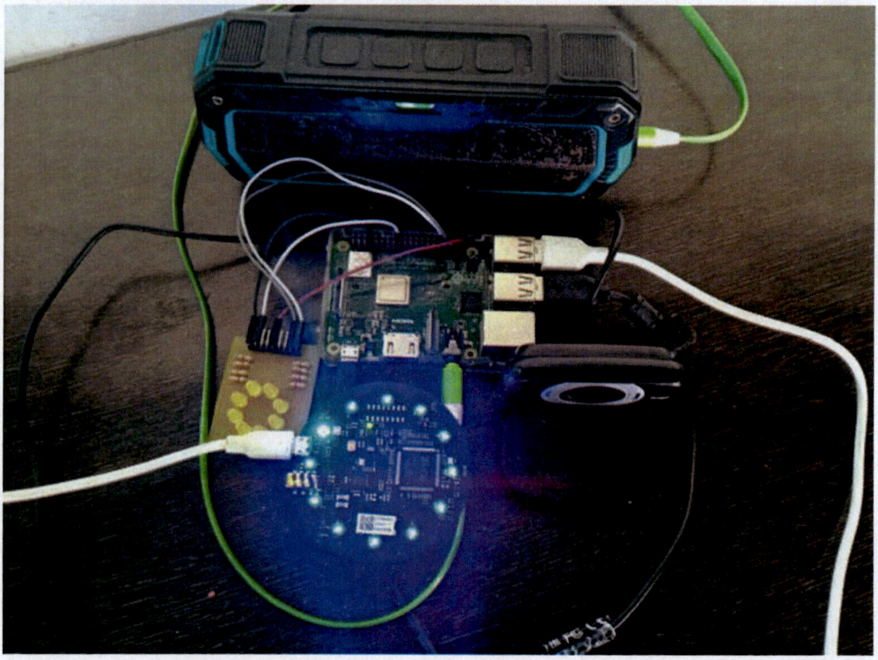

Fig. 7 Interconnection of all peripheral

5 Results and Discussion

The hardware of the system is implemented, and the output is taken into consideration. The system is intended to detect the voice and convert it into text using Google Cloud Speech API for the STT. The visual sensor is integrated to monitor the children and the speaker is added to the system to ensure a better speaking output in the

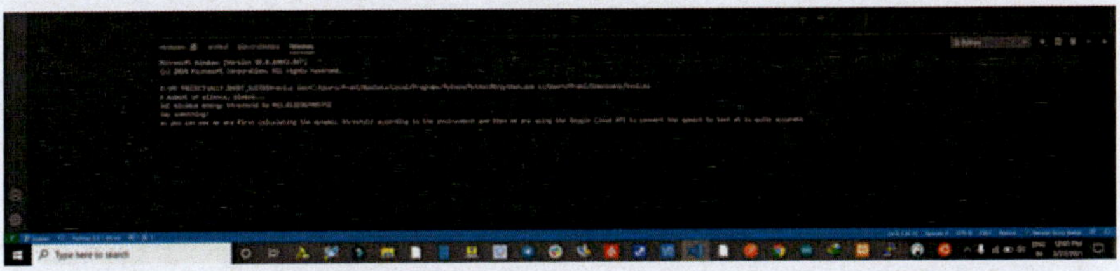

Fig. 8 Result of basic implementation

system. The speaker is used in the other way to provide feedback to the children. The microphone used has four microphones in different directions. The system is enabled to detect the child's position using a different microphone. The indication lights in the module indicate the same. The system has a high-end core processor to ensure the better working of the system. The interfacing of the microphone, speaker, display, motor, and cloud is added. The smooth running of the system requires a proper processor and that motivated in using Raspberry Pi. The system is developed with the features and the work is tested. The results of the basic implementation are shown in Fig. 8.

6 Recommendation and Conclusion

The energy of the nation, children are taken into consideration. Focusing on health and emotions forced us into the education methodologies. The problem statement on tutoring is stated and the solution is proposed. The Intelligent Tutor System (ITS) is the basic system or domain that provides various solutions to solve problems for children. The ITS has lots of applications in the education domain for preschool children. The implementation of ITS gives a brief knowledge on the principle of the ITS but the literature part stands high showing the experiments of different authors. The system is designed and the implementation of the same is proposed in this paper. The further implementation of the modules on cloud computing and machine learning on domain models is specified. Review on related work is done and the knowledge gap is considered to propose the idea for implementation. The inclusion of edge computing, vision node architecture, modules in cloud computing, deep learning, Artificial Intelligence to enhance the performance is to be enabled in further research.

References

1. Ramachandran A, Huang CM, Gartland E and Scassellati B (2018) Thinking aloud with a tutoring robot to enhance learning. In: ACM/IEEE Int. Conf. Human-Robot Interact, pp 59–68
2. Guardia JJ et al. (2019) Innovation in the teaching-learning process : the cas of Kahoot !

3. Yang J, Zhang B (2019) Applied sciences artificial intelligence in intelligent tutoring robots : a systematic revi and design guidelines
4. Scassellati B et al. (2018) Improving social skills in children with ASD using a long-term, in-home social robot 7544
5. Lambert A, Norouzi N, Bruder G, Welch G (2020) A systematic review of ten years of research on human interaction with social robots. Int J Hum Comput Interact 36(19):1804–1817
6. Johal W (2020) Research trends in social robots for learning
7. Suárez-Rodríguez J, Almerich G, Orellana N, Díaz-García I (2018) A basic model of integration of ICT by teachers: competence and use. Educ Technol Res Dev 66(5):1165–1187
8. Adamson T et al., Why we should build robots that both teach and learn
9. Aberšek B, Popov V (2004) Intelligent tutoring system for training in design and manufacturing. Adv Eng Softw 35(7):461–471
10. Corbett S (2017) From teacher to manager: expectations and challenge in the further education sector. a relationship model. Res Post-Compulsory Educ 22(2):208–220
11. Rosé CP, McLaughlin EA, Liu R, Koedinger KR (2019) Explanatory learner models: why machine learning (alone) is not the answer. Br J Educ Technol 50(6):2943–2958
12. Ramachandran A, Huang CM, Scassellati B (2017) Give me a break! Personalized timing strategies to promote learning in robot-child tutoring. In: ACM/IEEE Int. Conf. Human-Robot Interact., vol. Part F1271, pp 146–155
13. Das A, Deb K, Bajerjee S, Bag R (2017) A new method for tutorial gap identification towards students modeling. Math Model Eng Probl 4(2):80–83
14. Xt X, X D, X DX, and X LDX (2017) Emotion, age, D1 X X and gender D1 2X X D1 3X X classification in children's D1 4X X D1 5X X speech by D1 6X X humans and machines D1 7X X," Comput Speech Lang
15. Russo C, Madani K, Rinaldi AM (2020) Knowledge acquisition and design using semantics and perception: a case study for autonomous robots. Neural Process Lett (Ea 3956)
16. Almasri A, Ahmed A (2019) Intelligent tutoring systems survey for the period 2000–2018. Int J Acad Eng Res 3(5):21–37
17. Smakman M, Konijn EA (2020) Robot tutors: welcome or ethically questionable? Vol 1023. Springer International Publishing
18. Leyzberg D, Ramachandran A, Scassellati B (2018) The effect of personalization in longer-term robot tutoring. In: ACM Trans Human-Robot Interact 7(3)
19. Belpaeme T, Kennedy J, Ramachandran A, Scassellati B, Tanaka F (2018) Social robots for education: a review. Sci Robot 3(21):1–10
20. Schodde T, Hoffmann L, Kopp S, How to manage affective state in child-robot tutoring interactions?
21. S. E. E. Profile and S. E. E. Profile (2014) Applying ideas from intelligent tutoring systems for teaching programming in game based learning. No. October 2013
22. Lawrence JE, Tar UA (2018) Factors that influence teachers' adoption and integration of ICT in teaching/learning process. EMI Educ Media Int 3987:1–27
23. Ramachandran A, Huang C-M, Scassellati B (2019) Toward effective robot-child tutoring. ACM Trans Interact Intell Syst 9(1):1–23
24. Lehmann H, Rossi PG (2019) Social robots in educational contexts: developing an application in enactive didactics. J E-Learning Knowl Soc 15(2):27–41
25. Cangelosi A, Schlesinger M (2018) From babies to robots: the contribution of developmental robotics to developmental psychology. Child Dev Perspect 12(3):183–188
26. Jones A, Bull S, Castellano G (2017) I know that now, I'm going to learn this next. Promoting self-regulated learning with a robotic tutor. Int J Soc Robot
27. Vogt P et al.(2019) Second language tutoring using social robots: a large-scale study, pp 497505
28. Serholt S (2016) Robots tutoring children: longitudinal evaluation of social engagement in child-robot interaction
29. Konijn EA, Hoorn JF (2020) Computers & education robot tutor and pupils' educational ability : teaching the times tables. Comput Edu 157:103970

30. Chen H, Park HW, Zhang X and Breazeal C (2020) Impact of interaction context on the student affect-learning relationship in child-robot interaction. In: ACM/IEEE Int. Conf. Human-Robot Interact., pp 389–397

Effective Heart Disease Classification for Telehealth Systems

Deepa Jose, Arya Rajesh, P. Jaisharmila, Jeba M. Jasvine, and V. Andal

Abstract When left unchecked, arrhythmia is considered a life-threatening condition that causes severe health problems in patients. Arrhythmias can be diagnosed early in order to save lives. Electrocardiogram (ECG) signal is a vital role in the identification of arrhythmia. Because of the low data quality obtained by wearable devices and unprofessional consumers, automatic analysis and reliable identification of ECG signals remain unresolved problems. This raises the difficulty of hand-crafted feature extraction, affecting feature extraction performance and detection precision. As a reason, we need to build a more precise and effective automated method for the early diagnosis of arrhythmia. For that, the proposed solution used a machine learning algorithm for identification with the raw ECG signal in a wearable telehealth system to solve this problem and increase detection accuracy. For arrhythmia detection, machine learning algorithms such as support vector machine, Naive Bayes, and random forest are used to analyze the ECG signal. The experimental results show that our prototype solution is feasible and efficient in real-world use and that by comparing their accuracy, we can determine which machine learning algorithm is the best fit. The unique feature of the project is that it would classify the patient into one of the 16 arrhythmia classes.

Keywords Arrhythmia prediction · SVM · Naïve Bayes · Random forest · Feature selection · Extra trees classifier · And machine learning

D. Jose (✉) · A. Rajesh · P. Jaisharmila · J. M. Jasvine · V. Andal
Depatment of Electronics and Communication, KCG College of Technology, Karapakkam, Chennai 600097, TamilNadu, India
e-mail: deepa.ece@kcgcollege.com

V. Andal
Depatment of Science and Humanities, KCG College of Technology, Rajiv Gandhi Street, Karapakkam, Chennai 600097, Tamilnadu, India

N. Marriwala et al. (eds.), *Emergent Converging Technologies and Biomedical Systems*, Lecture Notes in Electrical Engineering 841,
https://doi.org/10.1007/978-981-16-8774-7_23

1 Introduction

People in today's world suffer from a number of chronic diseases. Heart disorders, for example, are found to affect a significant proportion of the population. Since coronary diseases can be life-threatening and cause accidental mortality, early diagnosis and precision medical aid to heart attack patients could save lives. The electrocardiogram (ECG), which is monitored based on electrodes mounted on the body and generates a graphical pattern of the heart electrical impulses, is the most commonly used method for diagnosing heart activity [1–3]. T waves, P waves, and the QRS complex are the most common ECG signals. Time length, form, and the interaction between P wave, QRS complex, T wave, and R-R interval are all important parameters to consider when examining cardiac patients. Any sudden change in these parameters signals a heart problem that may be caused by a variety of factors [4].

Arrhythmia is a type of erratic heart rhythm that can lead to heart failure, which presents a significant danger to people's lives. It must be properly diagnosed as soon as possible to minimize the chance of premature death, as it can even cause a heart attack if left untreated. Arrhythmia is a condition that disrupts the heart's electrical system's smooth rhythm, causing the heart to beat too slowly or too quickly, run, and miss beats, as well as heart signals nonsequential movement. Arrhythmia is usually diagnosed and analyzed by ECG records, as well as symptoms such as inadequate cardiac pumping, shortness of breath, chest pain, exhaustion, and unconsciousness. As a consequence, arrhythmia creates an atypical and sudden ECG signal [5].

Arrhythmias are classified into two types: bradycardia and tachycardia. Bradycardia occurs when the heart beats too slowly, typically less than 60 beats per minute (bpm), while tachycardia occurs when the heart beats too quickly, up to 100 bpm [6]. The importance of an effective, intelligent, and comprehensive arrhythmia detection model is being increasingly recognized with the implementation of various remote healthcare services for heart patients. Different ML (machine learning) methods have been used in the past to increase the precision of ECG signals based cardiac arrhythmia classification in order to create a reliable diagnostic method [7, 8]. The choosing of an effective methodology for arrhythmia classification is a challenging task since it is based on the application's context, data interpretation, prior encounters, and the needs of the individual patients.

In this article, we suggest an appropriate system for classifying ECG reports into normal and diseased types, i.e., distinguishing between the occurrence and absence of arrhythmia. The dataset was taken from the machine learning library at the University of California at Irvine (UCI), and classification was used to organize the data into one of 16 categories. A large feature collection is present in the dataset, which is minimized using a better feature selection method [9, 10]. To pick the most important features from the given dataset, the proposed feature selection process uses an Extra Trees Classifier algorithm. The following are the paper's main contributions:

(1) For choosing the most appropriate features, an optimized feature selection process based on extra trees classifier is suggested.

(2) On the UCI-arrhythmia dataset, machine learning algorithms are used with the chosen parameters to achieve high classification accuracy.

2 Previous Works

Many approaches for developing an intelligent classification model for arrhythmia diagnosis have been suggested. To identify cardiac arrhythmia patients, a learning vector quantization base NN (neural network) was applied to the ECG dataset. To define instants as regular or have arrhythmia, the characteristics are reduced by means of principal component analysis (PCA), followed through six NNs.

Another analysis uses automated artificial neural networks to identify arrhythmia patients based on data from a typical 12-lead ECG. The missing data is treated by substituting the nearest value from the concerned class for attribute values. For arrhythmia classification, a multilayer perceptron (MLP) with static backpropagation approach is utilized after missing values are replaced.

To classify cardiac arrhythmia into 16 distinct groups, researchers have used a generalized feed forward neural network, MLP with one-against-all approach, Bayesian artificial neural networks, and modular neural networks, proposes a new method for cardiac arrhythmia classification that employs a correlation-based feature filtering strategy for choosing the most important features from the UCI dataset, as well as an incremental back propagation neural network and Levenberg–Marquardt for early and accurate arrhythmia identification. Decision trees have also been used to design a computer aided diagnostic method for successfully classifying cardiac arrhythmia. These diagnostic and decision support services will assist doctors in quickly diagnosing diseases and reducing workload at the hospital's end.

3 Proposed Work

This paper proposes the three machine algorithms such as Support Vector Machine, Naïve Bayes, and Random Forest for prediction arrhythmia centered on medical data attributes from UCI. Figure 1 illustrates the workflow for arrhythmia prediction follow as,

i. The ECG dataset from the UCI-Machine Learning library is used to propose a novel model for classifying arrhythmia patients in this article.
ii. Using an improved feature selection strategy called Extra Trees Classifier; the suggested model first selects the most defining attributes.
iii. Then, modified dataset by feature selection is divided into 75% of training and 25% of testing data.
iv. Following the selection of important features, SVM, NB, and RF machine learning approaches are used to classify the patients into 16 arrhythmia subclasses using the selected features.

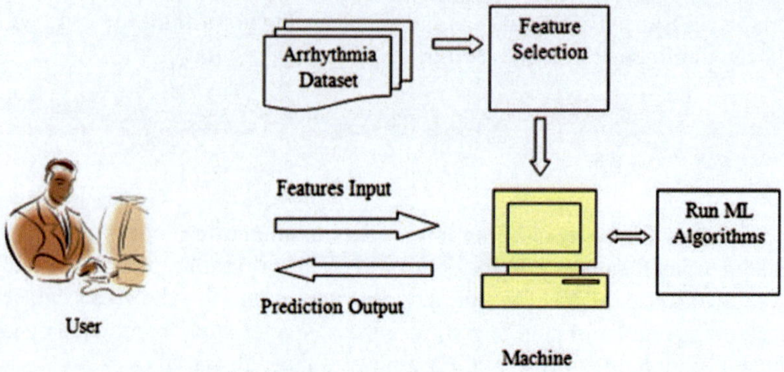

Fig. 1 Process for arrhythmia prediction

Prediction of Arrhythmia implemented by following modules

1. Data Visualization
2. Feature Selection
3. Data Splitting
4. Classification

1. **Data Visualization**

It's easier to grasp and interpret a vast volume of data when it's depicted graphically. Some employers demand that a data analyst be able to produce PowerPoint presentations, graphs, maps, and models. The histogram plot and feature extraction are seen as visualization in our approach (Fig. 2).

2. **Feature Selection**

In this module, the improved feature selection model like extra tress classifier is proposed for selecting the important features from a large features dataset.

Fig. 2 Data visualization

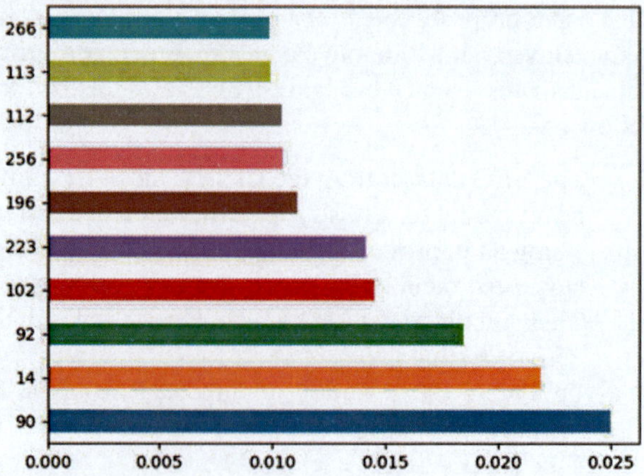

Extra Trees Classifier

The Extra Trees Classifier is a form of ensemble learning that works by fitting a number of randomized decision trees to the results. To ensure that the model does not overfit the results, random splits of all measurements are performed. A total of 50 features were chosen using this model.

3. **Data Splitting**

The modified dataset is divided into two parts: a train set and a test set, with a 75 percent and a 25 percent break, respectively.

4. **Classification**

In classification, machine learning models are used to evaluate split training and testing data. To build the prediction, three machine learning models are proposed. First, three ML models, Support Vector Machine (SVM), Naïve Bayes (NB), and Random Forest (RF) is used to train training data, and then testing data is predicted using the learned learn model. Finally, certain parameters such as Mean Squared Error (MSE), Mean Absolute Error (MAE), Root Mean Squared Error (RMSE), R-squared, and Accuracy are used to compare the above algorithms. The following are the descriptions of three related algorithms:

A. **Support Vector Machine (SVM)**

Support Vector Machine (SVM) is a set of similar supervised learning methods for classification and regression in medical diagnosis. SVM maximizes the geometric margin while minimizing the empirical classification error. SVM stands for Maximum Margin Classifiers, and it uses the kernel trick to effectively perform non-linear classification. An SVM model is an illustration of the examples as points in space, mapped such that the examples of the different groups are separated by a wide margin distance. As data points of the type, named training data is provided. After transforming the input vectors into a decision value, the SVM classifier performs classification using an acceptable threshold value (Fig. 3).

Fig. 3 SVM

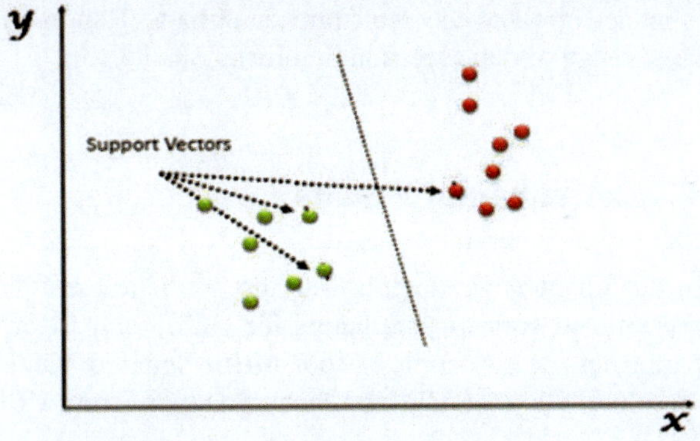

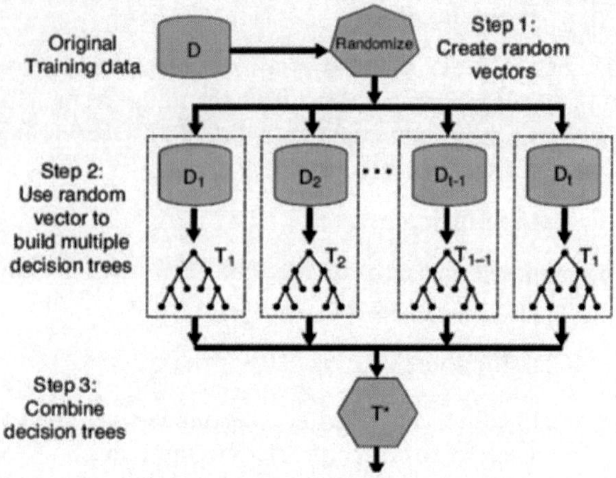

Fig. 4 Flow of random forest

B. **Naïve Bayes (NB)**

Naive Bayes classifiers are a family of basic "probabilistic classifiers" based on applying Bayes' theorem with strict (naive) independence assumptions between the features in machine learning. It's a classification method based on Bayes' Theorem and the predictor independence principle. A NB classifier, in basic words, implies that the existence of one function in a class is irrelevant to the presence of any other feature. The NB model is easy to construct and is particularly useful for large dimensionality data sets. NB is considered to better even the most advanced categorization methods because of their simplicity.

C. **Random Forest**

Random Forest is another common paradigm of supervised machine learning. Although RF can be used for both classification and regression, it is best for classification. Until having the output or outcome, often decision trees are used in random forests. As a result, the term "random forest" refers to the joining of many decision trees. In RF, a large number of trees will provide a reasonable outcome. In grouping, a voting scheme is used to determine the class, while in regression, the mean estimate is made for all of the decision tree outputs. Random forest performed well with a large range of datasets of high dimensionality (Fig. 4).

4 Experimental Results

In this chapter, we demonstrate the prediction results from different ML models. We utilized various parameters for build comparison with three ML models; the parameters are Accuracy, Root Mean Squared Value (RMSE), R-squared, Mean Absolute Value (MAE), and Mean Squared Error (MSE) Value.

Table 1 Accuracy analysis with three different models

Algorithm	Accuracy (%)
Support vector machine	47.82
Naïve Bayes	23.45
Random forest	68.18

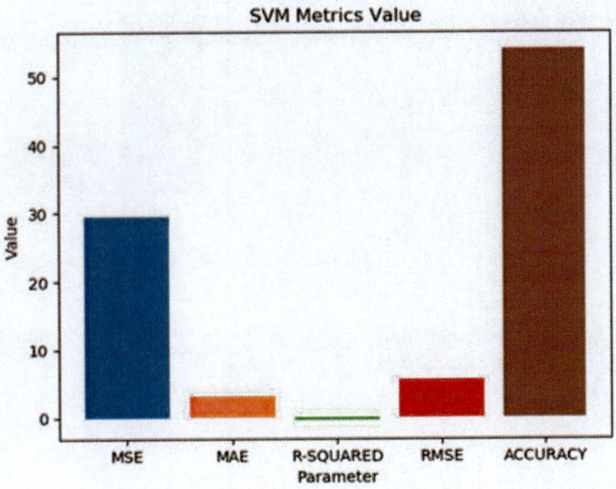

Fig. 5 Performance metrics of support vector machine algorithm

The dataset is being gathered from the UCI-Machine Learning library. There are 279 attributes in this database, 206 of which are linearly valued and the rest are trivial. Class 01 denotes a "normal" ECG, while classes 02 through 5 denote various types of arrhythmias, and class 15 denotes the majority of the unclassified ones.

From the prediction results in Table 1, we can conclude the random forest (RF) model provides high accuracy is 68.18% than the other two models.

Figures 5, 6, and 7 shows the performance analysis of three machine learning models.

5 Conclusion

This paper suggests three related three machine learning based methods, i.e., Support Vector Machine (SVM), naïve Bayes (NB), and random forest (RF) for classification of arrhythmias using ECG records. To reduce the dimensions of files, an improved feature selection approach is implemented for selecting the most important features which are done by an extra tress classifier. To prevent problems caused by the inclusion of binary values, the data is often standardized. On the normalized data, machine learning algorithms are used to identify the presence or nonappearance of disease and group the records into one of 16 categories. The synthesis of feature selection and classification techniques has yielded positive classification results. By comparing

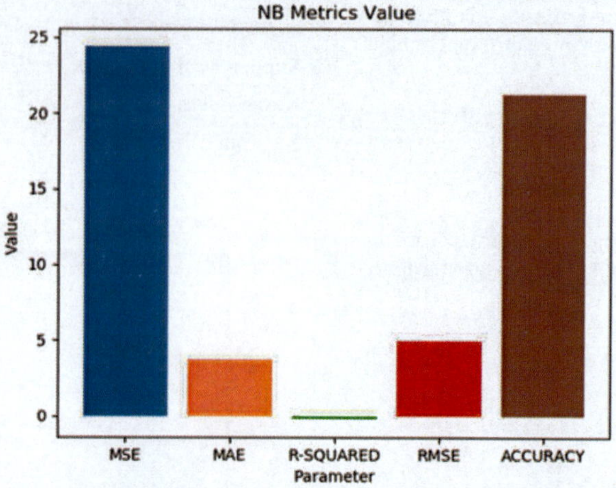

Fig. 6 Performance metrics of Naive Bayes algorithm

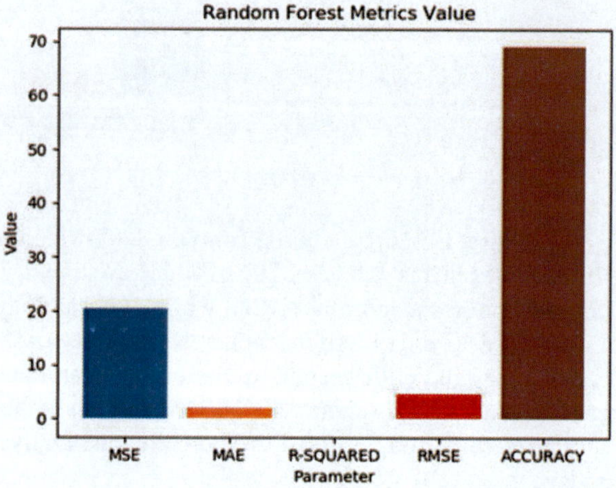

Fig. 7 Performance metrics of random forest algorithm

their accuracy, the classification results revealed which approach is better suited for classification on the ECG dataset taken from the UCI repository.

References

1. Heart Disease and Stroke|At A Glance Reports|Publications|Chronic Disease Prevention and Health Promotion|CDC, https://www.cdc.gov/chronicdisease/resources/publications/aag/heart-disease-stroke.html
2. Anderson C, Vasan RS (2017) Epidemiology of cardiovascular disease in young individuals. Nat Rev Cordial
3. Zuo WM, Lu WG, Wang KQ, Zhang H (2008) Diagnosis of cardiac arrhythmia using kernel difference weighted KNN classifier. In: Proceedings of the computers in cardiology (CAR'08),

vol 35. View at: Publisher Site | Google Scholar, pp 253–256
4. Alickovic E, Subasi A (2016) Medical decision support system for diagnosis of heart arrhythmia using DWT and random forests classifier. J Med Syst 40, article 108:1–12. View at: Publisher Site | Google Scholar
5. Kumar SU, Inbarani HH (2017) Neighborhood rough set based ECG signal classification for diagnosis of cardiac diseases. Soft Comput 21(16):4721–4733. View at: Publisher Site | Google Scholar
6. Özbay Y, Karlik B (2001) A recognition of ECG arrhythmias using artificial neural networks. Selcuk University, Electrical and electronics engineering
7. Rahhal MMA, Bazi Y, Alhichri H, Alajlan N, Melgani F, Yager RR (2016) Deep learning approach for active classification of electrocardiogram signals. Inf Sci 345:340–354. View at: Publisher Site | Google Scholar
8. Nayak CG, Seshikala G, Desai U, Nayak SG (2016) Identification of arrhythmia classes using machine-learning techniques. Int J Biol Biomed 1:48–53. View at: Google Scholar
9. Peter TJ, Somasundaram K (2012) An empirical study on prediction of heart disease using classification data mining techniques. In: IEEE-International conference on advances in engineering, science and management, ICAESM-2012, pp 514–518
10. Wankhede J, Kumar M, Sambandam P (2020) Efficient heart disease prediction-based on optimal feature selection using DFCSS and classification by improved Elman-SFO. IET Syst Biol 14(6):380–390

Effective Plant Leaf Disease Detection for Farmers

Deepa Jose, M. Pavithra, S. Sasipriya, M. Satya Venkata Santosh, and Jhonatan Fabricio Meza Cartegana

Abstract Agriculture is backbone of India, more than half of the population depends on agriculture as source of income and India's economy is also depends on agriculture. This industry needs more attention for automated software. Artificial intelligence is more powerful when applied to agriculture industry. The proposed system discusses plant leaf detection through deep learning algorithm. Plants when affected by pests, it highly affect production and thus continuous monitoring is needed to avoid this problem. The proposed system uses images to capture and analyze the leaf whether infected or not. The deep learning algorithm, Convolution neural network is used for analysis. The model used images from mobile phones are loaded to Raspberry PI and applied deep learning algorithm. The dataset with infected leaf images and normal leaf images is considered for training. This involves image pre-processing techniques such as segmentation and grayscale conversions and then training and detection. Plant leaves are classified as normal and infected in the proposed work. Experimental results show that the accuracy of plant leaf disease is more accurate through our proposed model.

Keywords Artificial Intelligence · Image segmentation · Grayscale conversion · CNN algorithm · Raspberry Pi

1 Introduction

Agriculture plays an important for our economy. The plant disease identification is important for productivity for farmers. Plant disease if diagnosed at right time, may prevent severe damage to crops and production. The usage of pesticides without

D. Jose (✉) · M. Pavithra · S. Sasipriya · M. Satya Venkata Santosh
Department of ECE, KCG College of Technology, Karapakkam, Chennai, Tamil Nadu 600097, India
e-mail: deepa.ece@kcgcollege.com

J. F. M. Cartegana
Instituto Superior Tecnológico 17 de Julio, Ibarra, Ecuador
e-mail: jmeza@ist17dejulio.edu.ec

N. Marriwala et al. (eds.), *Emergent Converging Technologies and Biomedical Systems*, Lecture Notes in Electrical Engineering 841,
https://doi.org/10.1007/978-981-16-8774-7_24

proper training may cause reduce immunity of plants to fight against any disease. Thus the disease identified on time is important to prevent loss in agriculture and give high productivity. Changes in climatic conditions may also affect the plant and be monitored continuously. Sometimes, experienced farmers can only identify the disease others may not notice, thus causing huge damage. To avoid this problem, an effective solution for plant disease diagnosis is preferred.

Visible symptoms through naked eye may not be seen in some of the plant diseases, if those are unattended or lately notice may cause severe damage to plants. The computer vision monitoring system may be effective to solve this problem. Advancement in artificial intelligence domain has paved way for proper diagnosis of plant disease. Earlier machine learning was used for training diseased and non-diseased leaves then used for monitoring. In this proposed work deep learning was used. Commercializing agriculture these days is creating negative impact on environment, soil nature, and plant's healthiness. Usage of high pesticides level may bring spoil of underwater, soil, and nature. Though they can give productivity in short term, the impact on a higher time frame is dangerous.

India has the largest farming land and many vary are cultivated, there are many techniques developed for smart farming. Expansion of computer vision in the forming has largest scope in the future for artificial intelligence field. Whenever the plants are getting disease, the leaves are eventual part which shows early signs of disease, it these are detected on time, can help farmers with production and reduces loss. Due to industrialization and due to globalization, farming is affected a lot in our country. When the farmers get benefited through smart techniques, with less expenses, the economy grows eventually.

There are many researchers who proposed plant leaf disease detection through different analyses and methods, some of them included machine learning classification such as Support Vector Machine (SVM) and clustering techniques such as k-means algorithm was proposed. These models give less accuracy on prediction. Thus an effective algorithm and implementation are required for leaf disease detection (Fig. 1).

The main objective of proposed work is to identify plant leaf disease by an automated disease diagnosis system based on Deep learning algorithm. We use Convolutional Neural Network (CNN) model, which gives best performance on plant leaf disease prediction. This proposed work can be achieved on real time detection with the hardware kit and monitoring stations. This model gives us better detection results based on both deep learning algorithm, which is considered for the implementations.

Implemented a plan leaf disease classification system through an automated machine vision and deep learning diagnosis model. The dataset used for training contains diseased and healthy leaves. Healthy leaves of 388 instances and disease leaves of 364 images. The motive of work is to classify leaf as a binary classification type 0(healthy leaf) to 1 (diseased leaf). User or farmers can go for input of image to get the leaf classified as healthy and unhealthy. The implemented application helps farmers in making advance decisions for treating the plants early without damage.

The proposed work carried out in three phases, the first phase is to design a hardware architecture, where the input from mobile phone is taken and given to

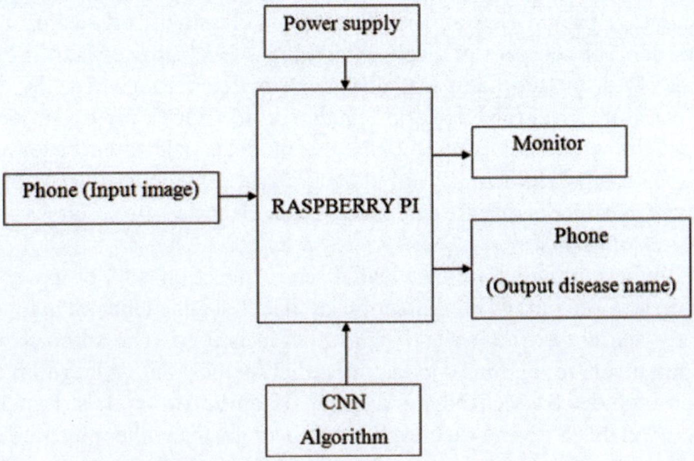

Fig. 1 Overview of plant leaf disease prediction

Raspberry model, the second phase contains training the CNN algorithm for a given dataset and making a trained model. The third phase, get input from mobile phone and use the trained model for detection of plant leaf disease in the given sample.

2 Related Work

There are several researchers who worked on plant leaf disease predictions and analysis. Machine vision and artificial intelligence are growing areas for agricultural industry, thus the research on this field is increasing dramatically. Some of such works are addressed below.

Diagnosis of plant leaf disease is proposed in [1] using a neural network algorithm. Author used grape leaves for the study. Back propagation neural network is used for detection. Pre-process of images are handled with k-means clustering and GLCM feature extraction modules. However, this work on BPNN has achieved less accuracy compared to our proposed model.

Watermelon leaf disease detection was studied in [2] with neural network algorithm of binary classification with Anthracnos, Downey Mildew are the two classes for detection. The dataset with 200 images on each class type is studied in this work. Implementation is carried out in Matlab. The accuracy achieved in this work 75% to 76% only. However, the work handled with real-time image detection, the accuracy of detection is less compared to CNN.

Some of the work on supervised machine learning algorithm is carried out, in which [3] used with Tomato leaf images with multiple classifications such as healthy, early blight, bacterial infection, and curl virus infections. Implementation is done with

Matlab with image pre-processing with GLCM and classifier as K-nearest neighbor (KNN) classifier. The accuracy of machine learning is less than deep learning models.

The work [4] discussed plant leaf disease detection through R-CNN, Region-Based Convolutional Neural Networks. Author used COCO for object detection, which is a pre-trained model using R-CNN, this model can detect more leaves based on pre-trained architecture from PlantVillage dataset. The author also proposed F-RCNN, Fast RCNN model disease detection, which identified more classes of disease in more species of plants.

A novel, hybrid model for plant leaf disease detection was proposed in [5], for capsicum leaf on binary classification as healthy and unhealthy. Image pre-processing for feature extraction and segmentation is used. The authors evaluated more than one machine learning model, to predict the best one. Algorithm used for classification includes SVM, KNN, and linear Discriminant models. Experimental results concluded that SVM has achieved good accuracy than other machine learning algorithms.

A review of plant disease classification through different classifications is analyzed in [6]. The work suggested other pattern recognition and also considered front and back views of leaves for accurate analysis. This also suggested finding severity of the disease.

It is inferred from the analysis of existing studies, there is a demand for highly effective model, which brings more accuracy to plant leaf disease prediction. Through this literature, it is observed that many researchers are proposed leaf disease detection through machine learning and deep learning neural network algorithm. However, the work was achieved around 75 to 76% on accuracy. Thus, in our proposed work, CNN algorithm is proposed for implementation, which is given high accuracy than existing models [7–13].

3 Proposed Work

The proposed implementation includes Raspberry Pi device install Raspberry software with Python 3.6.4 with libraries Tensor flow, Keras, matplotlib, and other needed libraries. We downloaded dataset from kaggle.com. The image dataset downloaded has binary types of data such as healthy and diseased. Deep learning algorithm is applied for detection of plant leaf disease.

The proposed work used Convolutional Neural Network (CNN) algorithm for train and detection of plan leaf images taken from kaggle.com of plant village dataset. The camera module captures images using raspberry pi then image pre-processing applied to prediction leaf is diseased or healthy. The image processing technique involved here includes color and feature extraction processes [14–16].

The above figure represents proposed architecture of plant leaf disease detection through deep learning, CNN algorithm, which is briefly explained here. Deep learning is a part of artificial intelligence and this learns similar to human brain through activated neurons. There are three layers represented in deep learning are input layer, hidden layer, and output layer. The algorithm input is given in the put layer are the features of images here. The hidden layer is activated with neurons and Adam optimizer. Output layers save the learned model as h5 file in the system. Deep learning models can themselves learn features automatically by input of images (Fig. 2).

The implementation is done with the below methodologies.

a. Dataset collection from kaggle.com
b. Image pre-processing
c. Split dataset into training set and testing set
d. Apply Deep learning CNN algorithm for training and analysis
e. Train the model with CNN
f. Get input from mobile phone to Raspberry pi
g. Given test set to trained model and predict disease.

PlantVillage dataset considered for study purpose, this image dataset is divided into training data and testing data. Around 70% images are considered for training algorithms for deep learning algorithms and to create a fit model. The remaining around 30% of image dataset is taken for testing data for Plant leaf disease prediction.

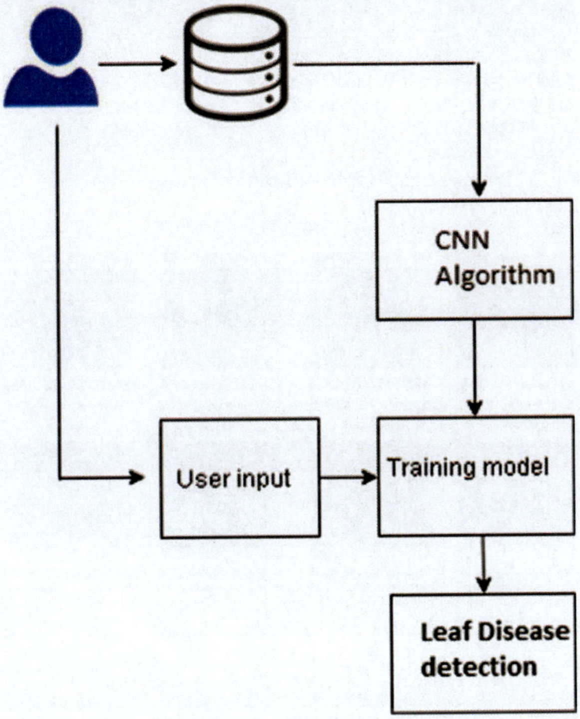

Fig. 2 Architecture of plant leaf disease prediction

3.1 Dataset Details

The dataset collected with binary values of 0 means healthy and 1-means diseased. The number of images in each class is 388 and 364 respectively. Sample of image dataset considered for the study is shown in below image for healthy leaves (Fig. 3).

The below figure shows the sample dataset view of disease leaves used for training (Fig. 4).

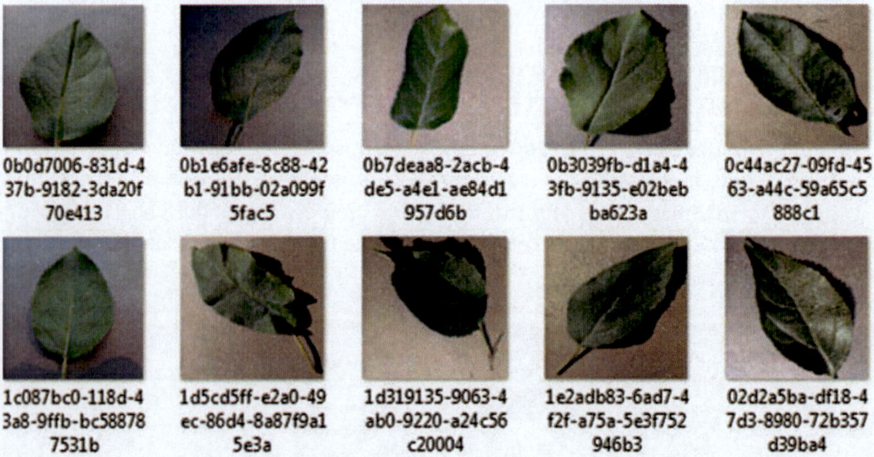

Fig. 3 Data set sample view of healthy leaves

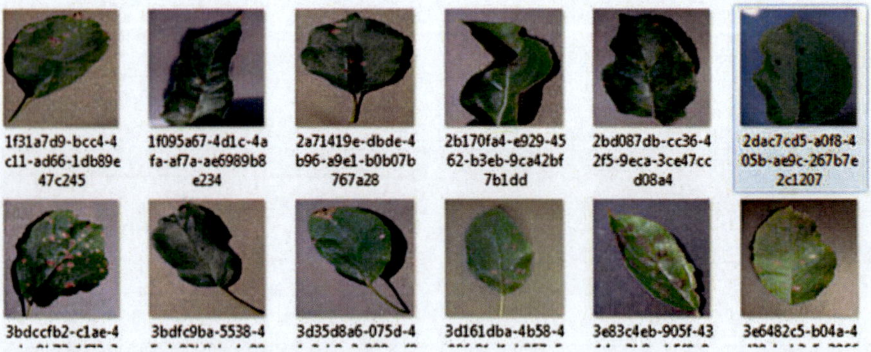

Fig. 4 Data set sample view of diseased leaves

3.2 Image Pre-processing

Data pre-processing involves converting the image dataset to features in CSV (Comma-separated values). Data pre-processing is handled in two phases. One is segmentation and other is feature extraction. Under the segmentation, the image path and image status (healthy or diseased) are given as input. The input image is converted to grayscale image for the first step. The grayscale converted image is shown below (Fig. 5).

The next level in pre-processing is thresholding with help of OTSU. In this process, a value of the threshold is identified automatically. This method considers two different values with two peaks to identify the threshold value of middle level. The next process would be noise removal on images. OpenCV enables background detection can be done through distanceTransform for binary value. The below figure shows the pre-processing output once segmentation is completed (Fig. 6).

The next level of pre-processing is done image feature extraction. The segmentation image is taken input for feature extraction process, we used KAZE extraction from OpenCV, this detects key point from image and extracted as CSV data file. The following image represents the output of segmentation on plant leaf image (Fig. 7).

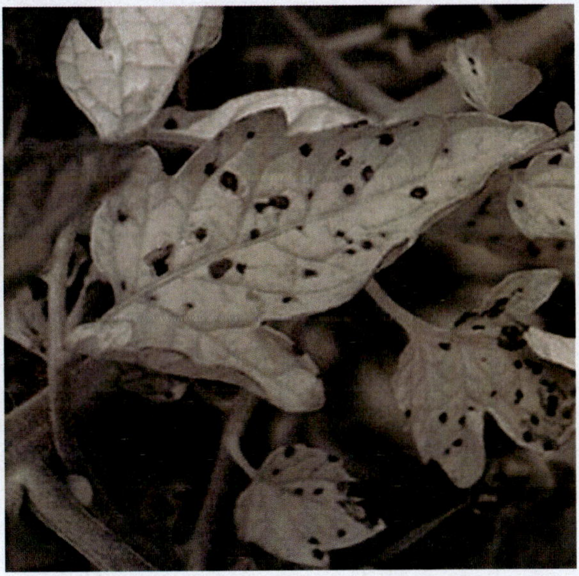

Fig. 5 Grayscale image after pre-processing

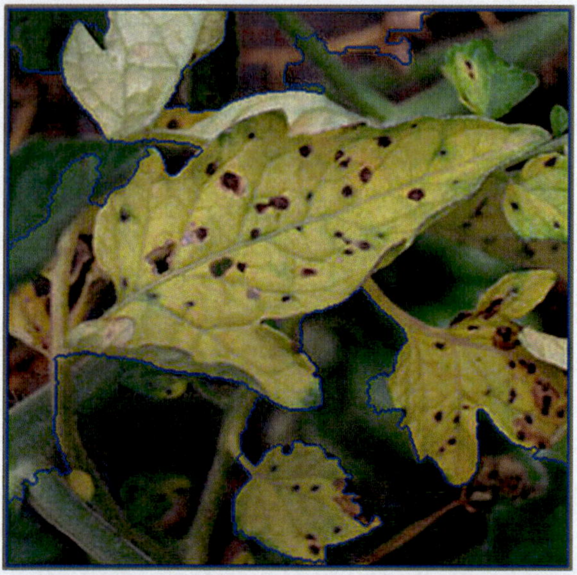

Fig. 6 Pre-processing output after segmentation

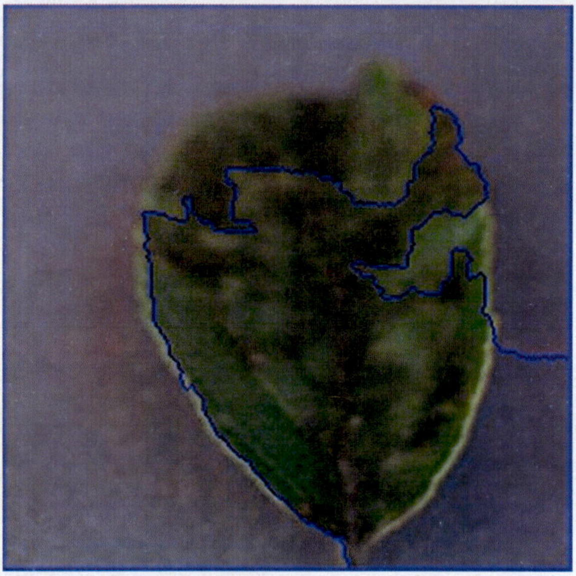

Fig. 7 Image segmentation on leaf

3.3 Convolutional Neural Network Algorithm

The proposed Convolution neural network (CNN) algorithm's architecture is shown below. Two Dimensional Convolutional Neural Network (Conv2D) is used for implementation. In the convolutional layer, each point on input data is given as leaf image

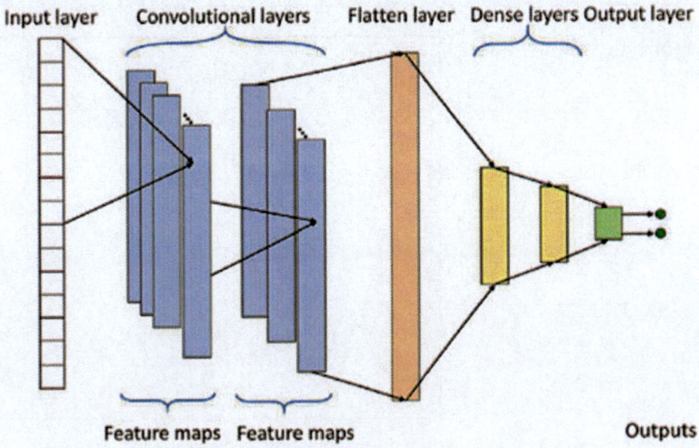

Fig. 8 Convolutional neural network architecture

features as input. The number of epoch given in the hidden layer is 25 number to optimize the learning (Fig. 8).

As per the shown architecture, input layer of the algorithm is given as dense layer with 128 neurons for activation. Rectified linear Unit (Relu) is an activation function used in hidden layer. Maxpooling with pool size 2. The hidden layer gets the feature vectors of images as input. Epoch 25 is given for iterated learning in hidden layer, which increases accuracy and decreases loss. Thus optimized epoch value is preferred which can be tested on development time. Adam optimizer utilized for optimization this reduces noise and gradient problems.

4 Results and Discussions

The proposed plant leaf disease classification is implemented Raspberry Pi and on Rasbion OS with Python and mandatory libraries Keras, Tesorflow, pandas, matplotlib. Plant leaf dataset with binary class healthy and diseased downloaded from kaggle.com is taken for study. Deep learning algorithm, CNN is implemented for disease detection. Experimental result shows that Convolutional Neural Network (CNN) is outperforming n disease detection with good accuracy. The following table shows the accuracy achieved in our proposed work (Table 1).

Table 1 Experimental results

Algorithm	Accuracy (%)
Convolutional neural network (CNN)	96%

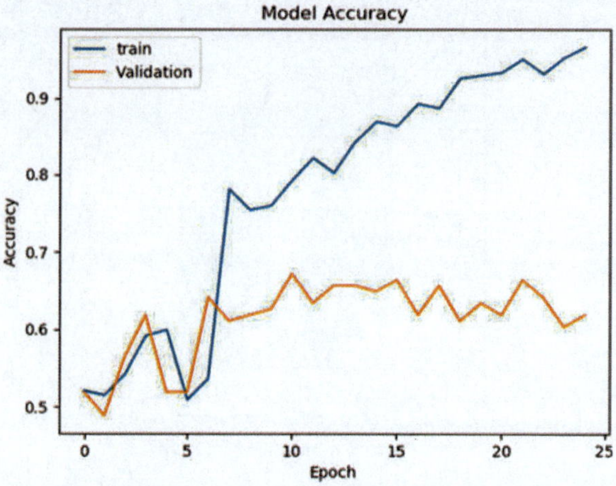

Fig. 9 Accuracy of plant leaf disease prediction through CNN

The below figure shows the experimental learning loss MSE (mean square error) error data on the training set and validation sets as shown below for the CNN model (Fig. 9).

5 Conclusion

Plant leaf disease detection is considered in this proposed work with deep learning algorithm, Convolutional Neural Networks (CNN). Plant leaf disease when identified early, proper measures can be taken by farmers to resolve this problem, thus their productivity increases. Machine vision and artificial intelligence growth enhance to achieve this work with simple hardware and less maintenance. Plant leaf can be taken through surveillance camera in real time or through mobile phone, given as input to the trained CNN model to identify whether the leaf is healthy or diseased. Experimental results show that the deep learning model achieved good accuracy on detection (Fig. 10).

Future work is to be carried out for classification of diseases in different plant species and to improve the classification accuracy.

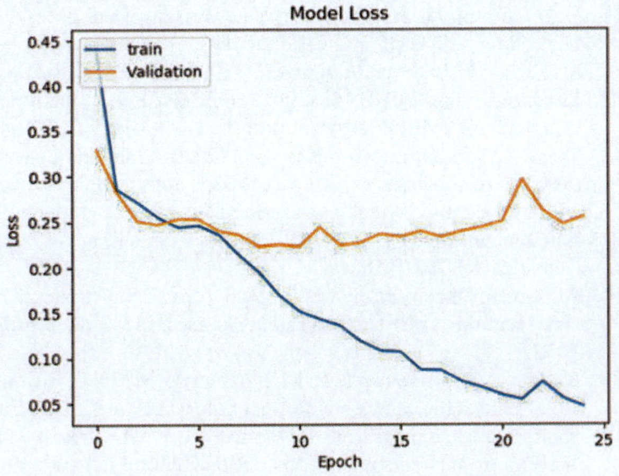

Fig. 10 Model loss—plant leaf disease prediction through CNN

References

1. Sannakki SS (eds) (2013) Diagnosis and classification of grape leaf diseases using neural networks. In: Proceedings of fourth international conference on computing, communications and networking technologies (ICCCNT). Tiruchengode, India, pp 1–5. https://doi.org/10.1109/ICCCNT.2013.6726616.
2. Kutty (eds) (2013) Classification of watermelon leaf diseases using neural network analysis. 2013 IEEE Business Engineering and Industrial Applications Colloquium (BEIAC). Langkawi, Malaysia, pp 459–464. https://doi.org/10.1109/BEIAC.2013.6560170
3. Geetha G (eds) (2020) Plant leaf disease classification and detection system using machine learning. J Phys: Conf Ser 1712 012012. https://doi.org/10.1088/1742-6596/1712/1/012012
4. Saleem M, Khanchi S, Potgieter J, Arif K (2020) Image-based plant disease identification by deep learning meta-architectures. Plants 9:1451. https://doi.org/10.3390/plants9111451
5. Anjna, Sood M, Kumar Singh P (2020) Hybrid system for detection and classification of plant disease using qualitative texture features analysis. Procedia Comput Sci 167:1056–1065. ISSN 1877-0509
6. Sandhu G, Kumar V, Joshi H (2018) Study of digital image processing techniques for leaf disease detection and classification. Multimed Tools Appl 77:1–50. https://doi.org/10.1007/s11042-017-5445-8
7. Sharma P, Hans P, Gupta SC (2020) Classification of plant leaf diseases using machine learning and image preprocessing techniques. In: Proceedings of 10th International conference on cloud computing, data science & engineering (Confluence). Noida, India, pp 480–484. https://doi.org/10.1109/Confluence47617.2020.9057889
8. Madhulatha G, Ramadevi O (2020) Recognition of plant diseases using convolutional neural network. In: Proceedings of 2020 fourth international conference on I-SMAC (IoT in Social, Mobile, Analytics and Cloud) (I-SMAC). Palladam, India, pp 738–743. https://doi.org/10.1109/I-SMAC49090.2020.9243422
9. Kumar S (eds) (2020) Leaf disease detection and classification based on machine learning. In: Proceedings of 2020 international conference on smart technologies in computing, electrical and electronics (ICSTCEE). Bengaluru, India, pp 361–365. https://doi.org/10.1109/ICSTCEE49637.2020.9277379.
10. Tiwari D (eds) (2020) Potato leaf diseases detection using deep learning. In: Proceedings of 2020 4th international conference on intelligent computing and control systems (ICICCS). Madurai, India, pp 461–466. https://doi.org/10.1109/ICICCS48265.2020.9121067.

11. Dai Q, Cheng X, Qiao Y, Zhang Y (2020) Crop leaf disease image super-resolution and identification with dual attention and topology fusion generative adversarial network. IEEE Access 8:55724–55735. https://doi.org/10.1109/ACCESS.2020.2982055
12. Sundarraj (eds) (2018) Identification of diseases in plant parts using image processing. Int J Eng Technol 7(461). https://doi.org/10.14419/ijet.v7i2.8.10485.
13. Trang K, Tonthat L, Minh Thao NG (2020) Plant leaf disease identification by deep convolutional autoencoder as a feature extraction approach. In: Proceedings of 2020 17th international conference on electrical engineering/electronics, computer, telecommunications and information Technology (ECTI-CON). Phuket, Thailand, pp 522–526. https://doi.org/10.1109/ECTI-CON49241.2020.9158218.
14. Albashish, Dheeb, Braik, Malik, Bani-Ahmad Sulieman (2011) A framework for detection and classification of plant leaf and stem diseases. 113–118. https://doi.org/10.1109/ICSIP.2010.5697452.
15. Kanipriya M, Krishnaveni R, Krishnamurthy M (2020) Recognizing audience feedback through facial expression using convolutional neural networks. Int J Eng Res Technol 13(12):4230–4235
16. Kanipriya M, Krishnaveni R, Bairavel S, Krishnamurthy M (2020) Aspect based sentiment analysis from tweets using convolutional neural network model. J Adv Res Dyn Control Syst 12(4):106–114.

Analysis of Various Non-invasive Methods for Pulmonary Cancer Identification

S. V. Banabakode and Swati R. Dixit

Abstract This Paper represents the various methods of pulmonary cancer detection and comparison of various methods of cancer detection. The main objective behind this study is to select the method which can be able to detect pulmonary cancer at an early stage. There are different methods available for detection of pulmonary cancer. These methods are mainly classified as invasive and non-invasive methods. The invasive methods which are available for detection of pulmonary cancer are not able to detect pulmonary cancer at early stages. The main reason behind this is signs of pulmonary cancer typically do not occur until the disease is reasonably in advanced stage and in non-curable stage. So even after detection, there are less chances of positive results because disease is already in advance stage and the treatment for this is also very costly which is beyond the capacity of common man. The invasive methods are also very dangerous. So there is only one option left to cure pulmonary cancer and that is to detect pulmonary cancer at an early stage then only from proper treatment pulmonary cancer can be cured.

1 Introduction

There are total 18.1 million new cases of cancer in the year 2018 out of which 9.6 million people were dead due to cancer worldwide. Out of these new cases, 2.1 million people deal with pulmonary cancer which is 11.6% of all cancer which is highest among all types of cancer and death due to pulmonary cancer are 1.76 million which is 18.4% of all the deaths is also highest (Figs. 1 and 2).

S. V. Banabakode (✉) · S. R. Dixit
Electronics & Telecommunication Engg Department, G H Raisoni University, Amaravati, Amaravati, India
e-mail: sanket.banabakode@raisoni.net

S. R. Dixit
e-mail: swati.dixit@raisoni.net

N. Marriwala et al. (eds.), *Emergent Converging Technologies and Biomedical Systems*, Lecture Notes in Electrical Engineering 841,
https://doi.org/10.1007/978-981-16-8774-7_25

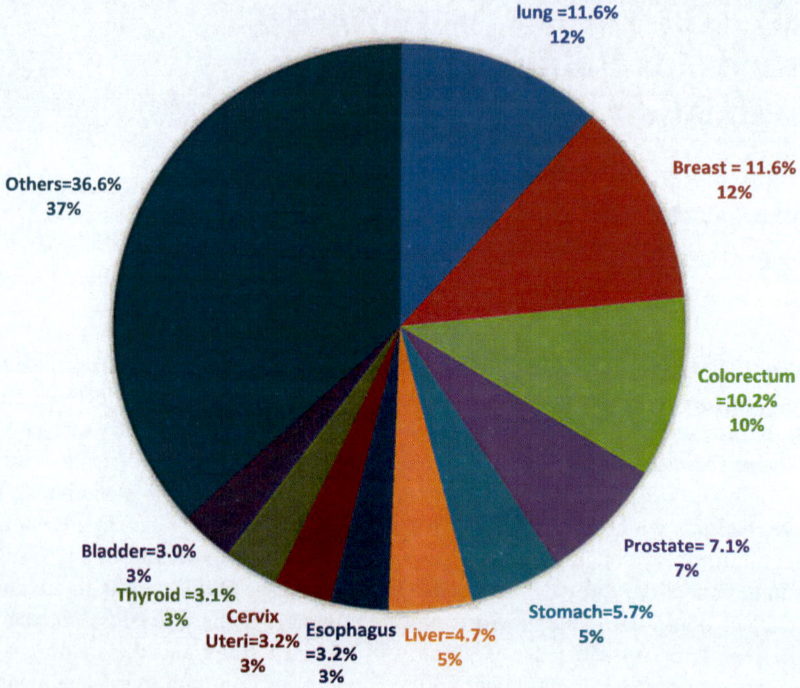

Fig. 1 Incidence of new cancer cases

The main reason behind large numbers of death is the symptoms of pulmonary cancer typically do not occur until the disease is reasonably advanced and in non-curable stage. Thus early detection of pulmonary cancer is a key issue to recover from pulmonary cancer. So for early detection as a screening tool, low dose chest computed tomography (CT) scanning has been proposed. This type of procedure should be carried out every year by person which is likely to be infected from pulmonary cancer which increases the probability of early-stage tumour diagnosis which increases the percentage of Survival of a person. The primary drawback of this approach is that it increases the risk of developing cancer as body is regularly exposed to the ionizing radiation of low dose computed tomography (CT). So for premature detection non-invasive methods are required which have no disadvantages on human body.

2 Cancer Detection Methods

There are various cancer detection techniques that are divided into two categories which are as follows.

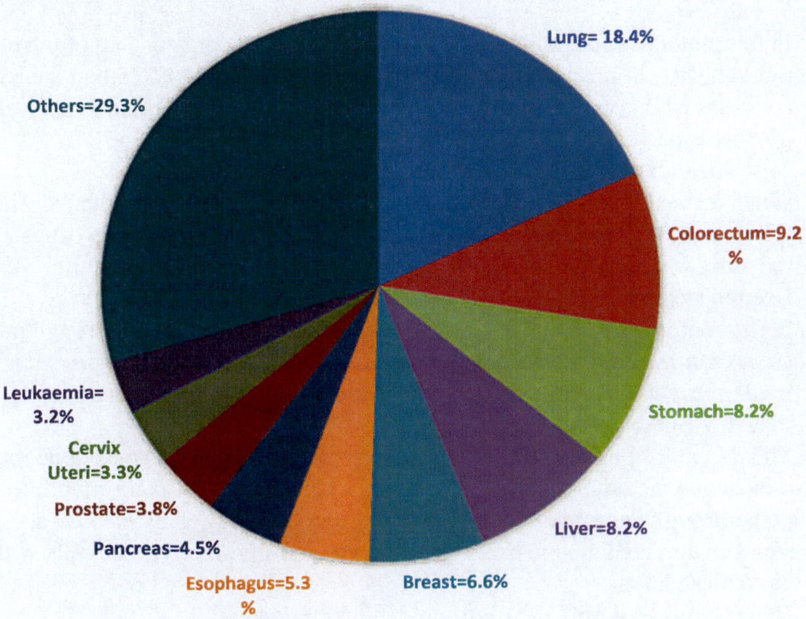

Fig. 2 Mortality rate due to cancer

(a) Invasive Method
(b) Non-invasive Method.

2.1 *Invasive Method*

In an invasive method, some part of body (infected) tissue is taken out from the body for testing using machine or exposed body to radiation, these methods are dangerous and costly and there is a chance of transmission of cancerous cells. Important thing is that using this method it is not possible to find pulmonary cancer at an early stage because signs of pulmonary cancer typically appear when the disease is at a very advanced stage. There are various invasive methods which are as follows,

(1) Needle Biopsy.
(2) Chest X-Ray.
(3) Low Does Spiral CT Scan.
(4) Bronchoscopy.
(5) PET Scan (Positron Emission Tomography).
(6) Sputum Cytology.
(7) Detection Based on Convolution Neural Network.
(8) Detection using Support Vector Machine (SVM).
(9) Detection using ASIC Based fluoroscopic capsule.

(1) **Needle Biopsy**:
In this method, a long thin needle is inserted in the suspicious part of the body through skin. Some cells from the suspicious area are extracted and analyzed and decided the status of cells. The disadvantage of this method is that it may give false-positive or false-negative results.

(3) **Low dose CT scan**:
When the results of chest X-ray is not sufficient to detect cancer then low dose CT scan method is used for screening. In this method, the body is exposed to radiation which may be dangerous.

(4) **Bronchoscopy**:
In this method, a bronchoscope tube is inserted inside the body through lungs airways or through mouth which consists of light and lens. This procedure is used to reveal the areas of tumours that can be sampled for diagnosis.

(5) **PET CT Scan**:
This is called positron Emission Tomography which uses small amount of radioactive material which is called a tracer. This tracer was inserted into the body through veins and required 1 h to absorb by body. This method decides whether tumour tissue actively grow or not and find the type of cells within particular tumour.

(6) **Detection Based on Convolutional Neural Network**:
The above-mentioned method is deep learning-based method for detection of pulmonary cancer which uses histopathology images. Two CNN architectures were employed for sampling histopathology images. This method is good but classification of histopathological images need more accuracy.

(7) **Detection using Support Vector Machine (SVM)**:
The above method uses CT images for detection of pulmonary cancer. After collecting CT images, image enhancement operation and segmentation is performed on images separately and then detection and prediction algorithm is applied using multiclass support vector machine (SVM).

(8) **Detection using ASIC Based fluoroscopic capsule**:
The above method uses ASIC based fluorescence capsule for early detection. The sensitivity of the ASIC based capsule is very high which detect very low photocurrent so that system is able to detect low concentration of the biomarker present in the cells. In this method, external instrument is required to receive the signal.

2.2 *Non-invasive Method*

In this method for testing any disease, there is no need to involve any instrument. In this method, exhaled gas of humans is used to detect the disease. Concentration of various compounds is different in exhaled gas of a normal person and an infected person. So by examination of exhaled gas one can determine the disease as well as severity of disease. Using this method premature detection of disease is also possible and there is no chance of spreading the cancerous tissues when someone used this technique.

Techniques.
There are various Non-Invasive techniques that are used for detection of pulmonary cancer which is as follows,

(a) Nucleic Acid-based detection
(b) Protein-based Detection
(c) Cell-Based Detection
(d) VOCs Based Detection (Breath Analysis).

Out of the above four detection techniques, VOCs based detection has some advantages over others. VOC based detection is done using breath analysis which has some advantages over above-mentioned techniques. There are different types of breath analysis techniques which are as follows,

(1) Gas Chromatography Mass Spectrometry
(2) Proton Transfer Reaction Mass Spectrometry
(3) Ion Mobility Spectrometry
(4) Selected Ion Flow Tube Mass Spectrometry
(5) Chemical Sensor Platform
(6) MEMS Microstructure.

(1) Gas Chromatography Mass Spectrometry:

It is an analytical method that is carried out to find different samples within a substance. This method considers as a gold standard for identification of different types of samples in a substance because the result of this test is very accurate. Breath analysis is carried out to find the particular biomarker from VOCs. After finding specific biomarkers from VOCs use mass spectroscopy to find the concentration of that particular biomarker. After finding concentration one can decide the extremity of disease. Concentration of biomarkers is different for normal people and infected people. The advantage of this technique is sensitivity. Reactivity of this technique is in ppb range. There are also some advantages like the system which is used in this technique is not handy and mobile and real-time measurement is not also possible using this technique.

(2) Proton Transfer Reaction Mass Spectrometry:

This technique is used for chemical evolution of VOCs. This technique is used to detect gaseous organic compounds in air. VOCs in air have both natural and manmade sources. Natural sources include VOCs exhaled by both plants and animals. The VOCs present in the air constitutes a very small percentage of air. The most common VOC found is methane which is present at the level of two parts per million by volume. After methane, ethane, propane, iso propane such VOCs are found but they are also at the level of parts per billion or parts per trillion but such a small quantity is also not good for humans which may cause the problem. So if some of the above mentioned VOCs are found in human respiration then it can be dangerous and may be caused serious disease. So if we are able to detect such VOCs from human breath then it is possible to detect the disease from such VOCs. Proton transfer is performed in this system via the soft ionization mechanism that fragments the analyte molecules. The first step of the Proton Transfer Reaction Mass Spectrometry is the Proton Transfer Reaction ionization source where gas-phase VOCs molecules are ionized by the transfer of a proton from to VOC molecules. The VOCs ions produced in this reaction are subsequently detected by mass analyzer. Following are the main components of Proton Transfer Reaction Mass Spectrometry,

(a) Sampling Inlet.
(b) Ion Source.
(c) Proton transfer reaction cell.
(d) Ion processing Interface.
(e) Mass Analyzer.

There are some benefits of the above-said technique like real-time measurement possible, sensitivity in parts per billion. The disadvantages are like VOCs chemical identification not possible.

(3) **Ion Mobility Spectrometry:**

It is an analytical technique that distinguishes and recognizes the ionized molecules in the gas based on their mobility. The main consideration for this process is mobility of different ions which totally depends on charge, mass, shape and size of the biomarker. Separated ions or biomarkers from VOCs are transferred to the drift tube. Drift tube is a hollow cylindrical structure that is operated with an electric field and buffer gas. Buffer gas flow in the opposite direction of ion flow. Different ions or biomarkers have different mobility's based on the size and mass. These ions or biomarkers are then collected and sent for spectrometry. After spectrometry, each ion or biomarker is analyzed and characterized. The advantage of this process is that it is movable system having low cost sensitivity in parts per million range but the main disadvantage is that real-time measurement is not possible.

(4) **Selected Ion Flow Tube Mass Spectrometry:**

For gas analysis, it is a quantitative method. The chemical ionization of selected volatile compounds by selected positive precursor ions along a flow tube involves this process. From the precursor and product ion signal ratios absolute concentration of selected compounds present in exhaled breath can be calculated. Real-time detection is also possible with the technique. The range of this process extends up to parts per trillion. There are three elements of these techniques which are as follows,

(a) Reagent ion generation and selection
(b) Analyte ionization
(c) Analyte Quantitation.

The eight reagents H_3O, NO^+ , O_2+ , $O-$, $OH-$, NO_2- and NO_3- are formed using microwave. Then selected reagent ions are injected into the flow tube. Then Sample is introduced at a known flow rate and reactive compounds it contains are ionized by the reagent to form well-characterized product ions and unreacted reagent ions analytes absolute concentration can be found using software. The drawback of this technique is that VOCs chemical identification is not possible.

(5) **Chemical Sensor Platform:**

The ideal chemical sensor is a low cost, easily movable, foolproof device that responds with perfect instantaneous selectivity to a particular target chemical substance present in any desired medium but in reality, chemical sensors are complex devices. The complexity of chemical sensor is based on the material which is to be analyzed. In this process, highly sensitive chemical compounds can be used to detect the specific analyzer that detailed VOCs are obtained from human breathing. Then analytes and chemical compounds are left for chemical reaction for a few hours. After that pre-concentration is processed and characterization of various chemicals present in VOCs are found through which we can detect the disease and severity of disease. The primary benefits of this process are that it is very easy to use and has less cost but the drawback is to design a chemical sensor if very difficult task.

(2) **MEMS Microstructure:**

In above technique, micro cantilever or array of micro cantilevers will be designed using CMOS Technology. This structure is very reactive to particular biomarkers. Various sensitive layers of various compounds are designed and these sensitive layers are allowed to respond directly to VOCs. These sensitive layers are formed in such a way that they are reacted only with the particular biomarkers present in VOCs. The concentration of acetone, methanol and toluene are found to be increased in the VOCs of the person who is infected from pulmonary cancer which is collected from the exhaled breath of that person. So we will need to find the concentration of the above-said elements from the VOCs. So compounds that are reactive only to acetone, Methanol and toluene are deposited in the microstructure cantilever to get the required result.

Table 1 shows the comparison of above techniques.

There are various parameters such as deflection of cantilever, pressure, voltage which are to be considered to check the seriousness of disease The benefits of this method are as follows,

(a) Real-time measurement is possible
(b) Very Simple and portable
(c) Sensitivity lies from parts per billion to parts per trillion
(d) Having less cost
(e) Time to produce result is less as compared to other methods.

Table 1 Comparison of various parameters of non-invasive methods

Methods	Parameters					
	Real-time measurement	Sensitivity range	VOC's chemical identification	Cost	Portable system	Time to produce result
Gas Chromatography Mass Spectrometry	Not possible	ppm	Possible	High	No	High
Proton Transfer Reaction Mass Spectrometry	Possible	ppb	Not possible	High	No	High
Ion Mobility Spectrometry	Not possible	ppb	Not POSSIBLE	Low	Yes	High
Tube Mass Spectrometry	Possible	ppb	Not possible	Low	Yes	High
Chemical Sensor Platform	Not possible	ppb	Not possible	Low	Yes	Less
MEMS Microstructure	Possible	ppb-ppt	Possible	Low	Yes	Less

As we saw all the different methods of breath analysis and from the above comparison MEMS Microstructure technique has more advantages compared to others. Also using these methods we can avoid false positive and false negative results and get accurate results at early stages which helps in treatment of patients.

3 Conclusion

This paper includes comparison of various techniques which are used for the detection of cancer. From the above research work, we can find that non-invasive methods are more reliable and promising for detection of cancer at early stage as compared to various invasive methods which are currently used for the detection of cancer. Out of above mentioned non-invasive techniques, MEMS Microstructure technique is more useful because of the advantages like accuracy, sensitivity, low cost and real-time measurement. It is possible to detect cancer at early stage using above-said technique so diagnosis of disease like cancer can be advanced with MEMS.

Bibliography

1. Amal H, Ding L, Liu BB, Tisch U, Xu ZQ, Shi DY, Zhao Y, Chen J, Sun RX, Liu H et al (2012) The scent fingerprint of hepato carcinoma: in-vitro metastasis prediction with volatile organic compounds (VOCs). In: IEEE transactions instrumentation and measurement, 2005
2. Wang S, Wang J, Zhu Y, Yang J, Yang F (2015) A new device for liver cancer biomarker detection with high accuracy. Sens Bio-Sens Res 4:40–45
3. Bray F, Ren JS, Masuyer E et al (2013) Estimates of global cancer prevalence for 27 sites in the adult population in 2008. Int J Cancer 132(5):1133–1145
4. .Rabbani S, Brishbhan P (2011) Cantilever embedded MOSFET for biosensing. In: IEEE 24th Canadian conference on electrical and computer engineering (CCECE), Canada, pp 489–492
5. Loizeau F, Lang HP, Akiyama T, Gautsch S, Vettiger P, Yoshikawa G, de Rooij N (2015) Comparing membrane- and cantilever based surface stress sensors for reproducibility. Sens Actuators A 228:9–15. Elsevier
6. Singh P, Chua GL (2014) Anchor-free NEMS non-volatile memory cell for harsh environment data storage. J Micromech Microeng 24:115007
7. Chua GL, Singh P, Soon BW (2014) Molecular adhesion controlled micro electromechanical memory device for harsh environment data storage. Appl Phys Lett 105:113503
8. Vashist SK, Luong JHT (2018) Microcantilever-based sensors IDS Immunodiagnostic Systems Deutschland GmbH, Frankfurt am Main, Germany; University College Cork, Cork, Ireland
9. Bhure V, Sumathi M (2019) Study of different methods for characterizing benign & cancerous breast tissue. In: 2019 9th international conference on emerging trends in engineering and technology—signal and information processing (ICETET-SIP-19)
10. Fenske JD, Paulson SE (1999) Human breath emissions of VOCs. J Air Waste Manag Assoc 49:594–598
11. Bhattacharya D, Rathore PK, Mujumdar S (2018) Non invasive piezoelectric sensor for detection of lung cancer. In: 2018, proceedings of international conference on communication and electronics systems (ICCES-18)
12. Race CM, Kwon LE, Foreman MT (2018) An automated microfluidic assay for photonic crystal enhanced detection and analysis of an antiviral antibody cancer biomarker in serum. IEEE Sens J 18(4)
13. Saríc M, Russo M, Stella M, Sikora M, CNN-based method for lung cancer detection in whole slide histopathology images. University of split Croatia
14. Varnava G, Demosthenous P, Koulaouzidis A, Georgiou J (2018) Towards an ASIC-based fluoroscopic capsule for the early cancer detection in the small intestine. 978-1-5386-3646-6/18/$31.00 ©2018 IEEE
15. Timurdogan E, Erdem Alaca B, Halil Kavakli I, Urey H (2011) MEMS biosensor for detection of Hepatitis A and C viruses in serum. Bio sensor and bio electronics. Elsevier

Agriculture Assistant for Crop Prediction and Farming Selection Using Machine Learning Model with Real-Time Data Using Imaging Through UAV Drone

Muskan Jain, Manpreet Singh Bajwa, and Hemant Kumar

Abstract Agriculture, as an income source, plays an important role in the economy of a country like India for its holistic growth. For better results, we need to improve the quality of products and predict the yield. which leads us to our problem statement, we will be designing a machine learning model to predict yield depending upon various features like soil moisture, fertilizers, and weather forecasting, etc. Farmers are facing problems related to better yield due to multiple constraint dependencies like rainfall, soil, weather prediction, the effect of natural calamities, timing. In this model, we will be predicting and representing the ideal scenario of unexpected devastating outcomes. Hence, we are proposing a model based on machine learning using image processing to predict the best yield possible to the farmers with the help of a drone. We are training our model using the dataset of the past few years and training our model accordingly. There are various techniques available that make the machines more optimized, but no technology works on finding the co-relation between the crops and the conditions required for better yield of crops. There will be no benefit to optimizing the machines until the crops will be provided with the best conditions to prosper. These existing techniques only make farming optimal but do not optimize productivity. There are many factors which affect the growth of crops but there are two most important out of them: The soil in which our crop is grown & weather. Other factors affecting will be water, fertilizers, manures, sunlight, weather forecasting, area of cultivation, and financial perspectives. Depending upon the factors discussed, we will predict the best outcomes and most suitable crop from all parameters after training the model with the most effective, simpler, cheaper, faster interface & efficient sensors with less requirement of labor and energy-efficient plus eco-friendly components with a proper quality check measures on water, fertilizers, manures, and soil. We will be focusing on the best prediction for market demand. This model is also optimized to even provide the best fertilizer to the farmer according to the requirement of the crop.

M. Jain · M. S. Bajwa (✉) · H. Kumar
Faculty of Engineering and Technology, SGT University, Gurugram, India
e-mail: manpreet_feat@sgtuniversity.org

N. Marriwala et al. (eds.), *Emergent Converging Technologies and Biomedical Systems*, Lecture Notes in Electrical Engineering 841,
https://doi.org/10.1007/978-981-16-8774-7_26

Keywords Agriculture monitoring · Precision agriculture · Prediction · Weather forecasting · Machine learning · E-agriculture

1 Introduction

Agriculture accommodates the staple to the industry that adds up to contribute to the rise in GDP in the overall growth of India. With the emerging population, the pressure on the need for agricultural productivity is additionally increasing. As the population is rising, the demand for its growth went up high at an exponential pace and the traditional methods using manpower aren't enough to serve the whole population. So, to satisfy the market demand and increasing needs, they need to determine the best possible soil for which farmers may not be able to use harmful pesticides and insecticides in excessive quantity. These pesticides may increase the productivity of crops in contrast to adverse effects on human health. The usage of UAVs will ensure the amount of pesticide spread evenly in the land thus reducing cost and increasing efficiency, making the model best for pest control. However, determining the patterns of movements of pesticides applied by air spraying is a difficult task. Based on Computational Fluid Dynamics (CFD). The UAVs give us the freedom to control the movement of pesticides as well as the drip distribution features based on Computational Fluid Dynamics (CFD). UAVs used for smart farming have important extracted features for their usage like payload, stabilization, flight time, and autonomous missions. This paper discusses a variety of UAV-based farming techniques including health screening and diagnosis of plant diseases, pest monitoring, and yield estimation [1]. Due to the stability of UAVs, we will be able to acquire high-resolution images very conveniently. As a result of using these harmful pesticides, the land gets barren with no fertility in the end. In the era of big data and AI [2], we will predict many factors like the soil during which our crop is grown, pH of the water, crop health, cropping pattern, and growth rate that will ultimately boost the productivity of the crop. Using machine learning in agriculture helps to detect the disease in crops and provide the immediate solution there too, aerial vehicles will monitor the crop and can provide us with accurate and precise data sets. Automated irrigation systems will use the weather outlook to predict the requirement of a crop to extend the typical yield. The problems faced with the agriculture field are weed management, lack of storage management, pesticide control, types of weed, crop diseases, and types of pests, these problems can be solved by the model proposed below [3].

2 Objective

The objective of this paper is to visualize the factors affecting the growth of crops like soil, nutrients, fertilizers, water and to observe the changes occurring in the climate. By collecting the data through user or UAVs, and then feeding this data to machine learning algorithms to predict the best fertilizer, find suitable climate and soil for the particular crop to get aware of the amount of sunlight needed by crops. Moreover, the amount of moisture and water required by the crop for maximum yield production is calculated. It is also essential to know the area of cultivation and financial outcomes obtained through it. The purpose of this qualitative study is to build a Machine Learning model to help identify a correlation between the crops and the conditions required by the crops to grow and give maximum yield with effect on plant diseases in less-economically-developed countries like India using drones. We explored the best method for the increase in agriculture productivity, with the help of machine learning and UAVs. UAVs can click and record multispectral photography but the interpretation of these high-resolution photographs are difficult without the help of machine learning algorithms. So, training the algorithms with proper data set obtained from different sources provide clarity to the farmers with what is best for their crop. The amount of water provided to the crop is sufficient or not, the soil moisture for the growth of the plant is correct or not, in what amount the sunlight to the crop should be provided, best fertilizer for that particular crop, etc. are some factors including others which would be taken care of.

We will be implementing this through the collection of details mentioning fields like the type of soil, environmental conditions, location, an investment he/she can make, and some other basic things and he/she will get the best possible results accordingly. It will be easily available to him/her in the form of the Android Application. The problem which our invention is solving is to how to increase the productivity of his/her field. It works on the root cause of all problems. This is because if a farmer is getting good productivity, he/she will not be trapped in the problem of debt. Moreover, it will make a farmer independent and provide freedom for experimentation on different varieties of crops.

3 An Overview on Machine Learning

Machine learning is considered the foundation of Artificial Intelligence through which computers use a large number of knowledge sets (training models) and apply algorithms to classify and predict. In other words, Machine learning is the ability for a program to find out something without having to be programmed to find out that specific knowledge. Machine Learning tasks are divided into broad categories, namely the type of training: supervised and unsupervised, the learning models: regression, clustering, etc. The data in supervised learning is represented with sample inputs and thus the corresponding outputs that means mapping input(s) to output(s), on the other hand, there's no discrepancy in training and test sets in unsupervised learning with unlabeled data. The learner processes the input file to discover hidden patterns. Inspiration for ANNs work on the human brain and represent a simplified model of the neural network emulating complex functions such as pattern production, comprehension, learning, and decision making. In agriculture, they must predict crop yield and quality.

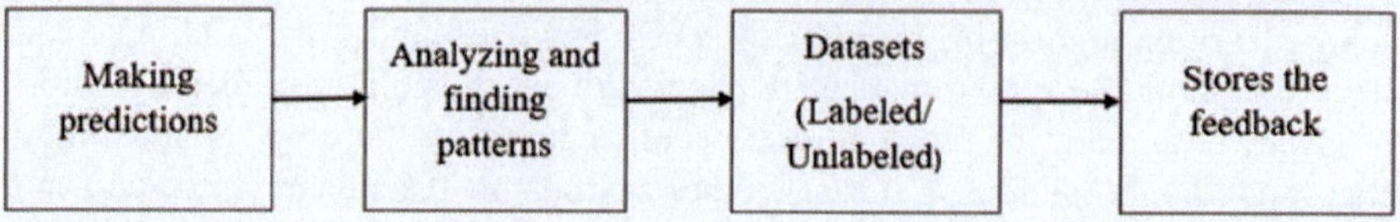

Fig. 1 Working of machine learning on datasets

ANN is used to calculate input, output energy to input rate, and also used to calculate energy productivity with the help of Life cycle Assessment [4]. Also, used to save the crop from extreme temperatures by providing a greenhouse environment [5]. With the help of Deep CNN, satellite images of crops can be recognized [6]. Plants also need a good quality of air to grow well which can be predicted by Deep Learning [7]. Machine Learning Techniques used to predict the photosynthetic capacity of a crop using Leaf Reflectance spectra, if increased, can increase the yield [8] (Fig. 1).

4 Background

Machine Learning is used in agricultural practices for several years [9] where we will be predicting crop yield, which depends mainly upon when, where, how, how much to grow. So, analysis of the field, crop, and environment can be done effortlessly using machine learning tools [10]. Apart from yield prediction, weed detection, disease detection, and crop quality are also analyzed using machine learning. The datasets provided to the machine learning algorithm are obtained from a variety of sensors equipped on the UAVs for a better understanding of the environment and weather conditions [11] (Table 1).

5 Literature Survey

With the advancement in technology, applications of agriculture UAVs have improved with time. From providing just image-based dataset [26] to the version of decision-making intelligent system helping farmers in making smart decisions by giving them intelligence-based oriented data processed from images with the assistance of machine learning tools and other technologies [27]. An illustration explaining it is multimodal plant identification developed with the help of datasets obtained from capturing images with the help of UAV drones using hyperspectral data [28]. Many global agricultural systems are present that uses satellite imagery and remote sensing that provides information regarding food production [29]. The data from the satellites and remote-sensing technology with machine learning calculates parameters like rainfall or Standardized Precipitation Index [30]. Also, for the prediction of crop pests, machine learning can be used [31] using various techniques. In the lessening

Table 1 Different machine learning tools used in agricultural practices

S. no.	Year of publication	Author name	Machine learning tool	Functionality	References
1	2019	Charoen-Ung and Mittrapiyanuruk	Random Forest	Crop yield prediction	[12]
2	2019	Ranjan and Parida	Linear Regression	Crop yield prediction	[13]
3	2019	Filippi et al.	Random Forest	Crop yield prediction	[14]
4	2019	Xu et al.	Support vector machine	Crop yield prediction	[15]
5	2019	Bo Jiang, Jinrong He	AlexNet-CNNs deep learning network	Crop yield prediction	[16]
6	2018	Shah et al.	Support vector machine, random forest, multivariate polynomial regression	Crop yield prediction	[17]
7	2018	Goldstein et al.	Gradient boosting tree, linear regression	Crop yield prediction	[18]
8	2018	Ferentinos	DNN/CNN	Disease detection	[19]
9	2017	Ali et al.	ANFIS, neural networks, multiple linear regression	Crop yield prediction	[20]
10	2017	Pantazi et al.	ANN/Clustering/one-class MOG	Weed detection	[21]
11	2017	Binch and Fox	SVN	Weed detection	[22]
12	2016	Maione et al.	EL/RF	Crop quality	[23]
13	2015	Paul et al.	Naïve Bayes, k-nearest neighbor	Crop yield prediction	[24]
14	2014	Mohsou et al.	SVM/LS-SVM	Disease detection	[25]

of crop yield, an aspect resulting in crop loss is plant disease, which can be overcome with algorithms of ANN or with image processing techniques in identifying crop diseases [32, 33]. Based on the needs of agricultural fields, various applications of UAVs can be put to use that we have thoroughly described. A farmer can make several decisions with the data provided by the UAVs to solve the problem(s) that are detected and to improve the harvest by assessing the yield.

5.1 Application of Using UAV in Agriculture

Some of the popular applications of using drones in Precision Agriculture, as listed in the literature, are mentioned below:

- **Analyses of soil and field.**

Soil is a very crucial parameter with important features contributing to the success rate of crop production. The analyses of soil and field should be at different times during crop growth which includes the start stage of planting, mid-way while the crop is growing, and at the time of gathering in of the crops. Analyses can be performed with the help of UAVs as they can provide us with the soil health, pattern in which the planting is done through precision cameras and thus providing with necessary data of the substances needed for irrigation [34]. Additionally, this data obtained through the UAV imagery can also help the farmers in knowing the quantity of nitrogen, fertilizer required for growing any particular crop. By this approach, overall yield can be improved, hence saving costs on fertilizers and pesticides [35]. A perfect soil profile data [36], including soil temperature [37] at multiple-depth is necessary for crop yield predictions based on crop modeling applications.

- **Planting crops.**

Crop planting is an expensive and difficult task that has traditionally relied on human ability. Modern advanced drone farming technology provides planting techniques that reduce planting costs up to 85%. The dramatic reduction in planting costs is probably the result of the drone's ability to perform many responsibilities including, planting within the soil, injecting pods with seeds, and making plants that can be grown and used, drone features are just not limited to this but many more. For a farmer it is very important to know the distance between roots and plants, number of plants grown per square meter of land as proper growth of plants is essential [38]. Also, to keep a check on the balance of the soil and the plant, the regeneration of nutrients, it is important to know the value of the plant.

- **Crop spraying application.**

Crop spraying has been an onerous and exhausting process for the farmers and producers as it is the main factor defining the yield production. To ensure the proper growth of plants, large areas of land are sprayed with fertilizers and chemicals. Often crop spraying uses many harsh chemicals present in pesticides, etc., with continued exposure to it may result in danger to human health. So, Drone technology can be a much safer alternate instead of traditional crop spraying. Due to its speed and accuracy, it can cover long distances in a short period. Using ultrasonic lasers, sensors, precision crop spraying can be achieved as UAV make sure the proper coverage of land with the spread of right amount of pesticide or insecticide for correct growth of plants, avoiding unnecessary waste. With UAVs it is important to accurately measure the height of the flying drone due to the constraints present in the flight environment and the amount of pesticide reaching the ground as if the height is more, the pesticide may flow with the wind, if the height is less, spraying may not impact much. Another such method similar to crop spraying is spot spraying which targets weeds. UAVs with help of resolution cameras, can identify weeds and can spray precisely on weeds, and can save up to 90% of the chemical herbicides [39].

- **Plant observation.**

One of the biggest problems faced by the farmers in farming is poor crop monitoring in large fields as the humans alone cannot monitor the whole field at a time. This problem is exacerbated by the increase in unpredictable weather conditions which can lead to an increase in the risks and the repair costs. Observation of the field is a very important task because if the boundary of the fields is not secured by fences, then they may be prone to animals, and birds disturbing the croplands. In traditional methods, the use of a scarecrow is generally done to discourage the birds from feeding on crops. Now drones can be used as surveillance on cropland, using multispectral photography UAV can differentiate between humans, animals, birds, and crops easily. Also, UAV remote sensory can provide us with crop stress maps generated with the help of UAV captured images, helping farmers in monitoring the field [40].

- **Crop irrigation.**

Irrigation of crops is important while preventing the crops from dry conditions that end up being dead due to absence of water. The most refined drone technology uses a wide range of sensors including thermal, multicolored, and hyperspectral types to research and identify specific dehydrated plants. In addition, these sensors are used to measure the density, temperature, and overall health of the sector to bring a holistic view of growers and producers. Also, UAVs can be used to detect areas that are waterlogged which in traditional farming is either inefficiently done or is very expensive. A lot of the time is consumed in the detection of precise crops or the exact location on the field which may result in less yield but, with the help of UAVs, farmers can do it themselves [41].

- **Plant health assessment.**

It is extremely important to access the health of plants and fields time to time, as it will turn in maximum yield production only if all the requirements that are, nutrients, water, needed by the crops are fulfilled. The medical examination will not only record dry, dead plants but will also perform important fungal and bacterial analyses of trees, plants, and fields. Using light sources like infrared, drones detect plants having spots that reflect sunshine indicating some disease or deterioration of plant health. As a result, farmers use agricultural drones to obtain real-time drawings of the fields to prevent losses and ensure the growth and success of their crops. Using machine learning algorithms with UAVs, the problem of agricultural pests in farmlands can be improved [42] (Table 2).

Nowadays, UAVs [46] are becoming effective sensing systems as they comprise specialized sensors that complement IoT that makes them reliable to use. These sensors capture high-resolution images, which in turn helps farmers in monitoring

Table 2 Some sensors used for particular application

S. no.	Application	Sensor used	Implementation
1	For detecting the type of crop	Raspberry pi Module + camera and TensorFlow Machine learning	On UAV
2	To calculate the dirt and PH of water	PH sensor and Turbidity sensor [43]	Water canal (field)
3	To calculate the humidity and temperature	DHT11 sensor	Root zone of crop
4	To check the raining condition	Rain sensor	On sprinkler system
5	To measure nutrient solution	Electrical conductivity	In soil
6	To detect the area of cultivation	AI and ML- Raspberry pi Module with a camera and TensorFlow Machine learning	On UAV
7	To check how acidic/basic is water	PH sensor	Water canal (field)
8	To determine the ability of water to disinfect itself	ORP	Water canal (field)
9	To detect the moisture in soil and electronic conductivity	Soil Moisture sensor	In soil
10	To calculate the air quality and the dust amount in the environment	Dust sensor	On UAV or suspended in air
11	For Air Quality Monitoring (Gases like NH_3, NO_x, alcohol, Benzene, smoke, CO_2)	MQ135 sensor + Arduino	On UAV
12	Sunlight sensor	LDR sensor	Field
13	Environmental sensor with temperature, barometric pressure, *and* humidity	BME280 sensor	Field
14	To obtain the ambient light data	BH1750FVI Is a Digital Light sensor	Field
15	To check if motor is providing water or not	Water flow sensor	Water pipe
16	To open pipeline of the certain area	Electronic gatewall	Water pipe (field)
17	To connect b/w the modules (to make connection totally wireless and mess free, also no Wi-Fi and GPS required for up to 40 km Range)	LORA Module	Nearby field

(continued)

Table 2 (continued)

S. no.	Application	Sensor used	Implementation
18	A depth sensor (distinguishing between crops, weeds, and soil, weed detection)	Kinect v2.0 [44]	On UAV
19	Crop spraying (dense vegetation environments)	Lightware SF11-C [45]	UAV or on sprinkler system
20	Crop spraying (sparser vegetation)	LeddarTech M16 [45]	UAV or on sprinkler system
21	Crop Observing	RGB camera	On UAV

crops and fields. Different sensors depending on the parameter for which the crop monitoring is used with an agricultural drone, these sensors are available in the market in a wide variety. However, a limitation is that the drones do not have high payload capacity and minimum space limits the selection of sensors equipped. The sensors applied to drones should meet the minimum requirement that they should be of low weight, small size, and should consume low energy. Sensors used for Precision Agriculture that surpasses the mentioned restrictions are Visible light sensors, Multispectral, Hyperspectral sensors, Light Detection and Ranging (LiDAR) sensors. Characteristics like color, texture and geometric outline of the vegetation are monitored with the help of sensors through high-resolution cameras. The data obtained through these sensors are further used to analyze soil and fields, monitor crop health, etc. at different crop growth stages.

5.2 *Types of Farming*

- **Subsistence Farming.**

Majority of the community in a country like India practice farming. As the farmers are poor, they suffer, due to less money they are not able to use proper fertilizers and seeds which provide maximum yield in their fields to the extent that they should. The main reason for low productivity can be the absence of necessities like electricity and water supply which are not available to them. Areas where the rainfall is low and irrigation facilities are inadequate, they practice dryland farming, where, with a focus on moisture conservation the plants such as Jowar, Bajra, and pulses are grown as they require less water. Only one crop is grown whole year in dry farming. In areas that receive high rainfall and are irrigated areas, they practice wetland farming, growing crops like Rice, sugarcane, and vegetables. In wet farming, in a year, minimum of two crops can be grown, in kharif and rabi seasons respectively.

The characteristics of this farming are: the whole family works on a farm, most of the work is done by hand, the farms are small, they follow the traditional farming methods, yet the yield is not very high [47].

a. *Intensive Farming.*

In areas where farmers have easy access to irrigate their farms, those farmers use fertilizers, pesticides, and insecticides on a large scale. They also need to bring their land under the most productive type for yielding seeds which require maximum nutrients. To make farming easy, they introduced machines in various farming systems thus reducing manpower and saving time. This helps in making the yield by unit area high and increasing cost.

b. *Primitive Farming.*

(1) Shifting Agriculture

In this sort of agriculture, the first set is to clear a small amount of forest land by cutting down trees and burning logs and branches. As soon as the land is cleared, the seeds are planted deep in the ground. This type of planting does not involve soil cultivation or other agricultural practices. The crops are planted for 2–3 years, then the clearing is abandoned because the production of the yield decreases due to weeds, erosion, and loss of soil fertility. Then a fresh clearing is formed, and therefore the community migrates to new areas and so the process is repeated again. This may be a wasteful method of cultivation. Dry paddy, maize, millets, and vegetables are the crops commonly grown during this sort of farming.

(2) Nomadic Herding

Nomadic herding is an ecological system of agriculture. It's carried on mainly to supply food for the family and to satisfy the requirements of clothing, shelter, and recreation. It's the only sort of pastoralism. The nomadic herders are hooked into sheep, cattle, goats, camels, horses, and reindeer for his or her livelihood. The composition of the herd varies from one region to the other, but throughout the arid zone sheep and goats are the most common animals used in nomadic herding and cattle are the least used in quantity as they do not like hot and dry areas.

- **Commercial Farming.**

  a. Plantation Agriculture.

  Plantation farming is to plant trees or shrubs. The Britishers introduced plantation farming in the middle of the nineteenth century. Plantation farming includes trees like rubber, tea, coffee, cocoa, spices, coconut, and fruit crops such as apples, grapes, oranges, etc. Good investment and management of the farm are required. Some fields, such as tea, coffee, and rubber, have a processing plant inside or on the edge of the farm. This type of farming is done in the hilly areas of north-eastern India and the Nilgiris.

b. Mixed and Multiple Agriculture.

Mixed farming is crop farming and animal husbandry at the same time. In multiple farming, two or more crops are grown together. In such cases, several crops with different times of maturity are planted at the same time. If any of the planted crops mature early, it means it is usually harvested before the long-term extension of the growing crop, therefore there is not much completion between the plant growth [48]. Mixed farming is practiced in areas receiving good rainfall or having better facilities for irrigation.

- **Precision Agriculture.**

Precision farming uses history, real-time data, and machine learning algorithms to make specific decisions for smaller application areas, rather than performing the same function on a wider area within the traditional model. For instance, instead of placing large amounts of pesticides over large areas, applying small amounts of pesticides over certain trees, shrubs, or even leaves, to cut costs and avoid waste while protecting the potential damage caused by chemicals when used in bulk [49]. Using a UAV to collect the data which is helpful in precision agriculture as the UAV is connected to an Android app where all back-end algorithms work simultaneously to provide maximum results [50] (Fig. 2).

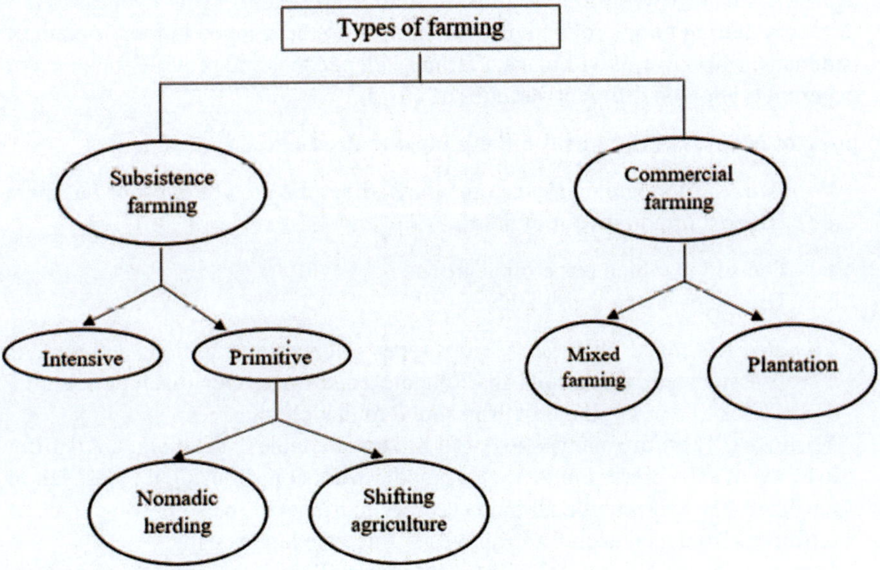

Fig. 2 Farming types

6 Procedure

We are using machine learning at the back end and android app development at the front end to provide this complete package to farmers. In machine learning, we are using Linear Regression (Multiclass), Logistic Regression, KNN, and Tensors. We will deploy this entire model into Android using Tensor Flow Lite. We are training our model using previous data of some years and training our model accordingly. A user just must provide some details regarding crops like which crop to grow, environmental conditions there, and many of the data will be collected from drone and he/she will get the best possible outcomes. Likewise, the details of fertilizer are provided to the farmer.

Difference Between Problems Solved and Benefits Over Existing Technology.

- *Existing Technology.* There are many techniques available that make the machines more optimized, but no technology works on finding the co-relation between the crops and the conditions required by the crops to grow well. There will be no benefit to optimizing the machines until the crops will be provided with the best conditions to grow. These existing techniques only make farming faster but do not optimize productivity.
- *Our Technology.* It solves a major problem on how to increase the productivity of his/her field. It works on the root cause of all problems. This is because if a farmer is getting good productivity, he/she will not be trapped in the problem of bad loans. Moreover, it will make a farmer independent and provide freedom for experimentation on different varieties of crops.

Important Measures Used as the Basis for our Prediction.

1. *Necessities.* There are many factors which affect the growth of crops but there are two most important out of them.
   a. The soil in which our crop is grown.
   b. The water which is used there.
2. *Climate conditions.* There are various types of climate conditions and there is a crop associated which suits that climate conditions. Our machine learning model tries to find out the best crop suited to that climate.
3. *Fertilizers.* There are many kinds of fertilizers available in the market. All differ in terms of salts present in them. Our model works on choosing the best salt of fertilizer that will provide all the necessary nutrients to the soil. The choice of fertilizer also depends on the crop we are interested in growing.
4. *Manures.* These are natural substances. We will find the amount of manure required for a crop.
5. *Sunlight.* Sunlight is a natural phenomenon that cannot be controlled by us, but we can find the intensity of sunlight in a season. By doing this we can find the best time period for crops to grow so that our crops can get adequate heat and light.

6. *Area of Cultivation.* We have also tried to find out the area factor impacting the growth of crop production so that to get the best outcome.
7. *Financial Perspective.* This is a very important factor that was taken into consideration while making this model. At last, our focus was only on increasing the output of the field and decreasing cost for the same. We are also calculating using various algorithms the cost which will be approximately used on the selected crop.
8. *UAVs.*

Results. Our output depends on the above factors discussed. In order to get the best outcomes, we have trained out our model in an efficient manner by adding on important factors and eliminating out useless features.

7 Experimental and Model Evaluation

This research paper focuses on how machine learning is often integrated with drone technology to supply solutions to identifying plant diseases. This project is focusing on: The constraints of building a cheap, easy-to manufacture drone; what materials should be used, and how machine learning has been a great tool in identifying plant diseases and the way this will be linked to drone spot-checking.

Throughout In the last ten years, there have been different companies trying to solve these agricultural problems but have failed due to costs and the project being inefficient. My report showcases the stages in starting with an idea, designing it, and then building it to a point where it can be used as a product. The product is often used, mainly, in less economically-developed countries to assist provide a simple solution to the issues of the farmers and crop yielders for many years. According to National Geographic, 'Agriculture is the art and science of cultivating the soil, growing crops and raising livestock. Smart Agriculture, a term that has not been heard of for a long time, we are hearing more use cases of drones and with the growing population, making crop yields more efficient.

8 Prototype

In this project, the drone with the use of machine learning helps us to detect plant diseases using images that it will take and with the use of crops, as a way of improving crop yield. So, to program a machine learning model in drone; IBM Watson is used as it is one of the most advanced machine learning computers in the world. The drone is programmed in a way that categorizes the crop as 'Healthy' and 'Diseased'. Then, by adding images to every category showing the machine learning model what a healthy plant seemed like and what a diseased plant seemed like. Furthermore, this would add credibility to the images that the machine learning algorithm would be processing. The drone is programmed in a way that every time it flies in a set path it captures the images at different stages of the flight. The drone autonomously takes the pictures, resizes all the pictures, and tests them within the machine learning model to output whether the image was 'healthy' or 'diseased' and therefore the confidence level of the model. This prototype Autonomous Agricultural drone can hold up to 2Ltrs. Of herbicides or pesticides and the field, mapping is done before the autonomous drone takes flight. Creating a plane map (for Autonomous missions) for the agriculture drone has never been so easy, a software program called Mission Planner (similar to Google Earth) provides a satellite image of the Farm or inventory and the edge is often drawn around the target field.

Mission Planner automatically sets up the waypoints for the functioning area. And this all communicated wirelessly from Mission Planner to the drone. We do not need to physically map the device as required by current agricultural drones. The drone automatically links up to the waypoints and begins its precision spray application, combined with a six-wheel UAV and spray actuator consisting of a tank, a pump, pressure gauge, and a meter to measure water flow for a flexible UAV spray device. The battery propels the entire drone flight and the spray application and the battery lasts up to 20 min and this drone can travel at a speed of 15 feet per second meaning that in a single run it can cover about 0.5 Acre (Figs. 3 and 4).

As it is a Prototype Agricultural UAV, an actual with a bigger size can also be made with less cost than the market.

Disadvantage in Present Scenario

- No such model.
- No Prediction yet.
- Loss of resources/time/money.
- Unwanted/Unpredictable weather change.
- Machine Automation is there but no optimization is there in way of farming.

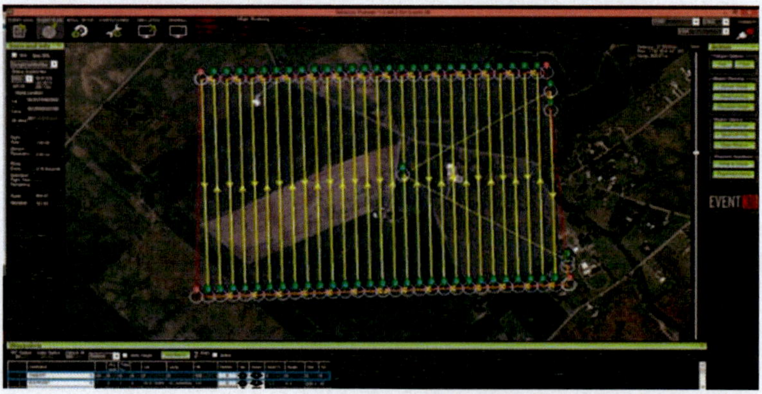

Fig. 3 Mapping of flight path before an actual flight on Mission Planner

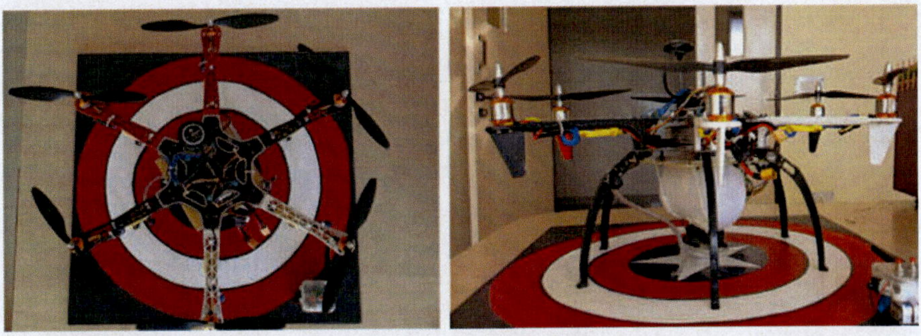

Fig. 4 Images of agricultural drone “AGRONE” from different Angles

S. no.	Existing state of art	Drawbacks in existing state of art	Overcome
1	No such Model	Not able to analyze without data	Developed such model to analyze
2	No Prediction	Not able to detect without prediction	Our model will predict the best possible outcomes
3	Loss of resources/time/money	Its only leads to wastage	We come up with our invention to tackle this by optimizing farming
4	Unwanted/Unpredictable weather change	This leads to damage of crops	We have analyzed these changes to make crops seasonal
5	Machine automation but no farming optimization	Machine automation only makes farming fast but don’t make it optimized to make it productive	Our invention will optimize the farming by best possible outcomes out of the data we have

Advantage

- It is time saving.
- It provides better results with time.
- It will work on root cause of how to increase productivity.
- It is a Machine Learning based model which is cost effective.
- It will be deployed into Android to make its access fast and simple.
- It will work better with time. As soon as this model work more data will be generated and we can try to optimize it as much as we can.

9 Conclusion

The agricultural field should be well monitored at all times without much human intervention. The day-by-day demand for food is increasing at a much higher pace than crop productivity so, without using the shortcuts in agriculture such as machinery, robots, it is very difficult to compete with the growing demand. Monitoring agriculture is a major concern as it helps to reduce labor work and increase production. Artificial Intelligence has been used to select crops and to assist the farmer in selecting fertilizers in accordance with the soil type and environmental conditions. With the help of a database that the user has collected and specified in the system, the machine interacts with them to determine which crop is suitable for harvesting and the fertilizer needed that promotes full growth. Using deep learning gives extra benefit in addition to machine learning as it adds depth to machine learning, providing wide reach and its application in the industry has made great strides. Using new technology, the farmers can ensure the betterment of their crops and field management, as food is what people most need and cannot live without, thus contributing to the overall growth of the world. Other than deep learning, IoT is widely used in intelligent irrigation systems as it highlights its importance in assisting real-time information monitoring. With these technological advancements, water crisis issue can be solved by effective use of the available fresh and salty water. Water scarcity and floods are both the major problems that farmers face using the traditional methods and these methods of irrigation have little effect in this modern time. There are a lot of gaps in this system so in this agricultural automation it is necessary to protect the agricultural land. This paper represents the idea of building a system that uses sensors, IoT, and machine learning to automate the common agricultural practices followed by farmers in rural areas.

10 Discussion

An android app is provided for monitoring environmental, soil, or climate conditions and increasing the productivity of the crops using the android app. The android app includes controlling various sensor devices for monitoring environmental conditions, soil, or climate and controlling the irrigation of the crop. The android system also provides a wireless sensor network that monitors the environment, soil, or climate conditions and controls the productivity and irrigation of a particular crop at the site.

The agricultural sector is focused on sustainable agriculture where management will be carried out according to the care required by the crop. The precision requirement means the requirement of a plant to grow efficiently and productivity's precision requirement depends on various factors that help to visualize the growth of a crop. The various factor includes but is not limited to the suitable climate and the weather required for a particular crop, prediction of the best fertilizer, soil, moisture level, water required, area of cultivation required for a particular crop to grow. On the basis of the favorable environmental conditions suitable for the sustainable development of the plant, farmers use expanded methods like deep learning to discover a variety of things such as the type of flower or plant. Eventually, resulting in the increased production of customized fruits and vegetables, leading to increased diversity of products and production methods. Technologies like Artificial Intelligence including, CNN, RNN, or other computer networks are growing at a higher pace which can be used to detect plant diseases and the growth of unwanted weeds on the farm. Nowadays greenhouse farming is widely used as they provide an environment for the plants to grow well, but it is not possible without human intervention. This led to the involvement of wireless technology, IoT, the latest communication protocols, and sensors which are used to implement systems like climate monitoring, water flow, and the farm can be automated without the presence of humans. Robots would do the harvesting of crops and fruits which is equivalent to 20 workers' manpower. The use of robots is great for farming as robots can also be used for sowing, planting, fertilizing, irrigating, weeding, spraying, and herding. Monitoring of the farm is done by drones which provide the information related to the land to the farmers so that they can work accordingly. For instance, if some part of the field is facing water scarcity, then the farmer starts the day by irrigating that area and providing the crops water. It not only prevents waterlogging or water shortages in the field but also makes sure that the correct amount of water is always available to the crops. The crops need a viable environment at all times which can be gained using different approaches but in end, the result obtained should be proper growth and maximum yield from the field.

References

1. Huang R, Huang JX, Zhang C, Ma HY, Zhuo W, Chen YY, Zhu DH, Wu Q, Mansaray LR (2020) Soil temperature estimation at different depths, using remotely-sensed data. J Integr Agric 19(1):277–290. https://doi.org/10.1016/S2095-3119(19)62657-2
2. Cruz A, Ampatzidis Y, Pierro R, Materazzi A, Panattoni A, Bellis LD, Luvisi A (2019) Detection of grapevine yellows symptoms in Vitis vinifera L. with artificial intelligence. Comput Electron Agric 157:63–76. https://doi.org/10.1016/j.compag.2018.12.028
3. Su YX, Xu H, Yan LJ (2017) Support vector machine-based open crop model (SBOCM): case of rice production in China. Saudi J Biol Sci 24:537–547. https://doi.org/10.1016/j.sjbs.2017.01.024
4. Elhami B, Khanali M, Akram A (2017) Combined application of Artificial Neural Networks and life cycle assessment in lentil farming in Iran. Inf Process Agric 4:18–32. https://doi.org/10.1016/j.inpa.2016.10.004
5. Taki M, Mehdizadeh SA, Rohani A, Rahnama M, Joneidabad MR (2018) Applied machine learning in greenhouse simulation; new application and analysis. Inf Process Agric 5:253–268. https://doi.org/10.1016/j.inpa.2018.01.003
6. Cevallos JP, Villagomez JM, Andryshchenko IS (2019) Convolutional neural network in the recognition of spatial images of sugarcane crops in the Troncal region of the coast of Ecuador. Procedia Comput Sci 150:757–763. https://doi.org/10.1016/j.procs.2019.02.001
7. Athira V, Geetha P, Vinayakumar R, Soman KP (2018) DeepAirNet: applying recurrent networks for air quality prediction. Procedia Comput Sci 132:1394–1403. https://doi.org/10.1016/j.procs.2018.05.068

8. David H, Urte S, Weber A (2017) Machine learning techniques for predicting crop photosynthetic capacity from leaf reflectance spectra. Mol Plant 10(6):878–890. Resource Article. https://doi.org/10.1016/j.molp.2017.04.009
9. McQueen RJ, Gamer SR, Manning CG, Witten IH (1995) Applying machine learning to agricultural data. Comput Electron Agric 12(4):275–293. https://doi.org/10.1016/0168-1699(95)98601-9
10. Klompenburga TV, Kassahuna A, Catalb C (2020) Crop yield prediction using machine learning: a systematic literature review. Comput Electron Agric V 177:105709. https://doi.org/10.1016/j.compag.2020.105709
11. Liakos KG, Busato P, Moshou D, Pearson S, Bochtis D (2018) Machine learning in agriculture: a review. Sensors 18(8):2674. https://doi.org/10.3390/s18082674
12. Charoen-Ung P, Mittrapiyanuruk P (2019) Sugarcane yield grade prediction using random forest with forward feature selection and hyper-parameter tuning. In: Unger H, Sodsee S, Meesad P (eds) Recent advances in information and communication technology 2018. IC2IT 2018. Advances in intelligent systems and computing, vol 769. Springer, Cham. https://doi.org/10.1007/978-3-319-93692-5_4
13. Ranjan AK, Parida BR (2019) Paddy acreage mapping and yield prediction using sentinel-based optical and SAR data in Sahibganj district, Jharkhand (India). Spat Inf Res 27:399–410. https://doi.org/10.1007/s41324-019-00246-4
14. Filippi P, Jones EJ, Wimalathunge NS et al (2019) An approach to forecast grain crop yield using multi-layered, multi-farm data sets and machine learning. Precis Agric 20:1015–1029. https://doi.org/10.1007/s11119-018-09628-4
15. Xu X, Gao P, Zhu X, Guo W, Ding J, Lia C, Zhu M, Wu X (2019) Design of an integrated climatic assessment indicator (ICAI) for wheat production: a case study in Jiangsu Province, China. Ecol Indic 101:943–953. https://doi.org/10.1016/j.ecolind.2019.01.059
16. Jiang B, He J, Yang S, Fu H, Li T, Song H, He D (2019) Fusion of machine vision technology and AlexNet-CNNs deep learning network for the detection of postharvest apple pesticide residues. Artif Intell Agric 1:1–8. https://doi.org/10.1016/j.aiia.2019.02.001
17. Shah A, Dubey A, Hemnani V, Gala D, Kalbande DR (2018) Smart farming system: crop yield prediction using regression techniques. In: Vasudevan H, Deshmukh A, Ray K (eds) Proceedings of international conference on wireless communication. Lecture notes on data engineering and communications technologies, vol 19. Springer, Singapore. https://doi.org/10.1007/978-981-10-8339-6_6
18. Goldstein A, Fink L, Meitin A, Bohadana S, Lutenberg O, Ravid G (2017) Applying machine learning on sensor data for irrigation recommendations: revealing the agronomist's tacit knowledge.https://doi.org/10.1007/s11119-017-9527-4
19. Ferentinos KP (2018) Deep learning models for plant disease detection and diagnosis. Comput Electron Agric 145:311–318. https://doi.org/10.1016/j.compag.2018.01.009
20. Ali I, Cawkwell F, Dwyer E, Green S (2017) Modeling managed grassland biomass estimation by using multitemporal remote sensing data—a machine learning approach. IEEE J Sel Top Appl Earth Obs Remote Sens 10(7):3254–3264. https://doi.org/10.1109/JSTARS.2016.2561618
21. Pantazi XE, Tamouridou AA, Alexandridis TK, Lagopodi AL, Kashefi J, Moshou D (2017) Evaluation of hierarchical self-organising maps for weed mapping using UAS multispectral imagery. Comput Electron Agric 139:224–230. https://doi.org/10.1016/j.compag.2017.05.026
22. Binch A, Fox CW (2017) Controlled comparison of machine vision algorithms for Rumex and Urtica detection in grassland. Comput Electron Agric 140:123–138. https://doi.org/10.1016/j.compag.2017.05.018
23. Maione C, Batista BL, Campiglia AD, Barbosa F Jr, Barbosa, RM (2016) Classification of geographic origin of rice by data mining and inductively coupled plasma mass spectrometry. Comput Electron Agric 121:101–107. https://doi.org/10.1016/j.compag.2015.11.009
24. Paul M, Vishwakarma SK, Verma A (2015) Analysis of soil behaviour and prediction of crop yield using data mining approach. In: 2015 international conference on computational intelligence and communication networks. IEEE. https://doi.org/10.1109/CICN.2015.156

25. Moshou D, Pantazi XE, Kateris D, Gravalos I (2013) Water stress detection based on optical multisensor fusion with a least squares support vector machine classifier. Biosyst Eng V 117:15–22. https://doi.org/10.1016/j.biosystemseng.2013.07.008
26. Aroraa J, Pandyaa U, Shaha S, Doshi N (2019) Survey—pollution monitoring using IoT. In: 2nd international procedia computer science vol 155, pp 710–715. https://doi.org/10.1016/j.procs.2019.08.102
27. Bacco M, Barsocchi P, Ferro E, Gotta A, Ruggeri M (2019) The digitisation of agriculture: a survey of research activities on smart farming. Array 3–4:100009. https://doi.org/10.1016/j.array.2019.100009
28. Salve P, Yannawar P, Sardesai M (2018) Multimodal plant recognition through hybrid feature fusion technique using imaging and non-imaging hyper-spectral data. J King Saud Univ Comput Inf Sci. https://doi.org/10.1016/j.procs.2019.08.102
29. Fritza S, Seea L, Bayasa JCL, Waldnerb F, Jacquesc D, Reshefd I, Whitcraftd A, Baruthe B, Bonifaciof R, Crutchfieldg J, Rembolde F, Rojash O, Schucknechti A, Veldee MV, Verdinj J (2019) A comparison of global agricultural monitoring systems and current gaps. Agric Syst 168:258–272. https://doi.org/10.1016/j.agsy.2018.05.010
30. Goyala H, Joshib N, Sharma C (2018) An empirical analysis of geospatial classification for agriculture monitoring. Procedia Comput Sci 132(2018):1102–1112. https://doi.org/10.1016/j.procs.2018.05.025
31. Kima YH, Yooa SH, Gua YH, Limb JH, Hana D, Baik SW (2013) Crop pests prediction method using regression and machine learning technology: survey. IERI Procedia 6(2014):52–56. https://doi.org/10.1016/j.ieri.2014.03.009
32. Mishraa S, Sachan R, Rajpal D (2020) Deep convolutional neural network based detection system for real-time corn plant disease recognition. Procedia Comput Sci 167(2020):2003–2010. https://doi.org/10.1016/j.procs.2020.03.236
33. Sethya PK, Barpandaa NK, Rath AK, Behera SK (2020) Image processing techniques for diagnosing rice plant disease: a survey. Procedia Comput Sci 167:516–530. https://doi.org/10.1016/j.procs.2020.03.308
34. Pathak A, Uddin A, Abedin J, Andersson K, Mustafa R, Hossain S (2019) IoT based smart system to support agricultural parameters: a case study. Procedia Comput Sci 155:648–653. https://doi.org/10.1016/j.procs.2019.08.092
35. Shannon HD, Motha RP (2015) Managing weather and climate risks to agriculture in North America, Central America and the Caribbean. Weather Clim Extremes 10(Part A):50–56. https://doi.org/10.1016/j.wace.2015.10.006
36. Han E, Ines AVM, Koo J (2019) Development of a 10-km resolution global soil profile dataset for crop modeling applications. Environ Model Softw 119:70–83. https://doi.org/10.1016/j.envsoft.2019.05.012
37. Samadianfard S, Ghorbani A, Mohammadi B (2018) Forecasting soil temperature at multiple-depth with a hybrid artificial neural network model coupled hybrid firefly optimizer algorithm. Inf Process Agric 5(4):465–476. https://doi.org/10.1016/j.inpa.2018.06.005
38. Shafian S, Rajan N, Schnell R, Bagavathiannan M, Valasek J, Shi Y, Olsenholler J (2018) Unmanned aerial systems-based remote sensing for monitoring sorghum growth and development.https://doi.org/10.1371/journal.pone.0196605
39. Yallappa D, Veerangouda M, Maski D, Palled V, Bheemanna M (2017) Development and evaluation of drone mounted sprayer for pesticide applications to crops. In: 2017 IEEE global humanitarian technology conference (GHTC), San Jose, CA, USA, pp 1–7. https://doi.org/10.1109/GHTC.2017.8239330
40. Guo T, Kujirai T, Watanabe T (2012) Mapping crop status from an unmanned aerial vehicle for precision agriculture applications. ISPRS Int Arch Photogramm Remote Sens Spat Inf Sci. https://doi.org/10.5194/isprsarchives-XXXIX-B1-485-2012
41. Banjo C, Ajayi O (2019) Sky-Farmers: applications of unmanned aerial vehicles (UAV) in agriculture. https://doi.org/10.5772/intechopen.89488
42. Sandino J, Pegg G, Gonzalez F, Smith G (2018) Aerial mapping of forests affected by pathogens using UAVs hyperspectral sensors, and artificial intelligence. Sensors 18(4):944. https://doi.org/10.3390/s18040944

43. Patil K, Patil S (2015) Monitoring of turbidity, PH & temperature of water based on GSM. Int J Res Emerg Sci Technol 2(3). https://www.researchgate.net/publication/328686469
44. Andújar D, Dorado J, Fernández-Quintanilla C, Ribeiro A (2016) An approach to the use of depth cameras for weed volume estimation. Sensors 16(7):972. https://doi.org/10.3390/s16 07097
45. Hentschke M, Pignaton de Freitas E, Hennig CH, Girardi da Veiga IC (2018) Evaluation of altitude sensors for a crop spraying drone. Drones 2(3):25. https://doi.org/10.3390/drones203 0025
46. Khan AI, Al-Mulla Y (2019) Unmanned aerial vehicle in the machine learning environment. Procedia Comput Sci 160:46–53. https://doi.org/10.1016/j.procs.2019.09.442
47. Baiphethi MN, Jacobs PT (2009) The contribution of subsistence farming to food security in South Africa. Agrekon Agric Econ Res Policy Pract South Afr 48(4):459–482. https://doi.org/10.1080/03031853.2009.9523836
48. Iizumi T, Ramankutty N (2014) How do weather and climate influence cropping area and intensity? Glob Food Sec 4(2015):46–50. https://doi.org/10.1016/j.gfs.2014.11.003
49. Tsouros DC, Bibi S, Sarigiannidis PG: A review on UAV-based applications for precision agriculture. Information 10(11):349. https://doi.org/10.3390/info10110349
50. Shamshiri RR, Hameed IA, Balasundram SK, Ahmad D, Weltzien C, Yamin M (2018) Fundamental research on unmanned aerial vehicles to support precision agriculture in oil palm plantations.https://doi.org/10.5772/intechopen.80936

Handling Security Issues in Fog Computing Environment Using Blowfish Encryption Algorithm

Sapna Gambhir, Parul Tomar, and Preeti Sharma

Abstract There are different applications for different IoTs, hence IoT is a technology that is diverse in terms of applications. IoT devices do not have their own capability of storage, processing or computing, so we use IoT with cloud computing, as cloud provides pay as per use services such as; on-demand, scalable and shared resources. But due to the enormous growth in IoT devices cloud computing has issues like; low latency, location awareness and immediate data processing. Another computing paradigm like cloud computing was introduced by Cisco, with the difference to provide services near to the end devices in the network, called fog computing. Fog computing introduces a new layer, called fog layer between cloud and end devices, which help to resolve the problems that occurred in cloud. Fog computing has its own issues which required to be explored. In this paper, the security issue of fog has been discussed. This paper proposes a security system for fog environment by using Blowfish algorithm, Third Party Auditor and Three-way hand shaking method.

Keywords IoT · Fog computing · Cloud computing

1 Introduction

Initially, IoT was introduced in 1999 [1], with this idea of minimizing human interaction. This idea proofs it's working in many fields such as: health care, transportation and many more. IoT does not have the capability of computation and storage as its own so it requires some computing paradigm that can work with IoT, Cloud, in order to provide resource pooling and elasticity [2] to work with IoT. Cloud is centralized in nature but the IoT devices are not. Due to the growing demand for IoT devices, the traditional cloud environment is insufficient to provide services that required immediate processing, for taking decisions, for time-sensitive data. A new concept in computing, called Fog Computing has come into existence to solve these issues and it is not evolved to do work without the cloud but to work together with cloud

S. Gambhir (✉) · P. Tomar · P. Sharma
Department of Computer Engineering, J. C. Bose University of Science and Technology, YMCA, Faridabad, India

N. Marriwala et al. (eds.), *Emergent Converging Technologies and Biomedical Systems*, Lecture Notes in Electrical Engineering 841,
https://doi.org/10.1007/978-981-16-8774-7_27

environment so that it can provide high-quality services. An approach called fog computing [3] was proposed by Cisco in 2015,

> A standard that defines how edge computing should work and it facilitates the operation of compute, storage and networking services between end devices and cloud computing data centers.

A foundation, by Cisco in 2015, called OpenFog Consortium [4] founded along with Dell, Intel, Microsoft Corp. and the Princeton University Edge Laboratory, whose first priority is to provide standardization in Fog computing. They focus on fog computing-related technologies, new innovations in fog and the potential market for fog [4] and have proposed a lot of technical and white papers on fog, specifically on its architecture, to give a view of fog architecture. As the focus is on the high-level view, that document does not address security issues. Focusing on security is started in last few years by researchers, yet to identify which security challenges are inherited by fog computing from cloud computing and also to address some other new ones that may be not in cloud.

2 Fog Computing

Like cloud, fog computing provides services required for users; data processing and storage. But the difference between cloud computing and fog computing is that fog computing provides services locally to end devices instead of sending data to cloud for storage or processing. The main motive of fog computing in IoT is to improve efficiency, performance and reduce the amount of data transferred to the cloud for processing, analysis and storage. Basically, fog computing is, a new layer introduced in between cloud and end devices, called fog layer. The fog layer has fog nodes that have the capacity for data processing and storage. A three-layer architecture for fog computing was given in [5–7]. And another architecture, which has six layer was introduced by Aazam et al. [8].

The characteristics [5, 9, 10] of fog that is different from cloud;

- *Location Awareness*
  In the field of fog computing, there is a possibility for tracing down the location of a particular fog node. The nodes can be used to provide information about the applications with an awareness of the geographical location of a terminal node. Therefore, the location of end devices can be known.
- *Geographical Distribution*
  In the area of fog, nodes can be spread widely over a geographical area and can be large in numbers. The nodes are deployed in a way that the quality of data transmission is guaranteed even in the case of mobile terminal nodes. In the situation where the latency with respect to services gets poor because of the mobility of the terminal nodes and the nodes have moved away from the fog node correspondingly, then to handle the situation the nodes are instructed to

get connected to another fog node that is available at that time and can provide improved latency.

- *Low Latency*
  Fog nodes have good storage and computational capabilities. The nodes can work on the data that is being received from the terminal nodes without interfering with the working of the cloud system. The time for getting a response is less as compared to the cloud system because the fog nodes are set closer to the edge of the network.
- *Large-Scale IoT Applications Support*
  Fog nodes have the ability to be used in a versatile range of fields and hence support IoT applications to a larger extent. This would deal with the problem of overhead if they had to be managed by the centralized system. They have a high degree of scalability and autonomy that can support terminal nodes.
- *Decentralization*
  The fog system or atmosphere is not managed in a centralized way to provide different services. The fog nodes have a high degree of autonomy and thus, cooperate with one other for providing services to the users.
- *Heterogeneity*
  Fog nodes can have versatility in various forms and hence, can be deployed in different environments.

3 Literature Survey

There are plenty of security issues in the atmosphere of fog computing. These issues are divided into two families, one is risks and other one is vulnerability.

3.1 Security Risks Encountered in Fog Computing

There is no predefined array of security risks encountered in fog computing. In recent years various researchers presented some risks that were encountered by them in their papers. This is different from that of cloud computing, where risk occurs in switches, routers or points of access.

Venomous malefactors/Forgery [6] can attempt to misguide other entities by forging their identities by generating false details. False data can cause exhaustion of network resources, such as memory and bandwidth. This is the case with Forgery. It can befall under the MitM category.

A malefactor/(Data) Tampering can meddle the information by performing various activities like altering, deleting or delaying it. This is frequently hard to identify since the remote idea of the fog system can once in a while bring about re-transmissions and deferrals. Alrawais et al. [11] utilize the expression "information modification" to allude to this assault. Successful altering endeavours can be misused into infusion assaults [9, 12].

Spam risks/jamming include the creation of a lot of pointless information so as to keep typical fog nodes from ordinary correspondence [6]. Spam information is any undesired data that is delivered by assailants so as to build asset utilization and flood the system, or even endeavour confidential information spills through phishing assaults.

Imitation is a risk aspect referenced by [6] and [13]. In computation of fog, there are two situations of imitation. In the primary situation, the malefactor imitates a real client (end gadget) so as to access data or utilize different administrations given by the nodes of fog. This situation can be the aftereffect of a savage power or phishing risk and is investigated by different papers as "suspicious insider" [5, 10]. In the secondary situation of imitation, the malefactor mimics a genuine node of fog, so as to offer phoney types of assistance and execute phishing and MitM risks. This is alluded to by most papers as a rogue hub risk or is utilized with regards to depicting the procedure behind a MitM risk.

In the family of potential danger, Sybil attack is one of them. Sybil attacks are normal in shared frameworks [14]. In such situations, a suspicious hub produces counterfeit characters and works with other attacking hubs so as to disturb the ordinary hub activity. A Sybil risk can include producing counterfeit cloud sensing reports so as to subvert the reliability of crowdsensing results. Papers [6] and [13] give some basic review of the Sybil assault, while [9] just notice it.

Other kind of risk is rogue hub, which is a device of fog that claims to be a typical hub of the system and attempts to deceive clients to interface with it. As Roman et al. [12] state, the open idea of edge and fog ideal models makes situations where the malefactor may convey his own rogue passage gadget. When viably associated, the malefactor can control approaching and active solicitations from the end clients or the cloud. Therefore, the malefactor can gain admittance to fog-cloud administrations, endeavour phishing assaults or any MitM related assault, which makes the fog hub an extreme risk to information security and protection.

3.2 *Security Vulnerability in Fog Computing*

Vulnerabilities of security in fog computing is a major concern, such as performing authentication or detecting the intruder, that has not been properly addressed yet in environments of fog, mostly due to lack of experience and standardization.

Trust is a significant security instrument for any edge worldview, for example, processing of fog. Notwithstanding, rather than cloud, fog figuring has almost no human mediation and absence of excess, implying that it is more probable for fog hubs to encounter vacation [15]. The eccentric status of fog hubs makes them harder to trust. Cloud-fog-IoT systems must offer secure and solid types of assistance to the end clients. Trust issues have been recognized in fog conditions [15]. Between the fog and the end-gadget layer, trust ought to be bi-directional. The fog hubs that offer administrations to IoT gadgets must confirm if the end gadget is genuine. Then again, the IoT gadgets that demand some help from the fog hubs, need to know whether the fog hub they connect with is secure.

System/Network security is a serious expansive term, yet with regards to the ebb and flow explore in fog registering, it is commonly used to allude to make sure about correspondence. Similarly, as with some other remote innovation worldview, fog registering is powerless against a great deal of remote empowered assaults, for example, sniffer, caricaturing, sticking and so on. Abbasi et al. [16] notice that fog organizes security is extremely significant since fog goes about as a middle of the road layer among cloud and IoT and traded off fog hubs or systems can influence the whole foundation, if not detached appropriately. [14] and [17] express that arranging security for the board can likewise be a difficult errand, as a result of the need to isolate the executives from standard traffic in circulated conditions of such huge scope and without simple access for support.

Privacy Spillage of private data has been a significant issue when benefits as cloud, remote network and IoT are utilized, which are all components of fog processing. Specialists [14, 18, 19] have distinguished three separate issues concerning protection in fog processing: information security, utilization designs, area protection.

We have studied about the Fog computing and also the differences between fog a cloud and the conclusion is that fog has many issues, as it is a new concept and also need standardization but it has lack of implementation issues. From the various issues of fog like; resource allocation, load balancing, optimization, security and some other issues are also existing, we work to choose on security of fog.

4 Proposed Work

After doing the literature survey we get to know there are many security challenges in fog computing. Under the security challenges, there are also many issues that can affect the security in fog computing like trust, authentication, privacy, access, access control, network security and some other issues. Among these issues of security challenges, privacy issue seems to be important from the user's point of view. So, in the proposed work, data privacy is handled by using Blowfish algorithm, Third Party Auditor and Three-way handshaking method. In our proposed work, we used Blowfish Algorithm for encryption reasons for enhancing data security and efficiency. Data travelling over fog is encrypted using blowfish algorithm. The proposed system specifies that users can access the data in a fog without worrying about the security and integrity of the data (Fig. 1).

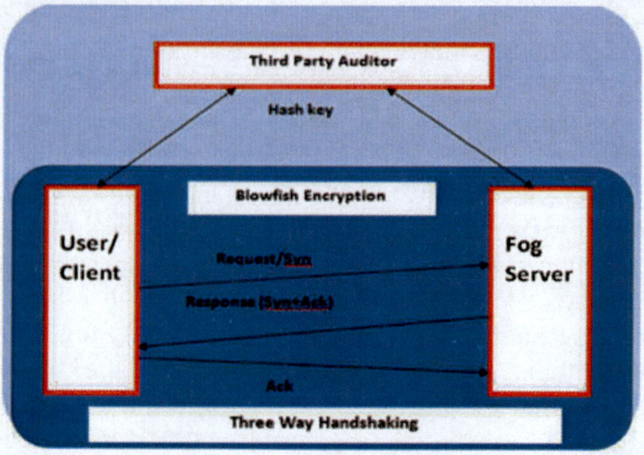

Fig. 1 Framework of proposed system

4.1 *Working of Proposed Framework*

For the communication between client and server, three-way handshaking process is used, the hash keys used by TPA (which has all the information about the files at the server with their hash values) to provide data integrity.

The process starts when the client wants to access the file for getting the data and sent the request to the server for communication. TPA check whether there is any request for data file. When it gets to know that there is a request, then it finds for which file the request has arrived. After that TPA compare the hash code for the requested file with the already saved hash code for that file, if both are the same, then the request for the file will be accepted, otherwise, the user cannot access the file. After the verification, the server allowed the communication by sending the acknowledgement. After getting the acknowledgement the user will take the file from the server and decrypt it and access the data.

4.2 *Terms Used in the Proposed System*

We use the concept of Blowfish algorithm for encryption, the Third Party Auditor, which use the hash key values for data integrity. And for the communication between client and server, we use three-way handshaking. Various terms used in proposed system are:

Third-Party Auditor (TPA):

TPA provides integrity to the proposed system. It will check the hash codes for the requested file. It ensures that the file had not to get affected by any malicious entity. This happens by checking the hash code of the file. It contains the hash code for those files, which are stored at the server. When the user wants a file for decryption it requests that file. TPA check that whether any request has arrived or not. If there is a request for data, it will check the hash code for that file and verify whether the hash code at the time of request is the same as the code when it was saved at the server. If both hash codes are the same the user allows to access the file otherwise not.

Hashing Algorithm:

Hashing algorithm uses a mathematical function, called hash function that converts a numerical input value into another compressed numerical value, values returned by a hash function are called message digest or simply hash values/keys. Has key can be used for integrity check. Here, in our proposed system we use hash key for data integrity check, which is the most common application of the hash functions. With the help of integrity check, the user is able to detect any changes made to original file.

Three-Way Handshaking:

It is a three-way process in which both the client and server exchange synchronization and acknowledgement before starting the real data transfer communication. For the communication between client and server, the three-way handshaking process is used. In this process, client requests the server to start the communication. Then after receiving the request the server sends the acknowledgement to the client. When the client gets the acknowledgement from the server, client can start the communication. It is designed in such a way that both ends can help in, to start the process, transfer the data and end the process.

Blowfish Algorithm:

Blowfish algorithm [20] is symmetric encryption technique which is proposed by Bruce Schneier in 1993. This algorithm has a block size of 64-bits and variable key size from 32-bits to 448-bits. The diagram which is shown below is for Blowfish's encryption routine. Each line represents 32 bits. There are five subkey-arrays: one 18-entry P-array, we mentioned P-array as K and P is the plain text and four 256-entry S-boxes (S0, S1, S2 and S3).

Every round r consists of four steps:

Step 1-XOR the left part (L) of the plaintext with the r th P-array entry

Step 2-Use the XORed result as input for Blowfish's F-function

Step 3- XOR the F-function's output with the right part (R) of the plaintext

Step4- Exchange L and R

Blowfish algorithm uses a function, called F -function which breaks the 32-bit input into four groups of 8-bit and uses them as input to the S-boxes (substitution-boxes). S-boxes takes 8-bit input and produce 32-bit output. The outputs are added modulo 2^{32} (addition will be divided by 2 and remainder will be taken) and XORed to produce the final 32-bit output. After the last round that is the 16th, undo the last swap and XOR L with K18 and R with K17.

The process for decryption is the same as the encryption, except P1, P2, …, P18 (K1, K2,.., K18 are used in the figure) are used in the reverse order. It is because XOR is commutative and associative. Or decryption, first XORing P17 and P18 to the ciphertext block, then using the P-entries in reverse.

4.3 How Is the Proposed Framework Help in Fog Security?

In our proposed framework, we used various concepts so that security in fog computing can be improved. We use Blowfish encryption algorithm to secure the data and the proposed framework has TPA, which is used for data integrity check, ensures that the file is not get affected by any malicious entity and for communication between client and server, three-way handshaking process is used, in which both client and server communicate in a synchronized way. So, in the proposed framework, we ensure that secure communication will be held and the user gets its data without any change in it. Hence data privacy can be improved by this proposed system.

5 Conclusion and Future Scope

In recent years the use of IoT devices is increased, hence the data generated by these dives also vast amount, which cannot be handled by cloud because of its centralized approach. So, a new computing paradigm introduced by Cisco, known as fog computing, add an extra layer between cloud and end devices to handle the enormous amount produced by the IoT devices. But this new paradigm also has some issues. Our paper focused on security challenges of fog, various papers were published on security in fog but many of them surveyed the security issues in fog. We also studied various security issues in fog environment, but in this paper, focus is on data privacy issues and we proposed a system, which can improve the data privacy issue in fog. We use encryption algorithm to decrypt the data and to provide more security we introduced TPA (Third Party Auditor) which takes care of the data integrity, by which user/client ensures the correctness of data. Our system tries to ensure the privacy of data, but as the IoT devices improved day by day and also working on fog is in progress we require more security aspects in fog, maybe we can use ECC for encryption so that minimum number of keys used to encrypt the data and data integrity check should be more for privacy, so this can be our future scope.

References

1. Shi W, Cao J, Zhang Q, Li Y, Xu L (2016) Edge computing: vision and challenges. IEEE Internet Things J 3(5):637–646
2. Mell P, Grance T (2011) The NIST definition of cloud computing, 2011. csrc.nist.gov/publications/detail/sp/800-145/final
3. Fog computing and the Internet of Things: extend the cloud wo Where the things are, Cisco.com, 2018. https://www.cisco.com/c/dam/en_us/solutions/trends/iot/docs/computing-overview.pdf
4. OpenFog Consortium, Openfogconsortium.org, 2018. https://www.openfogconsortium.org/
5. Mukherjee M et al (2017) Security and privacy in fog computing: challenges. IEEE Access 5:19293–19304
6. Ni J, Zhang K, Lin X, Shen XS (2018) Securing fog computing for Internet of Things applications: challenges and solutions. IEEE Commun Surv Tutor 20(1):601–628, Firstquarter 2018
7. Sarkar S, Chatterjee S, Misra S (2018) Assessment of the suitability of fog computing in the context of Internet of Things. IEEE Trans Cloud Comput 6(1): 46–59
8. Aazam M, Huh E (2016) Fog computing: the cloud-IoT\/IoE middleware paradigm. IEEE Potentials 35(3):40–44
9. Rauf A, Shaikh RA, Shah A (2018) Security and privacy for IoT and fog computing paradigm. In: 2018 15th learning and technology conference (L&T), Jeddah, 2018, pp 96–101
10. Roman R, Lopez J, Mambo M (2018) Mobile edge computing, Fog et al.: A survey and analysis of security threats and challenges. Future Gener Comput Syst 78:680–698
11. Alrawais A, Alhothaily A, Hu C, Xing X, Cheng X (2018) An attribute-based encryption scheme to secure fog communications. IEEE Access 5:9131–9138
12. Irwan S, Redesigning security for fog computing with blockchain | OpenFog Consortium, OpenFog Consortium |. http://www.openfogconsortium.org/redesigning-security-for-fog-computing-with-blockchain
13. Aljumah A, Ahanger TA (2018) Fog computing and security issues: a review. In: 2018 7th international conference on computers communications and control (ICCCC), Oradea, 2018, pp 237–239
14. Yi S, Qin Z, Li Q (2015) Security and privacy issues of fog computing: a survey WASA
15. Rahman FH, Au TW, Newaz SHS, Suhaili WS (2017) Trustworthiness in fog. In: Proceedings of the 2017 VI international conference on network, communication and computing—ICNCC 2017
16. Abbasi BZ, Shah MA (2017) Fog computing: security issues, solutions and robust practices. In: 2017 23rd international conference on automation and computing (ICAC), 2017
17. Kumar P, Zaidi N, Choudhury T (2016) Fog computing: common security issues and proposed countermeasures. In: 2016 international conference system modelling & advancement in research trends (SMART), 2016
18. Alrawais A, Alhothaily A, Hu C, Cheng X (2017) Fog computing for the Internet of Things: security and privacy issues. IEEE Internet Comput 21(2):34–42
19. Abubaker N, Dervishi L, Ayday E (2017) Privacy-preserving fog computing paradigm. In: 2017 IEEE conference on communications and network security (CNS), Las Vegas, NV, 2017, pp 502–509
20. https://en.wikipedia.org/wiki/Blowfish_(cipher)

Investigating Novel Coronavirus Through Statistical Methods for Biomedical Applications: An Engineering Student Perspective

Amit Kumar Shakya, Ayushman Ramola, and Anurag Vidyarthi

Abstract The World of today is suffering from novel coronavirus (nCOV2). This is a respiratory infectious disease that has affected the entire globe. This respiratory infection is first originated in Wuhan, China. Today, it has many variants like the "United Kingdom (UK) variant called B.1.1.7," "South African variant is called B.1.351," "Brazilian variant is known as P.1," etc. In this research work, we will discuss the Indian scenario to tackle nCOV2. We will also present an engineering student's perspective to detect changes developed in the patient's chest suffering from nCOV2 employing statistical methods. Among all the statistical techniques, GLCM-based texture analysis-based technique has gained popularity due to its diverse applications. It is used in many applications like remote sensing, image processing, biomedical applications, seismic data analysis. Thus in this research work, this methodology is used various changes in the before and after images of the patient suffering from the novel coronavirus.

Keywords Novel coronavirus (nCOV2) · B.1.1.7 · B.1.351 · P.1 · Statistical methods

1 Introduction

The World of today is infected from the "novel coronavirus SARS-CoV-2 (COVID-19)" [1]. This virus has stopped the fast-moving World all of a sudden [2]. Due to the spread of this infection, most World countries were in lockdown mode in 2020. Besides this, measures, like imposing curfews, deploying military personals to restrict peoples' physical movement, thermal scanning, avoiding social gatherings, identifying virus hotspots, etc., are some measures taken by the worldwide

A. K. Shakya (✉) · A. Ramola
Department of Electronics and Communication Engineering, Sant Longowal Institute of Engineering and Technology, Longowal, Sangrur, Punjab, India
e-mail: xlamitshakya.gate2014@ieee.org

A. Vidyarthi
Graphic Era (Deemed to be University), Dehradun, Uttarakhand, India

N. Marriwala et al. (eds.), *Emergent Converging Technologies and Biomedical Systems*, Lecture Notes in Electrical Engineering 841,
https://doi.org/10.1007/978-981-16-8774-7_28

government to prevent the spread of the virus. Wearing masks in public places, no handshakes, daily sanitization of offices, frequent hand wash, social distancing, etc., are some of the people's measures that become a necessity in 2020 [3]. Global superpowers like the China, United States of America (USA), the United Kingdom (UK), France, Italy, Spain are severely affected by this coronavirus [4]. The death toll in the World is increasing day by day. By the time, we write this paper, confirmed coronavirus cases reported globally are 119,220,681, and 2,642,826 deaths are reported due to this virus attack [5]. nCOV-2 has also put a brake on my country. Recently, after February second wave of coronavirus has struck our country. It is assumed that this second wave is more deadly and dangerous than the previous one. During the first strike of the coronavirus PM, Mr. Narendra Modi took several precautionary measures in 2020 to tackle this global epidemic.

Some of the crucial steps taken by India's government (GOI) as a preventive measure are as follows.

The first step was imposing Janta Curfew on March 22, 2020, in which no movement of the public was allowed. Schools, colleges, universities, government offices, private offices were all closed [6].

Declaration of the complete lockdown Phase 1 (March 25, 2020 –April 14, 2020). It lasted for 21 days [7].

Declaration of national lockdown Phase 2 (April 15, 2020 –May 3, 2020). It lasted for 18 days [7].

Declaration of national lockdown Phase 3 (May 4, 2020 –May 17, 2020). It lasted for 13 days [7].

Declaration of national lockdown Phase 4 (May 18, 2020 –May 31, 2020). It lasted for 14 days [7].

After that government started to unlock the country, unlock 1 to 10, which started from June 1, 2020, and still in progress. In India, there are currently 219262 active cases which are (1.93%), 11007352 discharged cases (96.68%), and 158725 deaths (1.39%) reported due to this deadly virus [8]. India has twenty-eight states and eight union territories, but coronavirus has spread in an entirely different way in every state and union territory. In the Indian states, Maharashtra is most severely affected by this epidermic, followed by Kerala and Andhra Pradesh [9]. Among all these alarming situations, a ray of hope "vaccination" is also started, and it is expected that in the coming years, nCOV-2 will become history all around the globe.

2 Experimental Results

Several methods, techniques, and algorithms are designed and developed in image processing through which the amount of statistical change developed in an image can be monitored. Some of the prominent techniques include gray level co-occurrence matrix (GLCM) [6, 7], content-based image query (CBIQ) [8], deep learning algorithms [9], supervised learning algorithms [10, 11, 12], unsupervised learning algorithms [10, 13], etc. Among all these algorithms, GLCM and deep learning methods are the most popular in image processing. *Robert M Haralick* invented GLCM [14]. He presented fourteen different features through which images can be classified and changes developed can be quantified. Four texture features, contrast, correlation, energy, and homogeneity [14], explain the change in the texture features' behavior as they are known as visual texture features. Thus, we have used these features in this work. While calculating the GLCM from the input image, one should take care of distance and orientation angle. They are the most important parameters while calculating the GLCM from an input image. In this research, digital images in communication and medicines (DICOM) images of human chest infected from nCOV2 are obtained from [15, 16]. The pre-COVID image is slightly lighter in color than the post-COVID image represented by Fig. 1a, b, respectively. The "gray level representation" of the pre-COVID and the post-COVID image are presented in Fig. 1c, d, respectively. Through these versions of the images, it can be easily identified that the chest is clear and responding effectively to the light signals. Thus, no un-usual behavior is observed shown in Fig. 1c. In Fig. 1d, excessive infection in the chest can be observed. The light signals cannot pass through them, and they behave like

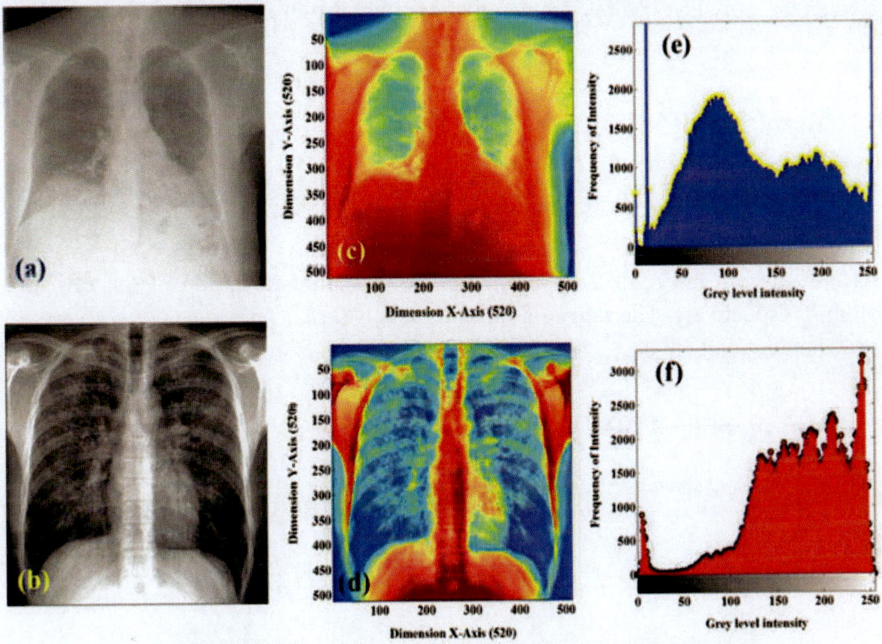

(a) Negative COVID (b) Positive COVID (c) Greyscale Negative COVID (d) Greyscale Positive COVID (e) Histogram signature Negative COVID (f) Histogram signature Negative COVID

Fig. 1 Result of the changes developed in the pre- and post-DICOM image human chest infected from nCOV2 a barrier surface toward the light signals. Histogram signature plots represented in Fig. 1e, f shows the different behavior in terms of variation in the frequency intensity.

Mathematical notations of the visual texture features and their operational range are expressed by Eq. (1–4). This range of numerical values belongs to the normalized GLCM. Let for an input image $I(m, n)$ having m number of rows and n numbers of columns. The number of total pixels present in the image is $m \times n$. Let a pixel of interest (PoI) be $P(q, r)$,Dg represents the number of unique gray levels present in the image. Then the visual texture features are expressed as follows.

3 Contrast [17]

$$f1 = \sum_{n=0}^{D_g-1} z^2 \times \left\{ \sum_{m=1}^{D_g} \sum_{n=1}^{D_g} P(q, r) \right\} \tag{1}$$

Here the difference between the $|q - r|$ is represented by z, which is the difference between the gray level pairs. The range of contrast is more significant than zero.

4 Correlation [18]

$$f2 = \sum_m \sum_n \frac{(m, n)P(q, r) - \mu_m \mu_n}{\sigma_m \sigma_n} \tag{2}$$

Here μ_m, μ_n and σ_m, σ_n are the mean and standard deviation of the row and column, respectively. The range of correlation is $[-1, 1]$.

5 Homogeneity [19]

$$f3 = \sum_m \sum_n \frac{1}{1 + (m - n)^2} P(q, r) \tag{3}$$

The normalized range of homogeneity for an input image is [0, 1].

6 Energy [20, 21]

$$f4 = \sum_m \sum_n (P(q, r))^2 \tag{4}$$

The normalized range of energy lies between [0, 1].

Table 1 Texture feature quantification of the "pre-COVID image"

S. no	Degree	Features	D = 1	D = 2	D = 3	D = 4	D = 5	D = 6	D = 7	D = 8
1	0°	Contrast	0.0873	0.1746	0.2342	0.2712	0.2912	0.3086	0.3285	0.3477
2		Correlation	0.9799	0.9599	0.9462	0.9378	0.9333	0.9294	0.9249	0.9026
3		Energy	0.6957	0.6908	0.6881	0.6864	0.6851	0.6838	0.6825	0.6812
4		Homogeneity	0.9655	0.9513	0.9449	0.9416	0.9397	0.9383	0.9368	09,350
5	45°	Contrast	0.1220	0.2208	0.2691	0.2916	0.3190	0.3465	0.3739	0.4007
6		Correlation	0.9720	0.9494	0.9384	0.9334	0.9273	0.9212	0.9151	0.9092
7		Energy	0.6933	0.6883	0.6857	0.6837	0.6816	0.6795	0.6775	0.6754
8		Homogeneity	0.9587	0.9460	0.9414	0.9395	0.9368	0.9344	0.9323	0.9301
9	90°	Contrast	0.0756	0.1507	0.2146	0.2687	0.3030	0.3221	0.3353	0.3499
10		Correlation	0.9826	0.9654	0.9507	0.9384	0.9306	0.9263	0.9233	0.9201
11		Energy	0.6965	0.6918	0.6887	0.6863	0.6847	0.6834	0.6821	0.6807
12		Homogeneity	0.9684	0.9545	0.9469	0.9418	0.9390	0.9375	0.9362	0.9347
13	135°	Contrast	0.1065	0.2060	0.2835	0.3224	0.3421	0.3631	0.3859	0.4087
14		Correlation	0.9755	0.9528	0.9351	0.9263	0.9220	0.9174	0.9124	0.9074
15		Energy	0.6941	0.6888	0.6854	0.6831	0.6813	0.6794	0.6773	0.6753
16		Homogeneity	0.9616	0.9479	0.9407	0.9374	0.9357	0.9339	0.9318	0.9299

The texture feature computation for the pre-COVID image is presented in Table 1 for eight different distances and four orientation angles.

The texture feature quantification for the post-COVID image is presented in Table 2 for eight different distances and four orientation angles. This quantifies the features of the image texture. We can predict the behavior of the COVID infected images. Like in Table 1, quantification for the pre-COVID image is present. Likewise, in Table 2, texture features of the post-COVID image quantification are present. Thus, we can quantify numbers of images to obtain a pattern of the changing texture.

Thus, similar texture visual features can be quantified and compared to obtain the amount of change developed in the "pre-COVID image" and "post-COVID images."

7 Conclusion

This research presents the image processing-based statistical techniques' efficiency to quantify and present the change developed due to COVID infection. The proposed GLCM-based technique presents the change in terms of visualization as well as in terms of quantification. Thus, GLCM can be considered as an effective tool to analyze the COVID images so that more interpretations can be obtained by analyzing these images.

Table 2 Texture feature quantification of the "post-COVID image"

S. no	Degree	Features	D = 1	D = 2	D = 3	D = 4	D = 5	D = 6	D = 7	D = 8
1	0°	Contrast	0.8663	2.2068	3.4531	4.5047	5.3648	6.0841	6.7005	7.2365
2		Correlation	0.9149	0.7834	0.6610	0.5579	0.4735	0.4030	0.3425	0.2900
3		Energy	0.1603	0.1316	0.1127	0.0990	0.0889	0.0811	0.0752	0.0706
4		Homogeneity	0.8073	0.7277	0.6773	0.6373	0.6084	0.5829	0.5611	0.5423
5	45°	Contrast	1.4847	3.3436	4.7794	5.8603	6.7269	7.4547	8.0684	8.5872
6		Correlation	0.8542	0.6717	0.5307	0.4245	0.3394	0.2679	0.2075	0.1565
7		Energy	0.1453	0.1148	0.0962	0.0839	0.0752	0.0689	0.0644	0.0612
8		Homogeneity	0.7647	0.6827	0.6306	0.5924	0.5611	0.5353	0.5142	0.4977
9	90°	Contrast	0.9896	2.4016	3.6267	4.6336	5.4449	6.1194	6.6967	7.2050
10		Correlation	0.9028	0.7641	0.6438	0.5448	0.4650	0.3987	0.3418	0.2917
11		Energy	0.1565	0.1277	0.1093	0.0963	0.0870	0.0800	0.0746	0.0703
12		Homogeneity	0.7953	0.7157	0.6658	0.6280	0.5984	0.5741	0.5538	0.5362
13	135°	Contrast	1.4941	3.3752	4.8295	5.9053	6.7502	7.4382	8.0133	8.4898
14		Correlation	0.8533	0.6686	0.5258	0.4201	0.3371	0.2695	0.2130	0.1661
15		Energy	0.1440	0.1125	0.0939	0.0823	0.0743	0.0686	0.0645	0.0615
16		Homogeneity	0.7600	0.6736	0.6198	0.5820	0.5530	0.5300	0.5117	0.4973

References

1. Organization WH (2020) Coronavirus disease 2019 (COVID-19). WHO, Geneva, Switzerland
2. Cohut M, Field P (2020) COVID-19 global impact: How the coronavirus is affecting the world. Healthline Media UK Ltd, Brighton, 24 April 2020. https://www.medicalnewstoday.com/articles/covid-19-global-impact-how-the-coronavirus-is-affecting-the-world#Hopes-for-the-future?. Accessed 27 May 2020
3. Organization WH (2020) Coronavirus disease (COVID-19) advice for the public: Myth busters. WHO, 24 March 2020. https://www.who.int/emergencies/diseases/novel-coronavirus-2019/advice-for-public/myth-busters. Accessed 27 May 2020
4. Organization WH (2020) WHO coronavirus disease (COVID-19) dashboard. WHO, 26 May 2020. https://covid19.who.int/?gclid=EAIaIQobChMI-KfOxaHT6QIVBVdgCh34oAsaEAAYASAAEgLjTfD_BwE. Accessed 27 May 2020
5. Worldometer (2020) COVID-19 coronavirus pandemic. 29 April 2020. https://www.worldometers.info/coronavirus/. Accessed 29 April 2020
6. Shakya AK, Ramola A, Kandwal A, Prakash R (2019) Change over time in grey levels of multispectral landsat 5TM/8OLI satellite images. Lecture notes in electrical engineering. Springer, Ranchi, pp 309–356
7. Ramola A, Shakya AK, Pham DV (2020) Study of statistical methods for texture analysis and their modern evolutions. Eng Rep: e12149
8. Shakya AK, Ramola A, Vidyarthi A (2020) Conversion of Landsat 8 multispectral data through modified private content-based image retrieval technique for secure transmission and privacy. Eng Rep: e12273
9. Aubreville M, Bertram CA, Marzahl C, Gurtner C, Dettwiler M, Schmidt A (2020) Deep learning algorithms out-perform veterinary pathologists in detecting the mitotically most active tumor region. Sci Rep: 16447

10. Shakya AK, Ramola A, Kandwal A, Prakash R (2018) Comparison of supervised classification techniques with ALOS PALSAR sensor for Roorkee region of Uttarakhand, India. Int Archiv Photogramm Remote Sens Spat Inf Sci XLII–V:639–701. https://doi.org/10.5194/isprs-archives-XLII-5-693-2018
11. Wang X, Lin X, Dang X (2020) Supervised learning in spiking neural networks: a review of algorithms and evaluations. Neural Netw: 258–280
12. Shakya AK, Ramola A, Sawant K, Kandwal A (2018) Comparison of supervised classification techniques for high-resolution optical aerial image. In: international conference on automation and computational engineering (ICACE), Noida
13. Sinaga KP, Yang M-S (2020) Unsupervised K-means clustering algorithm. IEEE Access: 80716–80727
14. Haralick R (1979) Statistical and structural approaches to texture. Proc IEEE: 786–804
15. Sharman BS (2021) High-accuracy Covid 19 prediction from chest X-ray images using pre-trained convolutional neural networks in PyTorch. Towards Data Science, 22 February 2021. https://towardsdatascience.com/high-accuracy-covid-19-prediction-from-chest-x-ray-images-using-pre-trained-convolutional-neural-2ec96484ce0. Accessed 15 March 2021
16. Shakya AK, Ramola A, Pandey DC (2017) Polygonal region of interest-based compression of DICOM images. In: International conference on computing, communication and automation (ICCCA), Noida
17. Shakya AK, Ramola A, Kashyap A, Pham DV, Vidyarthi A (2020) Susceptibility assessment of changes developed in the landcover caused due to the landslide disaster of Nepal from Multispectral LANDSAT Data. In: Communications in computer and information science, Mohali, Springer, pp 406–418
18. Shakya AK, Ramola A, Kashyap A, Vidyarthi A (2020) Susceptibility assessment of changes developed in the landcover caused due to the landslide disaster of Nepal from multispectral LANDSAT data. In: Communications in computer and information science, Mohali, Springer, pp 406–418
19. Shakya AK, Prakash R, Ramola A, Pandey DC (2017) Change detection from pre and posturbanisation LANDSAT 5TM multispectral images. In International conference on innovations in control, communication and information systems (ICICCI), Noida
20. Shakya AK, Ramola A, Kandwal A, Mittal P, Prakash R (2019) Morphological change detection in terror camps of area 3 and 4 by pre- and post-strike through MOAB: B. Lecture notes in electrical engineering. Springer, Sikkim, pp 265–275
21. Fauzi AA, Utaminingrum F, Ramdani F (2020) Road surface classification based on LBP and GLCM features using kNN classifier. Bull Elect Eng Inf 9(4):1446–1453

A Comprehensive Analysis on Technological Approaches in Sign Language Recognition

Kamaldeep Sharma, Brajesh Kumar, Deepti Sehgal, and Ayan Kaushik

Abstract Communication is one of the imperative sides of the twenty-first century. We as human being cannot even imagine this world without communicating with each other. For honest communication to happen two persons should agree on a common language that each of them understands. Keeping this context in mind, there will be a necessity for a translator in between a hearing/speech-impaired person and a normal person. But the translators or consultants who understand sign language do not seem to be simply and commonly offered all the days, if offered conjointly, they charge tons. To help the social interaction of hearing-impaired–speech debilitated individuals with the society economical interactive communication tools are made. As the importance of sign language interpretation is increasing day by day so several triple-crown applications for linguistic communication recognition comprise new forms of real-time interpretation with progressed artificial intelligence and image processing approaches. In this paper, we gave an entire outline of various methodologies and processes rooted in deep learning and discussed technological approaches for linguistic communication interpretation, also achieving 95.7% accuracy with two layers of CNN model classifier for the sign gestures of 26 English alphabets with readily available resources. This paper also provides current analysis and advances in this area and tends to distinguish openings and difficulties for future exploration.

Keywords Linguistic communication · Deep learning · Convolutional neural network · Image processing · Sign language recognition

K. Sharma · B. Kumar (✉) · D. Sehgal · A. Kaushik
Lovely Professional University, Phagwara, Punjab, India

K. Sharma
e-mail: kamaldeep.16958@lpu.co.in

N. Marriwala et al. (eds.), *Emergent Converging Technologies and Biomedical Systems*, Lecture Notes in Electrical Engineering 841,
https://doi.org/10.1007/978-981-16-8774-7_29

1 Introduction

Gesture-based communication is a remarkable kind of correspondence that regularly goes understudied. Deaf or speech-disabled people tend to communicate with others using gesture-based communication to convey their contemplations and emotions. Sign language is a little complicated language that involves the movement of hands, face, and different stances of the body. Each nation has its own local sign language [1]. Different sign languages have their own standard of language structure, different gestures for different words, and different pronunciations. Hearing/speech-impaired individuals are not self-reliant henceforth prepared gesture-based communication translators or consultants are required during clinical, legitimate arrangements, and instructional meetings. Though it is good to have access to translators, it very well can be seen as problematic for various reasons: first and foremost, hearing/speech-impaired individuals face quandaries in expressing themselves, so an interpreter needs to understand their gestures and represent them on their behalf, and second, the interpreter who is more than the judge of phonetic content acts as a medium between the signers and the non-signers [2]. Translators are masters of depiction but they are not commonly and easily offered all the days, if offered conjointly, they charge tons. The vast majority of ordinary people do not possess any knowledge of sign language. Thus, numerous corresponding hindrances exist for hearing/speech-impaired gesture-based communication users.

The number of deaf people has recently reached four hundred million [3], as per the data provided by World Health Organization. Following this cause, the latest experiments are being intensified to make it easier for disabled people to communicate [3]. Though there are several sign languages concerning other sign languages, American Sign Language (ASL) is more spoken. In contrast, we see that ASL which is used in the USA and English-speaking Canada has a vast variety of lingos. There are 22 handshapes related to the 26 alphabets in order, and one can sign the 10 digits on a single hand.

With the wish to accelerate the capacity of hearing/speech-deprived people to receive assistance in their own society without the aid of a skilled consultant in sign language. These kinds of virtual machines can address the unmet need for professional decoding facilities and increase the quality of living considerably.

The primary aim of this paper is to propose a two-layer CNN classifier model which can achieve significant accuracy with readily available resources and to provide a comprehensive analysis of different processes, methodologies for the understanding of sign language focused on deep learning and computational approaches. The recent developments in this field are further explored which helps to recognize prospects and obstacles for future research work.

2 Methodology

Decades after human–computer interaction (HCI) became popular in the industry, sign language recognition (SLR) has been explored. The standard and widespread methodology for the identification of vision-based SLR is depicted in Fig. 1, which involves user input, preprocessing, extraction of features, classification based on various methodologies of deep learning, and then output predictions. Sign gesture illustration covers the spot to represent the key data. One of the important parts of the whole framework is preprocessing because it involves different stages.

2.1 Preprocessing

Creation of histogram. The very initial step is hand gesture recognition, and for this, a threshold of the image is required. For the creation of the threshold of an image, a histogram is made. Graphical representation of the frequency of pixels in a grayscale image in which pixel value varies from 0 to 255 is known as histogram [4]. To get a good histogram of our hand with respect to surroundings, our hand should cover all

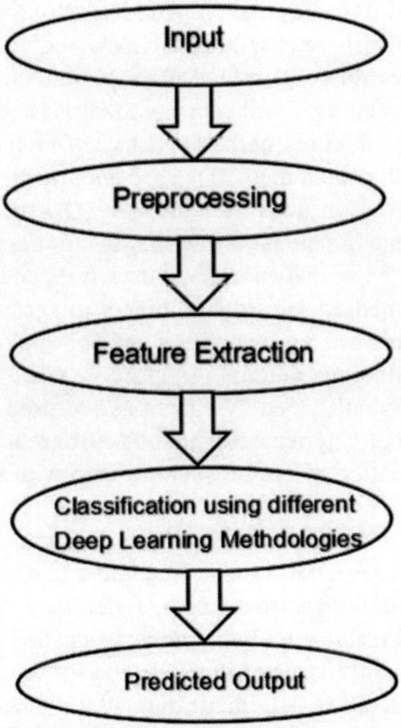

Fig. 1 General flow diagram for sign language recognition

Fig. 2 Hand covering all green spots to create a good histogram

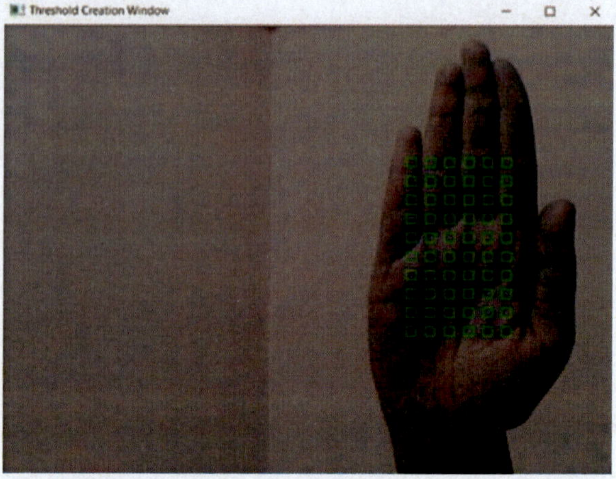

those small squares to get a good histogram as shown in Fig. 2. The histogram has a significant role in the calculation of the threshold value.

Separation of background and creation of the binary image. To facilitate the process of sign gesture recognition, the hand gesture region must be separated from the background. Hand and background have different pixel intensities; hence, differences in their pixel intensity are used to separate them out from each other [5]. Pixels representing the hand region are assigned with a value so that those pixels could be identified. If pixel value exceeds a threshold value, it is assigned with a value that will represent that it is white, else it is assigned any other value which will represent that it is black. To remove our hand from the background, an adaptive threshold method is used and images are scaled to 128 × 128 pixels.

Contour Detection using OpenCV. All the continuous points along the boundary, having the same intensity or color are joined which forms a curve called contour. For shape analysis, object detection, and its recognition, contours proved to be a useful method [6]. Filtered binary images are preferred for better accuracy. Threshold or canny edge detection should be applied before finding contours [6]. Point to note that finding contours in OpenCV is like detecting a white entity on black background. Inbuilt OpenCV functions are used to identify the shape of the hand through the contour detection method. Different contour properties are required for the identification of gestures and to map with their meaning therefore outline is being drawn [5].

Image Labeling. After the creation of grayscale images, those grayscale gesture images are assigned a number that is in sequence and can be considered as a gesture identification number. Later these images are mapped with their corresponding meaning, and this process is called image labeling. After this process, the labeled image is saved in the database.

Data Augmentation. While making gestures, restricting users to make gestures from one hand (either left hand or right hand) would not be convenient at all. If they are allowed to do so, it will affect the model accuracy. Therefore, data augmentation is one of the important aspects to get good accuracy. We can define data augmentation as the method by which slightly altered copies of pre-existing data are added to the already existing dataset in order to increase the amount of data which helps the model to learn from a different type of situation. This modification can be done by flipping images along horizontal or vertical axes or by rotating images by few angles. It behaves as a regulator and helps to bring down the extent of overfitting while training deep learning or a machine learning model [7].

2.2 Feature Extraction

The process to pull out condensed and discriminative descriptors which are further used as training data for the classifier for a stronger recognition purpose and to enhance accuracy is known as feature extraction. One of the difficult issues that are being faced is to pull out the discriminative feature from different kinds of videos or images exposed to different lighting conditions. For the proposed model, the red–green–blue (RGB) input images are converted to grayscale images and Gaussian blur is applied to minimize unwanted noise.

2.3 Model Training

The selection of a deep learning method among the pool of various deep learning methodologies which can give promising results over varied data is another considerable issue. Among various deep learning methodologies, convolutional neural network (CNN) gives promising results while making predictions in vision-based SLR. The architecture of CNN which is being followed is shown in Fig. 3.

128 × 128 pixels are the size of the input images. These are processed using 32 filter weights in the first convolutional layer (3 × 3 pixels each). This produces a 126 × 126 pixel representation for each of the filter weights.

Further, they are down-sampled using max-pooling of 2 × 2 resulting in images of 63 × 63 pixels. The input picture was subjected to max-pooling with a pool size of (2, 2) and to the rectified linear unit activation function. This decreases the number of parameters, lowering both the computing expense and the risk of overfitting. The resulting 63 × 63 images from the first pooling layer are then served to the second convolutional layer as an input. It is then processed in the second convolutional layer using 32 filter weights (3 × 3 pixels each). The resulting 60 × 60 pixels images are again down-sampled using a max pool of 2 × 2 and further reduced to 30 × 30 resolution of images. These images are fed into a 128-neuron which is a completely connected layer, and the output of the second convolutional layer is then reshaped into a 30 × 30x32 = 28,800-value array. This layer receives a 28,800-value array as input. The second densely connected layer receives the contribution of all these layers. To prevent overfitting, a dropout layer is used with a value of 0.5. The output from the first densely connected layer is fed into a 96-neuron entirely connected

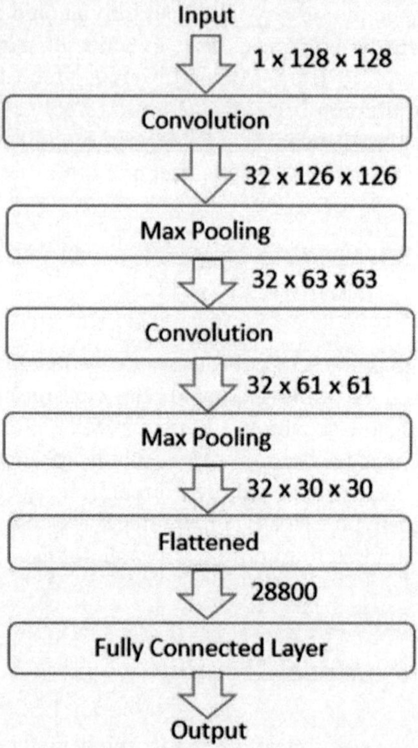

Fig. 3 CNN architecture

layer. The second densely connected layer's output is fed into the final layer, which would have the same number of neurons as the number of groups were classified (alphabets + blank symbol).

The prediction layer calculates the likelihood of the picture falling into one of the groups. As a result, the output is scaled between 0 and 1, and the sum of each class's values equals 1. We were able to accomplish this by using the softmax function. The prediction layer's contribution will initially be a little off from the actual value. To improve it, we used labeled data to train the networks. Cross-entropy is the performance measurement that is used in classification.

3 Results and Discussions

3.1 Project Outcome

The primary goal was to improve the model's performance with readily available resources while also improving its accuracy. Two layers of the CNN model algorithm were used for this. In the first layer, a threshold was generated using the histogram obtained, and then a Gaussian blur filter was used to extract features from the captured hand gesture. The data was then augmented to generate more inputs, allowing the model to identify movements from multiple angles and sides. The processed image input was then transferred to the layer 1 CNN model, which yielded the same results for a particular set of symbols. The symbols for which the model did not make sufficient predictions are described below.

- For D:U, R
- For U:R, D
- For T:I, K, D
- For S:N, M

Then such sets were categorized using four different CNN classifier designed specifically for each of them in layer 2. The principle behind layer 2 is that if the layer 1 model decides that the input belongs to one of those sets, the input would then proceed through the CNN classifier in layer 2, which was designed explicitly to distinguish ambiguous symbols.

We obtained 85.4% accuracy in our model using just layer 1 of our algorithm, and 95.7% accuracy using a mix of layer 1 and layer 2 of our algorithm, which is higher than most existing study papers on American Sign Language. The confusion matrix of our model is shown in Fig. 4. We used the Adam optimizer to update the model in response to the performance of the loss function. Adam integrates the advantages of extensions of two stochastic gradient descent algorithms which are adaptive gradient algorithm (ADA-GRAD) and root mean square descent algorithm (RMSD).

Predicted Values

Correct Values	A	B	C	D	E	F	G	H	I	J	K	L	M	N	O	P	Q	R	S	T	U	V	W	X	Y
A	147	0	0	0	0	0	0	0	0	0	0	0	1	2	0	0	0	0	0	0	0	0	2	0	0
B	0	139	0	0	0	0	0	0	0	0	0	0	0	0	0	0	0	0	0	0	0	11	0	0	0
C	0	0	152	0	0	0	0	0	0	0	0	0	0	0	0	0	0	0	0	0	0	0	0	0	0
D	0	0	0	153	0	0	0	0	0	0	0	0	0	0	0	0	0	0	0	0	0	0	0	0	0
E	0	0	0	0	152	0	0	0	0	0	0	0	0	0	0	0	0	0	0	0	0	0	0	0	0
F	0	0	0	0	0	135	0	0	0	0	0	4	0	0	0	0	0	0	0	0	3	10	0	0	0
G	0	0	0	0	0	0	150	0	0	0	0	0	0	0	0	1	0	0	0	0	0	0	0	0	0
H	1	0	0	0	0	0	7	143	0	0	0	0	0	1	0	0	0	0	1	0	0	0	0	0	1
I	0	0	0	0	0	0	0	0	150	0	0	0	0	0	0	0	0	0	0	0	1	0	0	0	0
J	0	0	0	0	0	0	0	0	0	153	0	0	0	0	0	0	0	0	0	0	0	0	0	0	0
K	0	0	0	0	0	0	0	0	0	0	153	0	0	0	0	0	0	0	0	0	0	0	0	0	0
L	0	0	0	0	0	0	0	0	0	0	0	153	0	0	0	0	0	0	0	0	0	0	0	0	0
M	0	0	0	0	0	0	0	0	0	0	2	0	152	0	0	0	0	0	0	0	0	0	0	0	0
N	0	0	0	0	0	0	0	0	0	0	0	0	0	152	0	0	0	0	0	0	0	0	0	0	0
O	0	0	0	0	0	0	0	0	0	0	0	0	0	0	154	0	0	0	0	0	0	0	0	0	0
P	0	0	0	0	0	0	0	0	0	0	0	0	0	0	0	153	0	0	0	0	0	0	0	0	0
Q	0	0	0	0	0	0	0	0	0	0	0	0	0	0	2	2	147	1	0	0	0	0	0	0	0
R	0	0	0	0	0	0	0	0	0	0	0	0	0	0	0	0	0	150	0	0	0	0	0	0	0
S	0	0	0	0	1	0	0	0	0	0	0	0	0	0	10	0	0	0	133	0	0	0	0	8	0
T	0	0	0	0	0	0	0	0	0	0	0	1	0	0	0	0	0	0	0	151	0	0	0	0	0
U	0	1	0	0	0	0	0	0	0	0	0	0	0	0	0	0	0	0	0	0	150	0	0	0	0
V	0	0	0	0	0	0	0	0	0	0	0	0	0	0	0	0	0	0	0	0	0	151	1	0	0
W	0	0	0	0	0	0	0	0	0	0	0	0	0	0	0	0	0	0	0	0	0	1	149	0	0
X	0	0	0	0	0	0	0	0	0	0	0	0	0	0	3	0	0	0	0	0	0	0	0	148	0
Y	0	0	0	0	0	0	0	0	0	0	0	0	0	0	0	0	0	0	0	0	0	0	0	0	151
Z	0	0	0	0	0	0	0	0	0	0	0	0	0	0	0	0	0	0	0	0	0	0	0	0	0

Fig. 4 Confusion matrix of the proposed model

3.2 Challenges Faced

Initially, a dataset containing raw images of all ASL characters was to be compiled; however, no fitting dataset could be identified in either of the public dataset repositories. As a result, a new dataset was developed. The next issue was to choose the filter for feature extraction. Various filters, such as Gaussian blur, binary threshold, canny edge detection, and others, were tested, with the Gaussian blur filter proving to be the most efficient. Aside from that, there were problems with the model's accuracy due to lighting conditions; the model did not have promising accuracy when lighting conditions were poor. However, the advances and other techniques in this area are discussed in further sections which have high cost and the resources used in these methodologies are not easily available.

3.3 Object Recognition Techniques

In the case of single object recognition, for its clear recognition, two-dimensional features like histogram of oriented gradient [8], scale-invariant feature transform (SIFT) [9], kernel descriptors [10] are used. All these methods are good only for single object detection. Therefore, these methods might not perform well when gestures involve multiple parts of the body as a part of the gesture. SIFT [9] can compute at the edges which will be invariant to scaling, rotation, the addition of noise. One of the advantages of depth images is that it is not get affected by illumination changes. Therefore, this advantage gives an edge to reduce the texture and color variability which occurs due to background, skin, and hair. Space–time occupancy pattern (STOP) [11] is proposed to resolve the problems like occlusions and noise in-depth images. Space–time occupancy pattern is focused on characterized space–time patterns of human gestures (which are four-dimensional in nature) to utilize the temporal and spatial contextual knowledge and permitting intra-class variations [3].

3.4 Sensor-Based Technologies

The category in which physical intervention of the user is required includes magnetic, visual, or acoustic sensor-based devices which need to be connected with hands or other body parts to locate their position. Few examples are: information gloves [12], accelerometer [13], digital camera sensor [14]. All these sensor-based technologies vary with different parameters like latency, resolution, accuracy, the vary of motion, price, and user comfort. In this category, individuals are required to wear a bulky gadget and to hold a load of wires or cables that link the device to a computer system. The ease and naturalness of user engagement are impeded by this. Also, when handling such instruments, a lot of precautions and calibration are required. Therefore, this class adds a layer of complexity to the user experience.

On the other hand, there is a category in which physical intervention is not required. This category gets much more appreciation than the previous one when Microsoft Kinect was first introduced. Google Tango Project [15], Microsoft Kinect [16], Leap motion controller [17] provide depth images or maps. As already discussed before, the advantage of depth images is that it does not get affected by illumination changes. Hence, the effect of illumination variability can be decreased to a larger extent. In the past recent years, it has been seen the increment in the studies carried out by researchers focused on human gesture-based recognition by utilizing depth information provided by different sensing devices. Google Tango Project [15] is a limited-run experimental device which has a Microsoft Kinect-like vision along with innovative system-on-chip (SoC) integrated inside. It has also a dedicated and very subtle 3D scanner. All these recent advances would make methods based on depth maps even more convenient and useful for signers [3].

3.5 *Different Sign Languages Across the Globe*

There is no specific standard for sign languages. Diverse gesture-based communications are utilized in numerous nations or locales. Table1 shows the most commonly used sign languages and their respective geographical region in which they are being spoken.

Table 1 Different sign languages and their respective countries/regions

Sign languages	Respective countries/Regions	References
British Sign Language (BSL)	UK	[18]
British, Australian, and New Zealand Sign Language (BANZSL)	UK, Australia, New Zealand	[18]
French Sign Language (LSF)	France and French-speaking areas of Switzerland	[19]
American Sign Language (ASL)	USA, Canada, West Africa, and Southeast Asia	[20]
Irish Sign Language (ISL)	Ireland	[18]
Chinese Sign Language (CSL or ZGS)	China	[18]
Brazilian Sign Language (Libras)	Brazil	[18]
Indian Sign Language	India	[21]
Thai Sign Language	Thailand	[22]
German Sign Language (DGS)	Germany	[23]
Arabic Sign Language	Arab Middle East	[24]

Table 2 Deep learning methodologies and their accuracy

Various deep learning methodologies	Accuracy (%)	References
Motion Sensor Information + SVM k-NN	79.83	[25]
Edge Orientation Histogram	88.26	[26]
DBN (3 RBM layers + 1 translation layer)	79	[27]
CNN	82	[28]
DNN + CRF	92	[29]
HMM + BLSTM-NN	96.2	[30]
PCA + HMM	89.10	[31]
Random Forest + Depth Comparison	90	[32]
Full Dimensional Feature + k-NN	99.6	[33]
SURF + SVM	97.13	[34]
AdaBoost + HAAR	98.7	[35]
GRNN + Ring Projection and Wavelet Transform	90.44	[36]
CNN + Convex Hull + Skin Detection	98.05	[37]
Edge Detection + Cross-Correlation	94	[38]
Hybrid CNN-HMM	92.6	[39]

3.6 Comparison of Various Deep Learning Methodologies

Deep neural network (DNN)-based methodologies can take in reasonable contextual information from crude pictures or video fragments straightway, which is sturdy and adaptable. The comparison between different deep learning methodologies based on their accuracy is shown in Table 2.

4 Conclusion and Future Scope

On the whole, this paper provides the different advances in sign language recognition. Experts in different disciplines have primarily performed past studies on sign language comprehension for numerous sign languages, reducing real-world utility. More than 25 studies were reviewed to get the knowledge of the past researches, and then the different works based on sign language recognition using various deep learning methodologies and other technological approaches are discussed. This paper also highlights the various terms and processes involved in this area.

From the various studies, it can be depicted that there is no universal sign language. Sign language changes with concerning countries and regions. Therefore, when a deaf- or speech-impaired person travels to another country or region, he/she might face the problem because the device in which SLR is integrated might not have the sign language of the region he/she belongs to. Also, deep neural network (DNN) shows promising performance in various practical aspects. But it can learn good features from multimodal histogram because these histograms can enhance the accuracy of recognition by providing more knowledge or features about sign gestures. So, further studies should be concerned about integrating all the sign languages used across the globe into one device with a convenient and customizable user interface to make it more robust and barrier breaker. In conjunction, in future research work, studying high-level functionality across deeper networks remains questionable to see the potential in terms of usability and accuracy development.

Conclusively, everyone is of value in society and has the right to communicate with others regardless of their physical impairments contemplating this, let us try to embrace hearing- and speech-impaired people in our everyday life and fostering them ahead in their life by incorporating innovation with their exigencies and other needs.

References

1. Islam MM, Siddiqua S, Afnan J (2017) Real time Hand Gesture Recognition using different algorithms based on American Sign Language. In: 2017 IEEE international conference on imaging, vision and pattern recognition, icIVPR 2017. https://doi.org/10.1109/ICIVPR.2017.7890854
2. Young A, Oram R, Napier J (2019) Hearing people perceiving deaf people through sign language interpreters at work: on the loss of self through interpreted communication. J Appl Commun Res 47(1):90–110. https://doi.org/10.1080/00909882.2019.1574018
3. Zheng L, Liang B, Jiang A (2017) Recent advances of deep learning for sign language recognition. In: DICTA 2017—2017 international conference on digital image computing: techniques and applications, vol 2017, pp 1–7. https://doi.org/10.1109/DICTA.2017.8227483
4. https://www.geeksforgeeks.org/opencv-python-program-analyze-image-using-histogram/. Accessed 22 Feb 2021
5. Manikandan K, Patidar A, Walia P, Roy AB (2018) Hand gesture detection and conversion to speech and text
6. Contours—OpenCv. https://docs.opencv.org/3.4/d4/d73/tutorial_py_contours_begin.html. Accessed 22 Feb 2021
7. Data Augmentation | How to use deep learning when you have limited data — Part 2. https://nanonets.com/blog/data-augmentation-how-to-use-deep-learning-when-you-have-limited-data-part-2/. Accessed 22 Feb 2021
8. Rai R, Shukla S, Singh B (2020) Reactive power based MRAS for speed estimation of solar fed induction motor with improved feedback linearization for water pumping. IEEE Trans Ind Inf 16(7):4714–4725. https://doi.org/10.1109/TII.2019.2950094
9. Lowe DG (2004) Distinctive image features from scale-invariant keypoints. Int J Comput Vis 60(2):91–110. https://doi.org/10.1023/B:VISI.0000029664.99615.94
10. Bo L, Lai K, Ren X, Fox D (2011) Object recognition with hierarchical kernel descriptors. In: Proceedings of the IEEE computer society conference on computer vision and pattern recognition, pp 1729–1736. https://doi.org/10.1109/CVPR.2011.5995719
11. Vieira AW, Nascimento ER, Oliveira GL, Liu Z, Campos MFM (2012) STOP: space-time occupancy patterns for 3D action recognition from depth map sequences. In: Lecture notes in computer science (including Subseries Lecture notes in artificial intelligence and lecture notes in bioinformatics), vol 7441, LNCS, pp 252–259. https://doi.org/10.1007/978-3-642-33275-3_31

12. Mohandes M, Aliyu SO (2017) (12) United States Patent, vol 2, no 12
13. Zhang X, Chen X, Li Y, Lantz V, Wang K, Yang J (2011) A framework for hand gesture recognition based on accelerometer and EMG sensors. IEEE Trans Syst Man Cybern Part A Syst Humans 41(6):1064–1076. https://doi.org/10.1109/TSMCA.2011.2116004
14. Hongo H, Ohya M, Yasumoto M, Niwa Y, Yamamoto K (2000) Focus of attention for face and hand gesture recognition using multiple cameras. In: Proceedings—4th IEEE international conference on automatic face and gesture recognition, FG 2000, pp 156–161. https://doi.org/10.1109/AFGR.2000.840627
15. https://en.wikipedia.org/wiki/Tango_(platform). Accessed 22 Feb 2021
16. Lai K, Konrad J, Ishwar P (2012) A gesture-driven computer interface using Kinect. In: Proceedings of IEEE Southwest symposium on image analysis and interpretation, pp 185–188. https://doi.org/10.1109/SSIAI.2012.6202484
17. Chuan CH, Regina E, Guardino C (2014) American sign language recognition using leap motion sensor. In: Proceedings—2014 13th international conference on machine learning and applications ICMLA 2014, pp 541–544. https://doi.org/10.1109/ICMLA.2014.110.
18. A guide to the different types of sign language around the world. https://k-international.com/blog/different-types-of-sign-language-around-the-world/. Accessed 22 Feb 2021
19. FrenchSign Language. https://www.tradonline.fr/en/blog/french-sign-language-a-language-in-its-own-right/. Accessed 22 Feb 2021
20. ASL—Wikipedia. https://en.wikipedia.org/wiki/American_Sign_Language. Accessed 22 Feb 2021
21. Welcome to Indian Sign Language Portal. https://indiansignlanguage.org/. Accessed 22 Feb 2021
22. Thai sign-language—Wikipedia. https://en.wikipedia.org/wiki/Thai_Sign_Language. accessed 22 Feb 2021
23. German sign-language—Wikipedia. https://en.wikipedia.org/wiki/German_Sign_Language. Accessed 22 Feb 2021
24. Arab sign-language family—Wikipedia. https://en.wikipedia.org/wiki/Arab_sign-language_family. Accessed 22 Feb 2021
25. Vaitkevičius A, Taroza M, Blažauskas T, Damaševičius R, Maskeliunas R, Woźniak M (2019) Recognition of American Sign Language gestures in a virtual reality using leap motion. Appl Sci 9(3):1–16. https://doi.org/10.3390/app9030445
26. Pansare JR, Ingle M (2016) Vision-based approach for American Sign Language recognition using edge orientation histogram. In: 2016 international conference on image, vision and computing ICIVC 2016, pp 86–90. https://doi.org/10.1109/ICIVC.2016.7571278
27. Rioux-Maldague L, Giguere P (2014) Sign language fingerspelling classification from depth and color images using a deep belief network. In: Proceedings—Conference on Computer and Robot Vision, CRV 2014, no May 2014, pp 92–97. https://doi.org/10.1109/CRV.2014.20
28. Ameen S, Vadera S (2017) A convolutional neural network to classify American Sign Language fingerspelling from depth and colour images. Expert Syst 34(3). https://doi.org/10.1111/exsy.12197
29. Kim T et al (2017) Lexicon-free fingerspelling recognition from video: data, models, and signer adaptation. Comput Speech Lang 46:209–232. https://doi.org/10.1016/j.csl.2017.05.009
30. Kumar P, Gauba H, Pratim Roy P, Prosad Dogra D (2017) A multimodal framework for sensor based sign language recognition. Neurocomputing 259(2017):21–38. https://doi.org/10.1016/j.neucom.2016.08.132
31. Zaki MM, Shaheen SI (2011) Sign language recognition using a combination of new vision based features. Pattern Recognit Lett 32(4):572–577. https://doi.org/10.1016/j.patrec.2010.11.013
32. Dong C, Leu MC, Yin Z (2015) American Sign Language alphabet recognition using Microsoft Kinect. In: IEEE computer society conference on computer vision and pattern recognition workshop, vol 2015, pp 44–52, 2015. https://doi.org/10.1109/CVPRW.2015.7301347
33. Aryanie D, Heryadi Y (2015) American sign language-based finger-spelling recognition using k-Nearest Neighbors classifier. In: 2015 3rd international conference on information

communication technology ICoICT 2015, pp 533–536. https://doi.org/10.1109/ICoICT.2015.7231481
34. Jin CM, Omar Z, Jaward MH (2016) A mobile application of American sign language translation via image processing algorithms. In: Proceedings—2016 IEEE region 10 symposium TENSYMP 2016, pp 104–109. https://doi.org/10.1109/TENCONSpring.2016.7519386
35. Truong VNT, Yang CK, Tran QV (2016) A translator for American sign language to text and speech. In: 2016 IEEE 5th global conference on consumer electronics GCCE 2016. https://doi.org/10.1109/GCCE.2016.7800427
36. Fiagbe Y (2020) World journal of engineering, no April
37. Taskiran M, Killioglu M, Kahraman N (2018) A real-time system for recognition of American Sign Language by using deep learning. In: 2018 41st international conference on telecommunications and signal processing TSP 2018, pp 1–5. https://doi.org/10.1109/TSP.2018.8441304
38. Joshi A, Sierra H, Arzuaga E (2017) American sign language translation using edge detection and cross correlation. In: 2017 IEEE Colombian conference on communications and computing COLCOM 2017—proceedings. https://doi.org/10.1109/ColComCon.2017.8088212
39. Koller O, Zargaran S, Ney H, Bowden R (2016) Deep sign: hybrid CNN-HMM for continuous sign language recognition. In: British machine vision conference 2016, BMVC 2016, vol 2016, no August, pp 136.1–136.12. https://doi.org/10.5244/C.30.136

Accurate Machine Learning-Based Automated Sleep Staging Using Clinical Subjects with Suspected Sleep Disorders

Santosh Kumar Satapathy, Ravisankar Malladi, and Hari Kishan Kondaveeti

Abstract Sleep is a basic requirement of human life. It is one of the vital roles in human life to maintain the proper mental health, physical health, and quality of life. In this proposed research work, we conduct an automated sleep staging classification system to a proper investigation of irregularities that occurred during sleep based on single-channel electroencephalography (EEG) signal using machine learning techniques. The major advantage of this proposed research work over the standard polysomnography method are: (1) It measures the sleep irregularities during sleep by considering three different medical condition subjects of different gender with different age groups. (2) One more important objective of this proposed sleep study is that here we obtain different session recordings to investigate sleep abnormality patterns, which can help to find better diagnosis toward the treatment of sleep-related disorder. (3) In the present work, we have obtained two different time-framework epochs from individual subjects to check which window size is more effective toward identification on sleep irregularities. The present research work based on a two-state sleep stage classification problem based on a single channel of EEG signal was performed in a different stepwise manner such as the acquisition of data from participated subjects, preprocessing, feature extraction, feature selection, and classification. We obtained the polysomnographic data from the ISRUC-Sleep data repository for measuring the performances of the proposed framework, where the sleep stages are visually labeled. The obtained results demonstrated that the proposed methodologies achieve a high classification accuracy of 99.46 and 97.46% using SVM and DT classifiers, respectively, and which support sleep experts to accurately measure the irregularities that occurred during sleep and also help the clinicians to evaluate the presence and criticality of sleep-related disorders.

S. K. Satapathy (✉)
Department of CSE, Pondicherry Engineering College, Puducherry, India
e-mail: Santosh.satapathy@pec.edu

R. Malladi
Department of CSE, Gudlavalleru Engineering College (A), Andhra Pradesh, India

H. K. Kondaveeti
School of Computer Science Engineering, VIT-AP University, Amaravati, Andhra Pradesh, India

N. Marriwala et al. (eds.), *Emergent Converging Technologies and Biomedical Systems*, Lecture Notes in Electrical Engineering 841,
https://doi.org/10.1007/978-981-16-8774-7_30

Keywords Sleep staging · Electroencephalogram · Feature screening · Machine learning

1 Introduction

Sleep is one of the important physiological activities for the human body, which directly controls memory consolidation, and it also decides the performance of the daily activities. Sleep plays an important role in the human body because it represents the primary functions of the human brain. One human individual is spending one-third of its duration as sleep. Proper quality of sleep maintains the physical and mental fitness of the human body, which is alternatively helpful to perform well in workplaces, control emotions, and be able to take proper decisions [1, 2]. Nowadays, it has seen that sleep diseases (SD) are becoming one of the major causes of death across the world. The main reason for this serious health issue is an imbalance of sleep patterns, and it has occurred due to job pressure, and rapid changes in lifestyles. Across the globe. It has been observed that the prevalence of sleep diseases has significantly increased over the past years. According to the report of the Center for Control of Disease and Prevention (CDC) of the US Government, around 9 million populations have difficulty maintaining good quality sleep [3]. According to a survey of the National Highway Traffic Safety Administration in the USA, it has been found that due to the drowsiness factor, around 56,000 to 100,000 car accidents have happened, which directly reported that more than 1500 have died and 71,000 are affected with injuries annually [4]. It has been found that sleep diseases are considered to be the most predominant death cause with the different age groups of populations across the globe. In general, different types of sleep disorders are categorized such as obstructive sleep apnea, insomnia, hypersomnia, narcolepsy, breathing-related disorders, stroke, stress, and cardiovascular diseases [5]. All these diseases progressively increased with age. So early diagnosis is helpful for the human being to prevent the severity of these diseases, and it helps to improve the subject's quality of life. The first most important step for sleep diseases is sleep scoring. The most popular test for analyzing sleep quality is the polysomnography (PSG) test. PSG tests include the signals such as electroencephalogram (EEG), electrocardiogram (ECG), electromyogram (EMG), and electrooculogram (EOG). The entire sleep staging procedures are analyzed according to two available sleep standards such as the Rechtschaffen and Kales (R&K) [6] and the American Academy of Sleep Medicine (AASM) [7]. According to R&K sleep guidelines, the whole sleep cycle is categorized into six sleep stages such as wake stage(W), non-rapid eye movement (NREM stage1 (N1), NREM stage2 (N2), NREM stage3 (N3), and NREM stage4 (N4)) and rapid eye movement (REM) stage. The only changes reflected with the AASM manual incomparable to R&K standards are NREM sleep stages. According to the AASM guidelines, the total sleep stages are five, the NREM stage 3 (N3) and the NREM stage 4 (N4) are combined into one sleep stage called the NREM stage3. Traditionally the sleep scoring procedure was conducted through the visual inspection method, where one clinician was monitoring the sleep behavior of the subject for 6–8 h. of sleep. This traditional sleep analysis method requires more human resources for monitoring the whole sleep recordings, and also, it consumes more time for analysis, due to more human interpretation, sometimes the results are erroneous [6]. Sometimes it is also one of the major causes of not achieving higher classification accuracy in the classification of sleep stages. With consideration of all these above-mentioned facts, the automated sleep scoring approach has gained a lot of attention in recent researches [7, 8]. Automated sleep scoring not only causes accuracy improvements but also provides quick diagnosis [9]. It has been observed that the PSG test is one of the costly experiments, and it also gives so many unpleasant scenarios for the subjects because of its so much connectivity of wires in the different parts of the body [10, 11]. Henceforth instead of PSG signals, most of the researchers preferred to EEG signal, because it directly provides the brain activities during sleep hours. This helps a lot for analyzing the sleep abnormality, and it is also more popular for its easier recording facility. In general, EEG signals are combinations of different waveforms, which help to characterize the different sleep stages with different frequency bands such as delta band (0–4 Hz), theta (4–8 Hz), alpha (8–13 Hz), beta (13–30 Hz), spindle(12–14 Hz), sawtooth (2–6 Hz), and k-complex (0.5–1.5 Hz). Finally, the scoring and decisions are taken by the sleep experts through proper interpretation of the quantitative and visual analysis of collected sleep recordings. In some cases, the sleep experts use an algorithm for pre-scoring the entire sleep recordings, and these successive representations of the sleep stages information called hypnograms, which is highly required during the diagnosis of the different types of sleep disorders. Sleep staging is generally a tedious job, which requires highly experienced technicians and experts. This other limitation with subject to sleep staging is variations on sleep scoring from experts to experts, which is also one of the major causes for diagnosing sleep diseases [12, 13].

In this paper, we have obtained a single-channel EEG signal for sleep staging analysis; this approach makes it more interesting because of its ease of operational deployments on mobile devices. It also makes more comfortable situations for the patients due to less cabling used during recordings. It has been observed that most of the contributions with single-channel EEG signals were executed two-step methodology. In the first step, the different hand-engineered features are extracted from the different waveforms, and in the second step, the extracted features are forwarded to a classifier for classifying the sleep stages based on the feature characteristics. In general, it has been seen that most of the authors obtained one of the three following domains of the features [14] (a) time-domain features, (b) frequency-domain features, (c) nonlinear features. It is a very difficult part for sleep experts to manually monitoring the recorded EEG signals, and it raises so many errors because during long 7–8 h. EEG recordings, its hectic situation for sleep experts to monitoring within the 30 s framework and fix the labeling of sleep stages. This approach consumed more time and required more manpower for hours of sleep recordings. To overcome difficulty from the manual approach, nowadays automated sleep stage classification is obtained to analyze the sleep-related disorder and real-time diagnosis, and the most important step is designing sleep stage classification. Currently, overnight sleep study through polysomnography is one of the standard procedures for measuring sleep irregularities during sleep [14].

1.1 Related Work

Several sleep analysis studies were proposed for characterization the sleep-related abnormalities based on the sleep standards recommended by R&K and AASM manuals. Various computational methodologies were proposed by researchers to support sleep experts for assisting sleep staging. Those carried steps were on the information extraction (polysomnography channel selection), on the preprocessing (removing the data artifacts and data normalization), on the feature extraction step (transformation of time- and frequency-domain features), on the feature selection technique (identifying the most relevant features) and finally on the classification algorithm. Here we have presented some comparative studies regarding sleep staging. In [15], the authors have obtained wavelet concept techniques for feature extraction and classified the selected features using the fuzzy algorithm. The classification model provided 85% accuracy. Güneş, K et al. [16] used K-means clustering and feature weighting techniques to design an ASSC system. Welch spectral transform was considered for feature extraction, and those selected features were forwarded to a decision tree (DT) and obtained with an overall accuracy of 83%. Aboalayon [17] used EEG signal and obtained Butterworth bandpass filters and used SVM classifiers and reported 90% classification accuracy.

In [18], extracted features form an empirical mode decomposition of the signal and use bootstrap-aggregating techniques for multi-class sleep staging classifications.

In [19] applied the EEMD algorithm for signal enhancement from single-channel EEG signal, and extracted statistical features are forwarded into boosting techniques, and the reported accuracy for two-six sleep stages is reported as 98.15%, 94.23%, 92.66%, 83.49%, and 88.07%, respectively.

Kristin M. Gunnarsdottir et al. have designed an automated sleep stage scoring system with overnight PSG data. Here the authors extracted both time- and frequency-domain properties from PSG signal, and considered healthy individual subjects with no prior sleep diseases and the extracted properties were classified through DT classifiers. The overall accuracy for test set data was reported as 80.70% [20].

Sriraam, N. et al. used a multi-channel EEG signal from ten healthy subjects. In this study, the author has proposed the automated sleep stage scoring in between wake and stage1 of sleep. In this research work, spectral entropy features are extracted from the input channels to distinguish the irregularities among the sleep states. The extracted features processed through a multilayer perceptron feedforward neural network and the overall accuracy with 20 hidden units were reported as 92.9%, and subsequently for 40,60, 80, and 100 hidden units in MLP, it was reported as 94.6, 97.2, 98.8, and 99.2, respectively [21].

In [22] proposed two-state sleep staging and the acquired signal decomposed into eight sub-bands, finally 13 features are extracted from each sub-band epoch. The suitable features are identified through the mRMR feature selection algorithm. The model achieved an overall accuracy of 95.31% through a random forest classifier. Da Silveira et al. used discrete wavelet transform (DWT) for signal segmentation. Skewness, kurtosis, and variance features were extracted from respective input channels. The extracted features were applied to a random forest classifier, and overall accuracy was reported as 90% [23]. Prochaska et al. [24] used polysomnography data features to identify the sleep abnormalities from three different medical conditions of subjects and used an SVM classifier for two-state classifications in between the Wake versus NREM stage and another one in between the Wake versus REM stage. The proposed study achieved an overall accuracy of classification between the Wake-NREM and Wake-REM stage as 85.6% and 97.5%, respectively. Xiaojin Li et al. introduced the hybrid model for identifying the irregularities that occurred in different stages of sleep during the night, and extracted features were forwarded into random forest classifiers. It has been reported that overall classification accuracy has reached 85.95% [25].

2 Experimental Data

To analyze the proposed methodology effectiveness, we have obtained the session-1 and session-2 sleep recordings from the subjects who were already affected by the different types of sleep-related disorders. These required recordings were retrieved from the subgroups of ISRUC-Sleep dataset, which is one of the public databases specifically available for sleep research. These recordings were prepared by the groups of domain experts at sleep center in the Hospital of Coimbra University. This dataset contained the recorded subject details from different age groups, gender categories, and medical conditions. All recordings were recorded through the sleep experts in the sleep laboratory at the Hospital of Coimbra University (CHUC). As per our proposed research objective, the first subject used for experimental work from Subgroup-I of ISRUC-sleep repository. The second category of a subject is taken for our proposed experimental work from Subgroup-II of the ISRUC-sleep database. The distribution of sleep stages epochs per individual subjects is presented in Table 1.

3 Methodology

In this work, we proposed a machine learning-based sleep scoring system using a single channel with subjects having different medical conditioned subjects. The main objective of this proposed work is to study the sleep stages behavior of the subjects who were already had some types of sleep diseases symptoms. Additionally, in this research work we also analyzed the sleep quality of the subjects by obtaining

Table 1 Detailed information of each subject sleep dataset records used in this study

Enrolled subjects	Wake	N-REM1	N-REM2	N3-REM3	REM
Subject-16 Subgroup I/ One Session	128	125	280	120	97
Subject-23 Subgroup I/ One Session	212	99	270	65	104
Subject-3 Subgroup-II/ One Session	68	126	271	175	110
Subject-3 Subgroup-II/ Two Session	76	127	236	168	143

the different session recordings on two different dates. The complete layout of this proposed work is described in Fig. 1.

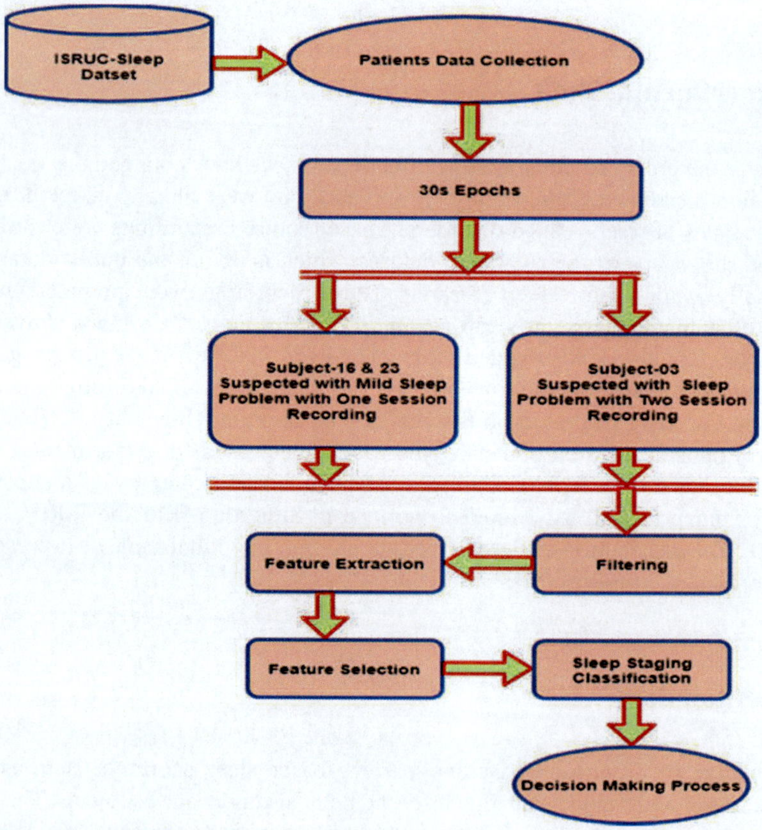

Fig. 1 Complete layout of the proposed sleep staging system

Table 2 Short explanation of the extracted features for this proposed study

Feature set	Feature no.	Feature set	Feature no.
Time-based			
Mean	1	Minimum	3
Maximum	2	Standard Deviation	4
Median	5	Variance	6
Zero Crossing Rate	7	75percentile	8
Signal Skewness	9	Signal Kurtosis	10
Signal Activity	11	Signal Mobility	12
Signal Complexity	13		
Frequency-based			
RSP in delta, theta, beta and alpha bands	14,15,16,17	Power Ratios	18,19,20,21 22,23,24
Band powers	25,26,27,28		

3.1 Feature Extraction

The selection of inputs for the classifier is the most valuable for identifying sleep pattern abnormality. Even if obtained highly effective classification model performed very poor performance, if proper inputs are to be identified. It can be found that the different classifiers performed different results for the same set of features; it indicates matching both may found results. On the other part, sometimes we have given some set of features that favors the classification process. It has been found that the sleep behavior of the subjects is highly unstable and non-stationary because the changes characteristics are directly linked with the time and frequency ranges. To properly discriminate the sleep stages, we need to analyze the signals by obtaining the time- and frequency-based parameters. In this study, we have as whole extracted 28 features from the input signal, out of those 13 features are time-based and the other 15 features are frequency-based [26–28]. The obtained features are described in Table 2.

3.2 Feature Selection

Next to feature extraction, the other important task with regard to classification problem is screening the relevant parameters which help to model for properly classifying the sleep stages. Sometimes it has been found that the extracted fall the features may not be more effective with respect to analyze of the sleep behavior, which directly put impacts on the classification performance of the models. In our study, we adopted the feature screening techniques as online streaming feature selection (OSFS) techniques to screen the suitable features from the pool of extracted features [29]. The selected features concerning the individual subject are presented in Table 3.

Table 3 Screened Feature Lists

Name/Gender	Selected features
Subject-16 MALE	$F1_{16}$,$F2_{16}$,$F3_{16}$,$F4_{16}$,$F5_{16}$,$F7_{16}$,$F9_{16}$,$F10_{16}$,$F11_{16}$,$F13_{16}$,$F14_{16}$, $F15_{16}$,$F22_{16}$,$F25_{16}$,$F27_{16}$,$F31_{16}$ (16 Features)
Subject-23 FEMALE	$F1_{23}$,$F2_{23}$,$F3_{23}$,$F4_{23}$,$F5_{23}$,$F7_{23}$,$F11_{23}$,$F12_{23}$,$F15_{23}$,$F16_{23}$,$F17_{23}$, $F20_{23}$,$F24_{23}$,$F26_{23}$,$F31_{23}$,$F33_{23}$,$F37_{23}$ (17 Features)
Subject-03 MALE (Session-1) Recording	$F1_{03S1}$,$F2_{03S1}$,$F3_{03S1}$,$F4_{03S1}$,$F5_{03S1}$,$F7_{03S1}$,$F8_{03S1}$,$F9_{03S1}$,$F11_{03S1}$, $F12_{03S1}$,$F13_{03S1}$,$F14_{03S1}$,$F21_{03S1}$,$F22_{03S1}$,$F25_{03S1}$ (15 Features)
Subject-03 MALE (Session-2) Recording	$F1_{03S2}$,$F2_{03S2}$,$F3_{03S2}$,$F4_{03S2}$,$F5_{03S2}$,$F7_{03S2}$,$F8_{03S2}$,$F9_{03S2}$,$F11_{03S2}$, $F12_{03S2}$,$F13_{03S2}$,$F14_{03S2}$,$F21_{03S2}$,$F22_{03S2}$,$F25_{03S2}$ (15 Features)

4 Experimental Results and Discussion

The main intention behind this research is to analyze the changes sleep stages and classifying the sleep stages using machine learning classification models. This entire procedure is called as sleep scoring. In this work, the entire experiments were performed on two different subgroups of sleep recordings one from ISRUC-Sleep subgroup-I and the other from ISRUC-Sleep subgroup-II dataset. The entire sleep staging experiments followed according to the AASM sleep standards. The proposed sleep scoring methodology is executed through four basic steps that are signal preprocessing, feature extraction, feature screening, and finally classification. In this work, we have considered only the single channel of EEG signal for acquisition of the signal recordings. Next to the acquisition, the required signals need to be processed for further eliminating the irrelevant noises and artifacts which are contaminated during recordings in the raw signal and eliminated these muscle artifacts and noisy portions from recorded signals through the Butterworth band-pass filter. In the next phase, a set of experiments were conducted to extract the features from both the time and frequency domains. As a whole 28 features were extracted from recorded signals of the subjects, and the same details are mentioned in Table 2. The size of the feature vectors for all enrolled subjects for 30 s epoch length is 28 × 750. Matrix dimension for feature vector is feature number x epoch number. The next task is the selection of the most efficient features from among the feature vector. To work out this selection experiment, we have applied OSFS feature selection techniques. The matrix representation for feature selection vectors is selected feature number x epoch number. These matrixes are 16 × 750, 17 × 750, 15 × 750, 15 × 750 for subject-16, subject-23, subject-03 (session-1 recording), and subject-03 (session-2 recording), respectively, for input length of epoch is 30 s. By implementations of tenfold cross-validation techniques on the SVM [30, 31] and DT [32] classifiers, the selected best features are fed as input to the model. We also conducted a comparative analysis with all these enrolled subjects and their session recordings, and finally, comparison experimental results are presented according to the single channel of EEG signals and two sleep classes (wake versus sleep). In this proposed study, we have used some criteria of evaluation metrics for measuring the performances of the proposed sleep scoring study. Here, we have considered six performance metrics for analyzing the performance of the proposed methodology such as classification accuracy [33], recall [34], specificity [35], precision [36], F1-score [37], and Kappa score [38]. Analysis of the comparative results from conducted experiments, and obtained results are presented below.

4.1 Classification Accuracy of Category-I Subject ISRUC-Sleep Database

In this experimental part, we have obtained two subjects who have been affected by some kind of sleep-related disorders and here from subject session-1 recording recorded by sleep experts for diagnosing the irregularities that happened during sleep hours. Table 4 presents the confusion matrix for two-state sleep stage classification problems for both the subjects 16 and 23 with time length of epoch is 30 s. It has been observed that the SVM depicts an overall classification accuracy of 95.62 and 91.20% achieved through DT classifiers for subject-16. For subject-23, the same classifiers SVM and DT reached overall accuracy of 91.46% and 87.73%, respectively, for epoch length 30 s.

The results achieved from the input of 30 s length epoch for subject-16 and subject-23 are specified in Table 5. Figure 2 displays performance statistics for 30 s epoch length for subject-16 and subject-23.

Table 4 Confusion matrix of subjects 16 and 23 according to AASM guidelines

Subject-16			
		W	S
SVM	W	133	30
	S	3	584
		W	S
DT	W	133	29
	S	37	551
Subject-23			
		W	S
SVM	W	174	38
	S	512	26
		W	S
DT	W	167	45
	S	29	509

Table 5 Performance of the proposed SleepEEG study using SVM and DT classifiers

	Subject enrolled epochs length-30s			
Channel	SVM classifier		DT classifier	
C3-A2	16	23	16	23
Accuracy (%)	95.62	91.46	91.20	87.73
Precision (%)	95.14	93.09	94.99	91.45
Recall (%)	99.59	95.17	93.70	91.45
Specificity (%)	81.64	82.08	82.21	78.30
F1-Score (%)	97.29	94.12	94.34	91.45

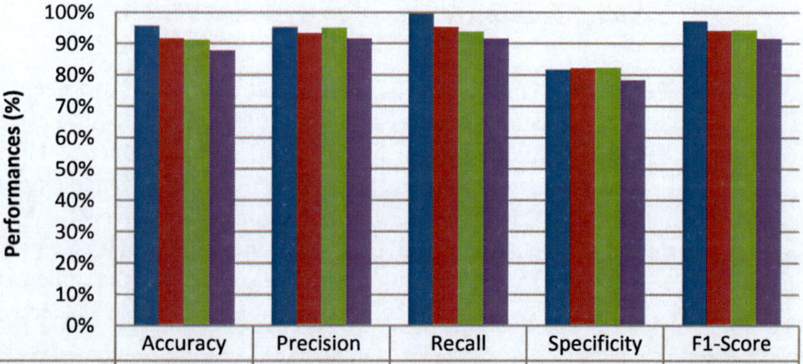

	Accuracy	Precision	Recall	Specificity	F1-Score
SVM Classifier 16	95.62%	95.14%	99.59%	81.64%	97.29%
SVM Classifier 23	91.46%	93.09%	95.17%	82.08%	94.12%
DT Classifier 16	91.20%	94.99%	93.70%	82.21%	94.34%
DT Classifier 23	87.73%	91.45%	91.45%	78.30%	91.45%

Fig. 2 Performance statistics of model with 30 s epoch duration for subject-16 and subject-23 using SVM and DT classifiers

The overall performance value of the proposed Category-I subject ISRUC-Sleep database is measured through the evaluation parameters that are recall, specificity, precision, and F1-score, and it reported for subject-16 as 99.59%, 81.64%, 95.14%, and 97.29% through SVM, 93.70%, 82.21%, 94.99%, and 94.34% through DT, respectively; similarly, the same parameters reached for subject-23 through SVM and DT are 95.17%, 82.08%, 93.09%, and 94.12%, and 91.45%, 78.30%, 87.73%, and 91.45%. The computation of score is of six levels of agreements:0.81–1, 0.61- 0.80, 0.41–0.60, 0.21–0.4,0.00–0.20, and less than 0 correspond to excellent, substantial, moderate, fair, slight agreement, and poor agreement [38]. Table 6 gives the kappa coefficient score concerning obtained classification techniques for both the subjects 16 and 23, and it has been found from results that all classification techniques are found excellent agreement with subject to best accuracy for investigation on sleep irregularities.

Table 6 Performance of the accuracy and Kappa score based on the two-state sleep classification problem for subjects 16 and 23

Classifiers	Subject-16		Subject-23	
	Accuracy (%)	Kappa score	Accuracy (%)	Kappa score
SVM	95.62	0.92	91.46	0.78
DT	91.20	0.73	87.73	0.69

4.2 *Classification Accuracy of Category-II Subject ISRUC-Sleep Database*

In the ISRUC-Sleep subgroup-II dataset experiment, the proposed sleep stage classification model has experimented based upon only a single channel with two different session recordings from one gender enrolled subject with suspected sleep-related disorder symptoms. Table 7 represents the confusion matrix for both session recordings of subject 03 with the duration of epoch 30 s.

The achieved results for subject-03 for both the sessions are shown in Table 8. The performance graph results for subject-03 for both session recordings of epoch length 30 s are displayed in Fig. 3.

Figure 3 presents the reported performances for the two-state sleep classification model, Subgroup-II with session-2 recordings for subject-03.

Table 7 Performance of the proposed SleepEEG study using SVM, and DT Classifiers for Subject-03 (session-2 Recordings)

30 s epoch length			
Subject-03			
Session1_Recording			
		W	S
SVM	W	20	47
	S	20	663
		W	S
DT	W	12	63
	S	55	620
30 s epoch length			
Subject-03			
Session2_Recording			
		W	S
SVM	W	20	69
	S	10	651
		W	S
DT	W	18	63
	S	40	629

Table 8 Performance of the proposed SleepEEG study using SVM and DT classifiers for Subject-03 (session-2 recordings)

30 s epoch length			
Subject-03			
Session1_Recording			
		W	S
SVM	W	20	47
	S	20	663
		W	S
DT	W	12	63
	S	55	620
30 s epoch length			
Subject-03			
Session2_Recording			
		W	S
SVM	W	20	69
	S	10	651
		W	S
DT	W	18	63
	S	40	629

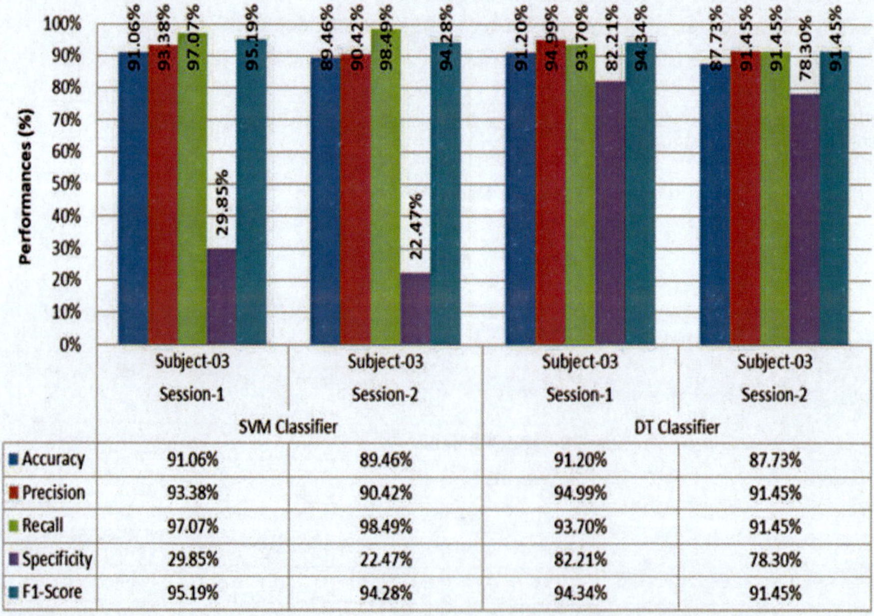

Fig. 3 Performance measures using SVM and DT classification techniques for the two-state sleep classification model with session-2 recordings for subject-03 (30 s epochs Length)

Table 9 Performance of the accuracy and Kappa score based on the two-state sleep classification problem for subject with mild sleep problem having session-2 recording for subject-03

Classifiers	Subject-03 (Session-1 Recording)		Subject-03 (Session-2 Recording)	
	Accuracy (%)	Kappa score	Accuracy (%)	Kappa score
SVM	91.06	0.87	89.46	0.86
DT	84.26	0.67	86.26	0.74

From each subject, here we have acquired two different session recordings; it has been observed that subject 03 with session-1 recording SVM classification model depicts an overall accuracy of 91.06% and 84.26% for DT, respectively. Similarly, it has been found that the classification results of subject 03 with session-2 recordings through SVM and DT were reported as 89.46% and 84.2%. The overall performance of recall, specificity, precision, and F1-score reported with the session-1 recording of ISRUC-Sleep Subgroup-II database of subject-03 through SVM as 97.07%, 29.85%, 93.38%, and 95.19%, similarly for DT classifier, the performances reached 93.70%, 82.21%, 94.99%, and 94.34%. Similarly, the performances with session-2 recordings are reported as 98.49%, 22.47%, 90.42%, and 94.28% through SVM, 91.45%, 78.30%, 91.45%, and 91.45% through DT. The results of the kappa coefficient for subject-03 with both session recordings are presented in Table 9.

For measuring the impact of session recordings for the classification of sleep stages, we have computed the Cohens kappa coefficient; according to session-1 recording for subject-03, the kappa score through SVM and DT is 0.87 and 0.67. From this kappa score, it concludes that DT is not up to the mark performance incomparable to the SVM classification techniques. Similarly for session-2 recording, the kappa performance for SVM and DT is 0.86 and 0.74, respectively.

4.3 *Comparative Analysis in Between Proposed Study and State-Of-The-Art Works*

Here we have made a comparison with other similar contributions work to measure the proposed research work effectiveness toward the identification of sleep disorder. Table 10 presents the comparison of the performances based on single-channel EEG acquisition among the proposed research work results with five contributed works.

Table 10 Comparison of performances of the proposed work with previously published works

Author	Year	Signal type	Method	Accuracy (%)
Eduardo T. Braun et al. Ref. [27]	2018	Single-channel EEG	FFT + Random forest classifier	97.1
Hassan, A. R. et al. Ref. [18]	2017		Tunable-Q wavelet transform (TQWT) +Bootstrap aggregating	92.43
Diykh, M. et al. Ref. [19]	2016		Structural graph similarity K-means (SGSKM) +SVM classifier	95.93
K. Aboalayon et al. Ref. [17]	2014		Frequency sub-bands features extraction + SVM classifier	92.5
Zhu, G. et al. Ref. [23]	2014		Graph domain features + SVM classifier	96.1
Proposed Work	**2020**		**SleepEEG study +SVM and DT classifier**	**99.46** **97.46**

5 Conclusion and Future Directions

The present proposed research work application showed the most effectiveness in the sleep stage scoring by using a single channel of EEG signal. This proposed SleepEEG study would provide an effective mechanism for handling different health conditions of the subjects with high accuracy of sleep abnormality identification from sleep recordings. The main objective of this application is to analyze the irregularities that occurred during sleep hours from various session recordings, and additionally, this application also successfully deals with the specially aged category of subjects with various disease conditions. The major part of this research work is to find the proper solutions based on irregularity's accuracy during sleep. Another important significance of this proposed SleepEEG study is that, according to our best knowledge, this proposed research work considered different session recordings from the participated subjects in these experimental processes.

This experimental research study provides new directions on scoring sleep stages to identify sleep abnormality through the extraction of different features from both domains such as frequency and time. The major changes are shown between the two different session recordings of sleep stages from two different days, and the general sleep stage classification problem is that annotations of sleep stages are another important source of information. These certain things support for discovering new concepts of investigation on sleep irregularities during sleep, and it may get more advantage for predicting the proper diagnosis plan for treating the disorder.

The proposed scheme automated sleep stage classification based on a single channel of EEG signal gives the benefits with the inclusion of different session recordings and obtained different health condition subjects. It has been observed from the experimental results that the proposed sleep analysis indicated an excellent agreement between automated sleep staging and the gold standard.

The present research work has certain disadvantages that the (1) data used for the experimental purpose from ISRUC-Sleep repository for statistical evaluation was relatively small, (2) only we have included single channel of EEG signal was used for classification, (3) we have not considered the subjects who were effects of diseases, such as narcolepsy and insomnia.

References

1. Aboalayon KAI, Faezipour M, Almuhammadi WS et al (2016) Sleep stage classification using EEG signal analysis: a comprehen-sive survey and new investigation. Entropy 18:272
2. Chung M-H, Kuo TB, Hsu N, Chu H, Chou K-R, Yang CC (2009) Sleep and autonomic nervous system changes? Enhanced car-diac sympathetic modulations during sleep in permanent night shift nurses. Scand J Work Environ Health: 180–187
3. Heyat MBB, Akhtar F, Azad S (2016) Comparative analysis of original wave & filtered wave of EEG signal used in the detection of bruxism medical sleep syndrome. Int J Trend Sci Res Develop 1(1):7–9
4. Heyat MBB, Akhtar SF, Azad S (2016) Power spectral density are used in the investigation of insomnia neurological disorder. In: Proceedings of pre-congress symposium of organized Indian Social Science Academy (ISSA) King George Medical University State Takmeelut-Tib College Hospital, Lucknow, Uttar Pradesh, 2016, pp 45–50
5. Rahman F, Heyat S (2016) An overview of narcolepsy. IARJSET 3:85–87
6. Kim T, Kim J, Lee K (2018) Detection of sleep disordered breathing severity using acoustic biomarker and machine learning techniques. BioMed Eng OnLine 17:16
7. Siddiqui M, Srivastava G, Saeed S (2016) Diagnosis of insomnia sleep disorder using short time frequency analysis of PSD approach applied on EEG signal using channel ROC-LOC. Sleep Science 9(3):186–191
8. Rechtschaffen A (1968) A manual for standardized terminology techniques and scoring system for sleep stages in human subjects. Brain Inf Serv
9. Iber C (2007) The AASM manual for the scoring of sleep and associated events: rules, terminology and technical specifications. American Academy of Sleep Medicine
10. Carskadon MA, Dement WC (2017) Normal human sleep: an overview. In: Principles and practice of sleep medicine. In: Kryger M, Roth T, Dement WC (eds) 6th edn. Elsevier, Amsterdam, The Netherlands, pp 15–24. https://doi.org/10.1016/B978-0-323-24288-2.00002-7
11. Acharya R, Faust O, Kannathal N, Chua T, Laxminarayan S (2008) Nonlinear analysis of EEG signals at various sleep stages. Comput Methods Progr Biomed 80(1):37–45
12. Holland JV, Dement WC, Raynal DM (1974) Polysomnography: a response to a need for improved communication. In: Presented at the 14th annual meeting association of psychophysiology study sleep
13. Acharya UR et al (2015) Nonlinear dynamics measures for automated EEG-based sleep stage detection. Eur Neurol 74(5–6):268–287
14. Spriggs WH (2014) Essentials of polysomnography. World Headquarter Jones & Bartlett Publishers, MA, United States
15. Obayya M, Abou-Chadi F (2014) Automatic classification of sleep stages using EEG records based on Fuzzy c-means (FCM) algorithm. In: Radio science conference (NRSC), 2014 31st national, 2014, pp 265–272
16. Güneş KP, Yosunkaya Ş (2010) Efficient sleep stage recognition system based on EEG signal using k-means clustering based feature weighting. Expert Syst Appl 37:7922–7928

17. Aboalayon K, Ocbagabir HT, Faezipour M (2014) Efficient sleep stage classification based on EEG signals. In: Systems, applications and technology conference (LISAT), 2014 IEEE Long Island, 2014, pp 1–6
18. Hassan AR, Subasi A (2017) A decision support system for automated identification of sleep stages from single-channel EEG signals. Knowl-Based Syst 128:115–124
19. Hassan AR, Hassan Bhuiyan MI (2016) Automatic sleep scoring using statistical features in the EMD domain and ensemble methods. Biocybern Biomed Eng 36(1):248–255
20. Gunnarsdottir KM, Gamaldo CE, Salas RME, Ewen JB, Allen RP, Sarma SV (2018) A novel sleep stage scoring system: combining expert-based rules with a decision tree classifier. In: 2018 40th annual international conference of the IEEE engineering in medicine and biology society (EMBC). https://doi.org/10.1109/embc.2018.8513039
21. Sriraam N, Padma Shri TK, Maheshwari U (2016) Recognition of wake-sleep stage 1 multichannel eeg patterns using spectral entropy features for drowsiness detection. Australas Phys Eng Sci Med 39(3):797–806. https://doi.org/10.1007/s13246-016-0472-8
22. Memar P, Faradji F (2018) A Novel Multi-Class EEG-Based Sleep Stage Classification System. IEEE Trans Neural Syst Rehabil Eng 26(1):84–95. https://doi.org/10.1109/tnsre.2017.2776149
23. Da Silveira TLT, Kozakevicius AJ, Rodrigues CR (2016) Single-channel EEG sleep stage classification based on a streamlined set of statistical features in wavelet domain. Med Biol Eng Compu 55(2):343–352. https://doi.org/10.1007/s11517-016-1519-4
24. Pernkopf F, O'Leary P (2001) Feature selection for classification using genetic algorithms with a novel encoding. In: Skarbek W (ed) Computer analysis of images and patterns. CAIP 2001. Lecture notes in computer science, vol 2124. Springer, Berlin, Heidelberg
25. Wutzl B, Leibnitz K, Rattay F, Kronbichler M, Murata M et al (2019) Genetic algorithms for feature selection when classifying severe chronic disorders of consciousness. PLoS ONE 14(7):e0219683. https://doi.org/10.1371/journal.pone.0219683
26. Zhu G, Li Y, Wen PP (2014) Analysis and classification of sleep stages based on difference visibility graphs from a single-channel EEG signal. IEEE J Biomed Health Inform 18(6):1813–1821
27. Braun ET, Kozakevicius ADJ, Da Silveira TLT, Rodrigues CR, Baratto G (2018) Sleep stages classification using spectral based statistical moments as features. Revista de Informática Teórica e Aplicada 25(1):11
28. Khalighi S, Sousa T, Santos JM, Nunes U (2016) ISRUC-sleep: a comprehensive public dataset for sleep researchers. Comput Methods Programs Biomed 124:180–192
29. Masaaki H, Masaki K, Haruaki Y (2001) Automated sleep stage scoring by decision tree learning. In: Proceedings of the 23rd annual EMBS international conference, October 25–28, Istanbul, Turkey
30. Cortes C, Vapnik V (1995) Support vector networks. Mach Learn 20(3):273–297; Kavzoglu T, Colkesen I (2010) Classification of satellite images using decision trees: Kocaeli case. Electron. J Map Technol 2(1):36–45
31. Ocak H (2013) A medical decision support system based on support vector machines and the genetic algorithm for the evaluation of fetal wellbeing. J Med Syst 37(2):1–9
32. Osman H, Gokhan B (2017) Sleep stage classification via ensemble and conventional machine learning methods using single channel EEG signals. Int J Intell Syst Appl Eng 5(4):174–184
33. Bajaj V, Pachori RB (2013) Automatic classification of sleep stages based on the time-frequency image of EEG signals. Comput Methods Programs Biomed 112(3):320–328
34. Hsu Y-L, Yang Y-T, Wang J-S, Hsu C-Y (2013) Automatic sleep stage recurrent neural classifier using energy features of EEG signals. Neurocomputing 104:105–114
35. Zibrandtsen I, Kidmose P, Otto M, Ibsen J, Kjaer TW (2016) Case comparison of sleep features from ear-EEG and scalp-EEG. Sleep Sci 9(2):69–72
36. Berry RB, Brooks R, Gamaldo CE, Hardsim SM, Lloyd RM, Marcus CL, Vaughn BV (2014) The AASM manual for the scoring of sleep and associated events: rules, terminology and technical specifications, version 2.1. American Academy of Sleep Medicine, Darien

37. Sim J, Wright CC (2005) The kappa statistic in reliability studies: use, interpretation, and sample size requirements. Phys Ther 85(3):257–268
38. Liang S-F, Kuo C-E, Hu Y-H, Cheng Y-S (2012) A rule-based automatic sleep staging method. J Neurosci Methods 205(1):169–176

Handwritten Multi-digit Recognition Using Convolutional Neural Networks with Par-Mod

Suraj Tiwari and Piyush Gupta

Abstract Since the dawn of AI, the ability to convert handwritten text to digital form has been an active area of research. Various models were introduced to perform electronic conversion of various types of images containing texts into machine-encoded text, also known as the OCR problem in technical community. Multi-digit numbers recognition is a sub-problem of the same OCR problem. In this paper, the performance of various deep convolution neural network architectures is compared for the task of recognizing arbitrary multi-digit numbers and a final model is proposed with state-of-the-art accuracy. The model will be tested against multiple datasets that include SVHN dataset and self-made dataset from MNIST handwritten images dataset. A comparison is held among the results, and it is shown that the use of ZFNet architecture of convolutional neural networks with par-mod led to significant improvements among other CNN architecture for the same task.

Keywords Convolution neural networks · LeNet · AlexNet · ZFNet · SVHN

1 Introduction

Numbers are everywhere around us. With so many handwritten numbers around, it becomes important for us to develop a mechanism to digitize these numbers. Recognizing multi-digit numbers from real-life images can be said to be a sub-problem of OCR [1]. The recognition problem is difficult because of a number of factors like improper lighting, shadows, specularities, occlusions low resolution, motion, and focus blurs [2].

A lot of work has been done earlier in the field. In Ref. [3], author introduces deep multilingual CNN for LVCSR. Author used the model to recognize real-time documents. In Ref. [4], Yan Lecunn et al. introduced graph transformer networks (GTNs) that allow training all the modules to optimize a global performance criterion. Later, Ian J. Goodfellow demonstrated how a convolution neural network can be used

S. Tiwari (✉) · P. Gupta
Department of Information Technology, JC Bose University of Science and Technology, YMCA, Faridabad, India

N. Marriwala et al. (eds.), *Emergent Converging Technologies and Biomedical Systems*, Lecture Notes in Electrical Engineering 841,
https://doi.org/10.1007/978-981-16-8774-7_31

to achieve a state-of-the-art accuracy of up to 97.84% per digit recognition task [5]. The model suggested by author took six days to train and had eleven hidden layers.

In this paper, we focus on creating a lightweight model which can be used to recognize multi-digit numbers, handwritten or printed with a good accuracy. The model presented in the paper took 4 h to train and had about 20–25 million parameters varying with implemented CNN architectures.

The identification process in any image is basically done in three steps that include localization, segmentation, and recognition steps [6]. We'll be implementing a unified model that integrates all these steps by using deep CNN [7] that operates directly on image pixels. The model consists of multiple hidden layers, and the model is itself divided into two parts—a CNN for feature extraction and par-mod or parallel module that consists of a set of parallel layers for classifying the value of each digit. The feature extraction module can be changed to various models. LeNet [8], AlexNet [9], and ZFNet [10] are examples of various models that can be implemented in feature extraction module. The best performance was achieved on a ZFNet model with nine hidden layers. The developed model was later tested on multiple challenging datasets, and an average test accuracy of 99.7% was obtained on self-made data set and 92.7% on SVHN dataset [11] in the best configuration. A best state-of-the-art accuracy of 99.3 can be obtained with it.

The paper demonstrates the unified approach to identify a complete multi-digit number by using a model consisting of feature extraction module followed by multiple parallel output layers. The results of applying model on multiple challenging datasets are also evaluated. Various architectures of CNN that includes LeNet, AlexNet, and ZFNet have also been tested, and their effect on model performance has been evaluated.

2 Convolution Neural Networks

The idea of the CNN was motivated by a concept of biology-Receptive Field [12]. Receptive field is an area present in sensory neurons, the presence of any stimulus in this area will alter the firing of that neuron, and the organ will respond differently. They are more like a detector for certain types of stimulus. Their key presence can be noticed across visual field. Depending upon the neuron fired the description of location of stimulus can be determined.

Similarly, in a CNN a filter kernel performs the work of receptive field. It senses various pixels of an image and assigns weights to them (Fig. 1).

CNNs unlike traditional neural networks take images as input. Artificial neural networks are used to take vectorized image as input, thus destroying the spatial structure of image. CNNs exploit the structure of image. They approximate the biological functions in form of convolution operations. They take as input, an image volume, and each layer outputs another 3D volume followed by convolution and pooling operations. The convolution operation [13] between any image i and a convolution filter kernel k can be defined as:

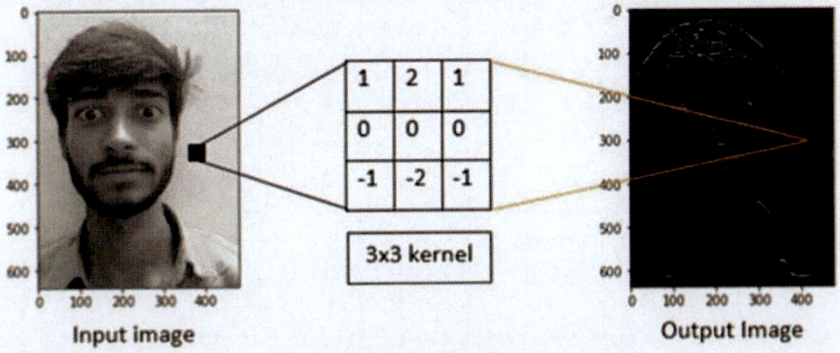

Fig. 1 Filter kernel operation on image to generate edges in an image

$$\phi[a, b] = i[a, b] * k[a, b] = \sum\sum i[x, y]k[a - x, b - y] \quad (1)$$

The dot product of the kernel k and matrix of sub-image Si of image i having dimensions same as k and center at A (a, b) produces the pixel value of ø at coordinates (a, b). The size of filter kernel can be changed for changing receptive field. This filter kernel is aligned with every sub-image matrix. Contrasts to ANN having large number of weights for neurons, CNN has parameter sharing that reduces number of weights and exploits local connectivity.

Pooling and Stride: It is also necessary to make model more acquiescent, and it will be a better step to reduce the size of activation map. The reduction of size is done on the deeper layers of network as require lesser information of exact spatial presence of patterns and more filter kernels to recognize high-level patterns. Thus, we reduce the size of activation maps to reduce computation to a reasonable level, keeping upper spatial patterns, and hidden patterns intact.

To achieve this, one of the ways is to define a pooling layer [14]. We define pooling layer following a convolution or a series of convolutions. The pooling layer downsamples the data volume. One can use max pool or average pool depending upon features of image. Another way to reduce size is to perform strided convolutions. The stride [15] parameter controls the convolution operation for every nth pixel (where n may range from 1 to image length) (Fig. 2).

The convolutional layers implement a nonlinear activation function [16], to produce a nonlinear decision boundary. Rectified linear (ReLU) activation function is the most common activation function used in CNN. Activation functions can sometimes be defined in a separate layer. The activation layer can be placed after convolution layer before performing pooling operation. Many architectures implement local response normalization in a different layer. Local response normalization is an efficient and commonly used regularization method. It decreases the activity of neighboring neurons as it mimics lateral inhibition.

The final layers of a CNN are usually fully connected layers followed by an output layer. These layers require very small volume of data to be practically possible.

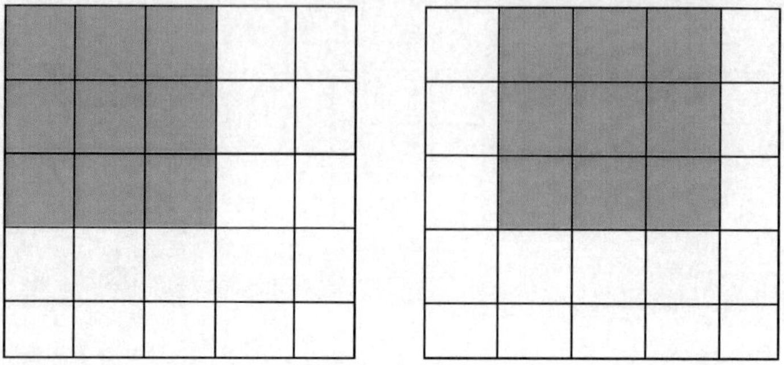

Fig. 2 Stride with one pixel

These layers capture patterns that are usually ignored by parameter-sharing convolutional layers. These fully connected layers are followed by SoftMax output layer for classification task.

Various architectures of CNN that have been worked upon are:

LeNet: LeNet-5 consists of seven layers. In addition to input, every other layer can train parameters. Layer1 is a conv layer with 5 × 5 kernels and 28 × 28 feature mapping followed by a 2 × 2 subsampling / pooling layer. It generates a 14 × 14 output. This is fed to conv layer with 5 × 5 kernel and obtained 10 × 10 feature mapping is further subsampled to 5 × 5 by next subsampling layer. The output of this layer is sent to a series of two fully connected layers after flattening. The SoftMax layer classifies the image into one of eleven classes.

AlexNet: The original AlexNet architecture accepted the input of size 227 × 227 × 3 and consists of 8 layers. It had more about 60 million parameters and was trained on multiple GPUs. It had five convolution and three fully connected layers. It used ReLU instead of tanh as activation which was the standard at that time. AlexNet also used the concept of overlapped pooling that reduced overall error by 0.5% and was harder to overfit. The architecture used dropout to avoid overfitting.

The AlexNet was originally designed for recognizing objects in ImageNet and produced the probability distribution of 1000 classes. The parameters of model are reduced specifically for making it compatible with our dataset and reducing the computation involved. The stride we'll be using will be of two instead of four used in original AlexNet, also the output will be a probability distribution of 11 classes that are numbers 0–9 and nan instead of 1000 classes seen in original design.

ZFNet: ZFNet has similar architecture to AlexNet. It was recreated same as AlexNet for ease of comparison. It addressed two major problems observed in first two layers of AlexNet. It reduced the filter size and the number of filters used. It reduced the filters of size 11 × 11 present in AlexNet to 7 × 7. It also replaced the strided convolutions of AlexNet from 4 to 2. This resulted in much cleaner features visible after first two layers in ZFNet than AlexNet. The ZFNet used filter kernels of size 512, 1024 and 512 instead of 384, 384, and 256 used in third, fourth, and fifth layers of AlexNet, respectively. The ZFNet was also designed for recognizing objects in ImageNet and original design had 1000 classes as final output. However, we reduced certain parameters of original structures, keeping basic design same. The final output will belong to one of 11 classes, and also, the stride is taken to be one in our case of ZFNet.

Remaining of work is organized in multiple sections. Section 3 discusses works related to multi-digit classification part in a chronological order. Afterward in Sect. 4, we define problem statement that is addressed in paper. Section 5 presents basic methodology that was implemented while solving the problem statement. Section 6 does the experimental analysis and is concluded by Sect. 7, followed by some useful references.

3 Related Work

In the paper "A Detailed Analysis of Optical Character Recognition Technology" [17], author defines OCR as the electronic or mechanical conversion of images of typed, handwritten or printed text into machine-encoded text, whether from a scanned document or from a photograph of a document. Initial approaches toward OCR include the implementation of various neural networks that were able to recognize characters but their accuracy was low and they were too slow to train.

The major breakthrough in OCR came when convolutional neural networks were introduced in paper "gradient-based learning applied to document recognition" [18]. The proposed model was able to extract more features from images than any other neural network of same depth. Author introduced graph transformer networks and finite state transducers for reading bank checks. The model had accuracy better than the best artificial neural network till that time, and paper was able to establish CNN as a better option over neural networks, in extracting features from images.

Later various improvements in CNN were done by many researchers. Next major contribution in recognizing multi-digit numbers was by Ian J Goodfellow. In the paper "Multi-digit Number Recognition from Street View Imagery using Deep Convolutional Neural Networks" [5], authors showed how deep CNNs can be used to recognize multi-digit numbers with high accuracy. The model served as a benchmark for various other multi-digit classification models for years. It was an eleven-layer deep model and was trained for six days over multiple GPUs. The final average accuracy achieved was about 97.84% in per digit recognition task.

In another paper "Convolutional neural networks applied to house numbers digit classification" [19], authors also demonstrated that CNNs can achieve high accuracy when it comes to recognize multi-digit numbers. Paper showed how a deep convolution neural network can extract important feature from images without any need to explicitly localizing and then recognition.

Other than constant progress in multi-digit number recognition task, a lot of work has been done on developing various CNN architectures. A network similar to LeNet was developed by Yann Lecun and was first introduced in his work "Generalization and network design strategies" [20]. Author also mentions weight space transformation in this paper and demonstrates the working of his network over 16 × 16 images of numbers created by a person over 16 by 13 bitmap using mouse.

Since then lot of enhancements have been done on CNNs. Capsule networks or CapsNet is also another form of network that is used for task of digit recognition. It was first introduced by Geoffrey E. Hinton et al. in the paper "Dynamic Routing between capsules" [21]. These models also preserve relative position of an object unlike CNNs giving them an edge over conventional CNNs.

4 Problem Statement

Given a set of images I, where each image consists of a multi-digit number N of length L and digits X1, X2... XL. Our aim is to define a probabilistic model of sequences and maximize the correctness of probability P (L' = L) and P (Xi' = Xi) for i in range 0 to L-1. We will also analyze the effect of changing CNN over LeNet, AlexNet and ZFNet architectures on accuracy of model. The criteria of error detection will be the average error E of E1 in determining length of number, $C(\Delta L)$ and E2 in determining value in each digit, $\sum C(\Delta X)$.

5 Methodology

5.1 Datasets

The model was trained on multiple datasets that include self-created multi-digit data set, that was created by joining random images from MNIST dataset [22] and then rescaling it to 64 × 64. In case of SVHN data, images were scaled to 64 × 64 after expanding boxes by 40% along x- and y-axes and cropping the image. Data augmentation was done on the dataset by making random crops and random rotation of up to 100. Color perturbations [23] can also be used but it'll not impact performance of model much (Fig. 3).

SVHN dataset image normalization is done by subtracting mean of pixel calculated over all images. The normalization can also be done by using local contrast normalization [24]. It operates on local patches in images instead of performing a global normalization based on the range of values of the entire image (Fig. 4).

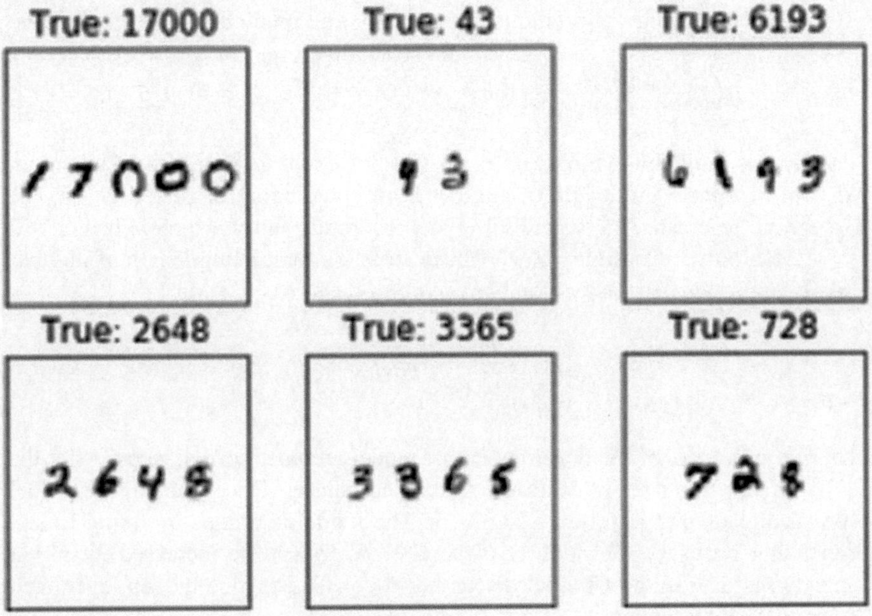

Fig. 3 Self-created MNIST multi-digit dataset

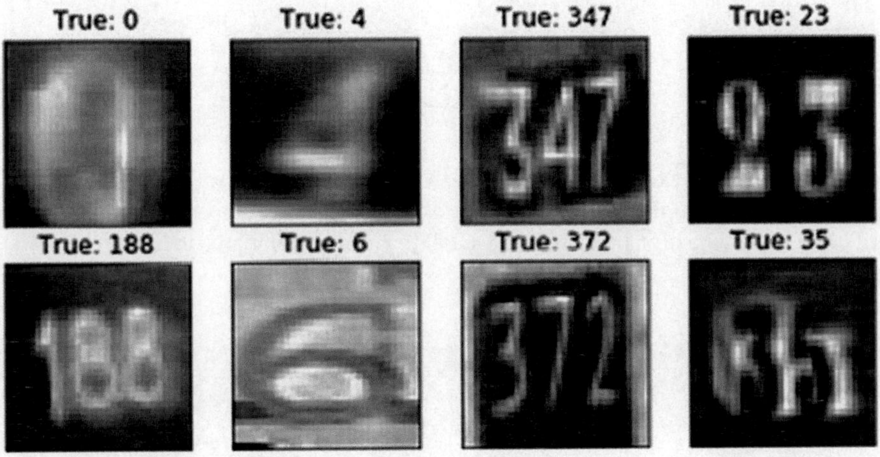

Fig. 4 SVHN dataset used for training the model

5.2 Architecture

Once the datasets are obtained, next step is to create a convolution model. We will create a probabilistic model of sequences. The objective will be to maximize the correctness of probability of prediction of length L and prediction for each digit Xi.

$$P\left(\hat{L} = L\right)\prod_{i=0}^{L-1} P\left(\hat{X}i = Xi\right), L \in [0, l], Xi \in [0, 9] \tag{2}$$

The input is provided to model in form of 64 × 64x1 image matrices. The output consists of two parts, the length of number L and prediction for each digit Xi. For this, we have to create Lmax parallel layers in output out of which L layers will give SoftMax output for digits [0, 9]. The accuracy in predicting length of number is equally important. The activation used in output layers is SoftMax.

$$\Re(z)_i = \frac{e^{(\partial zi)}}{\sum_{j=1}^{k} e^{(\partial zj)}} fori = 1, ..., K \tag{3}$$

The entire process of the development of model includes several steps. After the model is made, it is trained using the processed dataset. Once trained, the model can be used to predict multi-digit numbers. The model is trained by fixing Lmax, so depending on usage the number of parallel layers can be increased. Our best architecture is extension of model discussed; it consists of nine hidden layers and seven parallel output layers.

The parallel layers receive the output from dense D1 layer. The parallel layers consist of another dense layer with SoftMax activation. The categorical cross-entropy loss function is used to compute loss.

$$L(y, \hat{y}) = -\sum_{j=0}^{M}\sum_{i=0}^{N}(y_{ij} * log(\hat{y}_{ij})) \tag{4}$$

The metrics need to be evaluated for two sub-problems, the length of number and value of each digits. The output of detector is SoftMax activated, that makes it sufficient to achieve high precision and recall that can be compared to human labelers (Fig. 5).

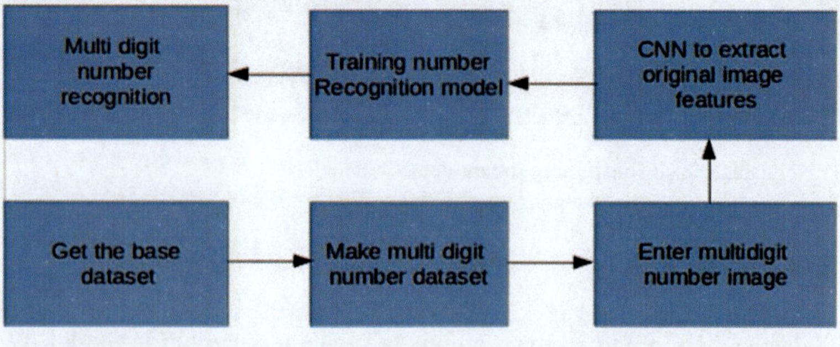

Fig. 5 Process of the development of CNN with par-mod model to recognize multi-digit numbers

The model can be extended to recognize RGB images. The input in the case is taken 128 × 128 × 3, and the model is extended up to eleven hidden layers for precise output. CNN with par-mod is a basic model that can be trained over any multi-digit number dataset with certain extensions to achieve a good accuracy in predicting the numbers. Since the model does not need explicit localization and segmentation, the training does not require localization entities or blob detection and hence is fast than any other model.

The model can be trained over a low GPU machine due to its ability to learn more features with lesser number of computations. A standard CNN with par-mod can be trained in a 4 GB RAM 2.2 Ghz processor system within hours, making it lightweight and efficient than other counterparts (Fig. 6).

The layers of feature extraction part are further changed in order to implement various CNN architectures. The layers are changed to one corresponding to LeNet, AlexNet, and ZFNet. The final layers of classification module are kept same.

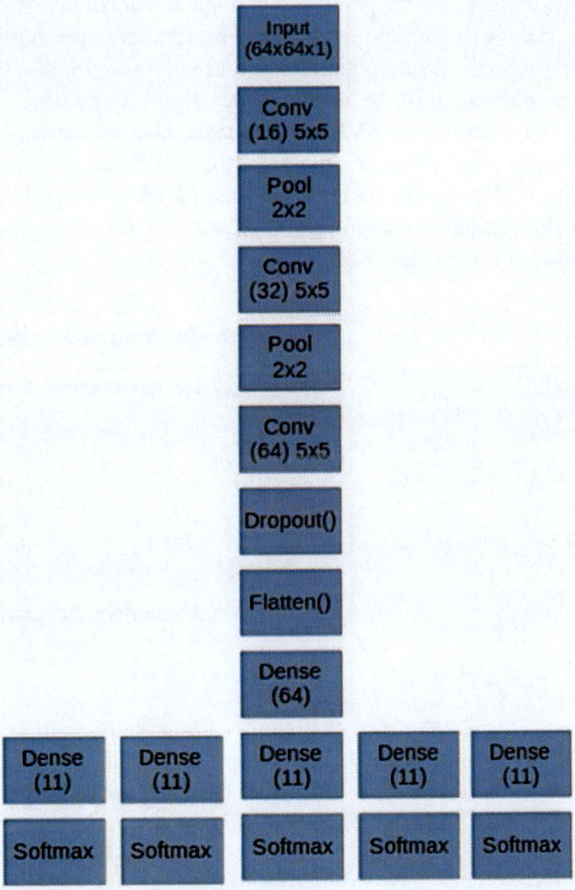

Fig. 6 Architecture of the basic CNN with par-mod to recognize multi-digit numbers from single-channel images

5.3 Environment

The model was built and trained over Intel core i3 processor with 2.2 Ghz clock speed and 4 GB RAM. No additional GPU was used. For RGB images, the model can be trained over any processor with base clock speed greater than 2.8 Ghz and RAM more than 8 GB. AlexNet and ZFNet being deeper than LeNet require more computation power to train. However once trained, the model can be deployed over any system with no high-end configuration required.

6 Experimental Evaluation

The CNN with par-mod model was tested on multiple datasets that include self-made MNIST multi-digit dataset and SVHN dataset. The results of model on MNIST self-made dataset were good. An average test accuracy of 98.9% was obtained on it. The accuracy in predicting the length of number was 99.89% while the average accuracy in predicting complete number correctly was 98.9%. This accuracy can be extended up to the state of the art 99.9% per digit recognition.

The results on SVHN dataset are also promising. An average test accuracy of 91.2% was achieved in predicting complete number correctly. The accuracy in predicting length of number was 98.9% while the maximum accuracy that was achieved on any position of digit was 99.6%. This is slightly better than the models introduced earlier (Fig. 7).

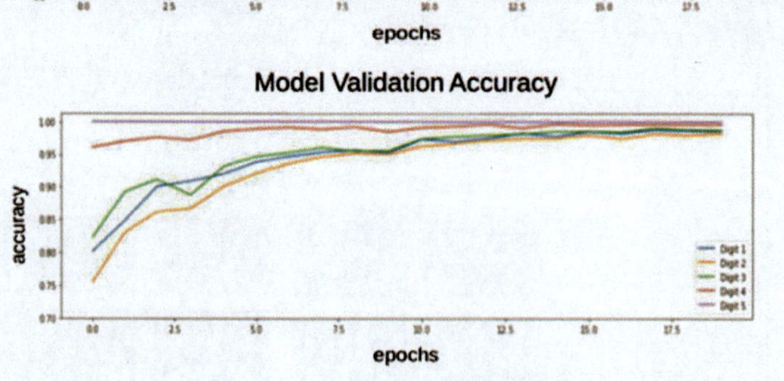

Fig. 7 Training and validation accuracy plot VS number of epochs per digit for SVHN dataset

The accuracy consists of accuracy in determining digit at every position as well as the accuracy in determining length of number correctly. The results for the same are better in case if MNIST self-made dataset because there less noise is present in images while in SVHN lot of extra features are present (Fig. 8 and Table 1).

The results on SVHN dataset on the other hand show a significant increase as the model architecture is changed from LeNet to AlexNet to ZFNet. The overall 1.5% increase in test accuracy is observed in SVHN dataset from LeNet to ZFNet. This means ZFNet is able to extract features better than any other architecture. The maximum accuracy per digit also increases significantly with change in architecture of CNN.

The results obtained on MNIST self-made dataset do not show significant increase with change in feature extraction part. An overall difference of 0.8% accuracy is observed between LeNet and ZFNet architectures (Tables 2 and 3).

A sanity check was also performed on model trained with SVHN dataset, and it gave an accuracy of 94.7% in predicting real-time multi-digit numbers on a dataset of 10,000 images.

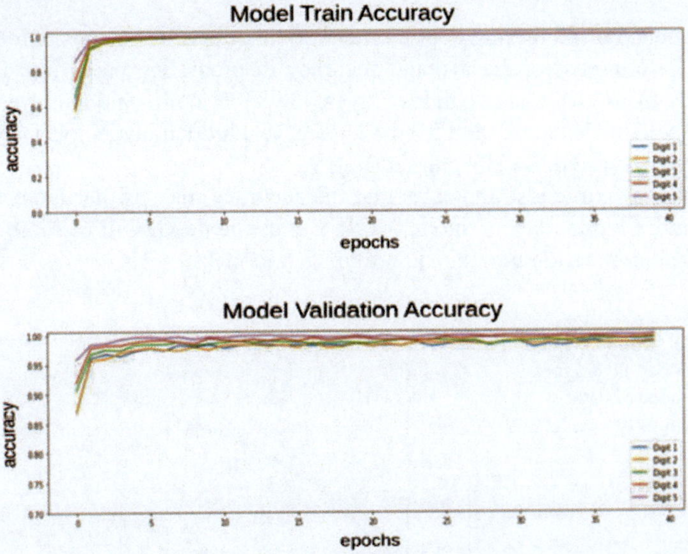

Fig. 8 Training and validation accuracy plot VS number of epochs per digit for MNIST self-created dataset

Table 1 Average accuracy of predicting multi-digit numbers of CNN with par-mod over various datasets

Dataset	Train accuracy	Validation accuracy	Test accuracy
MNIST self made	99.7	99.5	98.9
SVHN	97.2	98.1	91.2

Table 2 Comparison of performance of model with different CNN architectures and par-mod

CNN model	Train Accuracy MNIST	Validation Accuracy MNIST	Test Accuracy MNIST	Train Accuracy SVHN	Validation Accuracy SVHN	Test Accuracy SVHN
LeNet	99.7	99.5	98.9	97.2	98.1	91.2
AlexNet	99.8	99.7	99.2	98	98.4	92.3
ZFNet	100	99.8	99.7	98.9	98.7	92.7

Table 3 Comparison of average accuracy with different architectures and maximum value of accuracy obtained among digits

CNN Model	Mean accuracy MNIST	Max digit Accuracy MNIST	Mean Accuracy SVHN	Max digit Accuracy SVHN
LeNet	98.9	99.3	91.2	98.6
AlexNet	99.2	99.7	92.3	99.1
ZFNet	99.7	100	92.7	99.3

The influence of increasing depth in network should also be considered. As the depth of CNN increases, the average accuracy in predicting each digit increases significantly from 87.3% at two hidden layers to 98.9% at nine hidden layers in case of MNIST self-made dataset and from 82.1% at two hidden layers to 91.2% at nine hidden layers in case of SVHN dataset (Fig. 9).

The accuracy curve also indicates that the accuracy may further increase as we introduce more hidden layers into network. But as the depth will increase it'll also increase the computation power required to train model.

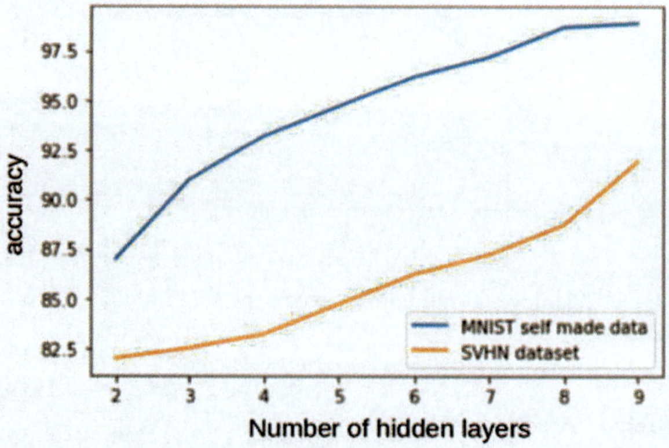

Fig. 9 Plot of accuracy VS number of hidden layers for MNIST self-created dataset and SVHN dataset

7 Conclusion

We consider that this model can be used to solve small-scale multi-digit handwritten number problems. The model up to nine hidden layers can easily be trained on any regular home PC, which further solves the problem of requirement of high GPU systems to train OCR models. One drawback of the model is that it can predict numbers up to a specific length Lmax for which the model is designed. Another problem that may occur is of numbers with large length, as we increase Lmax the same metrics may not be good enough. Consider SVHN dataset, for example, the entire dataset contains 0.01% of six-digit numbers, so if we consider the same matrix that we considered for par-mod with Lmax = 5 then, we'll be getting a better accuracy even if the model is not trained sufficiently for 6th position. Also, as the length of number increase, the capability of model with same number of hidden layers to correctly predict length decreases. One solution to the above-mentioned problem can be designing an adaptive network that determines the length of number first and then sequentially determines the value of each digit. Another solution can be designing a smart network that computes the length and fires parallel neurons, the number of such neurons is not hard coded but the model itself determines the number of parallel signals it requires and fire them accordingly.

The major finding of the paper was the utilization of low-weighted CNN's in recognizing multi-digit handwritten numbers. The concept can be extended to the superset OCR for document recognition as the CNNs are outperforming existing deep neural networks and human labelers in the task. Also, various models that were tested for performance for multi-digit recognition show that ZFNet is a better model for feature extraction than LeNet or AlexNet when it comes to multi-digit recognition task.

References

1. Mithe R, Indalkar S, Divekar N (2013) Optical character recognition. Int J Recent Technol Eng (IJRTE) 2(1):72–75
2. Impedovo S, Ottaviano L, Occhinegro S (1991) Optical character recognition—a survey. Int J Pattern Recognit Artif Intell 5.01n02:1–24
3. Sercu T et al (2016) Very deep multilingual convolutional neural networks for LVCSR. In: 2016 IEEE international conference on acoustics, speech and signal processing (ICASSP). IEEE
4. Bottou L, Bengio Y, Cun YL (1997) Global training of document processing systems using graph transformer networks. In: Proceedings of IEEE computer society conference on computer vision and pattern recognition. IEEE
5. Goodfellow Ian J et al (2013) Multi-digit number recognition from street view imagery using deep convolutional neural networks. arXiv:1312.6082
6. Neumann L, Matas J (2010) A method for text localization and recognition in real-world images. In: Asian conference on computer vision. Springer, Berlin, Heidelberg
7. Jaderberg M et al (2014) Deep structured output learning for unconstrained text recognition. arXiv:1412.5903

8. El-Sawy A, Hazem E-B, Loey M (2016) CNN for handwritten Arabic digits recognition based on LeNet-5. In: International conference on advanced intelligent systems and informatics. Springer, Cham
9. Almodfer R et al (2017) Enhancing AlexNet for arabic handwritten words recognition using incremental dropout. In: 2017 IEEE 29th international conference on tools with artificial intelligence (ICTAI). IEEE
10. Suresh R, Keshava N (2019) A survey of popular image and text analysis techniques. In: 2019 4th international conference on computational systems and information technology for sustainable solution (CSITSS), vol 4. IEEE
11. Netzer Y, Wang T, Coates A, Bissacco A, Wu B, Ng AY (2011) Reading digits in natural images with unsupervised feature learning. In: NIPS workshop on deep learning and unsupervised feature learning
12. Jia Y, Huang C, Darrell T (2012) Beyond spatial pyramids: receptive field learning for pooled image features. In: 2012 IEEE conference on computer vision and pattern recognition. IEEE
13. Hijazi S, Kumar R, Rowen C (2015) Using convolution neural networks for image recognition. Cadence Design Systems Inc., San Jose, CA, USA, pp 1–12
14. Graham B (2014) Fractional max-pooling. arXiv:1412.6071
15. Ayachi R et al (2018) Strided convolution instead of max pooling for memory efficiency of convolutional neural networks. In: International conference on the sciences of electronics, technologies of information and telecommunications. Springer, Cham
16. Nanni L et al (2020) Stochastic activation function layers for convolutional neural networks
17. Hamad KA, Kaya M (2016) A detailed analysis of optical character recognition technology. Int J Appl Math Electron Comput 4.1:244–249
18. LeCun Y et al (1998) Gradient-based learning applied to document recognition. In: Proceedings of the IEEE 86.11, pp 2278–2324
19. Sermanet P, Chintala S, LeCun Y (2012) Convolutional neural networks applied to house numbers digit classification. In: Proceedings of the 21st international conference on pattern recognition (ICPR2012). IEEE
20. LeCun Y (1989) Generalization and network design strategies. Connect Perspect 19:143–155
21. Sabour S, Frosst N, Hinton G (2017) Dynamic routing between capsules
22. LeCun Y, Cortes C (2010) MNIST handwritten digit database
23. Kim EK et al (2010) Data augmentation method by applying color perturbation of inverse PSNR and geometric transformations for object recognition based on deep learning. Appl Sci 10.11:3755
24. Veldkamp WJH, Karssemeijer N (2000) Normalization of local contrast in mammograms. IEEE Trans Med Imaging 19.7:731–738

Automated Detection of Cardiac Arrhythmia Based on a Hybrid CNN-LSTM Network

Shahriar Rahman, Shazzadur Rahman, and A. K. M. Bahalul Haque

Abstract Cardiac arrhythmia is an irregular sequence of electrical impulses which result in numerous shifts in heart rhythms. Such cardiac abnormalities can be observed using a standard medical examination known as electrocardiogram (ECG). However, with the drastic increase in heart disease patients, interpreting such pulsations on ECG can be time-consuming and a challenging task. Thus, the primary objective of this paper is to propose an automated system based on a hybrid model which consists of an amalgamation of convolutional neural networks (CNN) and long short-term memory (LSTM) in order to accurately detect and classify several cardiac arrhythmia ailments. The model incorporates a feature selection algorithm, principal component analysis (PCA), that ingresses the new features into 14-layers deep one-dimensional CNN-LSTM network. The experiment is conducted using PhysionNet's MIT-BIH and PTB diagnostics datasets and multiple strategies have been contemplated for evaluation purposes: firstly, using smooth ECG signals with filtered noise and alternatively, using signals that encompass artificially generated noise based on a Gaussian distribution. The proposed system achieved an accuracy of 99% with the denoised sets and 98% using the data with artificially generated noise, exhibiting a consistent and robust generalization performance and possesses the potential to be used as an auxiliary tool to assist clinicians in arrhythmia diagnoses.

Keywords Cardiac arrhythmia · Convolutional neural network · Long short-term memory · Principal component analysis

S. Rahman · S. Rahman (✉)
Department of Electrical and Computer Engineering, North South University, Dhaka, Bangladesh
e-mail: shazzadur.rahman01@northsouth.edu

S. Rahman
e-mail: shahriar.rahman10@northsouth.edu

A. K. M. Bahalul Haque
Software Engineering, LENS, LUT University, 53850 Lappeenranta, Finland
e-mail: bahalul.haque@northsouth.edu

N. Marriwala et al. (eds.), *Emergent Converging Technologies and Biomedical Systems*, Lecture Notes in Electrical Engineering 841,
https://doi.org/10.1007/978-981-16-8774-7_32

1 Introduction

Population aging is a global phenomenon. Between 2015 and 2050, the entire population is expected to increase by more than 2.1 billion, while the older population would expand by about 1.6 billion. Besides, the rate of the aged population is projected to escalate drastically, especially in southeastern Asia, North Africa, the Caribbean, and Latin America [1]. According to the 2019 National Institute report, adults with age over 60 are more likely to suffer from cardiovascular disease than the younger population. As the human body grows old over time, the functionality of the cardiovascular system starts to deteriorate and undergoes various alterations, affecting the heart and blood vessels, which leads to the body being more susceptible to heart diseases. In old age, the myocytes and apoptosis of the nearby tissue expand along with the left ventricle muscle wall, resulting in diastolic dysfunction [2], causing the primary chambers of the ventricle to become inelastic, and thus, obstructs the flow of the blood [3, 4]. Due to this blockage, the muscle tissues get damaged through the denial of oxygen, resulting in inefficient contractions, and, as a result, the heart's ability to pump blood impacts heavily as the sinus node starts to generate electrical impulses in an anomalous way, leading to cardiac arrhythmia disorder, which is often accountable for sudden deaths [5, 6].

Arrhythmias can be categorized into non-ectopic (N), ventricular tachycardia (V), supraventricular tachycardia (S), fusion (F), and unclassifiable (U) beats [7]. Table 1 demonstrates the five classifications of different ECG beats according to ANSI/AAMI EC57. For appropriate diagnosis of the aforementioned arrhythmia disorders, supervision by electrocardiogram (ECG) is employed to monitor the deviations in cardiac muscle depolarization and repolarization for every cardiac cycle. Treatment of each cardiac abnormality is non-identical and is incompatible with other classes. Therefore, it is imperative for cardiologists to accurately interpret the ECG signals before the administration of any medicament procedure. However, due

Table 1 Summarization of the categorized ECG beats [9]

Class	Group	Annotations
0	N	• Non-ectopic beats • Left bundle branch block (LBBB) • Right bundle branch block (RBBB) • Atrial Escape • Nodal (junctional) Escape
1	S	• Supra-ventricular tachycardia • Aberrant atrial premature • Nodal (junctional) premature
2	V	• Ventricular tachycardia • Premature ventricular contraction
3	F	• Fusion beats
4	U	• Paced beats • Fusion of paced and normal • Unclassifiable/unknown

to the exponential increase in the global population, especially adults having severe heart complications, undertaking such tasks can be tedious and time-consuming.

The primary incentive of this paper is to present an automated predictive model for ECG inspection, which will make signal classification much easier to comprehend with precision. Many healthcare systems have adopted deep learning (DL) algorithms [8] to classify arrhythmias accurately. The convolutional neural network (CNN) is an example of one of the widely used algorithms in finding a suitable solution for various complex tasks and diagnoses in the medical field and has achieved great success. Since the process of analyzing signals can be considered as a time-series problem, the long short-term memory (LSTM) undergoes various utilization as well, as it possesses the capacity to remember and pretermit knowledge depending on the significance of the processed information. The overall structure of the proposed model can be dissected into four phases: preprocessing, feature extraction, classification, and assessment.

2 Literature Review

In this section, various strategies, models, and techniques will be explored thoroughly and comparisons for each outcome will be examined in order to grasp a clear perception of the central mechanism applied for this problem.

2.1 Support Vector Machine

Developed by Vladimir Naumovich Vapnik, the support vector machine (SVM) is based on statistical learning frameworks. Although mostly used for classification purposes, SVM is also applied for tasks such as clustering and regression. The primary goal is to separate d-dimensional data on a $(d - 1)$ dimensional hyperplane. If the relationship distribution of a particular set exists as nonlinear, SVM can circumvent the obstacle by using a kernel trick, which increases the dimensionality to find a fitting separating decision boundary.

Kohli et al. proposed three models based on SVM: one-against-one (OAO), one-against-all (OAA), and fuzzy decision function (FDF) [10]. The plan is to distinguish and verify the presence of arrhythmia, categorizing them in a single class. Upon studying with all the aforementioned models, the OAA model performs adequately. It is argued that due to the complexity of the data, other models faced difficulties in generalizing accurately. In a different journal, a related examination has been carried out to confirm the appearance of an arrhythmia. Unlike the previous investigation, a feature selection method known as principal component analysis (PCA) is used [11]. Apart from the three models, a new approach, known as a decision-directed acyclic graph (DDAG), is considered. Despite introducing a different SVM model and PCA algorithm into the mix, the OAA model still gives a better result. A SVM classification algorithm is used along with a dimensionality reduction technique, independent component analysis (ICA) [12]. Using SVM quadratic kernel, the model attained an average accuracy of about 98.50%.

2.2 Artificial Neural Network

Also known as neural networks (NNs), the artificial neural network (ANN) is based on a set of neurons, which are interconnected with each other and operate similarly to a human brain. ANN embodies three diverse layers: input layer, hidden layers, and output layer. Each neuron carries weights that get adjusted as the information inside the neurons is processed in the hidden layer. ANN is one of the most popular algorithms in the field of artificial intelligent (AI) systems which gives consistent and reliable results.

A Bayesian ANN classifier is developed by Gao et al. for performance comparisons with other models such as decision trees (DT), random forest (RF), Naïve Bayes (NB), and so forth [13]. The use of logistic regression with the backpropagation algorithm is simulated using the noisy ECG data. The classification results prove that the Bayesian ANN gives decent results when compared to other contesting models, producing a sensitivity score of 0.76 ± 0.04. It is hoped that there is still potential for improvement on the recommended model. For classification of normal or abnormal class of arrhythmias, Jadhav et al. constructed three different ANN models and are able to achieve an accuracy of 86.67%, 93.75%, and 93.1% in specificity [14].

2.3 K-Nearest Neighbor

K-nearest neighbor (KNN) was first developed in 1951 by two well-known statisticians Evelyn Fix and Joseph Hodges. KNN classifies new cases by comparing with the given data that is accumulated and uses a similarity measure to find the veracious class member, where k is a parameter indicating the number of nearest neighbors to consider as the majority in the voting operation. KNN is mostly used for classification and is a nonparametric algorithm.

A kernel difference-weighted K-nearest neighbor (KDF-KNN) algorithm has been proposed by Zuo et al. in which a standard 12-lead ECG recordings are used for classifying arrhythmias. The model is considered distinct from the conventional KNN due to the computation of its weights by using the Lagrangian multiplier method [15]. Other models such as NBC, KNN, and VF-15 are used for performance observation, which provides an accuracy of around 60% while the KDF-KNN achieved 70%, proving that it performs better overall. Yang et al. also employed a modified version of KDF-KNN (MKDF-KNN) which is used to impute missing values inside an ECG dataset [16].

2.4 Convolution Neural Network

A convolutional neural network (CNN) is a deep learning algorithm that is popular for identifying various image patterns more precisely and effectively. A convolutional layer or a conv layer inside a CNN consists of filters that are responsible for extracting temporal and spatial information of an image or a signal. Although image analysis has been the widespread use of CNNs, they can also be used in other analyses such as time-series problems.

For this particular problem at hand, CNN is one of the widely and most commonly used algorithms. A voting mechanism has been performed for classifying myocardial infarction (MI) where for each lead out of the 12-lead ECG signals, a single CNN is applied [17]. However, a total of 12 CNNs would be impractical for realistic scenarios. A new approach, by Yıldırım et al., has proposed a 1D CNN model which comprises 17 ECG classes and is based on 10-s fragments of one lead ECG signal [18]. The overall accuracy obtained is 91.33% which has the potentiality to be used in telemedicine. Furthermore, Acharya et al. employed a CNN model for detecting MI from the ECG signals both with and without noise and achieved an accuracy of 93.53% and 95.22%, respectively [19]. Kachuee et al. built a CNN model for predicting the different types of arrhythmias and also suggested a model in which the knowledge can be transferred to accurately classify MI, achieving an accuracy of about 93% [20]. Liu et al. constructed a model based on denoising autoencoder (DAE) extracts and divide the sound of heartbeats to classify normal and abnormal beats [21]. Another related model is developed by Baloglu et al. in which a 12-lead ECG is processed with an end-to-end structure using CNN to diagnose MI [22]. Both the prior mentioned models manage to achieve 99% accuracy.

2.5 Recurrent Neural Network

Recurrent neural network (RNN) is well known for recognizing the temporal dynamic knowledge, whereas another class of networks has information based on static mapping. One of RNNs most advantageous functionality is their robustness during the analysis of time-series data to produce an accurate prediction. Furthermore, RNN can be merged with other models to effectively enhance the predictive capability [23].

There are various implementations of RNN regarding time-series predictions and classifications. RNN, gated recurrent unit (GRU), and long short-term memory (LSTM) models are recommended by Singh et al., which takes in the standard ECG time-series data and attempt to classify regular and irregular beats, attaining accuracy of 85.4%, 82.5%, and 88.1%, respectively [24]. Schwab et al. proposed a diverse RNN model where an annotated dataset is used to classify heart rhythm based on a single-lead ECG [25]. A convolutional recurrent neural network (CRNN) is applied to categorize ECG signals between 30 to 60 s by Limam et al. An SVM is used to evaluate the final decision [26].

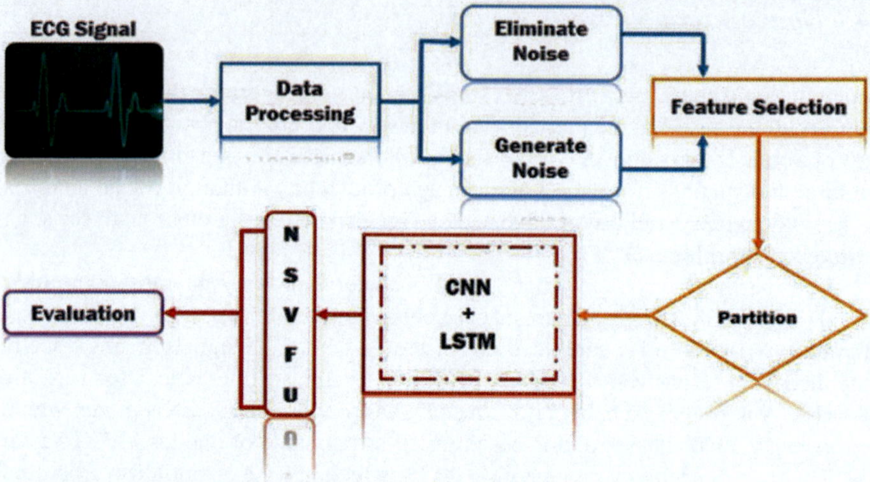

Fig. 1 Framework of the suggested model

3 Methodology

3.1 Methodology Overview

The ECG time-series data obtained is analyzed and processed by using various machine learning (ML) techniques to ensure stability and integrity. Multiple instances of the dataset are synthesized. The first set includes data that uses a peak enhancement technique to reduce and smoothen noise in the signals and the second data involves artificially generated noise based on Gaussian distribution applied to the raw dataset. A feature selection algorithm, PCA, is applied on both datasets, followed by a distribution procedure that segregates each dataset into training, validation, and test subsets. The partition strategy is illustrated in Fig. 5. The prepared data is applied in a series of CNN-LSTM layers with three layers of max pooling utilized. Figure 1 displays the overall framework of the CNN-LSTM model for arrhythmia classification.

3.2 Data Acquisition

The dataset utilized in this study is acquired from the Physiobank (PTB) database. To classify cardiac arrhythmia disease, an ECG dataset is designated from the source site [27]. Generally, the dataset was available to be used for experimentation purposes and was distributed publicly in 1980. The dataset encompasses the recordings of forty-seven patients which were recorded using two-lead ECG and were digitized at

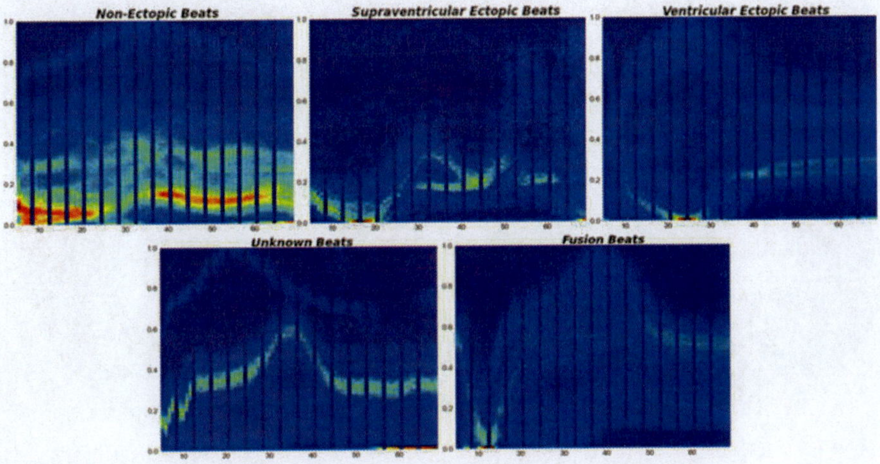

Fig. 2 Signal representation for each group on a two-dimensional histogram

360 Hz with 11-bit resolution over a range of 10 millivolts. Furthermore, the database included about forty-eight hour-long ECG signals and was annotated independently by multiple cardiologists. Figure 2 visualizes the silhouette of signals for each group.

3.3 Data Preprocessing

Before introducing the signal features to the suggested model, proper cleaning steps are required to perceive any errors and redundant records. Each required adjustment and modification to the dataset processing will be explored thoroughly below.

Monitor Anomalies. The assembled data might contain missing values, which would compile an error referred to as NaN, which implies that the recorded value is not a number. Thus, it is imperative to discard the redundant samples and has a clean set of features.

Data Sampling. Upon close inspection, the overall distribution of the data seems very skewed. Figure 3 displays each class pattern of the dataset. If the data is not properly calibrated, the classification algorithm will produce an artificial bias to the largest or majority class, thus hindering the model's performance as a result. To avoid such complications, the sample is restructured by under-sampling the majority and up-sampling the minority class to operate with about 20,000 data per class. The procedure applied is known as synthetic minority over-sampling technique (SMOTE) [28].

Table 2 displays the comparison of the amount of data before and after the sampling process. Samples for non-ectopic or normal beats take about 82.8% of the entire distribution, whereas fusion beats consist of only 0.7% data. Even though after sampling, around 8.6% of data are dropped, up-sampling the minority classes

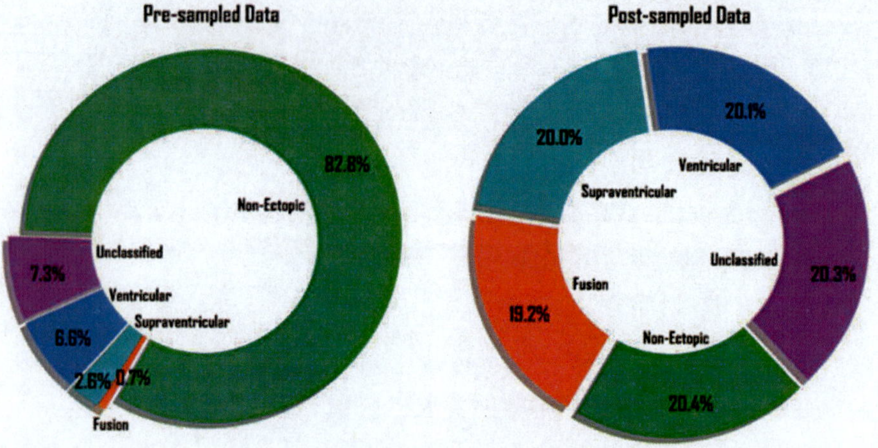

Fig. 3 Distribution comparison between pre- and post-sampled data using SMOTE

Table 2 Representation of sample quantification for the processed data

Class	Group	Pre-sampling	Post-sampling
0	N	90,589	19,184
1	S	2,779	20,123
2	V	7,236	20,301
3	F	803	20,040
4	U	8,039	20,352
Sum		109,446	100,000

and balancing the classes becomes a necessary task and far outweighs the small drawbacks.

Noise Suppression. For many signals processing applications, identifying peaks in a signal is a crucial measure. During various surveys, the signal quality can often be insufficient which could pose challenges for both clinicians and the algorithm used to perceive such patterns. In order to enhance the performance of the model and scrutinize its robustness on ideal set of features, the prudent approach is to filter out undesired noise. There is a multitude of ways of denoising a signal [29]. For this study, a peak enhancement technique has been considered which attempts to normalize the amplitude followed by an increase in the largest amplitude or R-peak by using linear transformations relative to the other portions of the signal. Thus, guaranteeing that the R-peaks are uninterrupted and undisturbed [30]. Figure 4 demonstrates the shape of the signal in contrast to the collective one.

Noise Generation. On the contrary, superimposing disturbance to the raw signal data is also a logical concern. While clean, noise-filtered data is essential for evaluating a model's performance on a faultless condition, it is equally imperative to take into consideration that in reality, and there is bound to be a few sporadicity in the

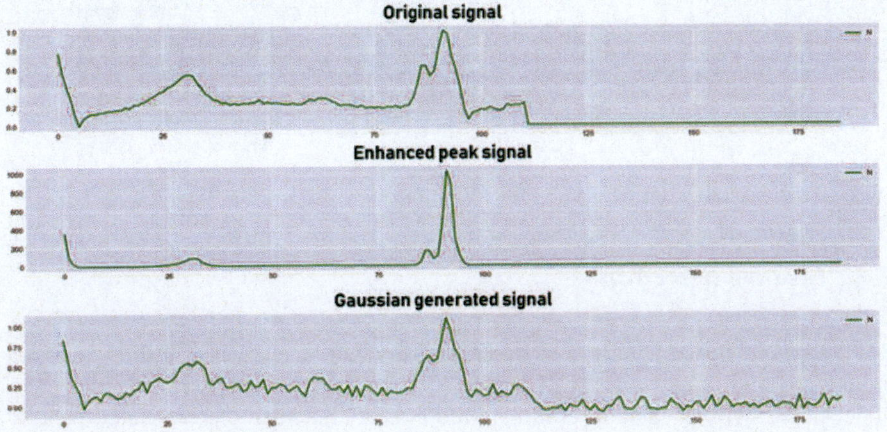

Fig. 4 Graphical comparison of different ECG signals for 'N' class

dataset. In most critical cases, the quality of data can deteriorate due to the presence of noise. Thus, it is also worth assessing the model's accuracy for the worst-case scenario, which would occur in practical circumstances. Furthermore, adding noise in the samples can also reduce the overfitting issue as the variance will be lower due to the increased training error. Therefore, a random value based on a Gaussian noise is generated on a scale of 0.05 to create more disruption to the signal.

Dimensional Transformation. In this research, the input of the hybrid model is two-dimensional. However, due to the nature of time-series data, the collected ECG signal is one-dimensional. Additionally, when considering noise generation, filtering and feature selection methods are involved in the preprocessing phase, it is essential to reconstruct the original input signal into two-dimensional data to ensure its integrity and avoid the data getting compromised [31]. Since the data are spatially distributed, the dimensional conversion is performed by formatting the initial dimension, which has a shape of AxB, into a new shape that represents a two-dimensional form of NxAxB, where A is the total samples, B is the features, and N is the number of channels involved.

Data Partition. According to the Pareto principle, the general rule of thumb is to fractionate the data into two subsets where the training and testing sets are divided into 80% and 20%, respectively [32]. However, an additional set is required to monitor the performance so that the system's hyperparameters can be tweaked and tuned to get a consistent outcome with miniature overfitting or underfitting. Thus, a validation set is considered as part of the partition strategy. The partition size for the training set is 70%, the validation set is 20%, and the testing set is 10%. It is also important to note that there were two separate datasets present, one for training and another for testing purposes explicitly. Each dataset is then concatenated and reshuffled afterward, then the partition procedure is applied. As a result, even though 10% for the test set might seem deficient on paper, but in contrast to the combined data, it is quantitative enough in this context (Fig. 5).

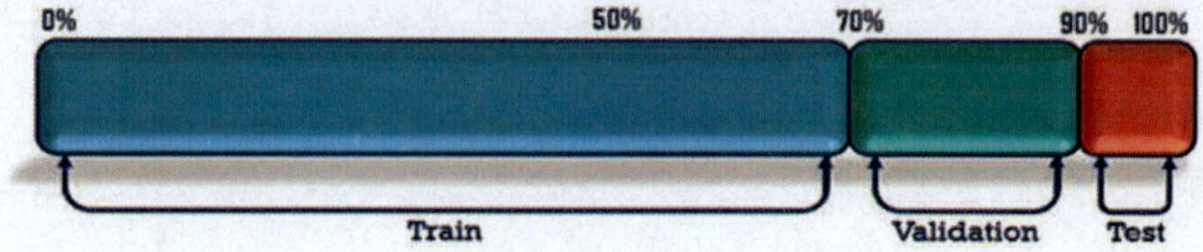

Fig. 5 Partition strategy for the data

3.4 Feature Selection

PCA is a widely used feature selection algorithm that benefits in identifying correct predictions and classifications [32]. The PCA is a technique used to reduce the dimensionality of the data to eliminate redundancy between the correlated data. It achieves by identifying the orthogonal of the entire input features, which are in linear combinations and combine them to form a new set of features that are smaller than the original size of the feature. Thus, reducing the computation power and time to train the model. In this study, the number of components is set to 50. Table 3 describes the computation time difference after applying PCA.

As displayed above, the model has 7.7% fewer parameters to deal with in the absence of hurting its overall accuracy. Additionally, while training without PCA, it takes about 262.5% more time than training time using PCA. Thus, the utilization of PCA makes the model quicker which is preferable when using it as a medical tool in realistic scenarios.

3.5 CNN-LSTM Network

The proposed model consists of five consecutive convolution layers, each with a single stride and a kernel size of five. Padding is applied to maintain the identical dimension as the input for the following convolution layers, which can be achieved by applying shorter length segments with zero padding. The number of filters for the first layer is 32, while the second and third layers include 64 filters and lastly, 128 for the fourth and fifth layers. A feature map can be obtained through the operation of convolving the input with the specified kernels or filters. For instance, considering

Table 3 Comparison of computational complexity

Comparison	Without PCA	With PCA
Input size	Nx187 × 32	Nx50 × 32
Total parameters	835,181	770,581
Average time per epoch	319 s	88 s
Time for 10 epochs	3194 s	909 s
Accuracy at 15th epoch	97.90%	97.78%

X as an input that comprises a list of n samples per beat, it can be expressed as:

$$X_i = [x_1, x_2, x_3, \ldots, x_n] \tag{1}$$

As a result, the output of a convolve operation can be stated as:

$$C_i^{L,j} = s\left(B_j + \sum_{f=1}^{F} W_f^j X_{i+f-1}^j\right) \tag{2}$$

where σ signifies the activation function, B_j is the bias for the jth feature map, L implies the index of the layer, and f represents the filter size [33]. The resultant convolution computation is then inserted into a leaky rectified linear unit (LReLU) activation function. A rectified linear unit (ReLU) can be applied to avoid the gradient from vanishing and can be less expensive computationally. However, LReLU solves a drawback that ReLU possesses where the weights for values less than zero stop adjusting during gradient descent and thus halts responding to error variations. This is known as a dying ReLU problem [34] which is why to avoid such impediments, LReLU is employed in this scenario and can be mathematically described as:

$$\sigma(z) = \begin{cases} z, z > 0 \\ \alpha z, z \leq 0 \end{cases} \tag{3}$$

Here, z is the variable that holds the convolved computations, α indicates the negative slope coefficient, and calculating σ *(z)* provides the subsequent feature map for the layer. The parameter is assigned as 0.001 for slope coefficient. Following the fifth convolutional layer, a subsampling layer is applied to reduce the input feature map of the preceding layer. This layer is known as max-pooling layer, which uses a max-pooling operation to fetch the maximum value and can be formulated as:

$$P_i^{L,j} = max\left(C_{i*S+r}^{L,j}\right); r \in R \tag{4}$$

where S represents the stride of the pooling layer and r dictates the size of the pooling. In this model, the strides for the max-pooling layer are two and the pool size designated is five. A dropout layer with a parameter of 0.45 is then followed afterward, which decides the activation of nodes during the training procedure on a dropout rate of 45%. The information is then directed to a series of LSTM layers. Figure 6 displays the hybrid architecture of the CNN-LSTM network. One limitation of using RNN is the appearance of exploding and vanishing gradients as the network migrates into the deep layers. LSTM helps by mitigating this problem as it can be used to regulate the amount of information the network can recollect over time. Thus, an LSTM layer is utilized in conjunction with the CNN layers. The extraction of spatial features is done by the series of convolution layers, while the succeeding LSTM

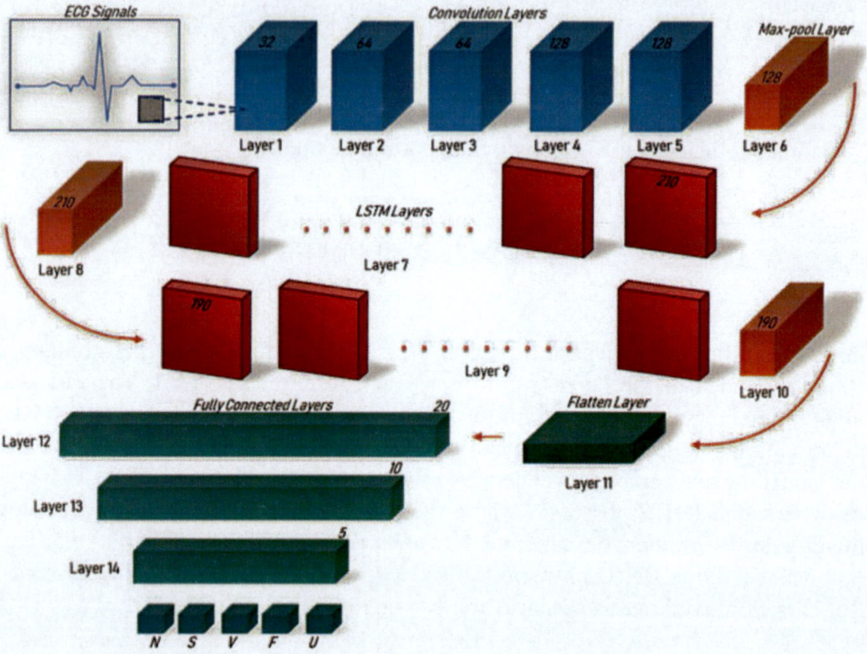

Fig. 6 An illustration of the proposed hybrid CNN-LSTM architecture

layers are used on the resulting feature maps to capture the temporal dynamics. A standard LSTM incorporates an input gate, output gate, a forget gate, and a cell, in which three of these gates regulate the flow of the information while the forget gate controls if the memory cell is reset to zero [35]. The activation for this gate L_t can be defined as:

$$L_t = \sigma(W\left[X_t,\ h_{t-1},\ C_{t-1}\right] + B_L) \tag{5}$$

where X_t represents the sequence of inputs, h_{t-1} can be dictated as the output of the previous block, C_{t-1} signifies the memory of the last LSTM block, W is the weights for each input, and lastly B_L is bias of the layer. The creation of new memory is attained by using a *tanh* activation function and the preceding memory of the blocks.

$$I_t = s\big(W\left[X_t,\ h_{t-1},\ C_{t-1}\right] + B_I\big) \tag{6}$$

$$C_t = L_t \odot C_{t-1} + I_t \odot tanh\left(\left[X_t,\ h_{t-1},\ C_{t-1}\right] + B_C\right) \tag{7}$$

$$s_t = s\big(W\left[X_t,\ h_{t-1},\ C_{t-1}\right] + B_0\big) \tag{8}$$

$$h_t = s_t \odot tanh\,(C_t) \tag{9}$$

Equations (6) and (7) are used for the calculation of the input operation and Eqs. (8) and (9) for the output operation [36], where I_t, C_t and σ_t represent the input gate, internal state and the output gate. Finally, h_t denotes the equivalent output.

Following each LSTM layer, another subsampling layer is implemented. The temporal sequence output of the individual LSTM layer is carried by the pooling layer which then, applies temporal Max-pooling and guides it to the subsequent layers. A flatten layer is used to perform a flattening operation that collapses the pooled feature map into a vector to be supplied into a series of fully connected layers. The data is compiled by extracting from the previous layer and then, process it by performing softmax operation in the final layer of the model, where probabilities for each of the classes are assigned to classify arrhythmia, which can be represented as 'N', 'S', 'V', 'F', or 'U'. Table 4 describes a detailed overview of the suggested structure.

However, overfitting can be a common issue as it can often result in poor performance when evaluating a particular model. As a result, three dropout regularization layers are employed to approximate training a comprehensive size of neural networks with various architectures. Dropout methods allow the training process to be noisy, forcing nodes in the layer to adjust probabilistically for the inputs and co-adapt in order to rectify mistakes from former layers [37]. Moreover, since portion of the output of a layer is affected by the dropout layer, it offers the effect of diminishing the capacity or reducing the size of the network during training. As a result, multiple schemes have been carried out for evaluation purposes. The dropout layer is utilized in plan A: one after the final convolution layer and two after each LSTM layer, whereas the model holds no dropout layer in plan B of the training procedure.

4 Result and Discussions

4.1 Simulation Specifications

All the aforementioned simulations are implemented using Python platform on Intel core-i7 processor with a memory of 16 gigabytes (GB) RAM and 500 GB solid-state drive (SSD) and are performed on a deep learning framework TensorFlow. In terms of graphics processing unit (GPU), NVIDIA GeForce RTX 2080 is used for the training operation.

Table 4 Detailed overview of the suggested architecture

Layers	Types	Activation	Filters	Kernel size	Strides	Output shape	Trainable parameters	Plan A	Plan B
0	Input	_	_	_	_	50 × 1	0	_	_
1	Conv1D	Leaky ReLU	32	5	1	50 × 32	192	_	_
2	Conv1D	Leaky ReLU	64	5	1	50 × 64	10,304	_	_
3	Conv1D	Leaky ReLU	64	5	1	50 × 64	20,544	_	_
4	Conv1D	Leaky ReLU	128	5	1	50 × 128	41,088	_	_
5	Conv1D	Leaky ReLU	128	5	1	50 × 128	82,048	Dropout 45%	_
6	Pool	_	128	5	2	25 × 128	0	_	_
7	LSTM	_	_	_	_	25 × 210	284,760	Dropout 45%	_
8	Pool	_	128	5	2	13 × 210	0	_	_
9	LSTM	_	_	_	_	13 × 190	304,760	Dropout 45%	_
10	Pool	_	128	5	2	7 × 190	0	_	_
11	Flatten	_	_	_	_	1330	0	_	_
12	Dense	ReLU	_	_	_	20	26,620	_	_
13	Dense	ReLU	_	_	_	10	210	_	_
14	Output	Softmax	_	_	_	5	55	_	_
Total trainable parameters							770,581		

4.2 Evaluation Measures

The performance of the model is examined at every epoch by using the criteria of precision (PR), sensitivity or recall (RC), f1-score (F1), and accuracy (ACC), which are determined based on true positive (TP), true negative (TF), false positive (FP), and false negative (FN), respectively. PR can be interpreted as positive predicted value, RC is the true positive rate, F1 is defined as the weighted average of the PR and RC values, and ACC is used to evaluate the model's overall performance. Whenever both the observation and prediction remain positive, TP is implied. On the contrary, TF is determined if both are concluded negative. Moreover, FP stands out if the observation is negative in contrast to the prediction being positive and similarly, FN is defined when the observation is positive but the prediction is negative. The equations for the metrics are stated as follows:

$$PR = \frac{TP}{TP + FP} * 100 \tag{10}$$

$$RC = \frac{TP}{TP + FN} * 100 \tag{11}$$

$$F1 = 2 * \frac{P * R}{P + R} * 100 \tag{12}$$

$$ACC = \frac{TP + TN}{TP + TN + FP + FN} * 100 \tag{13}$$

4.3 Performance Analysis

The experimental data in this work is derived from Physiobank (PTB) ECG database, where the partition size is 70%, 20%, and 10% for the training, validation, and testing set, respectively. Initially, the number of epochs used is 25, and an early stopping callback algorithm is applied to avoid overtraining the model, as soon as the degradation effect on the performance of the validation starts to form. One thing to note from Fig. 7 is the observation that beyond 15 epochs, the training accuracy continues to increase, however, the validation accuracy that begins to plateau.

The comparison in performance between plans A and B as illustrated in Fig. 7 is from using denoised signals data. In plan A, dropout regularization is implemented with a dropout rate of 0.45, as a result, 45% of information will be discarded, while the rest 55% will be retained. In plan B of the training procedure, no dropout regularization has been implemented, implying there will be no information loss during the entire training session.

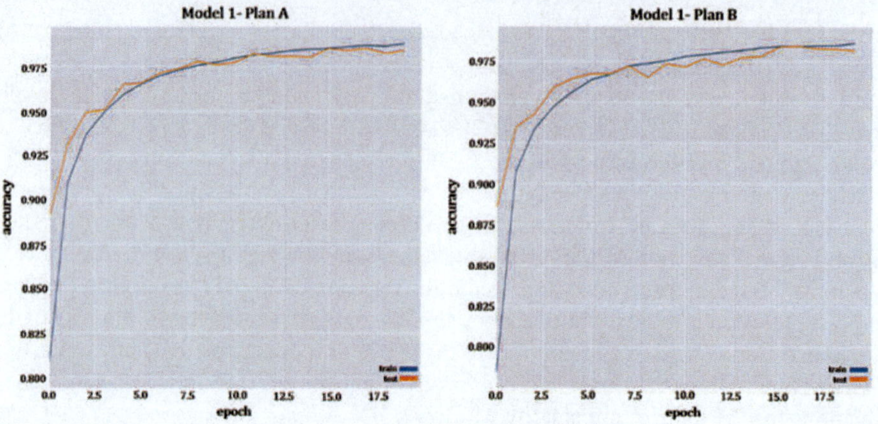

Fig. 7 Accuracy comparison of the models using denoised signals

From Fig. 8, it can be noticed that the validation accuracy of the model without dropout (plan B) starts to deteriorate faster than the model using dropout regularization. Thus, the training phase is stopped earlier than other comparative models. Nevertheless, the accuracy remains consistent across the entire models, obtaining around 98% to 99% accuracy overall. Tables 5 and 6 describe the accuracy of both the models for multiple experimental plans.

From Table 5, the overall PR, RC, F1, and ACC each show 99% when using dropout regularization, whereas each presents 98% when dropout is completely dismissed from the training model, depicting a reduction of accuracy by 1% when contrasted with plan A of the model. However, from Table 6, it can be interpreted that the presence of dropout does not affect the scores whatsoever when noise-generated data is applied. Figure 9 represents the confusion matrix of the models using separate datasets.

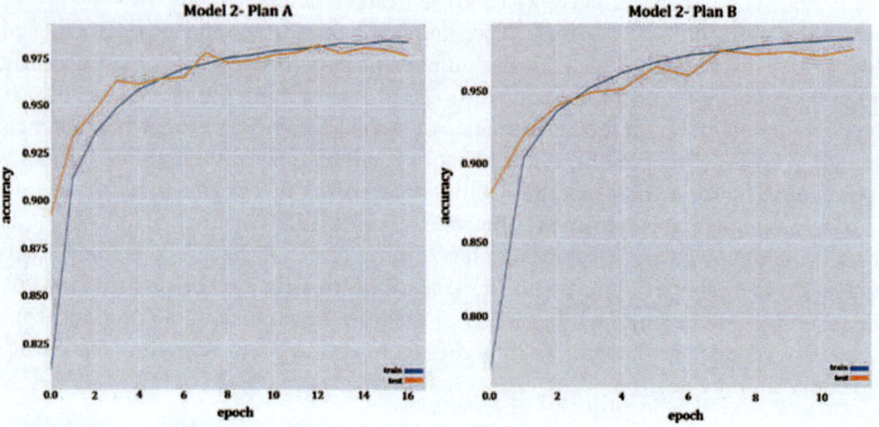

Fig. 8 Accuracy comparison of the models using noisy signals

Table 5 Classification performance for denoised signals

Classes	PR (%)		RC (%)		F1 (%)	
	Plan A	Plan B	Plan A	Plan B	Plan A	Plan B
N	98	98	96	95	97	96
S	98	98	99	99	98	98
V	98	98	99	98	98	98
F	99	98	100	100	100	99
U	100	100	99	100	100	100
Macroaverage (%)	99	98	99	98	99	98
Weighted average (%)	99	98	99	98	99	98
ACC (%)					99	98

Table 6 Classification performance for noise-generated signals

Classes	PR (%)		RC (%)		F1 (%)	
	Plan A	Plan B	Plan A	Plan B	Plan A	Plan B
N	93	96	96	95	95	95
S	98	97	97	99	98	98
V	99	98	97	98	98	98
F	98	99	98	98	98	99
U	100	100	99	99	99	99
Macroaverage (%)	98	98	98	98	98	98
Weighted average (%)	98	98	98	98	98	98
ACC (%)					98	98

In Model 1, approximately 3.81% of class 'N' fragments are misclassified, while model 2 has only 3.58% misclassifications. The best-predicted fragments for model 1 are Class 'F' as 99.7% are correctly predicted, which is a 1.36% improvement from model 2's classification for class 'F'. On the other hand, the best prediction accuracy for the second model would be class 'U' segments that have a misclassified segment of only 0.98%. However, in contrast to model 1's accuracy over class 'U', it performs 2.46% better making it the largest difference for the entire class. Despite having a comparatively bad result from model 2 when compared to model 1, it still manages to generalize considerably well, as the discrepancy between the two models is just 1%, demonstrating an overall robust representation for the entire architecture. The concept of extracting spatial features by CNN and selection of temporal dynamics by LSTM over a deep network serves strongly when compared to some of the prior mentioned ML and DL algorithms, making the proposed model remarkably consistent, as it succeeds to perform adequately when additional artificially generated noise is applied to the existing raw dataset, possessing the potential to be adopted in practical scenarios in various medical examinations.

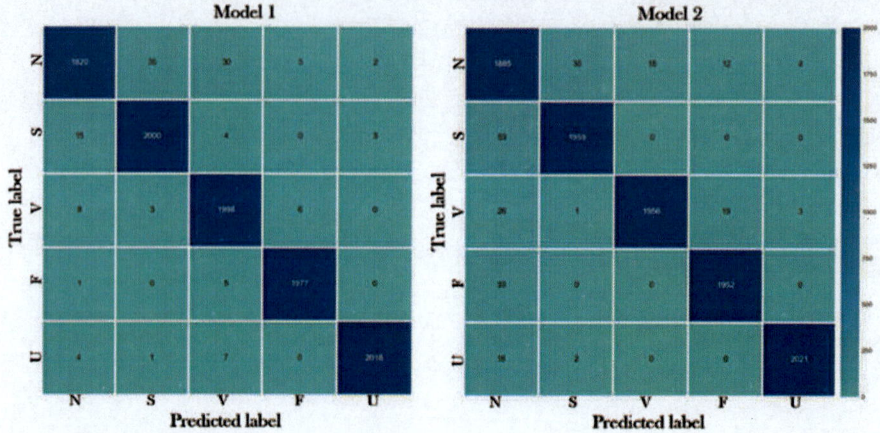

Fig. 9 Confusion matrix for the classified segments

5 Conclusion and Future Work

Identification and detection of arrhythmia are a critical step in the diagnosis of cardiovascular illnesses for diminishing the frequency of heart disease. This paper proposes an efficient computer-aided diagnosis system that encompasses a feature selection algorithm PCA and a classification technique based on CNN + LSTM network structure to accurately identify five fragments of arrhythmia ailments. One-dimensional signals acquired from ECG Physiobank (PTB) database are synthesized to create multiple instances for evaluating the model's performance under various circumstances. The accuracy of using smooth and denoised signals achieved 99% while the accuracy of using artificially generated noise signals achieved 98%, confirming a satisfactory and consistent generalization performance and could be a convenient tool for assisting clinicians to diagnose cardiovascular disease and reduce their workload significantly. Future work includes redesigning a simple but effective hybrid network structure without jeopardizing the accuracy. Furthermore, a transfer learning technique is strategized so that the necessary knowledge learned for arrhythmia detection from the hybrid architecture can be transferred for the identification of myocardial infarction which would be extremely beneficial in the field of medical science.

References

1. United Nation: Department of Economic and Social Affairs. Population Division. World Population Ageing: Highlights (ST/ESA/SER.A/430) (2019)
2. Zile M, Brutsaert D (2002) New concepts in diastolic dysfunction and diastolic heart failure: Part I: diagnosis, prognosis, and measurements of diastolic function. Circulation 105:1387–1393. American Heart Association

3. Thrainsdottir I, Hardarson T, Thorgeirsson G, Sigvaldason H, Sigfusson N (1993) The epidemiology of right bundle branch block and its association with cardiovascular morbidity—the reykjavik study. Eur Heart J 14(12):1590–1596. Oxford Academic
4. Fahy G, Pinski S, Miller D, McCabe N, Pye C, Walsh M, Robinson K (1996) Natural history of isolated bundle branch block. Am J Cardiol 77(14):1185–1190. ScienceDirect
5. Lown B, Wolf M (1971) Approaches to sudden death from coronary heart disease. Circulation 44(1):130–142. American Heart Association
6. Engström G, Hedblad B, Juul-Möller S, Tydén P, Janzon L (2000) Cardiac arrhythmias and stroke. Stroke 31(12):2925. National Library of Medicine
7. de Chazal P, O'Dwyer M, Reilly RB (2004) Automatic classification of heartbeats using ECG morphology and heartbeat interval features. Trans Biomed Eng 51(7):1196–1206. IEEE
8. Esteva A, Robicquet A, Ramsundar B, Kuleshov V, DePristo M, Chou K, Cui C, Corrado G, Thrun S, Dean J (2019) A guide to deep learning in healthcare. Nat Med 25(1). ResearchGate
9. For the Advancement of Medical Instrumentation, A.: Testing and reporting performance results of cardiac rhythm and ST segment measurement algorithms. 4301 N. Fairfax Dr., Suite 301. American National Standards Institute (2013)
10. Kohli N, Verma NK, Roy A (2010) SVM based methods for arrhythmia classification in ECG. In: International conference on computer and communication technology (ICCCT). IEEE
11. Kohli N, Verma NK (2011) Arrhythmia classification using SVM with selected features. Int J Eng Sci Technol 3(8). African Journals Online
12. Desai U, Martis RJ, Nayak CG, Sarika K, Seshikala G (2015) Machine intelligent diagnosis of ECG for arrhythmia classification using DWT, ICA and SVM techniques. In: Annual IEEE India conference (INDICON). IEEE
13. Gao D, Madden M, Chambers D, Lyons G (2005) Bayesian ANN classifier for ECG arrhythmia diagnostic system: a comparison study. In: Proceedings. IEEE international joint conference on neural networks. IEEE
14. Jadhav S, Nalbalwar SL, Ghatol A (2012) Artificial neural network models based cardiac arrhythmia disease diagnosis from ECG signal data. Int J Comput Appl 44(15):8–13. ResearchGate
15. Zuo WM, Lu WG, Wang KQ, Zhang H (2008) Diagnosis of cardiac arrhythmia using kernel difference weighted KNN classifier. In: Computers in cardiology. IEEE
16. Yang F, Du J, Lang J, Lu W, Liu L, Jin C, Kang Q (2020) Missing value estimation methods research for arrhythmia classification using the modified kernel difference-weighted KNN algorithms. BioMed Res Int: 1–9. Hindawi
17. Lodhi AM, Qureshi AN, Sharif U, Ashiq Z (2018) A novel approach using voting from ECG leads to detect myocardial infarction. In: Proceedings of SAI intelligent systems conference, IntelliSys: intelligent systems and applications. Springer, pp 337–352
18. Yıldırım Ö, Pławiak P, Tan R-S, Acharya UR (2018) Arrhythmia detection using deep convolutional neural network with long duration ECG signals. In: Computers in biology and medicine. ScienceDirect
19. Acharya UR, Fujita H, Oh SL, Hagiwara Y, Tan JH, Adam M (2017) Application of deep convolutional neural network for automated detection of myocardial infarction using ECG signals. Inf Sci: 415–416, 190–198. ResearchGate
20. Kachuee M, Fazeli S, Sarrafzadeh M (2018) ECG heartbeat classification: a deep transferable representation. In: IEEE international conference on healthcare informatics (ICHI). IEEE
21. Li F, Liu M, Zhao Y, Kong L, Dong L, Liu X, Hui M (2019) Feature extraction and classification of heart sound using 1D convolutional neural networks. EURASIP J Adv Sig Process (1):59. Springer
22. Baloglu UB, Talo M, Yildirim O, Tan RS, Acharya UR (2019) Classification of myocardial infarction with multi-lead ECG signals and deep CNN. In: Pattern recognition letters. ScienceDirect
23. Yin W, Kann K, Yu M, Schütze H (2017) Comparative study of CNN and RNN for natural language processing. ResearchGate

24. Singh S, Pandey SK, Pawar U, Janghel RR (2018) Classification of ECG arrhythmia using recurrent neural networks. Procedia Comput Sci 132:1290–1297. ScienceDirect
25. Schwab P, Scebba GC, Zhang J, Delai M, Karlen W (2017) Beat by beat: classifying cardiac arrhythmias with recurrent neural networks. In: Computing in cardiology conference (CinC). IEEE
26. Limam M, Precioso F (2017) AF detection and ECG classification based on convolutional recurrent neural network. In: 2017 computing in cardiology conference (CinC). IEEE
27. Goldberger AL, Amaral LAN, Glass L, Hausdorff JM, Ivanov PC, Mark RG, Stanley HE (2000) PhysioBank, PhysioToolkit, and PhysioNet: components of a new research resource for complex physiologic signals. Circulation 101(23):e215–e220. American Heart Association
28. Chawla NV, Bowyer KW, Hall LO, Kegelmeyer WP (2002) SMOTE: synthetic minority over-sampling technique. J Artif Intell Res 16(1):321–357. ResearchGate
29. Scholkmann F, Boss J, Wolf M (2012) An efficient algorithm for automatic peak detection in noisy periodic and quasi-periodic signals. Algorithms 5(4):588–603. MDPI
30. Gent PV, Farah H, Nes NV, Arem BV (2018) Analysing noisy driver physiology real-time using off-the-shelf sensors: heart rate analysis software from the taking the fast lane project. ResearchGate
31. Zheng Z, Chen Z, Hu F, Zhu J, Tang Q, Liang Y (2020) An automatic diagnosis of arrhythmias using a combination of CNN and LSTM technology. Electronics 9(1):121. MDPI
32. Dunford R, Su Q, Tamang E (2014) The pareto principle. Plymouth Stud Sci 7(1):140–148. University of Plymouth
33. Zubair M, Kim J, Yoon C (2016) An automated ECG beat classification system using convolutional neural networks. In: 2016 6th international conference on IT convergence and security (ICITCS). ResearchGate
34. Lu L, Shin Y, Su Y, Karniadakis GE (2019) Dying ReLU and initialization: theory and numerical examples. Cornell University
35. Hochreiter S, Schmidhuber J (1997) Long short-term memory. Neural Comput 9(8):1735–1780. MIT Press Direct
36. Yildirim Ö (2018) A novel wavelet sequence based on deep bidirectional LSTM network model for ECG signal classification. Comput Biol Med 96:189–202. ScienceDirect
37. Srivastava N, Hinton G, Krizhevsky A, Sutskever I, Salakhutdinov R (2014) Dropout: a simple way to prevent neural networks from overfitting. Department of Computer Science, University of Toronto. Journal of Machine Learning Research

Design of Visual-Image Classifier for Web Application

Shivani and Nidhi Gaur

Abstract In this paper, a self-designed model is put forward, in which a web application architecture interrelates with a self-designed classification-based image-retrieval search algorithm for electronic commerce grocery stores. This developed model for reference is named as "Search Images". The architecture of this model is designed in two segments—primarily the designing of convolutional neural network (CNN) and secondarily combining the CNN model with web application segment. Dataset of vegetables and fruits is used to train the CNN model also pre-processing, data augmentation, plots of training and testing of the model are obtained before assessing the accuracy of the designed model. Precise accuracies of the CNN model are obtained. This developed model makes use of a forward-thinking technological method which automatically classifies and retrieves the picture of desired vegetable and fruit commodity on the web application with the assistance of this designed visual-image search engine. This advanced visual search engine eradicates the requirement of manual grocery search in the web application. This model can classify 131 classes of fruits and vegetables based on the selected dataset. This paper encompasses the methodology and description for designing this search engine applying visual-image classifier.

Keywords Image processing · Visual-image search · Object recognition · Classification algorithm · Convolutional neural network · Vegetables classifier · Fruits classifier

Shivani (✉) · N. Gaur
Department of Electronics and Communication Engineering, Amity School of Engineering and Technology, Amity University Uttar Pradesh, Noida, India

N. Gaur
e-mail: ngaur@amity.edu

N. Marriwala et al. (eds.), *Emergent Converging Technologies and Biomedical Systems*, Lecture Notes in Electrical Engineering 841,
https://doi.org/10.1007/978-981-16-8774-7_33

1 Introduction

Marketing of groceries by the means of electronic commerce medium is levelling up immensely in recent times, and it also has been distinguished that for the reason that coronavirus disease-19 epidemic, there is a hastened change of consumers and vendors in the direction of electronic shopping [1, 2]. Grocery products are catalogued under everyday essential requirements for the population. In a contemporary digital survey stipulates that more than half of the consumers get hold of grocery products over the electronic commerce web application because of convenience and also occasionally disregard the charge [3]. This developed visual-image navigation engine for grocery products reinforces the local fruits and vegetables vendors extensively as they obligatory required to close down their shops or take it frontward through online approach amid the inflicted lockdown attributable to epidemic [4]. Mainstream of the population is taking apprehension about the origination of the fruits and vegetables, and so the inflated requests for organically harvested groceries are significantly multiplying which has identified boost among regional vendors. Present time search engines work with text query algorithms to come up with navigation results in web applications. The considerable restrictive characteristic of this manual product navigation primarily is that the information of the grocery product is being navigated by the consumer. The probability of a particular grocery item being precisely navigated in search engine by the way of text query is comparatively less than comparing it to the navigation in the search engines through an image, and the grounds in arrears are that the information confined in images is high and precise than text and so it assists in retrieving the grocery product efficiently and accurately [5]. Designing this model encompasses the integration of CNN architecture which has been verified to accomplish the multi-class classification of vegetables and fruits, to the web application to execute the visual classification of the grocery products [6].

2 Literature Review

Retail commerce in the present time has surface to be mainspring for object recognition and classification in supporting the advanced guard technologies, for example, implementation of image classification, object recognition and artificial intelligence in electronics commerce web application province. Mentioned domains provide multitudinous applications in web application architectures, navigation algorithm which is one of them [7]. For categorization of fruits and vegetables of single category with several classes in it, supervised learning procedure is used in the designed convolutional neural network model [8]. In the structure of this designed visual-image navigation algorithm for web application, two architectures are incorporated for fully functioning of model [9], and primary section comprises of a server end architecture designed with the support of Python's substructures—Rest and Django [10]. In the secondary section, client end which is the user/consumer side of this application manages the web application demonstrates data-specific information according to consumers provided input. Both image classification and electronic commerce web applications have significant demand in technological sector [11] in several provinces such as commercial, on public enterprise scale, private corporations along with others [12]. Designed search engine model can retrieve and categorize groceries of multi-class vegetables and fruits in web application architecture [13].

3 Contribution

This designed grocery product navigation algorithm accomplishes the function of visual-image search in electronic commerce web applications. Designed model can categorize and retrieve fruit and vegetable products in web application by selecting/uploading the picture of the desired grocery using the search engine window. This model eradicates the requirement of consumers to navigate the grocery items by smearing manual effort which is via typing the text and navigating in web application. While traditional search algorithms can mislead in product navigation sometimes in case of lack of product information, since this model provides navigation through picture of product, this lessens the probability of mislead in product search in web application. The existing local grocery ecommerce web applications do not contribute extensively in the domain of automatic/visual product navigation. This project connects this gap by developing an innovative design solution.

4 Designed Model

4.1 Design

A visual-image navigation model is designed to classify/categorize the grocery products—vegetables and fruits on web application. Programming segment is operated on visual studio code-editor tool and simulated utilizing windows terminal- power shell which allows to execute the programming codes through web browser- Google chrome and these tools befit for graphic image classification algorithms. The convolutional neural network prototype is combined with architecture of Django. Before integration, CNN prototype is trained on dataset and is acquired from Kaggle. Dataset is Fruits-360 of version 0.18.05.2020, and it is applied to compute the accuracy of training and accuracy of validation of the model. For training of data, overall quantity of images in the dataset is 90483. Training group has 67,692 pictures, and testing group has 22,688 pictures with one fruit or vegetable per image. It also has multi-fruit group having 103 pictures with more than one fruit each image. Dimension of all picture is [100 × 100] pixels. In succeeding phase, designing of web application with

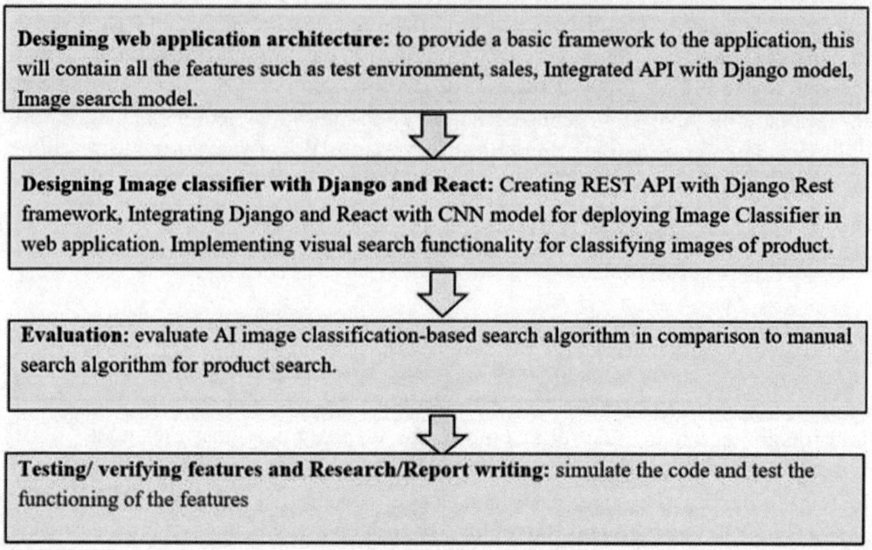

Fig. 1 Steps involved in designing fruits and vegetable image classifier

visual-image navigation engine. This CNN model is set aside in (.h5) arrangement and then is integrated with the web architecture which is discussed further. Figure 1 mentioned below designates the stages involving the designing procedure.

Designed web architecture functions on the interior of browser google chrome via uploading components in asynchronous technique while swapping information without simulating web-page screen. With assistance of application programmable interface (API), interaction between client end and server end is carried out, such as saving the picture information into database. Presentation and configuration of designed interface are performed across local server by means of http with certain distinct instructions. The architecture of client end comprises a rectangular design of picture drop window with magenta pink outline, and this visual grocery navigation engine specifies "Shivani drag n drop some files here, or click to select files" implying consumer has to search for grocery products from this section. Continuing in this section, this web architecture has navigation segment, having home page which is the product navigation page (navbar), it similarly has a section that shows picture or classification search history named as "Images". Moreover, client end section includes picture selection click-button, loader (spins while the picture uploads or result awaits). To extent this web architecture for consumer application across digital phone or electronic gadgets, designing of server end with a functioning constricted application programmable end-user interface is implemented. This section assists with consumer information such as signing in/signing out process, and it executes transaction of picture information with database when required. This section stores the picture classification details in database as well, for instance, classification status, date, product detail, time.

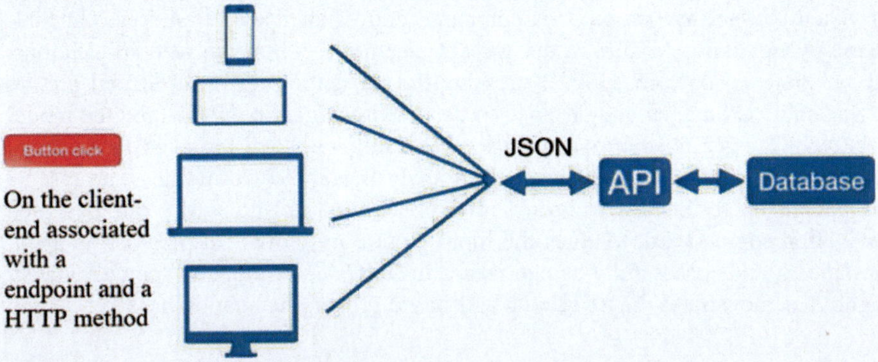

Fig. 2 Working scheme of visual-image navigation

4.2 *Working of Model*

Designing a web architecture with visual picture grocery navigation, server end (back end) is implemented utilizing- Django, rest substructure and client/consumer end (front end) is based on java-script substructure- react combined with rest interface. The CNN architecture is formed by stacking all the layers. The consumer end gets hold of input picture of desired fruit and vegetable from consumer and transfers it to the server end of Django's local server, then designed local server reserves the picture in its database and exchanges the address of the picture to the image classifier. The image classifier (designed CNN architecture) then generates the outcome, saves it in the database and then transfers it to the client end to render the result to the consumer. Figure 2 shows the functioning arrangement of this designed model. The consumer has to login to this grocery web application, "drag and drop or upload" the fruit/vegetable they require to purchase, then this designed visual-image navigation engine will classify the consumer's input image and display the navigated grocery item.

5 Results and Analysis

A visual grocery product navigation engine for web application architecture is designed by integrated CNN structure with web application architecture, which can categorize of 90,483 pictures of fruits and vegetables that are allocated into 131 groups. Evaluation of this model is accomplished by visually navigating and categorizing grocery products. Classification or product navigation accuracy is regulated by implemented CNN architecture, which delivers the training–accuracy of 99.14% and validation–accuracy of 96.06%. Designed model can successfully navigate and classify fruits and vegetables in web application architecture. Afterwards evaluation of visual product navigation, it is compared and equated with traditional manual-search navigation algorithm in the present electronic commerce web applications. Above attached outcome, Fig. 3 presents the navigation result, a desired picture of vegetable is dragged and dropped in designed navigation engine, and the model positively categorizes the input picture as "cauliflower" and retrieved its evidence on the web application. Another result of analysis is indicated in Fig. 4, it presents the navigation result of a fruit, a picture is selected and uploaded, this designed navigation engine acknowledges the input picture by individual pixel component, classifies it and successfully categorizes it in fruit picture input as "pomegranate". Figure 5 demonstrates the traditional text-based grocery navigation in self-designed

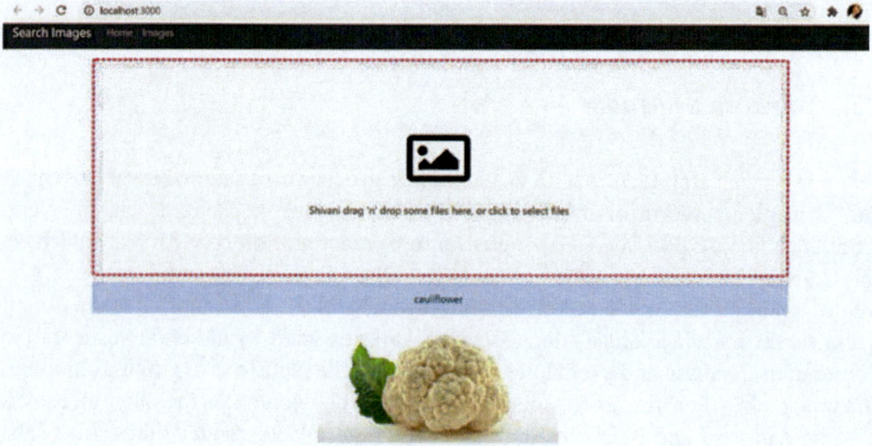

Fig. 3 Classification outcome of vegetable

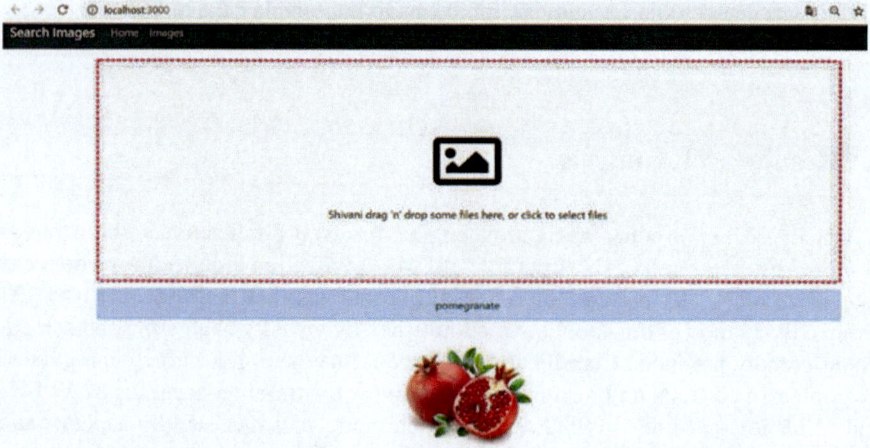

Fig. 4 Classification outcome of fruit

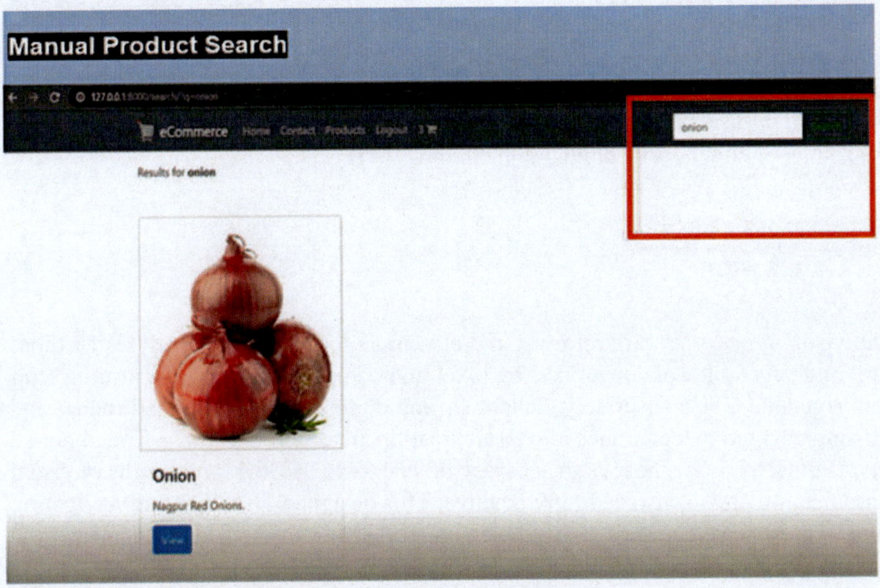

Fig. 5 Traditional manual navigation technique

web architecture, and Fig. 6 represents our recommended designed grocery picture retrieval and classification model for web application. This model has home page, navigation history page and consumers admin architecture for client applications.

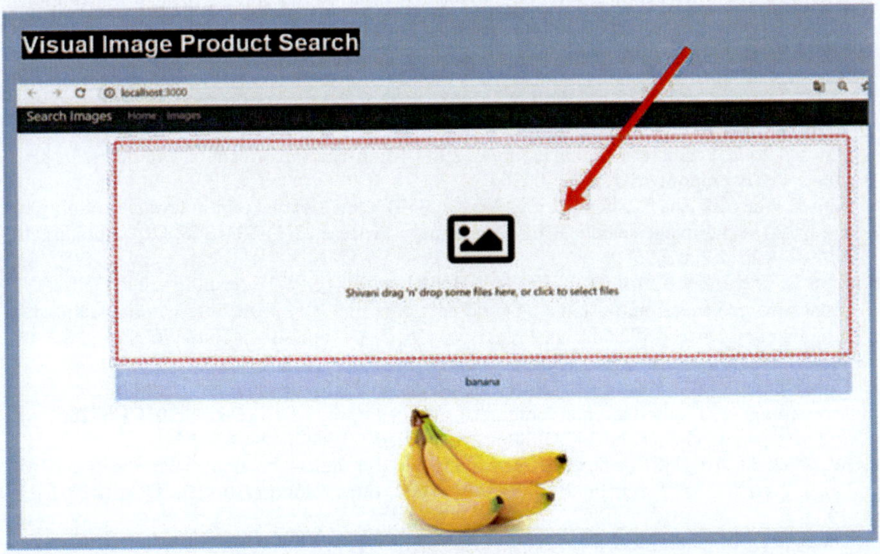

Fig. 6 Suggested visual-image navigation technique

Afterwards, comparison between traditional text grounded manual grocery navigation and designed visual picture-based grocery navigation is performed. The outcome turns out to be in approbation of visual navigation technique subsequently evaluating and determining advantages and drawbacks of both navigation techniques for grocery electronic commerce web application architectures.

6 Conclusion

The visual grocery picture retrieval and classification model can analyse the input fruit and vegetables pictures pixel by pixel and can represent the conforming fruit and vegetable labels accurately. Outcomes and comparison of designed model and existing navigation techniques in web application are discussed above. The obtained results of CNN model have high accuracy of 99.14 and 96.06%, and results of visual classification are also exceedingly positive. This designed visual picture navigation model can be scaled up and can be implemented separately or in addition with manual grocery product navigation technique in web applications.

References

1. Martin-Neuninger R, Ruby MB (2020) What does food retail research tell us about the implications of coronavirus (COVID-19) for grocery purchasing habits? Front Psychol 1:1448. https://doi.org/10.3389/fpsyg.2020.01448. PMID: 32581987; PMCID: PMC7292029
2. Krizhevsky A, Sutskever I, Hinton GE (2019) Imagenet classification with deep convolutional neural networks. Commun ACM 60(6):84–90
3. Xie B, Charness N, Fingerman K, Kaye J, Kim MT, Khurshid A (2020) When going digital becomes a necessity: ensuring older adults' needs for information, services, and social inclusion during COVID-19. J Aging Soc Policy 32:4–5, 460–470.https://doi.org/10.1080/08959420.2020.1771237
4. Hsu YC, Lv Z, Schlosser J, Odom P, Kira Z (2019) Multi-class classification without multi-class labels. arXiv preprint arXiv:1901.00544
5. Gao Y, Wang M, Zha Z, Shen J, Li X, Wu X (2013) Visual-textual joint relevance learning for tag-based social image search. IEEE Trans Image Process 22(1):363–376. https://doi.org/10.1109/TIP.2012.2202676
6. Shin D, Lee J, Lee J, Yoo H (2017) 14.2 DNPU: an 8.1TOPS/W reconfigurable CNN-RNN processor for general-purpose deep neural networks. In: 2017 IEEE international solid-state circuits conference (ISSCC). San Francisco, CA, USA, pp 240–241https://doi.org/10.1109/ISSCC.2017.7870350
7. Chen Y, Zhou XS, Huang TS (2001) One-class SVM for learning in image retrieval. In: Proceedings 2001 international conference on image processing (Cat. No.01CH37205), vol 1. Thessaloniki, Greece, pp 34–37. https://doi.org/10.1109/ICIP.2001.958946
8. Wei Y et al (2016) HCP: a flexible CNN framework for multi-label image classification. IEEE Trans Pattern Anal Mach Intell 38(9):1901–1907. https://doi.org/10.1109/TPAMI.2015.2491929
9. Dharani T, Aroquiaraj IL (2013) A survey on content-based image retrieval. In: 2013 international conference on pattern recognition, informatics and mobile engineering. Salem, India, pp 485–490. https://doi.org/10.1109/ICPRIME.2013.6496719

10. Ben-Haim N, Babenko B, Belongie S (2006) Improving web-based image search via content based clustering. In: 2006 conference on computer vision and pattern recognition workshop (CVPRW'06). New York, NY, USA, pp 106–106. https://doi.org/10.1109/CVPRW.2006.100
11. Chang S-F, Chen W, Meng HJ, Sundaram H, Zhong D (1998) A fully automated content-based video search engine supporting spatiotemporal queries. IEEE Trans Circuits Syst Video Technol 8(5):602–615. https://doi.org/10.1109/76.718507
12. Krapac J, Allan M, Verbeek J, Juried F (2010) Improving web image search results using query-relative classifiers. In: 2010 IEEE computer society conference on computer vision and pattern recognition. San Francisco, CA, USA, pp 1094–1101. https://doi.org/10.1109/CVPR.2010.5540092
13. Cui M, Hu S (2011) Search engine optimization research for website promotion. In: 2011 international conference of information technology, computer engineering and management sciences. Nanjing, China, pp 100-103.https://doi.org/10.1109/ICM.2011.308

A Comparative Analysis of Different Despeckling Filters Using Breast Ultrasonographic Images

Priyanshu Tripathi, Rajeshwar Dass, and Jyotsna Sen

Abstract Speckle noise is inherently present in breast ultrasonographic images, and it degrades the overall visual quality of these images which leads to complex interpretation and misdiagnosis of breast abnormalities. Hence to diminish its effect, different despeckling filters are employed. The breast ultrasonographic images are filtered using different despeckling filters, which are classified into two categories as linear despeckling filters and nonlinear despeckling filters. The performance of these despeckling filters is determined by computing PSNR, MSE, and SNR. Result of performance assessment indicates that Lee Sigma filter yields highest value of PSNR, SNR, and lowest value of MSE in linear category while SRAD filter yields highest value of PSNR, SNR and lowest value of MSE in nonlinear category and hence more suitable for despeckling of breast ultrasonographic images.

Keywords Speckle noise · Despeckling filters · Breast ultrasonographic images · SNR · PSNR · MSE

1 Introduction

Ultrasonographic imaging technique is widely employed in diagnosis of medical field due to its non-invasive property, lower cost, easily available, and non-radiant. Ultrasonography is used to capture real-time images of human body organs using sound wave having frequency greater than 20 kHz [1]. The visual quality of ultrasonographic images is highly desirable feature to detect any abnormal growth present in the inner part of breast. Speckle noise diminishes the visual quality of ultrasonographic images and leads to inaccurate diagnosis [2, 3]. Hence to diminish the effect of speckle noise, different despeckling filters are used [4].

P. Tripathi (✉) · R. Dass
D.C.R.U.S.T, Murthal, Haryana, India

J. Sen
PGIMS, Rohtak, Haryana, India

N. Marriwala et al. (eds.), *Emergent Converging Technologies and Biomedical Systems*, Lecture Notes in Electrical Engineering 841,
https://doi.org/10.1007/978-981-16-8774-7_34

Different linear and nonlinear despeckle filtering algorithms are implemented to reduce the effect of speckle noise. The assessment of different despeckling filters has been done by computing different performance evaluation parameters, e.g., signal-to-noise ratio (SNR), mean square error (MSE), peak signal-to-noise ratio (PSNR).

2 Methodology

2.1 Dataset

In this work, 25 benign and 25 malignant breast ultrasonographic images are utilized from benchmark dataset BUSI [5] and the filters are implemented using MATLAB.

2.2 Despeckling Techniques

Despeckling is a term which is used to reduce speckle noise. The despeckling algorithms can be classified into two main categories as linear despeckling filters and nonlinear despeckling filters as shown in Fig. 1.

2.3 Linear Despeckling Filters

Linear filters are based on equation which is given as

$$X_{\text{denoised}} = \overline{g_{s,t}} + \omega_{s,t}(g_{s,t} - \overline{g_{s,t}}) \quad (1)$$

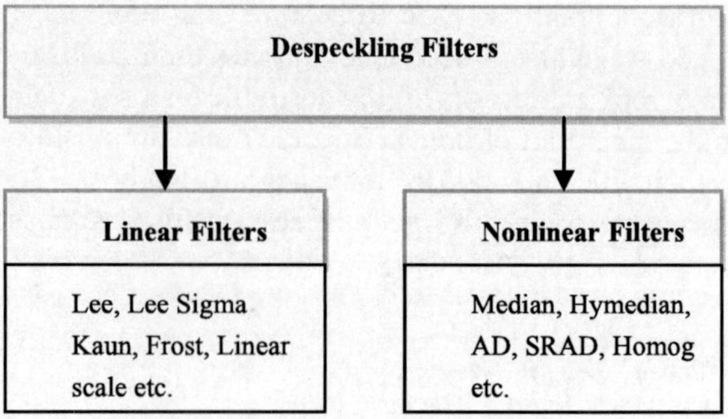

Fig. 1 Different despeckling filters

$g_{s,t}$ represents pixel value having noise, $\overline{g_{s,t}}$ represents mean pixel value, $X_{denoised}$ represents pixel value after filtering operation, and $\omega_{s,t}$ represents weighing factor, and s, t are coordinates of the pixel.

Lee [6], Kaun [7], Frost [8], Lee sigma, and linear scale filters are classified as linear filter [9].

2.4 Nonlinear Despeckling Filters

In this category, nonlinear iterative type filters are used such as median, hybrid median (Hymedian), maximum homogeneity (Homog), anisotropic diffusion (AD), and SRAD filters [10–12]. Nonlinear filters use increased neighborhood size and complex computation in comparison of linear filters.

The breast ultrasonographic images after filtering operation are depicted in Fig. 2. Blocking effect is noticed in breast ultrasonographic images using linear filters, and slight blur is observed in breast ultrasonographic images using nonlinear filters. Preprocessing of breast US images diminishes the effect of speckle noise but also there is a loss of some texture features [13, 14].

3 Performance Assessment of Different Despeckling Filters

The performance assessment of different despeckling filters has been done by calculating PSNR, SNR, and MSE. The standard value of SNR and PSNR must be greater than 20 dB, and value of MSE must be as low as possible. Lower value of MSE implies high value of PSNR which is the desirable feature. As we know that higher the value of SNR and PSNR, lower will be noise. High value of SNR implies that noise level is very low and high value of PSNR implies excellent quality of image [15].

MSE can be computed as follows:

$$\mathrm{MSE} = \frac{1}{\mathrm{mn}} \sum_{\mathrm{i}=1}^{\mathrm{m}} \sum_{\mathrm{j}=1}^{\mathrm{n}} (\mathrm{g}(\mathrm{i}, \mathrm{j}) - \mathrm{h}(\mathrm{i}, \mathrm{j}))^2 \tag{2}$$

g(i, j) & h(i, j) represent original and despeckled image.

SNR can be computed as follows:

$$\mathrm{SNR} = \frac{\sum_{\mathrm{i}=1}^{\mathrm{m}} \sum_{\mathrm{j}=1}^{\mathrm{n}} \mathrm{h}_{\mathrm{i,j}}^2}{\sum_{\mathrm{i}=1}^{\mathrm{m}} \sum_{\mathrm{j}=1}^{\mathrm{n}} (\mathrm{g}(\mathrm{i}, \mathrm{j}) - \mathrm{h}(\mathrm{i}, \mathrm{j}))^2} \tag{3}$$

$g(i, j)$ & $h(i, j)$ represent original and despeckled image.

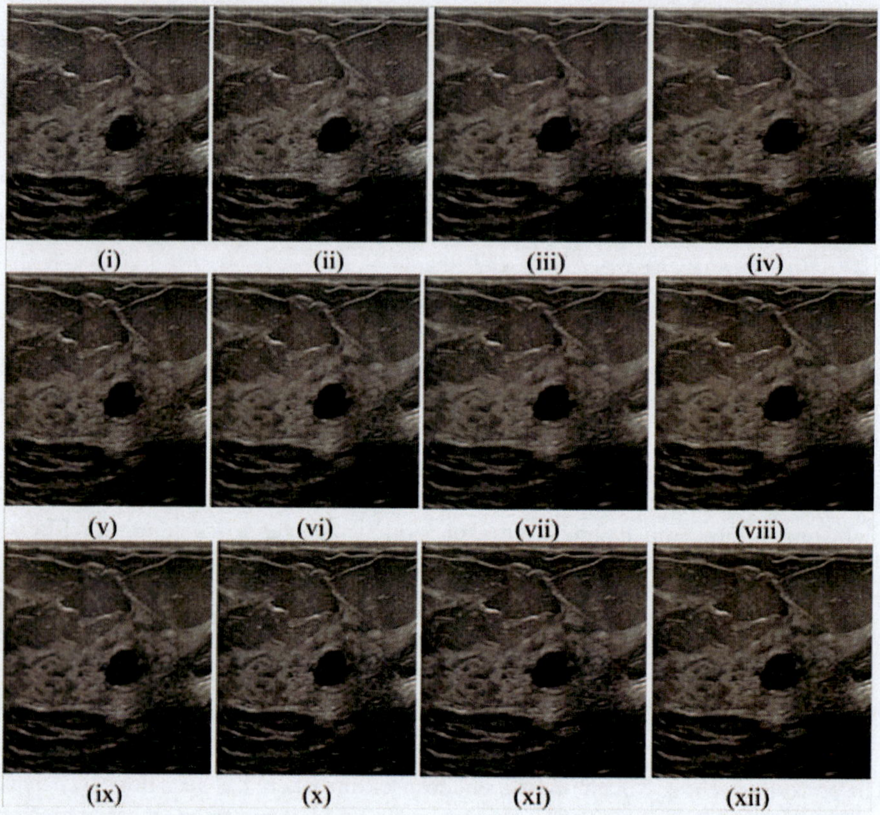

Fig. 2 Breast ultrasonographic images **i** original image, **ii** speckled image, image despeckled by **iii** lee filter, **iv** lee sigma filter, **v** frost filter, **vi** Kaun filter, **vii** linear scale, **viii** Homog filter, **ix** AD filter, **x** median filter, **xi** hymedian filter, **xii** SRAD filter

PSNR can be computed as follows:

$$\text{PSNR} = 20\log_{10}(255) - 10.\log_{10}(\text{MSE}) \tag{4}$$

MSE is mean squared error.

4 Results

The numeric values of MSE, SNR, and PSNR of different despeckle filters are computed using Eqs. 2, 3, and 4, respectively. The numeric value of different linear filters and nonlinear filters is given in Tables 1 and 2, respectively. The different values of SNR and PSNR of different linear as well as nonlinear filters are also represented graphically in Fig. 3.

Table 1 SNR, PSNR, and MSE values for ultrasonographic images using linear filters

Filter	SNR(dB)	PSNR(dB)	MSE
Lee	22.85	31.60	89.82
Kuan	21.38	30.14	125.81
Frost	21.69	30.43	117.68
Lee Sigma	**22.97**	**31.74**	**86.99**
Linear scale	21.77	30.48	116.25

Table 2 SNR, PSNR, and MSE values for ultrasonographic images using nonlinear filters

Filter	SNR(dB)	PSNR(dB)	MSE
Hymedian	24.81	33.58	56.95
SRAD	**36.84**	**46.53**	**12.24**
AD	23.95	32.74	69.16
Homog	21.11	29.91	132.71
Median	22.76	31.53	91.30

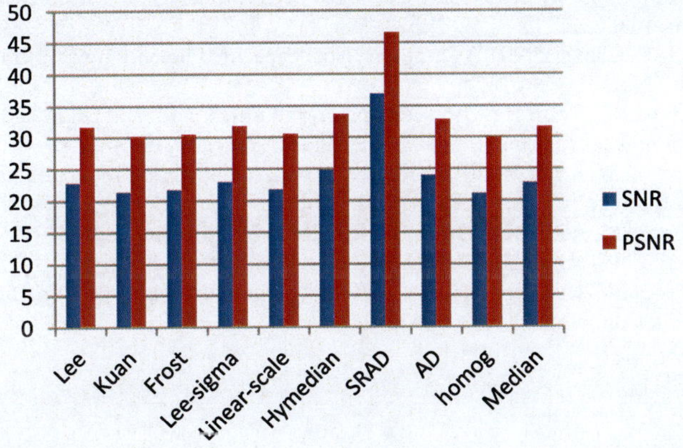

Fig. 3 SNR and PSNR values for breast ultrasonographic images using different filters

5 Conclusion

In the proposed work, the comparative analysis of different linear and nonlinear despeckling filters has been carried out on the basis of computation of MSE, SNR, and PSNR. As we know higher the value of SNR and PSNR, lower is noise and hence excellent quality of despeckled images. In linear category, Lee Sigma filter is considered as most effective filter since it has lowest value of MSE and highest value of SNR and PSNR and in nonlinear category, SRAD filter is considered as most appropriate filter since it has very low value of MSE and highest value of SNR and PSNR. Nonlinear filters have higher value of SNR and PSNR. High value of PSNR implies low value of mean squared error (MSE) and hence provides excellent quality.

References

1. Virmani J, Agarwal R (2019) Assessment of despeckle filtering algorithms for segmentation of breast tumours from ultrasound images. Biocybern Biomed Eng 39(1):100–121
2. Dass R (2018) speckle noise reduction of ultrasound images using BFO cascaded with wiener filter and discrete wavelet transform in homomorphic region. ICCIDS-2018. Procedia Comput Sci 132:1543–1551
3. Dass R, Devi S (2012) Effect of Wiener-Helstrom filtering cascaded with bacterial foraging optimization to despeckle the ultrasound images. Int J Comput Sci Issues (IJCSI) 9(4):372–392
4. Devi S, Dass R (2011) Speckle noise reduction techniques. IJEEE 16(1):47–57
5. https://scholar.cu.edu.eg/?q=afahmy/pages/dataset. Accessed 20 Jan 2021
6. Lee JS (1981) Speckle analysis and smoothing of synthetic aperture radar images. Comput Graph Image Process 17(1):24–32
7. Kuan DT, Sawchuk AA, Strand TC, Chavel P (1985) Adaptive noise smoothing filter for images with signal-dependent noise. IEEE Trans Pattern Anal Mach Intell 7(2):165–177
8. Frost VS, Stiles JA, Shanmugan KS, Holtzman JC (1982) A model for radar images and its application to adaptive digital filtering of multiplicative noise. IEEE Trans Pattern Anal Mach Intell 4(2):157–166
9. Osman FM, Yap MH (2018) The effect of filtering algorithms for breast ultrasound lesions segmentation. Inform Med Unlocked 12:14–20
10. Perona P, Malik J (1990) Scale-space and edge detection using anisotropic diffusion. IEEE Trans Pattern Anal Mach Intell 12(7):629–639
11. Zhang J, Wang C, Cheng Y (2014) Comparison of despeckle filters for breast ultrasound images. Circuits Syst Signal Process 1–24
12. Gupta D, Anand RS, Tyagi B (2015) Despeckling of ultrasound medical images using ripplet domain and nonlinear filtering. Signal, Image Video Process 9:1093–1100
13. Biradar N, Dewal M, Rohit M (2014) Edge preserved speckle noise reduction using integrated fuzzy filters. Int Scholarly Res Notices 1–11
14. Biradar N, Dewal M, Rohit M (2014) Speckle noise reduction using hybrid TMAV based fuzzy filter. Int J Res Eng Technol 3(3):113–118
15. Dass R, Yadav N (2020) Image quality assessment parameters for despeckling filters. ICCIDS-2019. Procedia Comput Sci 167:2382–2392

Sign Language Recognition Using Hand Mark Analysis for Vision-Based System (HMASL)

Akansha Tyagi and Sandhya Bansal

Abstract Sign language recognition (SLR) is an essential study area that allows us to provide a better communicating environment between humans and computers. Some prevailing and standard features extracted from sign language gestures include scale-invariant feature transform (SIFT), speeded-up robust feature (SURF), features from the accelerated segment (FAST), and oriented FAST and rotated Brief (ORB) are used. However, these element vectors contain a few highlights that are insignificant or excess, subsequently expanding the generally computational time just as acknowledgment error of a classification framework. To counter this issue, we have proposed another object detection calculation dependent on profound hand math. A novel approach called Hand mark analysis of sign language (HMASL) has been used in this concern. It combines the concept of feature extraction and hand geometry to reduce the computation and computes only and region in complex background. HMASL is compared to other classical feature extraction method and tested on several classifiers. The experimental results show that the HMASL eases the feature aspcct to a mcaningful amount as well as surges the recognition accuracy.

Keywords Indian sign language · Computer vision · Feature extraction · Hand geometry · Deep learning · SVM

1 Introduction

Sign language recognition (SLR) applies to many domains featured for the deaf-mute community. Even though various device-based recognition systems like sensors, gloves have been recently used, but vision-based recognition is more approachable. Vision-based recognition is becoming widespread due to the significant scope of application areas as found in the literature [1]. However, Indian Sign Language (ISL) comprises of 6000 words which are commonly used in Indian country.

A. Tyagi (✉) · S. Bansal
Department of Computer Science and Engineering, Maharishi Markandeshwar(Deemed to be) University, Ambala, Haryana, India

N. Marriwala et al. (eds.), *Emergent Converging Technologies and Biomedical Systems*, Lecture Notes in Electrical Engineering 841,
https://doi.org/10.1007/978-981-16-8774-7_35

SLR using machine learning and soft computing has been a ground of interest for a long time. Scientists have utilized a few methodologies and have made a ton of progress in preparing distinctive machine and profound learning models that can perceive signs comparing to various words. Most of the study that has been done is for American Sign Language (ASL), and the systems require the utilization of some sort of movement sensors or hand gloves to distinguish the places of various fingers precisely. The way that these methodologies are no uncertainty successful and can represent pretty much every sign, except these require the utilization of some exceptionally delicate equipment that cannot be utilized by everybody and commonly require explicit climate. Some different ways to deal with perceive communications through signing incorporate the utilization of deep learning models that work on skin enclosed images. Skin veiled pictures are framed by portioning out the part from the picture which coordinates with the shade of the skin. That area is given a particular tone (white), and all the rest pixels in the picture are doled out in another tone (dark). In such methodologies after skin veiling, significant highlights are extricated from the pictures utilizing a few strategies like SIFT, SURF, FAST, ORB, and profound learning models are prepared for arranging various signs. These methodologies have demonstrated to be quick progressively, yet the utilization of profound learning models requires the utilization of more assets, and they probably will not have the option to perform so well on basic devices having restricted resources [2–4].

The recent success of deep learning approaches in a task like an image classification [5] has been extended to the problem of sign language recognition [6]. Unlike other traditional soft computing methods such as neural network, KNN, or genetic algorithm (GA) where features were extracted manually, while neural network models learn features from the training database [7]. These networks save the spatial design of the issue and were created for object recognition roles, for example, manually written digit acknowledgment. They are famous because individuals are accomplishing cutting edge results on troublesome computer vision and normal language training tasks.

Another approach is that researchers have popularly started using this hand mark analysis methods; that is, hand geometry parameters are combined with graphical properties such as open pose and hand pose. The analysis of the shape and geometry of the hand provides the essential features of the hand. These methods have shown an impeccable result and giving an elevated recognition accuracy without using any sensor devices. These methods follow the state-of-the-art techniques, that is, to locate a set of essential key points representing the position of coordinates with the help of some neural network models. The sole issue with this technique is that even though it can work progressively, it requires a decent number of the dataset, and it gives a speed of 0.1 to 0.3 frames each second for the video input which is not acceptable in any way. It cannot handle outlines easily continuously.

Our methodology integrated the distances between the 0th central key point (the central key point at the extremely base in the palm) and the remainder of the 20 central key point as highlights. A hand geometry model is utilized to return the standardized directions for these central points; i.e., it returns the central key point by partitioning the x arranged by the width of the frame and y by the height of the frame, however, for a superior standardization, the new coordinates are determined by moving the root to the 0th point itself. Presently, we have the situation of central key points concerning the 0th central key points. Accordingly, the area of the hand will not have a lot of impact on the directions of these central features, and the model wants to deal with a broader scale.

This paper is composed of six sections: Sect. 2 discusses the literature review. Section 3 discusses the dataset used in this paper. Proposed work is discussed in Sect. 4. Experimental work and results are discussed in Sect. 5. Lastly, Sects. 6 and 7 highlight the conclusion and future scope of this work, respectively.

2 Literature Review

The communication between human beings is carried out in spoken form by speech and non-verbal through gestures. Generally, people make gestures either consciously or unconsciously while communicating with others. Non-verbal communication among the deaf and mute community is known as sign language. They use their two hands for making gestures to communicate among themselves. The sign language among the community who live in India is known as Indian Sign Language (ISL). ISL is composed of static and dynamic gestures precisely. Indian Sign Language recognition (ISLR) is a better approach for devolving a vision-based gesture recognition system that can help the above community to bridge the communication gap. The concept of computer vision has facilitated the ISLR area for research [8–10]. Various feature extraction and soft computing algorithms have been developed to train a model by using the above steps. Most of these techniques are deployed in content-based image retrieval (CBIR) features followed by classifier such as support vector machine (SVM) [11, 12], linear discriminant analysis (LDA) [13], neural network [14–16], and convolution neural network (CNN) [17–20].

In ISLR, the research work has undertaken from pre-processing of gestures to recognize gestures directly through CNN, while SIFT has evolved as the most promising technique in terms of feature extraction [21]. Here, [22] has used SIFT algorithm for feature detection and object matching on real-time images and achieved 60% more accurate results without performing pre-processing of images. To overcome the challenges in ISLR such as the requirement of constant illumination and wearing long attire sleeves for natural background constraint, an ISLR based on pixel-based segmentation and advanced SIFT is proposed [23]. Further, due to the invariant characteristic of SIFT, over-illumination, rotation, translation, scaling, and slightly to viewpoint [24] have implemented various phases of SIFT to extract features from ISL gestures. Each image has more than 400 features with the highest peak of 80% in the bag of visual words (BOG) providing a reliable matching between disrupted images. Instead of using conventional methods which take more computation time, an improved SIFT with a fuzzy closed-loop control method has been used for object recognition in the cluttered environment [3]. Another study [25] has elaborated on SIFT and CNN-based image retrieval processes and how they enhance the system's performance. CNN works on a large dataset and extracts features from images as by layers increase, but applying SIFT for refining of features reduces the model layers and improves accuracy in few epochs.

Bedregal et al. [26] used fuzzy for recognition of LIBRAS (Brazilian Sign Language) gestures. Hand gestures are classified using a set of angles of finger joints and their segmentation. A set of finite automata is created for the segmented gestures which are classified using fuzzy rule which enhances the classification accuracy of the system. Christian Zimmermann and Thomas Brox [27] uses a deep network for the classification of 3D hand pose using RGB pose estimation using low-cost customer depth cameras for 35 static German Sign Language (GSL) symbols. Albanie et al. [28] followed the co-articulation method to classify the British Sign Language (BSL) signs. A dataset of 1000 keywords in 1000 h of video is also created to automatically localize the sign-instances keywords. Kang et al. [29] proposed an efficient method using a depth map to recognize the fingerspelling gestures. Images were captured using the depth sensors following by some image pre-processing techniques that are then classified using the convolution neural network (CNN). The proposed system achieved an accuracy of 99.99%. Li et al. [30] proposed a vision-based sign language recognition system for 2000 words/glosses. Two deep learning models were approached, one is based on visual appearance, and another is based on a 2D human pose. The proposed model has achieved an accuracy of 62.63% at top-ten words.

From the literature survey, it can be concluded that hand mark analysis or hand geometry is an important part of the ISLR. Feature extraction and selection of essential key points considering redundancy and relevancy of features can do better performance. This has motivated us to develop hand mark analysis which can be hybridized with feature extraction technique FAST-SIFT to form HMASL. The evaluation of our HMASL model is done on several classification models.

3 Dataset and Pre-processing

Sign Language Dataset: The two-hand gesture ISL words (“afraid,” “agree,” “bad,” “become,” “chat,” “college,” “from,” “today,” “which,” “you”) images are captured in uniform background as no standard dataset is available. This dataset is extended by superimposing on complex backgrounds. The samples of the dataset are shown in Fig. 1. It contains a total number of 3000 images of 300 for each class. The images are in RGB mode. This dataset is also made publicly available for further usage of ISLR.

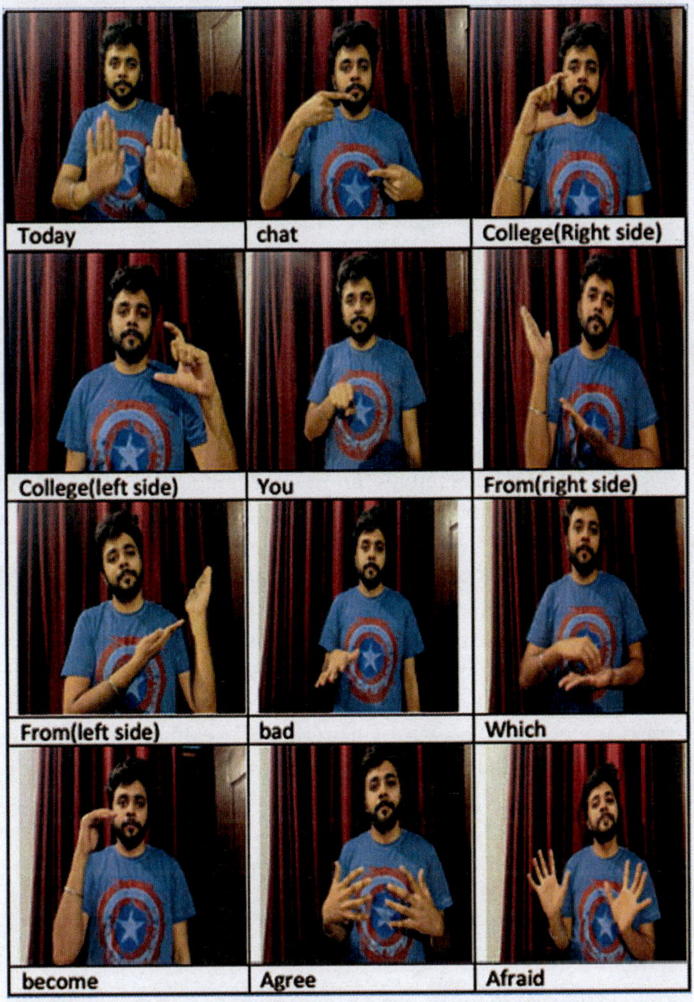

Fig. 1 Sample images from the ISL word dataset

4 Methodology

The necessary task is to extract features that are pertinent to any model and to eliminate or dispose of the ineffective pixels inside each picture test preventing the hand region. Thus, HMASL is utilized to distinguish the area of interest, that is, the area containing fundamental features called key points.

The model used for performing sign language recognition is to first process the images from the dataset. Then, we extract the features using the FAST-SIFT (FiST) algorithm from the training set. Other tools of hand geometry such as the bounding box are also used to perform the background segmentation. These images are then

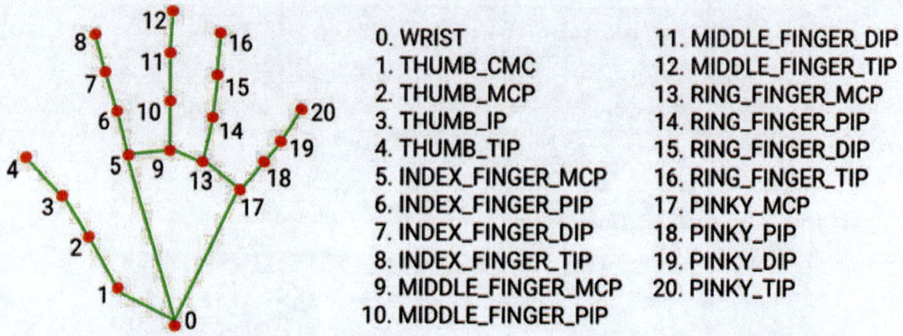

Fig. 2 Key points detected by HMASL

passed to the hand mark analysis model to detect the 21 3D hand knuckle coordinates inside the region of interest detected by the FiST. The detected hand landmarks are then passed to two separate functions. Twenty-one landmarks detected by HMASL are shown in Fig. 2.

The first function computes coordinated after the hand is moved to the 0th central points, and the subsequent capacity determines the Euclidean distance between the 0th central points and the remainder of the fundamental points. The model learns a reliable interior hand position representation and is powerful to halfway visible hands and self-impediment. To all the more likely that cover the feasible hand motions and give extra oversight on the idea of hand math, we likewise utilized complex foundations and guide it to the comparing 3D directions. At that point, this cropped area is given as aid to a second model that perceives the situation of hand landmarks. Presently, the new coordinates, distances, and the handedness (left or right) are given as a contribution to the classifier model which predicts and returns the class relating to the sign. The model can likewise have the option to effectively choose whether it is the right or the left hand.

The working of the HMASL is discussed in the above steps:

1. Capture image using the web camera of laptop.
2. Semantic segmentation is done to detect the different regions in an image and locate their respective labels. Constrained our focus here is to segment hand from the image. There are two stages to perform it:
   a. Detect the hand region from the image and segment it.
   b. Compute the number of fingers in the detected hand region.
3. Background subtraction: Compute the running average time over the current frame and previous frame using Eq. (1).

$$R_t = \frac{C_F}{P_F} \tag{1}$$

where R_t is the average running time, C_F is the current frame, and P_F is the previous frame.

4. The object in the background will be transformed into black, and only the hand gesture will appear in the foreground by applying the mask on the background objects. After figuring out the background B_k model using running averages R_t, now, we will use C_F which holds the foreground object F_O in addition to the background.
5. An absolute difference is calculated between the background model and the current frame to find the foreground object using Eq. (2).

$$F_O(I) = B_k - C_F \tag{2}$$

6. Thresholding: Thresholding is an assigning process of pixel intensities to 0's and 1's based on a certain threshold value, so that an individual object can be detected from an image using Eq. (3).

$$D_T(I) = T[F_O(I)] \tag{3}$$

where $D_T(I)$ is the threshold image, T is the threshold value applied to the image, and $[F_O(I)]$ is the image that contains the object. The threshold will convert unwanted regions into black.

7. Contour extraction: Result from Step 4 $D_T(I)$ is used to find the contour (C), which is an enclosed boundary of the gesture with the pixel structure that has the highest intensity. Let $D_T(I) = (x_i, y_i)$ be the edge coordinate in the edge list, and k is the angle between the direction vector and k edges. Suppose that there are n edge points (x_i, y_i), ..., $(x_n\text{'}y_n)$ in the edge list. The length of a digital curve can be approximated by adding the lengths of the individual segments between pixels using Eq. (4):

$$\mathrm{C} = \sum_{i=2}^{n} \sqrt{(x_i - x_{i-1})^2 + (y_i - y_{i-1})^2} \tag{4}$$

8. Find the approximation contour (C_{DT}), the total distance between the endpoints using Eq. (5):

$$C_{DT} = \sqrt{(x_n - x_1)^2 + (y_n - y_1)^2} \tag{5}$$

9. Find the moments, that is, pixel intensity and their corresponding location using Eqs. (6) and (7).

$$M_{ij} = \sum_x \sum\nolimits_y x^i y^i I(x, y) \tag{6}$$

$$M_{ij} = m_{00}, m_{01}, m_{02}, m_{03}, m_{04}, m_{05} \ldots\ldots\ldots . m_{30} \tag{7}$$

10. Find the area of the contour and its perimeter using the moments, it will help in the case of oriented gesture and the gestures which have different dimensions, and recognition can be done using the area. The area will be a composite analysis of contour moments as shown in Eqs. (8) and (9):

$$\text{Area(A)} = C_{DTM_{ij}}. \tag{8}$$

$$\text{Perimeter(P)} = AR_{LT}.C_{DT} \tag{9}$$

where AR_{LT} is the arc length of the contour curve.

11. A convex hull is now created over the detected object to check the curve for convexity defects and correct them. It will help us to find out the bulged-out or the flat hand regions by using Eq. (10):

$$H_C = Co_H.[C_{DT}] \tag{10}$$

where H_C is the hull, Co_H is the convex hull, and C_{DT} is the contour moments.

12. A bounding box is then created over the H_C region, and further feature extraction methods are applied.
13. Non-max suppression or FiST is used to locate and compute the key points (K_p) using Eqs. (11) and (12):

$$DoG = DoG + \frac{\partial DoG^T}{\partial x}x + \frac{1}{2}x^T\frac{\partial^2 DoG^T}{\partial x^2}x \tag{11}$$

$$K_p = \sum_{i,j=0}^{I=t} DoG \tag{12}$$

where DoG is the difference of Gaussian used to compute values of K_p, while K_p is the key points calculated from each image.

14. The resultant K_p is then located on the $F_O(I)$ image, the result from H_C is combined, and a graph is formed to link all the essential features and store them according to their coordinates values determined for all training images.
15. The resultant data are then provided to the classifier in array, and classification will be performed.
16. The models are saved for prediction.
17. Results are analyzed based on confusion matrix, recall, precision, and F1-score calculated from experiments.

These steps are repeated for all the training images, and further results are generated over testing images. Our HMASL model has acquired a remarkable accuracy over ISL words gestures. The flowchart of the HMASL is shown in Fig. 3. The sample image of the word "college" is taken in the flowchart.

Flowchart:

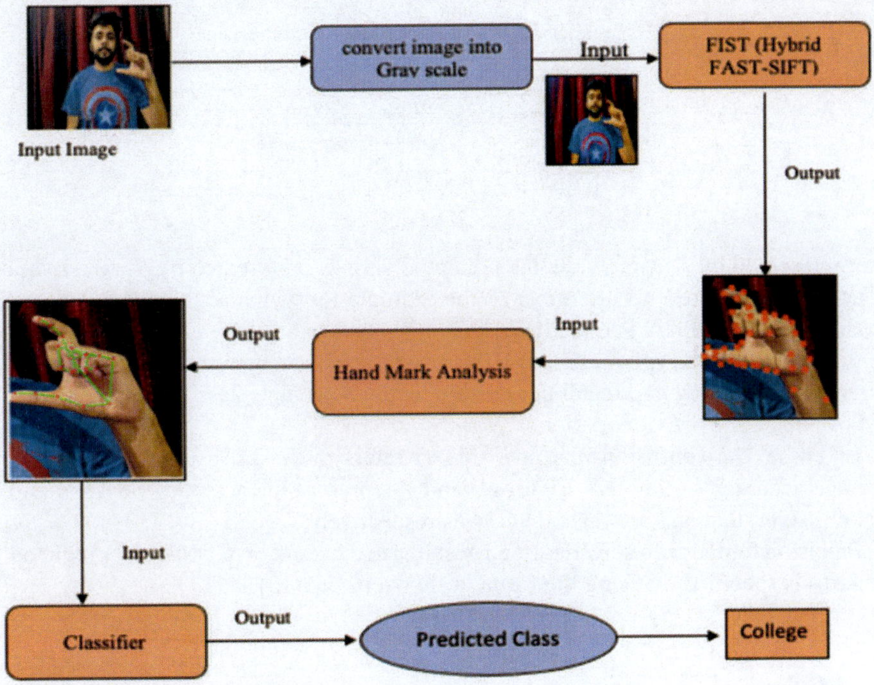

Fig. 3 Flowchart for the process

5 Experiment and Result

5.1 Experimental Setup

Python 3 Jupyter Notebook has been used for performing the experiments presented in this article. Specifications of the system are: Intel® Core™ i5-@1.8 GHz, 8 GB RAM, and 256 cache per core, 3MB cache in total. Graphics with GPU type with VRAM 1536 MB. TensorFlow is used as the backend for the CNN model. To store FAST-SIFT key points, NumPy commands have been used. VLFeat, CuPy, Scikit-learn, and CUDA can also be used on Windows or Linux platform. These experiments are performed on the macOS platform.

All the models are trained on 2600 images present in the dataset. The public dataset is used for the validation of the model. Each network is trained for 20 epochs with a batch size of 128. An accuracy of 96.74 is achieved by the proposed model on the deep learning models. The proposed methodology is tested on several other classifier such as SVM, MLP, and KNN. The results of HMASL on several classifiers are shown in Table 1.

The confusion matrix here is used to summarize the performance at classification stage. A good classifier represents a sparse matrix in the form of graph. Symbols

Table 1 Results of HMASL on different classifiers

Classifier	Accuracy	Precision	Recall
SVM	96.73	99	99
MLP	95.65	97	98
KNN	93.47	96	98
NN	96.34	98	96

are represented by X-axis, while the predicted class is represented by Y-axis. Label to point (X,Y) represents a number of the example for which actual class is X and predicted is Y. When X is equal to Y, then it shows the accurate classification. The confusion matrix in Fig. 4 represents the misclassification between gestures (1–10) in terms of precision and recall per gesture, with an average classification accuracy of 96.73% on the SVM classifier.

Likewise, the confusion matrix in Fig. 5 refers to the MLP classifier with an average accuracy of 95.65%. Figures 6 and 7 represent the accuracy of KNN and NN classifier, that is, 93.47% and 96.34%, respectively.

Precision for the precisely identified gestures to the number of particular predicted gestures is specified by using the formula shown in Eq. (13).

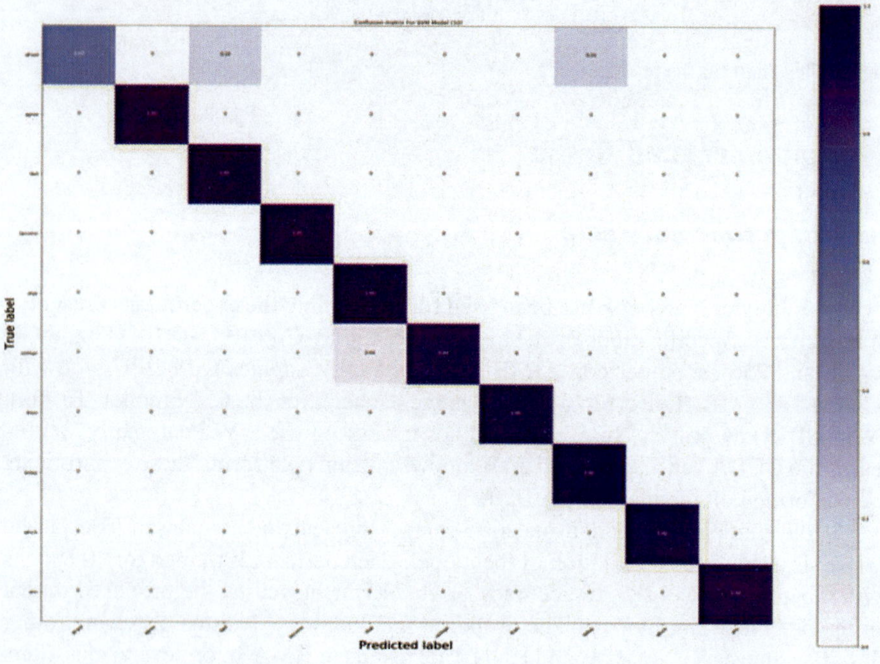

Fig. 4 Confusion matrix for SVM

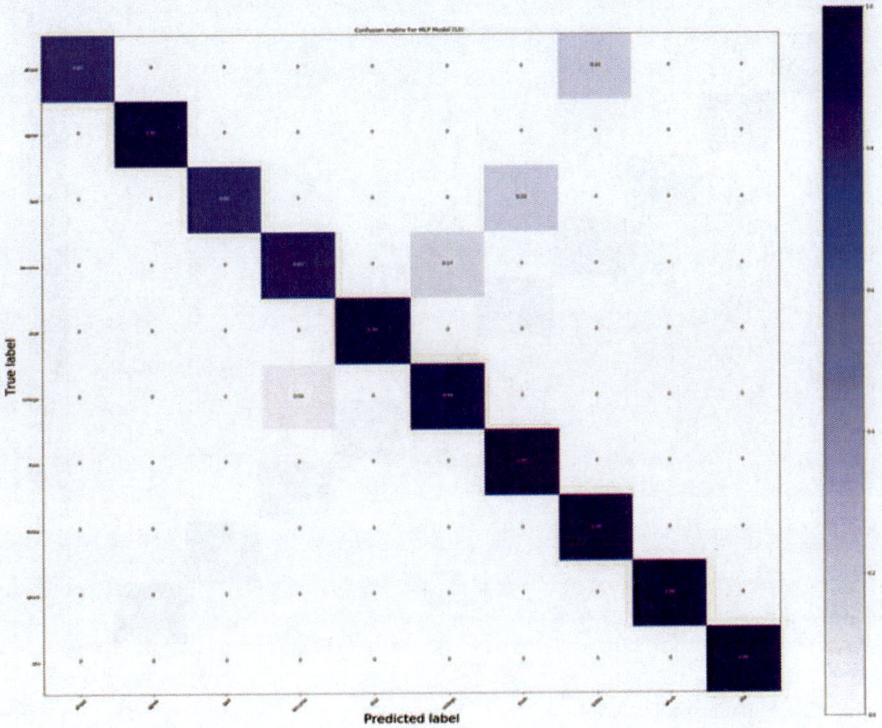

Fig. 5 Confusion matrix for MLP

$$\text{Precision} = \frac{CF_{ii}}{\sum_1^n CF_{ij}} \quad (13)$$

where CF_{ii} is (i, i)th entry in the confusion matrix, CF_{ij} is (i, j)th entry in the confusion matrix, and n is the total number of classes. Further to calculate the ratio of correctly matched gestures to the number of gestures available for that class, recall function is used as shown in Eq. (14).

$$\text{Recall} = \frac{CF_{ii}}{\sum_1^n CF_{ji}} \quad (14)$$

where CF_{ii} is (i, i)th entry in the confusion matrix, CF_{ji} is (j, i)th entry in the confusion matrix, and n is the total number of classes.

To seek a balance between recall and precision, the F1-score is also calculated using Eq. (15).

$$f1 = 2 * \frac{\text{Precsion} * \text{Recall}}{\text{Precision} + \text{Recall}} \quad (15)$$

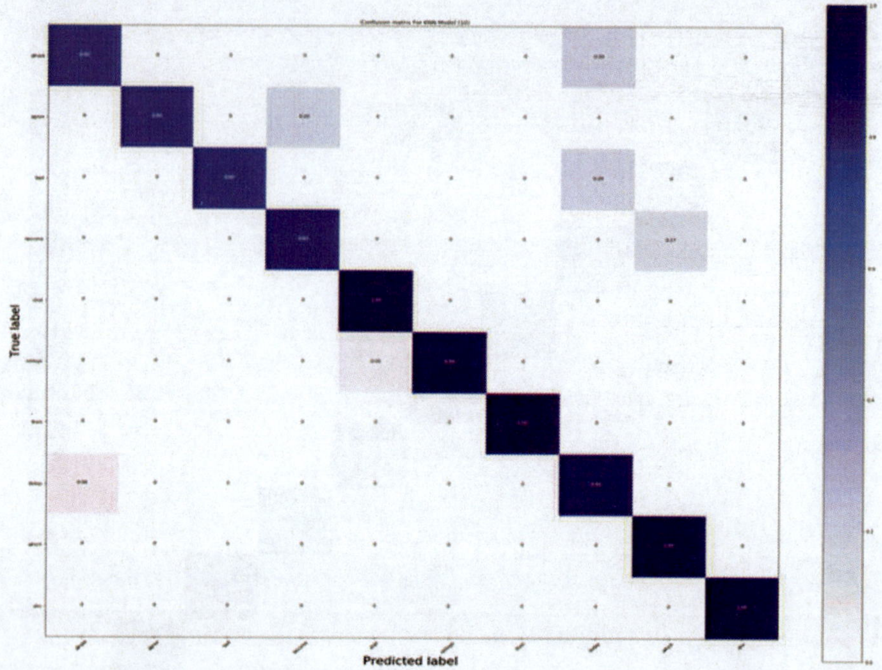

Fig. 6 Confusion matrix for KNN

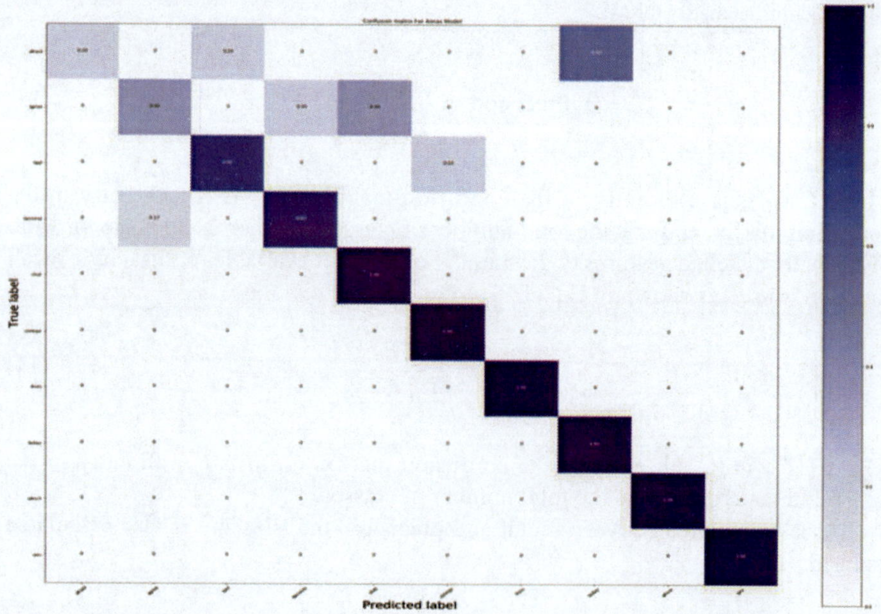

Fig. 7 Confusion matrix for NN

Table 2 Precision, recall, and F1-score obtained by HMASL for SVM

Sign	Precision	Recall	F1-score
Afraid	100	100	100
Agree	100	100	100
Bad	98	100	97
Become	100	97	98
Chat	100	100	100
College	98	100	99
From	100	100	100
Today	100	98	100
Which	100	100	100
You	97	96	98

All values were calculated for a multiclass classifier using the above equations. Table 2 shows the precision, recall, and F1-score obtained from the SVM classifier, and all the parameters were calculated for other classifiers also.

6 Conclusion

An HMASL has been proposed for a vision-based system for complex background gestures. Hand mark analysis-based features are capable of representing the main points representing the hand, and they do not require any image pre-processing. Therefore, in multiclass, shape classification hand mark analysis has been proved effective and efficient. Hybridization of FAST-SIFT is also done to detect and compute the main features from the hand. These features along with features detected by applying hand mark analysis are stored. The stored dataset values are then used for classification. This work is important in that robust hand gesture recognition system with the complex background is recognized with an accuracy of 96.34%. The dataset in this paper contains only ten ISL words.

7 Future Scope

Further work can be done to increase the number of signs as well as images per sign. In the future, more real-world gestures can be used. HMASL can also be implemented for motion-based Indian signs. In the future, the proposed system work may include dynamic gestures based on some real-world problem using soft computing techniques that can be implemented for real-time usage.

References

1. Tyagi A, Bansal S (2021) Feature extraction technique for vision-based Indian sign language recognition system: a review. In: Computational methods and data engineering, pp 39–53
2. Pisharady PK, Saerbeck M (2015) Recent methods and databases in vision-based hand gesture recognition: a review. Comput Vis Image Underst 141(December):152–165
3. Nie H, Long K, Jun M, Yue D, Liu J (2015) Using an improved sift algorithm and fuzzy closed-loop control strategy for object recognition in cluttered scenes. PLoS ONE 10(2):1–15
4. Gangrade J, Bharti J, Mulye A (2020) Recognition of Indian sign language using ORB with bag of visual words by Kinect sensor. IETE J Res 2020:1–15
5. He K, Zhang X, Ren S, Sun J (2016) Deep residual learning for image recognition. In: Proceedings of the IEEE conference on computer vision and pattern recognition, pp 770–778
6. Huang J, Zhou W, Li H, Li W (2015) Sign language recognition using 3D convolutional neural networks. In: 2015 IEEE international conference on multimedia expo, pp 1–6
7. Zhang J, Tao C, Wang P (2017) A review of soft computing based on deep learning. In: Proceedings—2016 international conference on industrial informatics-computing technology, intelligent technology, industrial information integration (ICIICII 2016), pp 136–144
8. Adaloglou N et al (2020) A comprehensive study on sign language recognition methods. arXiv, pp 1–12
9. Bragg D et al (2019) Sign language recognition, generation, and translation: an interdisciplinary perspective. In: ASSETS 2019—21st international ACM SIGACCESS conference on computers and accessibility, pp 16–31
10. Tyagi A, Bansal S, Kashyap A (2020) Comparative analysis of feature detection and extraction techniques for vision-based ISLR system. 2020 sixth international conference parallel, distributed and grid computing, pp 515–520
11. Huang D, Hu W, Chang S (2009) Vision-based hand gesture recognition using PCA+Gabor filters and SVM. In: 2009 Fifth international conference on intelligent information hiding and multimedia signal processing, pp 1–4
12. Raheja JL, Mishra A, Chaudhary A (2016) Indian sign language recognition using SVM. Pattern Recognit. Image Anal 26(2):434–441
13. Kumar N (2017) Sign language recognition for hearing impaired people based on hands symbols classification. In: Proceeding—IEEE international conference on computing communication and automation (ICCCA 2017), pp 244–249
14. Sharma M, Pal R, Sahoo AK (2014) Indian sign language recognition using neural networks 9(8):1255–1259
15. Bhavsar H (2018) Image based sign language recognition using neuro - fuzzy approach 3(1):487–491
16. Theodorakis S et al (2016) Recognition of alphabets of Indian sign language by Sugeno type fuzzy neural network. Pattern Recognit Lett 30(December 2012):737–742
17. Dudhal A, Mathkar H, Jain A, Kadam O, Shirole M (2018) Hybrid sift feature extraction approach for indian sign language recognition system based on CNN. In: International conference on ISMAC in computational vision and bio-engineering, pp 727–738
18. Sun X, Lv M (2019) Facial expression recognition based on a hybrid model combining deep and shallow features. Cognit Comput 587–597
19. Rao GA, Syamala K, Kishore PVV, Sastry ASCS (2018) Deep convolutional neural networks for sign language recognition. In: 2018 conference on signal processing and communication engineering systems (SPACES), pp 194–197
20. Kishore PVV, Anantha Rao G, Kiran Kumar E, Teja Kiran Kumar M, Anil Kumar D (2018) Selfie sign language recognition with convolutional neural networks. Int J Intell Syst Appl 10(10):63–71
21. Elouariachi I, Benouini R, Zenkouar K, Zarghili A (2020) Robust hand gesture recognition system based on a new set of quaternion Tchebichef moment invariants. Pattern Anal Appl 23(3):1337–1353

22. Alhwarin F, Wang C, Ristić-Durrant D, Gräser A (2008) Improved SIFT-features matching for object recognition. In: Visions of computer science-BCS international academic conference, pp 179–190
23. Abraham A, Krömer P, Snášel V (2015) Afro-European conference for industrial advancement: proceedings of the first international Afro-European conference for industrial advancement AECIA 2014. Adv Intell Syst Comput 334:359–360
24. Patil SB, Sinha GR (2017) Distinctive feature extraction for Indian sign language (ISL) gesture using scale invariant feature transform (SIFT). J Inst Eng Ser B 98(1):19–26
25. Zheng L, Yang Y, Tian Q (2018) SIFT meets CNN: a decade survey of instance retrieval. IEEE Trans Pattern Anal Mach Intell 40(5):1224–1244
26. Bedregal BC, Costa ACR, Dimuro GP (2006) Fuzzy rule-based hand gesture recognition. In: IFIP international conference on artificial intelligence in theory and practice. Springer, Boston, MA
27. Zimmermann C, Brox T (2017) Zimmermann, Brox - 2017—learning to estimate 3D hand pose from single RGB images (2).pdf. ICCV, pp 4903–4911
28. Albanie S et al (2020) BSL-1K: scaling up co-articulated sign language recognition using mouthing cues. arXiv, pp 1–18
29. Kang B, Tripathi S, Nguyen TQ (2016) Real-time sign language fingerspelling recognition using convolutional neural networks from depth map. In: Proceedings—3rd IAPR Asian conference on pattern recognition, ACPR 2015, pp 136–140
30. Li D, Opazo CR, Yu X, Li H (2020) Word-level deep sign language recognition from video: a new large-scale dataset and methods comparison. In: Proceedings—2020 IEEE winter conference on applications of computer vision, WACV 2020, pp 1448–1458

Factors Affecting Memory Retention in K-12 Students for the Development of AR-Based Learning Application

Shubham Gargrish, Archana Mantri, Deepti Prit Kaur, Bhanu Sharma, and Gurwinder Singh

Abstract Retention is an important aspect not only for students but also for teachers. The main aim of the paper is to identify such principles that affect memory retention in students and then considering those factors while developing an educational application. For designing an application, some of the key aspects have been supported by literature such as usability and learnability. However, no studies were found in the literature which discuss the most suitable memory retention principles to follow while designing an augmented reality (AR)-based application for students. The study aims the development of the memory retention principles for designing AR-based learning application. The paper proposes 32 memory retention factors through the existing literature based on retention. The principles will then be checked for the degree of importance so that in the future it can help developers to build an easy to use, interactive, and effective learning application for students.

Keywords Memory retention · Augmented reality · Retention factors · Interactive

S. Gargrish (✉) · A. Mantri · D. P. Kaur · B. Sharma · G. Singh
Institute of Engineering and Technology, Chitkara University, Chitkara University, Rajpura, Punjab, India
e-mail: shubham.gargrish@chitkara.edu.in

A. Mantri
e-mail: archana.mantri@chitkara.edu.in

D. P. Kaur
e-mail: deeptiprit.kaur@chitkara.edu.in

B. Sharma
e-mail: bhanu.sharma@chitkara.edu.in

G. Singh
e-mail: gurwinder55@chitkara.edu.in

N. Marriwala et al. (eds.), *Emergent Converging Technologies and Biomedical Systems*, Lecture Notes in Electrical Engineering 841,
https://doi.org/10.1007/978-981-16-8774-7_36

1 Introduction

The success of any educational institute depends on the success rate of its students and the knowledge/ skills they grab [1]. It becomes really important to retain the acquired information at the correct time whenever required. For this reason, an institution's capability to retain the knowledge of the students becomes a vital component. The retention among students depends on various factors, i.e., attention, self-efficacy, relevance, satisfaction, mnemonics, testing, and rewards. So to have long-term retention, the students need to pay complete attention while learning process.

Working memory (WM) is defined as a part of human memory that takes care of temporarily storing and manipulating information. It works as a physiological workspace that can be used flexibly to sustain everyday activities that need storage as well as processing. Memory is divided into two parts short-term memory (STM) and long-term memory (LTM). STM is a component of WM as it stores the original information, i.e., with no manipulation. WM is different from LTM as it is a unique part of memory that has a huge capacity for storage holding data in relatively much stable form.

An example of an everyday activity that makes use of WM is mental calculation. Imagine, an example, trying to get a product of two numbers (e.g., 29, 55) given to you by some other person, using paper and pen or phone. Firstly, you would need to carry two numbers in WM. In the next step, you would be using the learning multiplication rules of calculating the multiplication of two consecutive numbers, by adding the new product in the WM. So, to do these steps and get the results correctly it is necessary to use WM for storage and then methodically apply arithmetic rules. If while carrying such mental calculations, a distraction occurs or you lose your attention you would not be able to continue the process error-prone. As the lost data will not be recalled again, the only action to be taken then would be to start the entire calculation again. If a student gets distracted due to irrelevant thoughts springing in mind or someone else distraction, it will result in a total loss of the entire information and the student will not be able to concentrate in the lecture again. There the retention rate will also decrease. But if the content of the lecture is delivered differently by using technology-enhanced learning, it can help in better understanding and concentration.

This research focuses on finding and developing various memory retention principles suitable and required for designing an AR application for educational purposes. Then the identified principles will be arranged in order of their priorities. The degree of importance will be decided based on the literature review; a comparison analysis will be done to arrange the principles.

2 Literature Review

2.1 AR and Memory Retention

AR had been proved out to have a positive impact on students learning. It had also been found that the students learning using AR scored more marks in the testing phase [2] and also shows an increased retention rate. Research had revealed that only the scores of the tests are not enough to justify that the student perceives a higher and better understanding of the subject [3, 4]. Short-term memory is the most important principle which had been identified to be improved by using AR but, does AR helps in increasing long-term memory is still doubtful [3, 4]. Therefore, the outcome of the above-mentioned research suggests that usage of AR can correlate in deep understanding, only if the system successfully meets the emotional and cognitive needs to correctly encourage the user [5].

2.2 How Effective is Augmented Reality in Classroom Environments?

AR in the classroom have given the advantage of self-sufficiency within learning; students can manage and control progress and learning according to their pace [6–9]. AR gives a positive effect on education by providing an independent catering to every student, without worrying about the speed of the content delivery students are comfortablc with.

2.3 Traditional Learning and Attention

Based on the research, there is an imbalance between the roles of students and teachers while going through the learning process [10]. Educators targets delivering the teaching content, whereas the students focus on taking notes and hearing. Sabatini is one of the research revealed that most of the educators follow a traditional way of learning where educators act as a source of information. This way of learning results in a monotonous environment and boring situation in a classroom. The findings say that some of the students cannot pay attention and focus on learning.

Confirm that attention of students' in the classroom decline after 10–20 min of the lecture. The studies say that the student cannot learn by just sitting and listening to the teacher [11]. One should talk on the topic of what they are learning and connect it to the past work and apply where ever required. Students who have been involved actively in the process of learning tend to retain the content for a longer duration [12]. Table 1 covers the existing literature focusing on memory retention factors.

Table 1 Identified memory retention principles

Author/Year	Identified principles according to the level of importance	Justification
Ausubel [14]	Meaningful Learning and Motivation	The literature review paper targeted two factors; meaningful learning which helps in easily relating the content with the previously attend knowledge and motivation that gives positive energy toward learning
Miah [15]	Attention	The paper aims to find out the factors that affect college-level students memory retention. It has been concluded that retention and attention have a direct effect on students' educational performance
Tinajero [16]	Attention, Motivation	The regression analysis has been done to shortlist the principles required while learning Motivation targets to assess volitional and motivational control strategies, that is, strength and self-discipline to work with complete determination
Amin [17]	Attention, Testing effect, Rewards, and Mnemonics	Attention increases long-term retention and memory recall. Fractional attention results in decreased recall performance Testing helps in recalling the stored knowledge from memory. Rewards provide a positive enthusiasm to the students
Kizito [18]	Motivation, Self-Efficacy	Factors affecting the memory retention of students in the mathematics classroom were identified by using a questioner Motivation helps in increasing the level of interest among students. Whereas self-Esteem will help in enhancing the learning outcome
Velazquez [19]	Motivation, Interest	The use of AR-based learning has been done to achieve better engagement during the learning process. AR showed better learning outcomes as compared to traditional learning
Kitchel [20]	Relevance and Self-Efficacy	A research framework has been designed which clearly shows how relevance and self-efficacy are connected to help students in better retention
Birch [21]	Student Satisfaction, Student Motivation, and Self-Efficacy	The textbook has shortlisted a few principles which are important and affect the retention in students the most

(continued)

Table 1 (continued)

Author/Year	Identified principles according to the level of importance	Justification
Alshehri [22]	Usability	The usage of any application also affects the retention factor in students. If the application is easy to use will result in better engagement which further will affect retention

These identified problems should be overcome to attain the learning outcomes with the best results as Table 1 discusses the identified memory retention factors. Somatic, auditory, visual, and intellectual (SAVI) were another approach that mixes intellectual creativity with physical movement while learning [13]. Attention was considered the most important aspect of learning. When the student uses the SAVI approach, he/she would be able to engage and would actively participate in learning. It also helps in enhancing the students' memory retention by providing memorable and vivid learning.

3 Method for Identifying Memory Retention Factors

A random sample pre-experimental study has been chosen in the current research design [23]. As only a few studies have been investigated for retention of high school students this research comes under exploratory type. This research will be carried into two stages; the qualitative phase will elicit the factors of retention for peer form, and the second is the quantitative stage of the research. This shows a triangulated design of a study that blends quantitative and qualitative data that allows the information to be collected from two different perspectives and escalating the construct validity [23].

A total of 42 articles were selected for reviewing and selecting the parameters affecting memory retention in students while learning in a classroom. Out of which 36 articles were found which supports the research and match with the keywords searched as shown in Fig. 1. The keywords used were "memory retention, short-term memory, long-term memory, classroom-based education, principles of memory retention." From the selected articles, total of 32 principles were identified that affect retention of students in learning.

3.1 *Factors Affecting Memory Recall and Retention*

Various studies have shown that the process of recall and retention is related to each other and is associated with some concepts as learning, the complexity of the

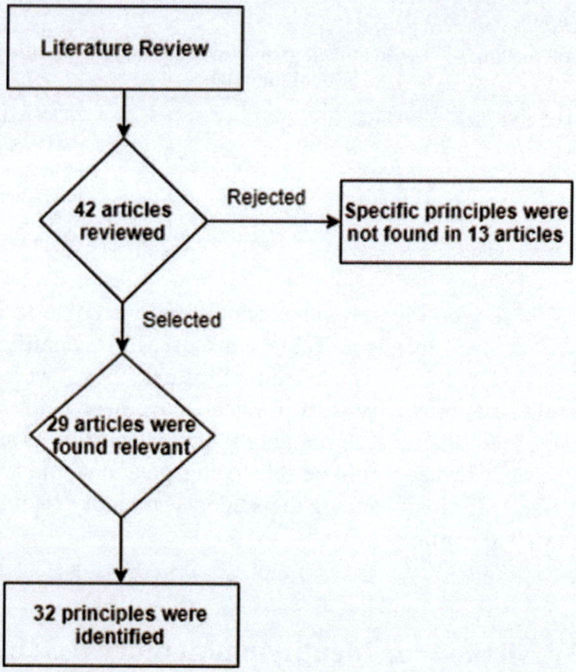

Fig. 1 Method of extracting retention factors

material, capacity limit of memory, and testing [24]. Nonetheless, few factors had been identified such as attention, mnemonics, testing, presence, usability, and rewards as discussed in Table 2. The process of retrieval and learning is that knowledge takes place while studying, whereas retrieval helps in assessing the learned information.

After reviewing the present literature and identified 10 memory retention factors, a discussion was done with 42 expert teachers with a minimum of 2–3 years of experience to clear and sort a few of the factors that affect retention the most. All the duplicate entries were deleted while selecting the valid factors. The finalized retention factors after discussion and deleting the duplicate entries are motivation, self-efficacy, relevance, testing effect, mnemonics, rewards, satisfaction, usability, interest, and presence.

Subsequently, we used a principal axis factoring for extraction. Forty-two teachers from different diplomas and schools were part of the process. The rotation method deployed was varimax rotation without Kaiser normalization as shown in Fig. 2 [29]. In this study, factors with eigenvalues greater than 1 and the loading factor in terms of extraction rule, >0.7 have been considered as shown in Table 3 [29]. Out of 32 principles, 4 constructs were identified after removing the duplicates as shown in Table 4.

Table 2 Summary of factors depending affecting retention

Factor	Affect	Reasons
Attention [25]	Full attention enhances memory recall and longer retention. Partial attention results in reduced recall performance	Partial attention cannot hold the knowledge which is desired while learning. That ultimately results in reduced retention
Satisfaction [21]	Student satisfaction has a strong positive impact on retention	Satisfaction among the students comes when the delivered content is presented uniquely. If the delivery of the content is smooth and presented in a way the students want will make students more satisfied
Self-efficacy [20]	The confidence of a student can increase memory retention and can help in better learning	Confidence can help in giving a positive impact on learning. Confidence can be increased by making the learning interesting as once the student starts learning will eager to learn more
Mnemonics [26]	Mnemonics help encode difficult-to-remember information in such a way that it becomes much easier to recall correctly	It strengthens network interactions and makes it easy to retain and retrieve difficult information
Testing effect [27]	Testing allows recalling of stored data from memory	Repeated testing allows the same neurons involved initially in learning to fire repeatedly. The neuronal networks become more stable and synchronized, and recollection of stored information becomes easy
Reward [28]	Reward-based training or learning leads to better results than non-reward learning or punishment situation	Rewards may attract more attention during the process of learning and also continue neuronal relations, which provide the stable memory performance

Table 3 Factors with the loading factor value

Principle	Components			
	Motivation	Relevance	Confidence	Satisfaction
Rewards	0.692			
Enjoyment	0.776			
Association	0.762			
Environment	0.713			

(continued)

Table 3 (continued)

Principle	Components			
	Motivation	Relevance	Confidence	Satisfaction
Visualization	0.752			
Satisfaction	0.824			
Learnability	0.675			
Relevant Data	0.797			
UI Design		0.853		
Real Time Examples		0.864		
Context-Based		0.844		
Consistency		0.902		
Low Physical Efforts		0.776		
Organized Data		0.813		
Appearance		0.825		
Early-Test		0.744		
Relevant Data		0.797		
UI Design		0.853		
Real Time Examples		0.864		
Context-Based		0.844		
Consistency		0.902		
Low Physical Efforts			0.776	
Organized Data			0.813	
Appearance			0.825	
Early-Test			0.744	
Efficiency				0.717
Interactive				0.848
Simplicity				0.814
Error-Tolerance				0.832
Respond Time				0.839
Easy to Use				0.813
Skipable Content				0.856

Table 4 Constructs assigned after factor analysis

S. no	Memory retention principles	Constructs assigned
1	Rewards, Enjoyment, Association, Environment, Visualization, Satisfaction, Learnability	Motivation
2	Relevant Data, UI Design, Real-Time Examples, Context-Based, Consistency	Relevance
3	Low Physical Efforts, Organized Data, Appearance, Early Test	Confidence
4	Efficiency, Interactive, Simplicity, Error Tolerance, Responsiveness, Easy to Use, Skip able Content	Satisfaction

4 Conclusion

The purpose of the study is to find already available literature for factors affecting memory retention to build an AR application. In this work, 32 memory retention factors were found out to be relevant according to the literature and teachers' perception. Varimax rotations without Kaiser normalization have been used to arrange the factors according to their level of importance in terms of retention. In our future work, the development of AR-based application by using the anticipated factors and the validation of them by heuristic evaluation would be done.

Conflict of Interest The authors declare that they have no conflict of interest.

References

1. Cawsey A (1999) Rethinking career development in an era of portfolio careers. Career Dev Int Conf 4:70–76
2. Billinghurst M, Dünser A (2012) Augmented reality in the classroom. Computer 45:56–63
3. Rosenbaum E, Klopfer E, Perry J (2007) On location learning: authentic applied science with networked augmented realities. J Sci Educ Technol 16(7):31–45
4. Chang Y, Hou H, Sung T, Chang K (2015) Apply an augmented reality in a mobile guidance to increase sense of place for heritage places. J Educ Technol 18(4):166–178
5. Santos M, Chen A, Taketomi T, Yamamoto G, Miyazaki J, Kato H (2013) Augmented reality learning experiences: survey of prototype design and evaluation. IEEE Trans Learn Technol 7:38–56
6. Wojciechowski R, Cellary W (2013)https://doi.org/10.1016/j.compedu.2013.02.014
7. Bujak R, Radu I, Catrambone R, MacIntyre B, Zheng R, Golubski G (2013)https://doi.org/10.1016/j.compedu.2013.02.017
8. Serio A, Ibáñez M, Kloos C (2013)https://doi.org/10.1016/j.compedu.2012.03.002
9. Bekele M, Pierdicca R, Frontoni E, Malinverni E, Gain J (2018) A survey of augmented, virtual, and mixed reality for cultural heritage. J Comput Cult Heritage 11(23):1–36
10. Lester S (2011) Mentoring impact on leader efficacy development: A field experiment. Acad Manage Learn Educ 10:409–429
11. Lujan L (2006) First-year medical students prefer multiple learning styles. Adv Physiol Educ 30(12):13–16

12. Ohshika K (2005) The continuity of convex cores with respect to the geometric topology. Commun Anal Geometry 34(1):479–510
13. Meier P (2000) Apoptosis in development. Nature 407(78):796–801
14. Ausubel V (2001) The acquisition and retention of knowledge: a cognitive view/response. Br J Educ Psychol 71(11):668–670
15. Miah I (2018) How being a commuter student affects social and academic engagement. Student Engage in Higher Educ J 2:2–7
16. Tinajero S (2012) Cognitive style and learning strategies as factors which affect academic achievement of Brazilian university students. Psicologia: Reflexão e Crítica 25(12):105–113
17. Amin A (2014) Brain behavior in learning and memory recall process: a high-resolution EEG analysis.https://doi.org/10.1007/978-3-319-02913-9_174
18. Kizito J (2016) Factors affecting student success in a first-year mathematics course: a South African experience. Int J Math Educ Sci Technol 47(9):100–119
19. Velazquez C (2020) Business model of learning platforms in sharing economy. Electron J e-Learning 18(2):102–113
20. Kitchel A (2018) Agriculture teachers' integrated belief systems and its influence on their pedagogical content knowledge. J Agric Educ 59(3):51–69
21. Birch D (2002) Strategies to improve retention of postgraduate business students in distance education courses: an Australian case. Turkish Online J Dist Educ 14(10):140–153
22. Alshehri A (2019) Assessing the relative importance of an e-learning system's usability design characteristics based on students' preferences. Eur J Educ Res 8(2):839–855
23. Leedy M (1997) Gender equity in mathematics: beliefs of students, parents, and teachers. School Sci Math 103(6):285–292
24. Parker E (2002) The cognitive neuroscience of memory: encoding and retrieval. Psychology Press, New York
25. Browne M (2007) Interactions between attention and memory. Curr Opin Neurobiol 17(9):177–184
26. Bellezza F (1987) https://doi.org/10.1007/978-1-4612-4676-3_2.
27. Butler H (2011) The critical role of retrieval practice in long-term retention. Trends in Cognitive Sci 15(5):20–27
28. Abe M (2011) Reward improves long-term retention of a motor memory through induction of offline memory gains. Curr Biol 21(2):557–562
29. Testa L (2020) Factorial invariance and orthogonal rotationhttps://doi.org/10.1080/00273171.2020.1770571

An Advanced VGG16 Architecture-Based Deep Learning Model to Detect Pneumonia from Medical Images

Mohit Chhabra and Rajneesh Kumar

Abstract In today's scenario, deep learning is considered as a powerful and popular way to detect diseases using pattern recognition. The computer-assisted method for more accurate interpretation of images has been an older issue in the area of medical images, so deep learning could impact a vital role in the diagnosis of X-ray images. In this research work, the authors have proposed a fine-tuned advanced VGG16 transfer learning-based convolutional neural network model to identify pneumonia disease from X-ray images. The publicly available pneumonia X-ray images standard dataset downloaded from the Kaggle repository have been used for experimental analysis. Data augmentation techniques such as flip, rotation, brightness, enhancement had been used for the betterment of classification and validation accuracy, which further minimize the loss and maximize the accuracy and also other performance measures. By properly applying the fine-tuning methods, the authors achieved an accuracy of 93.6% which is more than some of the recent literature work. Results suggest that the proposed model had provided better accuracy and can be used as a screening test for pneumonia disease detection.

Keywords Pneumonia · Convolution neural network · Deep learning · Data augmentation · X-ray images · VGG16

1 Introduction

Today, pneumonia is considered as a fatal lung infection disease and can be life-threatening due to several possible reasons. This can cause inflammation in the lungs and can cause fluid to fill in the lungs. This infection can be present in one lung or both lungs [1]. The main causes of this disease are bacteria, fungus, and viruses. Alveoli

M. Chhabra (✉) · R. Kumar
CSE Department, MMEC, Maharishi Markandeshwar Deemed to be University, Mullana, Ambala 133207, India
e-mail: Chhabra108@mmumullana.org

R. Kumar
e-mail: drrajneeshgujral@mmumullana.org

N. Marriwala et al. (eds.), *Emergent Converging Technologies and Biomedical Systems*, Lecture Notes in Electrical Engineering 841,
https://doi.org/10.1007/978-981-16-8774-7_37

is an infection that causes air sacs in the lungs. Due to this deadly alveoli virus, it is difficult for humans to breathe. The microbes which are responsible for pneumonia are transmittable; it can spread from human to human. This virus can spread in different ways such as inhalation of airborne droplets by sneezing or coughing, a person may also be affected by exposure to objects or substances that may be contaminated with viruses and bacteria [2]. The severity of the disease can be affected by numerous factors such as the age of the patient, type of germ which causes infection of the lung [3]. Due to this disease, the patient has to be hospitalized and millions of people die of pneumonia every year [4].

By early diagnosis, managing the disease using various antibiotics and antiviral drugs can secure the patient's life [5]. The common and best diagnostic method for diagnosis of this disease is a chest X-ray. However, this is considered as a tougher and challenging job even for expert radiologists [6]. The presence of pneumonia in X-ray images is unclear and may also act like other altruistic abnormalities. Therefore, these discrepancies during diagnosis can lead to significant subjective findings and variations among radiologists [7]. Hence, there is a scope for a computerized support system that can help detectors to easily diagnosis pneumonia from chest X-ray dataset images [8, 9]. The method of reading X-ray images to detect pneumonia can be considered less accurate and time-consuming. The reason behind this is many more medical problems that show the same ambiguity in the images [10].

1.1 Introduction to Deep Learning

Deep learning is a combination of structured learning, machine learning, and hierarchical learning. It relies on some specified algorithm that tries to modify the intelligence of different levels in the data using different processing layers using compound formats and multiple constructs nonlinear transformations [11]. This learning technique can be represented as an integral set of different types of machine learning processes that depend on learning the display method of data [12]. The picture can be viewed in many different ways such as values per pixel intensity, set of edges, areas of a particular size [13]. The most important capability of this technique is replacing some variants with effective processes for various feature learning and structural feature extraction [14, 15].

Due to technological advancement, deep learning and machine learning techniques play an important role in building a disease diagnostic tool. This is the major motivation behind this research work because health care services are very limitedly available in developing countries like India [16]. Authors have proposed an advanced deep learning-based VGG model to detect pneumonia using chest X-ray images [17]. The main focus of this research work is to develop an accurate and reliable pneumonia detection method. By the help of deep learning, disease prediction can be done accurately using pattern recognition [18]. Multiple types of disease prediction can be done by applying appropriate algorithm [19, 20].

2 Related Works

Yousef and Abdelmunim [1] in this paper formulated a problem based on global optimization solution whose purpose is to allow the use of an optimization solver; the author executed two different enhanced versions of the solution which can combine the pattern search solver and the objective function. Zhang et al. [2] in this chapter introduced applications, technologies, advantages, and disadvantages of the theory of learning and expert system, and also, the author introduces the concept of fuzzy logic, data mining, statistical analysis. They also analyze the structural algorithm of data mining technologies such that how e-commerce can be impacted by artificial intelligence and fuzzy sets. Zerdoumi et al. [3] focus on the convention of feature pattern recognition in the area of big data applications; also in that part, different applications such as biometrics, multimedia are highlighted. A pattern-based feature reduction algorithm was also discussed, and different techniques based on machine learning were presented. Wu et al. [4] proposed a method that can be used in the diagnosis of non-small cell lung cancer (NSCLC). Through the method of PET-CT, 640 images of each patient were generated for scanning. The author in this study collects the information of 2,789,675 patients from three hospitals in china, then by combining images and diagnosis parameters, an algorithm is developed named as machine decision diagnosis auxiliary algorithm where accuracy can be extended up to 77%.

Zhao et al. [5] in this study presented a method that depends on filtering, string mapping, and grasping of local interest points with PCA-SIFT descriptors. The author in the pattern matching presented a one-to-one symmetric matching (OOS) algorithm used for recognition of NDK, because of its expertise in neglecting wrong LIP matches linked with other identical strategies. Two issues are addressed here which are speed efficiency and search effectiveness, so propose a new system structure LIP-BS, then compare the two systems in terms of speed and accuracy. Srinivas et al. [6] presented a clustering method based on dictionary learning. In this method, similar types of images to be grouped into a cluster can be represented by learning dictionaries methods. The author proposed an orthogonal matching pursuit algorithm in which an input query picture is toned with the standing phrasebooks needed to recognize the contents of lexicon with the sparest demonstration. No training data are required and work well on medical databases which can be visualized on IRMA test image database showing better performance. Sotiropoulou et al. [7] presented a real-time pattern matching embedded system in which a complex system is developed for image processing. The focus is to find features of the imaging system which works as an identifier. It depends on perceptive image processing, so in resultant, it produces precise data reduction and faster pattern matching. Results can be shown on FPGA device chosen on a complex training algorithm. Sharmila and Sakthi [8] formed a medical pattern by character collection. The pattern length can differ for different types of diseases, so it will vary for all patients. So, the author here discussed a method that can be used to find the irregular arrangement by grasping the properties of the dataset, and by this perceiving and finding, an irregular pattern is much easy.

This research can be executed in MATLAB and investigated on the DNA dataset and RNA dataset. Rao and Viswanadha [10] proposed a concurrent information retrieval system (IRS) with multiple patterns for which shaft sequential and parallel string matching algorithms are proposed. To manage it, a large quantity of data information retrieval is required. The planned method simultaneously retrieves the user data information from the data warehouse which consists of huge unfiltered data. Output results have presented that the applied advanced string matching algorithms will decrease the time of searching in both parallel and sequential situations. Zhou et al. [11] worked on convolutional neural networks (CNNs) based on 3D medical images. In this paper, the author presented an innovative and effectual three-dimensional convolutional neural network that includes a deep training mechanism needed to address these encounters. This proposed three-dimensional approach was proficient in guiding volume-by-volume instruction and implication, and also, this algorithm performed well on two tasks: (i) 3D CT scans of liver segmentation and (ii) getting segmentation from 3D images of heart and vessels. The author finds that the speed is more accurate as compared to conventional methods.

3 Materials and Methods

By analyzing the work done by the different researchers in the literature survey, it has been observed that more work is required for the detection of pneumonia disease with more accuracy and precision while observing the different X-ray images. So, we had developed an advanced VGG16 model as shown in Fig. 1 to provide better accuracy and can be used as a screening test for pneumonia disease detection.

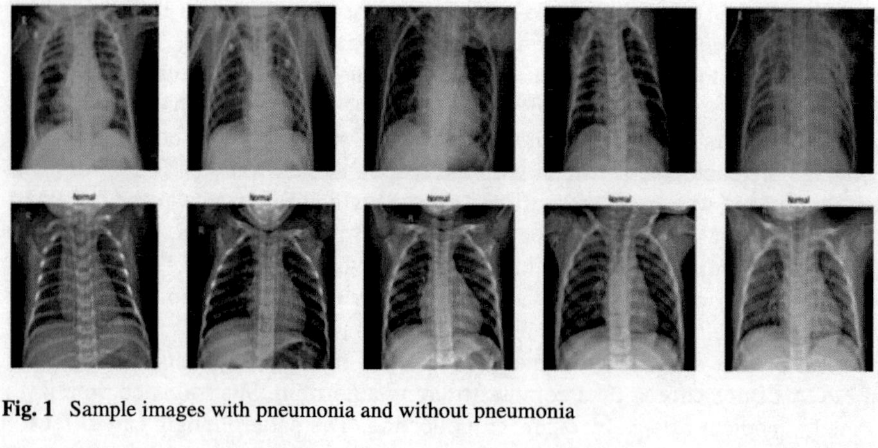

Fig. 1 Sample images with pneumonia and without pneumonia

3.1 Pneumonia Chest X-Ray Dataset and Specification

The dataset provided here is divided and grouped into three different segments which are classified as train dataset, test dataset, and validation dataset. Out of a total of around 6000 images of the dataset which are in jpeg format are available but when we apply data augmentation, then the number of images will increase by a huge margin. Then, it will be classified into two categories as pneumonia and normal as shown in Fig. 1. This dataset of chest X-ray was used for the diagnosis of pneumonia. For a better view, all the images of the chest radiograph were examined by neglecting the low-quality unreadable scans. Some of the scans cannot be removed as they were difficult to figure out. After this step, the diagnosis of the images was graded with the help of expert physicians before being cleared for further diagnosis by the artificial intelligence system. If there exists any type of grading error, their evaluation can be checked by a third expert. Some of the different sets of images with pneumonia and normal are shown below in Fig. 1. The sigma operator used below in the architecture model will sort out the images in two different categories according to disease prediction.

3.2 Data Augmentation

It is a technique that helps us to use deep learning when the images dataset is limited. Most datasets today contain millions of images, but if the provided dataset is not adequate, so here data augmentation can be used. Data augmentation is a very important feature by which we can generate different images from the given dataset of images by applying certain characteristics like flipping the image horizontally and vertically, zooming, brightness, rotation, width shift, height shift, rescale as shown in Table 1.

Table 1 Image augmentation parameters

S. no	Method	Value
1	Flip	Yes (horizontal)
2	Zoom range	0.2
3	Shear range	0.2
4	Rotation range	40
5	Width shift	0.2
6	Height shift	0.2
7	Rescale	1/255

3.3 Model Deployment

Figure 2 shows the overall architecture of the advanced VGG16-based model which consists of multiple different segments. In each of its layers, feature extraction takes its immediate preceding layer as an input, and its output is provided as an input to the succeeding layers. In the implementation part, firstly, we mount the dataset on the given model; further, we will use data augmentation techniques to multiply these images, then the advanced VGG16 model is categorized into three fields labeled as test, train, and validation. In the test dataset part, sample data tend to produce an unbiased assessment of the concluding model fitted on the training dataset. This model is the sampled part of data that is used for model fitting. The validation set is required for evaluating a given model. So, the directory will be required to categorize the data in these three different fields, then data will be categorized as normal (0) and pneumonia (1). Samples of the labeled images are given above in Fig. 1.

Model as shown in Fig. 2 consists of the proposed VGG16 model. The architecture model consists of different layers such as a convolutional layer, max-pooling layer, batch normalization, separable convolutional layer along with flattening, dropout, and dense layers. The developed model consists of different convolutional layers with different dimensions and a ReLU activator. After assembling all of them and after applying operation, their output is stored as feature maps of different dimensions. The dense layer is the artificial neural network placed at the end of the advanced VGG16 model which can be used in the final step. Separable convolutional layer is placed between dense layer and flattened layer. The flattened layer is contained in classification value with 0.5 dropout; after this, sigmoid function is activated whose task is to divide the data into two different categories pneumonia and normal.

In this approach, dataset consists of around 6000 images dataset taken from Kaggle. The image contained in the dataset has different resolutions from 705*429 to 2331*2012. The set contains both types of images such that normal case and pneumonia case images are represented by 0 and 1, respectively. Then, authors perform the

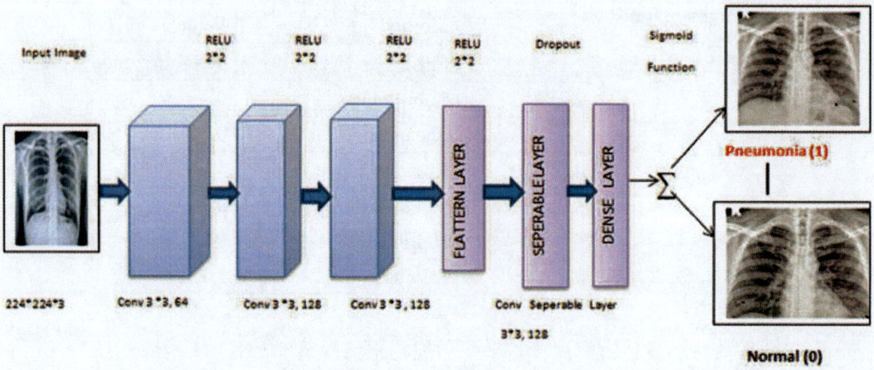

Fig. 2 Advanced VGG16 architecture model

distribution of data in form of training, validation, and testing phases. We implement the model by firstly visualizing the data, segmentation, and finally data augmentation to be applied, and we need it if the dataset size is limited. This will generate multiple images from the given dataset by applying certain characteristics like brightness, flipping the image, further, flipping can be consisted of two parts vertical flipping and horizontal flipping and zooming.

The proposed advanced VGG16 model is divided into three main segments as training, testing, and validation as shown in Fig. 3. The purpose of division into three segments is to find the best model with high accuracy. In the first segment, the dataset was trained; after that, we had applied the data augmentation technique to build an advanced VGG16 model for detection of pneumonia disease. In the testing part of the model, weighted load and forward propagation were applied to test data to improve the accuracy. In the validation segment, we are finding the accuracy of our model by increasing the number of epochs from 1 to 20. After applying that step, multiple models are developed, so out of all these models, we can save the advanced VGG16 model to predict pneumonia disease.

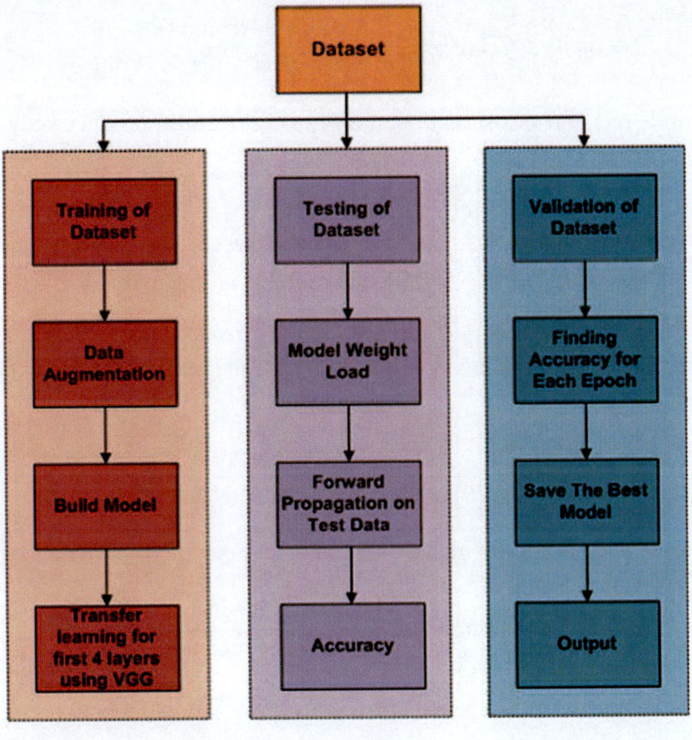

Fig. 3 Advanced VGG16 model for pneumonia disease

3.4 Performance Parameters

Performance parameters can be used to find the performance of different classifiers. After calculating the different fields from confusion matrix, we are able find the different parameters such as accuracy, specificity, precision, recall, and F-measure. In confusion matrix, we construct a matrix of 2*2 with the rows and columns. By visualizing that, we can find the values of a true positive, true negative, false positive, and false negative based on the true label and predicted labels. Provided a test dataset and a specific classifier, different parameters decisions can be obtained as

Accuracy: Accuracy can be measured as the correct predictions out of total predictions performed.

$$\text{Accuracy} = \frac{\text{Correct Predictions}}{\text{Total Predictions}}$$

Specificity: Specificity measures the ability of a system to make correct negative predictions. It is also known as true negative rate (TNR).

$$\text{Specificity or TNR} = \frac{\text{True Negatives}}{\text{True Negatives} + \text{False Positives}}$$

Precision: Precision measures the ability of a system to produce only relevant results and can be found by ratio of total positives to the summation of true positives and false positives.

$$\text{Precision} = \frac{\text{True Positives}}{\text{True Positives} + \text{False Positives}}$$

Recall: Recall measures the ability of a system to produce all relevant results. Mathematically, it can be equivalent to ratio of true positives to addition of true positives and false negatives.

$$\text{Recall} = \frac{\text{True Positives}}{\text{True Positives} + \text{False Negatives}}$$

F-measure: F-measure calculates the harmonic mean of precision and recall.

$$\text{FMeasure} = 2 * \frac{\text{Recall} * \text{Precision}}{\text{Recall} + \text{Precision}}$$

4 Results and Discussions

After deploying the advanced VGG16 model, the different results of accuracy, specificity, precision, recall, and F-measure are obtained as shown in Table 3; it shows the different types of cases where we distinguish the normal cases and cases with pneumonia as shown in Fig. 4. A further result of our advanced VGG16 model is shown in the form as described in Table 2 with different layer types, output shape, and parameters. As discussed above, different techniques are deployed into the advanced VGG16 model. As a final result, we obtain different parameters with the help of data augmentation and epochs. As we increase the number of epochs from 0 to 20, we see a decline in the loss curve, and similarly, the accuracy increases as shown in Figs. 5 and 6. As a collective mean, the result showing both the accuracy and loss is shown in Fig. 7. The performance parameters also obtain some substantial results, where accuracy, specificity, precision, F-measure, recall are calculated.

The output of the proposed advanced VGG16 model including layer type(), output shape(), and parameter shown above in Table 2. Different parameters are obtained for different layers with different values which are used for creating the advanced VGG16 model and further used for the detection of pneumonia disease.

The graph plotted above as shown in Fig. 5 shows the curve between loss and epoch. As the number of epochs is increasing, the curve for the loss is decreasing.

The graph plotted above as shown in Fig. 6 shows the curve between accuracy and epoch. As the number of epochs is increasing, the accuracy curve is increasing.

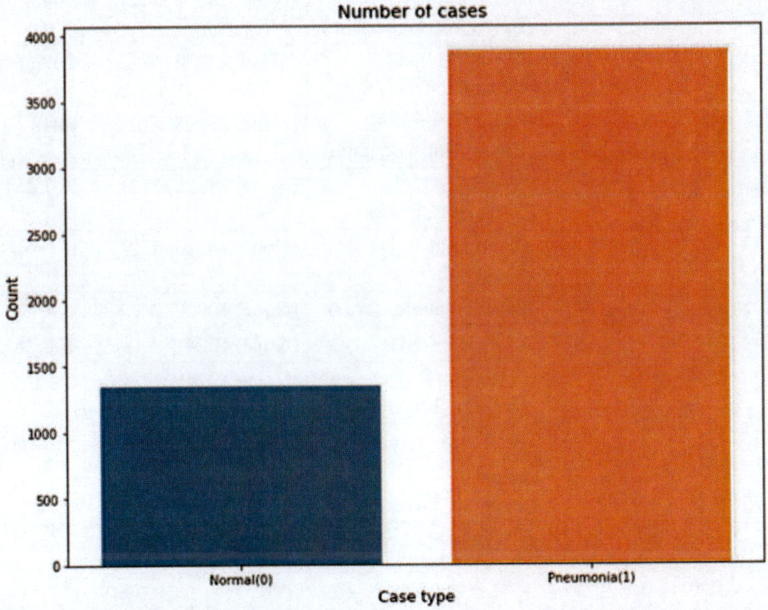

Fig. 4 Normal versus pneumonia cases

Table 2 Output of the proposed advanced VGG16 model

Layer type()	Output shape()	Parameters
Image input (Input Layer)	(None 224,224,3)	0
Conv1d_1(Conv2)	(None 224,224,64)	1784
Conv1d_2 (Conv2)	(None, 224, 224, 64)	36,928
Max_pool1 (MaxPooling2)	(None, 112, 112, 64)	0
Conv2d_1 (SeparableConv2)	(None, 112, 112, 128)	8896
Conv2d_2 (SeparableConv2)	(None, 112, 112, 128)	17,664
Max_pool2 (MaxPooling2)	(None, 56, 56, 128)	0
Conv3d_1 (Separable_Conv2)	(None, 56, 56, 256)	34,176
Conv3d_2 (Separable_Conv2)	(None, 56, 56, 256)	68,096
b.n2 (Batch_Normalization)	(None, 56, 56, 256)	1024
Conv3d_3 (SeparableConv2)	(None, 56, 56, 256)	68,096
Conv4d_1 (SeparableConv2)	(None, 28, 28, 512)	133,888
b.n3 (Batch_Normalization)	(None, 28, 28, 512)	2048
Conv4d_2 (SeparableConv2)	(None, 28, 28, 512)	267,264
b.n4 (Batch_Normalization)	(None, 28, 28, 512)	2048
Conv4d_3 (SeparableConv2)	(None, 28, 28, 512)	267,264
Max_pool4 (MaxPooling2)	(None, 14, 14, 512)	0
flatten (Flatten_Layer)	(None, 100,352)	0
fc1.1 (Dense_Layer)	(None, 1024)	102,761,472
dropout1 (Dropout_Layer)	(None, 1024)	0
fc2 (Dense_Layer)	(None, 512)	524,800
dropout2 (Dropout_Layer)	(None, 512)	0
fc3 (Dense_Layer)	(None, 2)	1026

Table 3 Comparison with existing methods

Study (Year)	Name of model	Accuracy	Specificity	Precision	Recall	F-measure
Mohit (2021)	Advanced VGG16 model	0.936	0.918	0.931	0.935	0.942
Rajaraman (2018)	Baseline customized VGG16 model	0.886	0.814	0.887	0.901	0.913
Zhang (2020)	Cropped sequential residual model	0.809	0.861	0.753	0.848	0.875

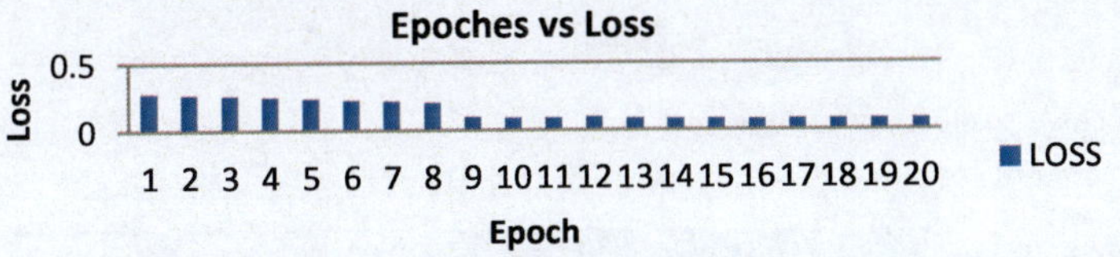

Fig. 5 Loss versus epoch

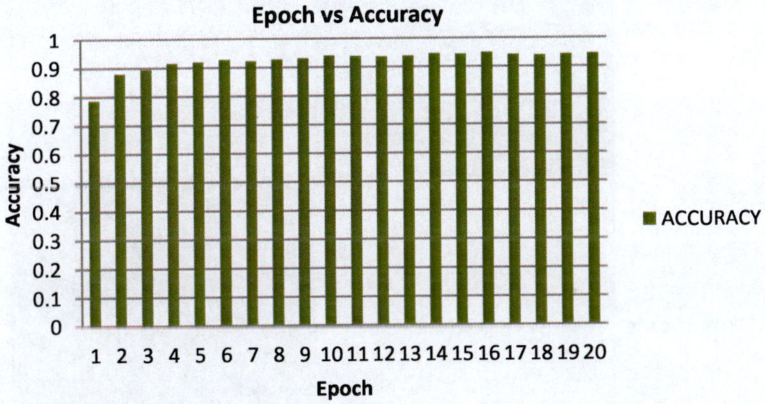

Fig. 6 Accuracy versus epoch

The graph plotted above as shown in Fig. 7 shows the curve between loss and accuracy measured and epoch. As the number of epochs is increasing, the curve for the loss is decreasing, and simultaneously, curve for the accuracy is increasing.

Figure 8 shows below a matrix of 2*2 having different axis true label and predicted label. So, from these values, different predicted values are true positive, true negative, false negative, false positive. These values show as true positive **(195),** true negative **(39)**, false positive **(25),** and false negative **(365)** for a particular set of implementation.

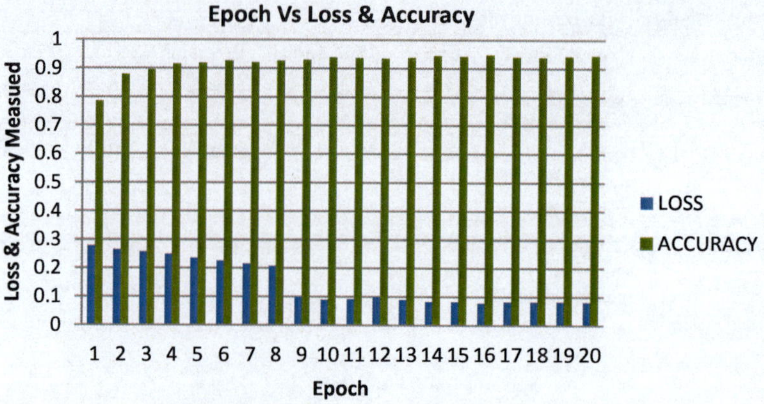

Fig. 7 Epoch versus loss and accuracy

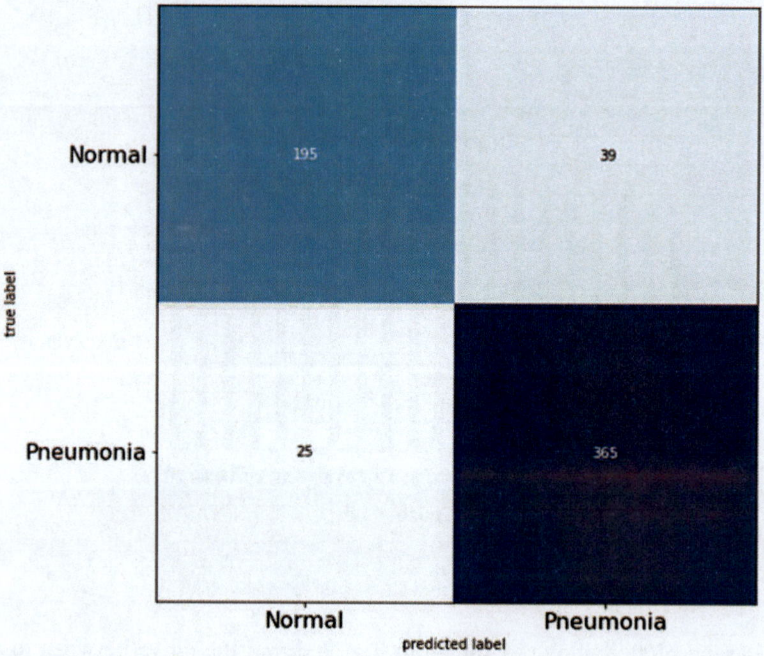

Fig. 8 Confusion matrix showing the true label and predicted label

True Positive: When a positive instance is predicted as positive, it is known as true positive (TP).

False Positive: When a negative instance is predicted as positive, it is known as false positive (TP).

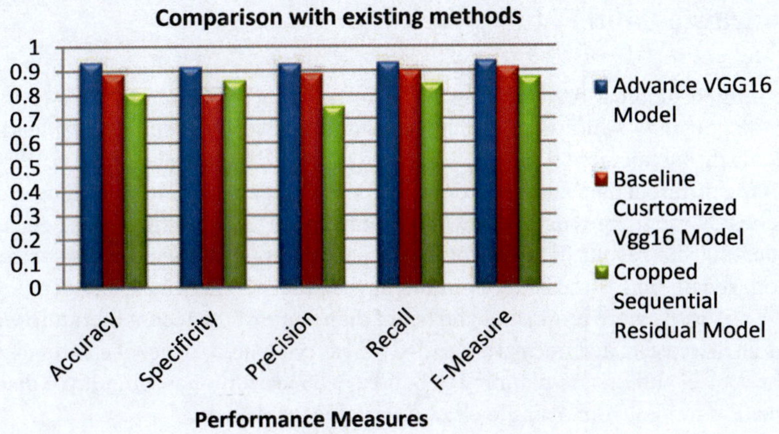

Fig. 9 Comparison with existing methods

True Negative: When a negative instance is predicted as negative, it is known as true negative (TN).

False Negative: When a positive instance is predicted as negative, it is known as false negative (FN).

All these parameters values are obtained as per the formulas given above in the form of true label and predicted label, and after finding the value of all these performance parameters, author tries to compare their values with the existing models who worked on pneumonia and compare the values of these models as shown below in the result section.

In the next step, we compared the performance of advanced VGG16 model with the other models such as (baseline customized VGG16 model and cropped sequential residual model) in terms of different performance parameters, and it was concluded that the results of advanced VGG16 models were better as compared to other models as shown in Table 3, and further, their parameters are shown below in Fig. 9. The value predicted from our advanced VGG16 model is as follows: accuracy: **0.936**, specificity: **0.918**, precision: **0.931**, recall: **0.935,** and F-measure: **0.942**.

5 Discussions

In this study, authors focus on the advanced VGG16-based model with some of its additional features such as augmentation, shearing, zooming, and here, the main aim of authors is to develop an advance diagnostic system for prediction of pneumonia from the X-ray images dataset. By using this model, different parameters can be obtained. Our model actually uses three types of values such as test the model, train the model, and validate the model. By providing the input values, we can easily distinguish the data into two categories such as normal (0) and pneumonia (1).

6 Conclusion and Future Work

Due to limited medical resources available in the developing countries like India, disease diagnosis is still a major concern. Authors have proposed a deep learning pneumonia disease detection model. An advanced VGG16 model has been developed by applying different data augmentation techniques and fine-tuning technique. Pneumonia chest X-ray images dataset downloaded from Kaggle repository has been used for evaluating the results. The performance parameters were accuracy, specificity, precision, recall, and F-measure. Authors have achieved classification accuracy of 93.6%. The results were promising and better than some of the recent literature work. There is an increase in accuracy around (5–15%) as compared to recent existing work.

In the future, authors are planning to build a deep learning-based multiple disease classification model from a single chest X-ray images dataset.

References

1. Yousef A, Abdelmunim H (2018) An accelerated shape-based segmentation approach adopting the pattern search optimizer. Ain Shams Eng J 9(4):1497–1505
2. Zhang J, Williams S, Wang H (2018) Intelligent computing system based on pattern recognition and data mining algorithms. Sustain Comput: Inform Syst 20:192–202
3. Zerdoumi S, Sabri A, Kamsin A, Hashem I, Gani A, Hakak S, Al-garadi M, Chang V (2017) Image pattern recognition in big data: taxonomy and open challenges: a survey. Multimedia Tools Appl 77(8):10091–10121
4. Wu J, Tan Y, Chen Z, Zhao M (2018) Decision-based on big data research for non-small cell lung cancer in medical artificial system in developing country. Comput Methods Programs Biomed 159:87–101
5. Zhao W, Ngo C, Tan H, Wu X (2017) Near-duplicate key frame identification with interest point matching and pattern learning. IEEE Trans Multimedia 9(5):1037–1048
6. Srinivas M, Naidu R, Sastry C, Mohan C (2015) Content based medical image retrieval using dictionary learning. Neuro Comput 16(8):880–895
7. Sotiropoulou C, Luciano P, Gkaitatzis S, Citraro S, Giannetti P, Dell M (2017) High performance embedded system for real-time pattern matching. Nucl Instrum Methods Phys Res, Sect A 845:628–632
8. Sharmila L, Sakthi U (2018) An artificial immune system-based algorithm for abnormal pattern in medical domain. The J Supercomput 76(6):4272–4286
9. Pneumonia Chest X-ray images dataset link. https://www.kaggle.com/madz2000/pneumonia-detection-using-cnn-92-6-accuracy. Accessed 15 Jan 2021
10. Rao C, Viswanadha S (2016) Concurrent information retrieval system (IRS) for large volume of data with multiple pattern multiple shaft parallel string matching. Ann Data Sci 3(2):175–203
11. Zhou S, Greenspan H, Shen D (2017) Deep learning for medical image analysis. Elsevier Inc. (433)
12. Lundervold A (2019) An overview of deep learning in medical imaging focusing on MRI. Zeitschriftfür Medizinische Physik 29(2):102–127
13. Syeda-Mahmood T (2018) Role of big data and machine learning in diagnostic decision support in radiology. J Am Coll Radiol 15(3):569–576
14. Chhabra M, Gujral R (2019) Image pattern recognition for an intelligent healthcare system: an application area of machine learning and big data. J Comput Theor Nanosci 16(9):3932–3937

15. Chhabra M, Kumar R (2020) Comparison of different edge detection techniques to improve quality of medical images. J Comput Theor Nanosci 17(6):2496–2507
16. Malik M, Abdallah S, Alaraj M (2016) Data mining and predictive analytics applications for the delivery of healthcare services: a systematic literature review. Ann Oper Res 270(1–2):287–312
17. Minaee S, Kafieh R, Sonka M, Yazdani S, Jamalipour Soufi G (2020) Deep-COVID: predicting COVID-19 from chest X-ray images using deep transfer learning. Med Image Anal 65:101794
18. Menger V, Scheepers F, van Wijk L, Spruit M (2018) DEDUCE: a pattern matching method for automatic de-identification of Dutch medical text. Telematics Inform 35(4):727–736
19. Kalyankar GD, Poojara SR, Dharwadkar N (2017) Predictive analysis of diabetic patient data using machine learning and Hadoop. In: International conference on I-SMAC (IoT in social, mobile, analytics and cloud) (I-SMAC), pp 619–624
20. Al Kindhi B, Sardjono T (2015) Pattern matching performance comparisons as big data analysis recommendations for hepatitis C virus (HCV) sequence DNA. In: 2015 3rd international conference on artificial intelligence, modelling and simulation (AIMS), pp 99–104

Experimental Study of the Robotically Controlled Surgical Needle Insertion for Analysis of the Minimum Invasive Process

Ranjit Barua, Surajit Das, Sudipto Datta, Amit Roy Chowdhury, and Pallab Datta

Abstract Needle insertion practice is needed in numerous medical and analysis techniques, for example, micro-surgery of kidney stone, brachytherapy, neurosurgery, biopsy. The main intention of this research is to study the different phenomenon (force, material properties, deflection, vibrational effects, etc.) of the surgical needle-tissue interaction process, in which presently micro-surgery mostly dependent. We study and do research on this kind of experimental and simulation analysis (FEM), in order to modify the instruments and program coding of robots. In this current experimentation, the influence of dissimilar insertion speed and the different types of vibrational frequencies on surgical needle insertion force has been evaluated by 2 DOF robotically linear control investigational system. The precision of this experimentation was established by robotically controlled surgical needle penetration into gel. The surgical needle insertion tests were completed by different types of speed such as 10 and 5 mm/s; different types of frequencies, i.e., 150 and 60 Hz; different percentage of hydrogel compositions (10 and 5% PVA); and also different diameter of bevel needle (0.4 and 0.64 mm); the highest forces were chosen for evaluating the outcome of speed and vibration frequency on surgical needle insert force. In this experiment, the surgical needle's highest insertion force was identified at the speed of 10 mm/s and 150 Hz frequency.

Keywords Needle insertion · Surgical needle · Micro-surgery · Toughness · Vibration · Nonlinear · Tissue

---

R. Barua (✉) · S. Datta · A. Roy Chowdhury
Indian Institute of Engineering Science and Technology, Shibpur, Howrah 711103, India

S. Das
R G Kar Medical College and Hospital, Kolkata 700004, India

P. Datta
National Institute of Pharmaceutical Education and Research-Kolkata, Kolkata 700054, India

N. Marriwala et al. (eds.), *Emergent Converging Technologies and Biomedical Systems*, Lecture Notes in Electrical Engineering 841,
https://doi.org/10.1007/978-981-16-8774-7_38

1 Introduction

Several crucial medical cures and diagnoses processes are effectively conducted by surgical needle attachment practice. Flexible surgical needles are desperately advantageous to influence any difficult human organ position like any inner curved vascular networks or any internal anatomical section [1, 2]. Hence, it is significant to observe and analysis the procedure of surgical needle insertion technique and also study the different restrictions of insertion process like the deflection phenomenon of needle and the distortion of sample tissue mimic bio-gel material or living tissue. Barua et al., 2019, [3] have clarified that the cutting force of surgical needle throughout the insertion practice is also varies on additional forces, such as needle-tissue/gel friction force, cutting force of surgical needle, and also the stiffness force. During the insertion process, surgical needle steering also comprises with different forms of mechanism [4, 5], having with horizontal guidance [6], surgical needle tip oriented direction, and applying the forces to the interaction zone where the surgical needle will interact [7]. There are numerous benefits of conventional approaches of vibratory cutting similar to exact surface finish and least cutting force [8]. In this experiment, the sample gel material deforms with the experimental surgical needle tip edge. With the analysis of Voigt model, dynamic model is considered to examine the relationship between the surgical needle tip penetration force and also the velocity of surgical needle tip. This model is useful to illuminate the effect of vibration on surgical needle insertion force. Here, two different insertion velocities were accomplished to ratify this experiment.

2 Work Proposal

In this experimentation, a robotically controlled surgical needle insertion method has been examined by experimentation and simulation and by way of two dissimilar speed (5 and 10 mm/s) and two dissimilar vibration frequencies (60 and 150 Hz); so that in micro-surgery, the result of the minimum invasive procedure can be analyzed properly, which is also considered to investigate the effect of needle speed and impact of the vibrational frequency on surgical needle insertion practice. In this experiment, we have used PVA hydrogel, as PVA hydrogel properties mimics the porcine liver [3]. Abaqus software by Dassault Systèmes® was used to analyze the force estimation, and we will compare the experimental result with simulation result.

Surgical Needle Insertion Model. Surgical needle insertion method has been applied in various surgical procedures, for example, ureteroscopic lithotripsy (URSL), biopsies [9, 10], brachytherapy [11], and neurosurgery [12]. To examine the surgical needle insertion method, the surgical needle steering [13] and the surface contact mechanism [14] of surgical needle are significant constraints to evaluate the associate forces [15]. Needle penetration force is mainly the summary of the frictional force and tip force of the needle [16]. In this research, a 10% PVA gel has been

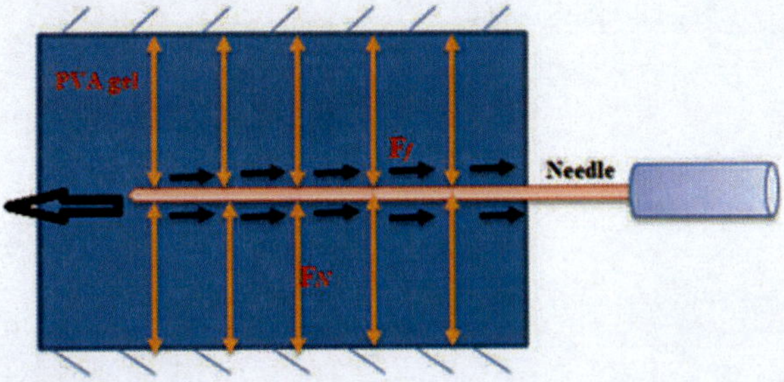

Fig. 1 Surgical needle insertion model

developed as an experimental gel material, such as there have no film on the outer gel surface area. So, we are not bearing in mind the stiffness force of the surgical needle for this present investigation (see Fig. 1).

The total surgical needle insertion force is defined below:

$$F_i = f_f + f_t \tag{1}$$

Here, F_i defines the surgical needle insertion force, f_f defines frictional force, and f_t is the tip force of surgical needle.

For the period of this insertion procedure, the element of frictional force is raised as a result of the surgical needle shaft slithering into the tissue mimic bio-gel material which is also influenced by the normal force of the needle.

$$f_f = \mu f_N \tag{2}$$

f_N defines the normal force of the surgical needle, which is also influenced by the diameter (d) and contact length (l) of the needle and also the foundation modulus.

$$f_N = kld/2 \tag{3}$$

"k" signifies the foundation modulus.

Frictional force of the surgical needle during the insertion process is also governed by the outer diameter of needle (D_n), the physical properties needle material, and tissue mimic bio-gel, i.e., the Young's modulus of needle (ϵ_N) and gel (ϵ_G), insertion distance (L), and the Poisson's ratio (υ_n) (see Fig. 2).

$$f_f = -\frac{\mu D_n 0.65\varepsilon_N}{2(1-\vartheta_n^2)}\left(\sqrt[12]{\frac{\varepsilon_N \pi d^4}{\varepsilon_G I(1-\vartheta_n^2)}}\right)L \tag{4}$$

In this research, a robotically controlled vibrational surgical needle is applied for needle penetration procedure, if the tip velocity is defined V_t, which can be determined by the vibrational surgical needle velocity (V_v) and surgical needle penetrating

Fig. 2 Gel bending model

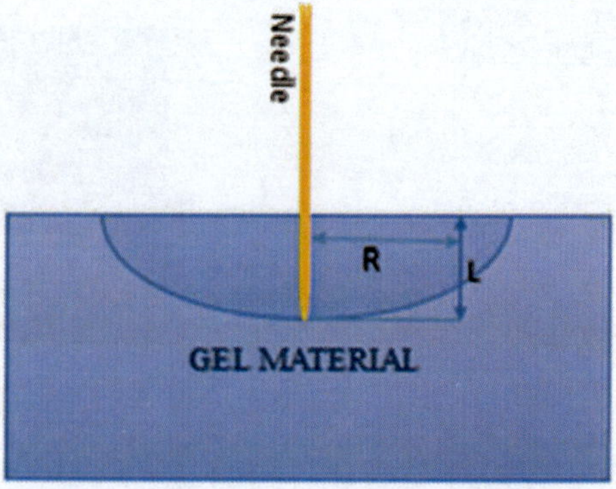

velocity (V_i).

$$V_v = 2\pi f_t A_t \cos(2\pi t/T) \tag{5}$$

Here, the frequency and amplitude of surgical needle tip are defined by $f_t and A_t$.

At the stable situations, the surgical needle cutting force is continual, and the total insertion force will be:

$$F_i = \begin{cases} f_f + f_c \\ f_f \end{cases} = \begin{cases} -\frac{\mu D_n 0.65\varepsilon_N}{2(1-\vartheta_n^2)}\left(\sqrt[12]{\frac{\varepsilon_N \pi D_n^4}{\varepsilon_G I(1-\vartheta_n^2)}}\right)L + C & i_{\max}^{\text{deform}} \le i \le i_{\max}^{\text{insrt}} \\ -\frac{\mu D_n 0.65\varepsilon_N}{2(1-\vartheta_n^2)}\left(\sqrt[12]{\frac{\varepsilon_N \pi D_n^4}{E_G I(1-\vartheta_n^2)}}\right)L & i_{\max}^{\text{insrt}} \le i \le i_{\text{exit}} \end{cases} \tag{6}$$

Experimental Model. In this experimentation, we practiced 16 G bevel tip needle (length 70 mm) and two different percentage of experimental PVA gels (5 and 10%) which are basically tissue mimic. The surgical needle is fixed to 2 DOF robotically controlled experimental setup (Fig. 3). In the beginning, we applied dissimilar feed deviation, and at that time, variant the frequency and every single difference are

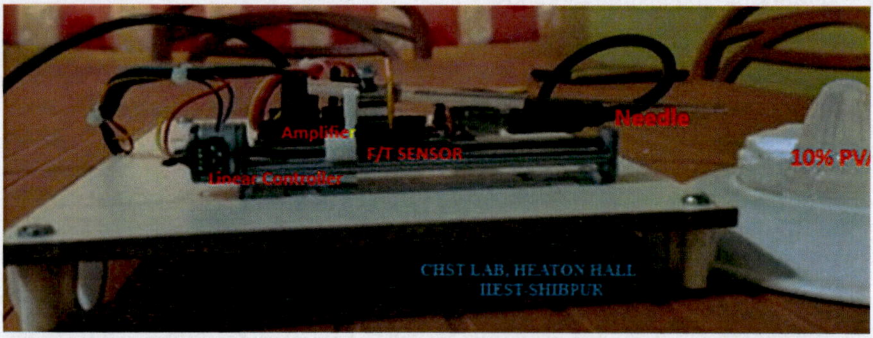

Fig. 3 Experimental arrangement

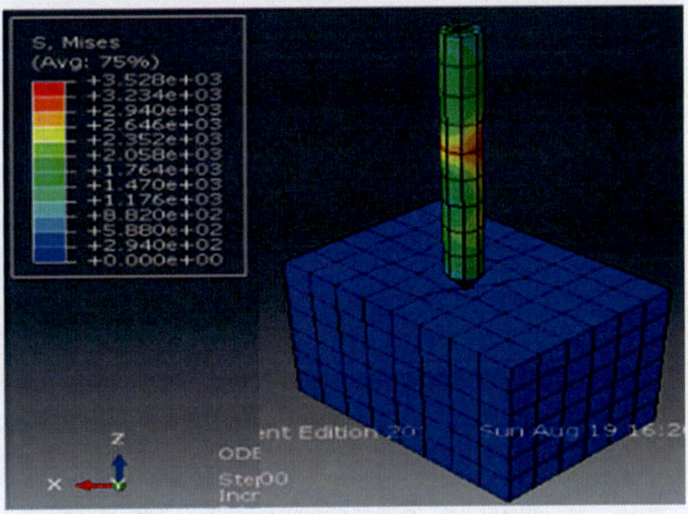

Fig. 4 Simulation model

verified for five times. The measurement of the experimental tissue mimic gel sample is $40 \times 50 \times 20$ mm $(h \times l \times w)$. F/T sensor (6 DOF) was fixed with the investigational prototypical which have a basically the force range 25 N and the accuracy ≈ 5.75 mN.

A data acquisition card was applied to alter the analog to digital signal on the screen of computer monitor. A pizeo-actuator was fixed with experimental surgical needle for producing the vibration, and the vibration amplitude varies 0–100 µm. In this experimentation process, two dissimilar forms of velocity, i.e., 5 and 10 mm/s and two dissimilar vibrational frequency, i.e., 60 and 150 Hz were examined, and also, two different types of gel material were used for force estimation like 5 and 10% PVA gel. Simulation process is being analyzed by Abaqus software by Dassault Systèmes® (see Fig. 4).

3 Results and Discussions

Analysis of insertion force and velocity. Figure 5 displays that the surgical needle insertion force increases for both experimental cases (5 and 10 mm/s), and also, it is noticed that the insertion forces for both precipitously elevated between 30 and 40 mm of insertion depth. In this experiment, the gel has viscoelastic properties (as the gel is tissue mimic), and the maximum force was detected for the period of the concentrated speed of the surgical needle. Total experimental surgical needle insertion force increases with the velocity of experimental needle, in addition to the

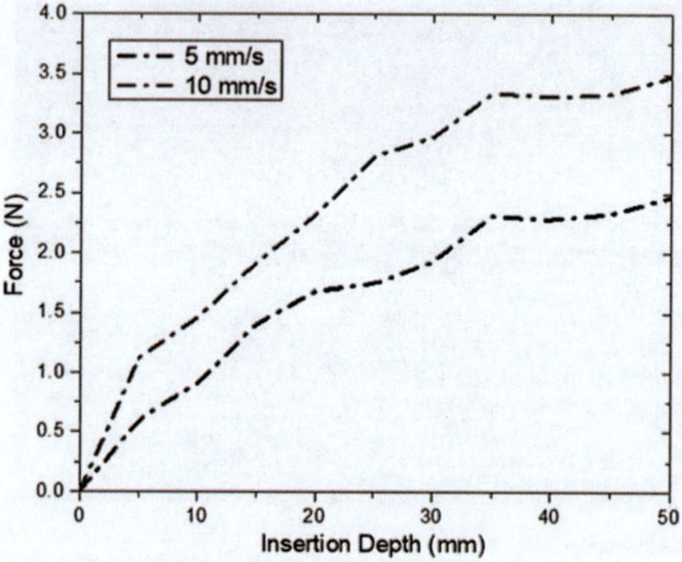

Fig. 5 Force summary of surgical needle insertion by two altered speed: 5 and 10 mm/s

needle insertion depth. Hence, it can be understood that the both surgical needle velocities and the penetration forces are relational and influenced by each other.

Analysis of insertion force and vibration frequencies. Figure 6 displays the influence of dissimilar vibration frequencies on surgical needle penetration force at fixed amplitude 1.5 μm. At 150 Hz, the maximum force was observed, but the gradient of the surgical needle insertion forces was equivalent as a result of const. speed and amplitude.

Fig.6 Force summary of surgical needle insertion by two altered frequencies: 150 and 60 Hz

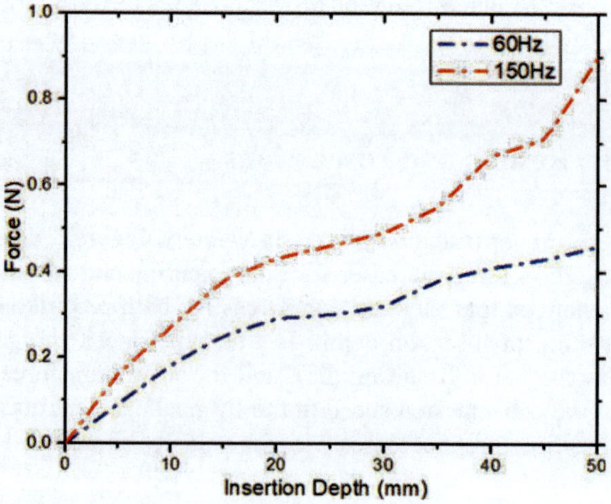

Fig.7 Force profile during different gel materials: 5 and 10% PVA

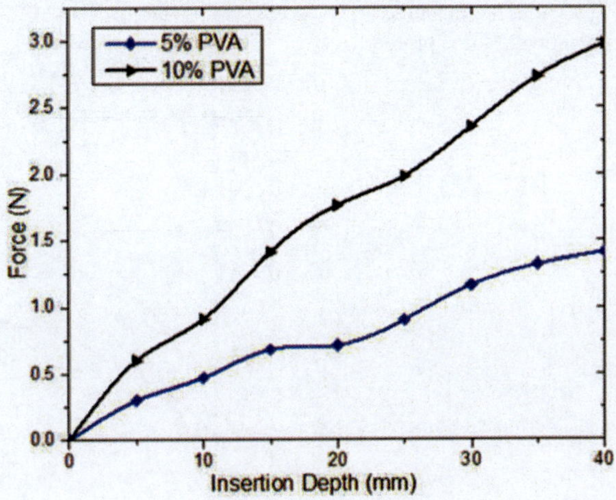

Analysis of force characteristics with gel material properties. Figure 7 displays that the surgical needle insertion force is increasing for both gel materials during the experimental practice; however, the determined force was observed at the insertion experiment with 10% PVA, as the nonlinear viscoelastic properties of 10% PVA gel (viscous and elastic properties) are more than 5% PVA gel. Therefore, the insertion force depends on material properties; maximum insertion force will be required for more density material.

Analysis of needle deflection at needle insertion experiment. In Fig. 8, it shows that both the needles are deflected from their own path. In this experiment, two different types of diameters like 0.4 and 0.64 mm bevel tip needle are used to observe the needle deflection variation. The experimental gel is viscoelastic gel; when needle

Fig.8 Needle deflection profile during different gel materials: 5 and 10% PVA

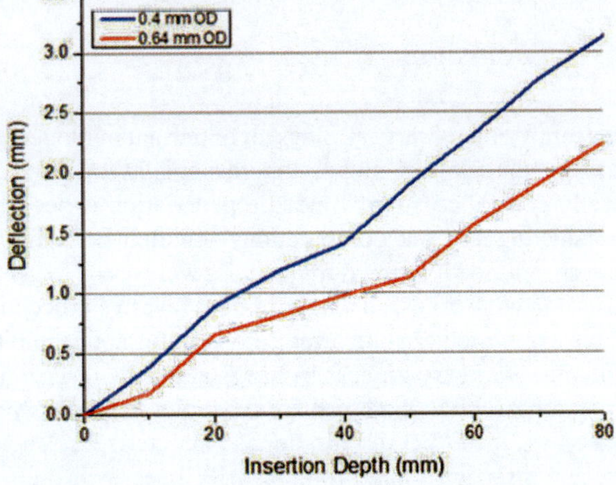

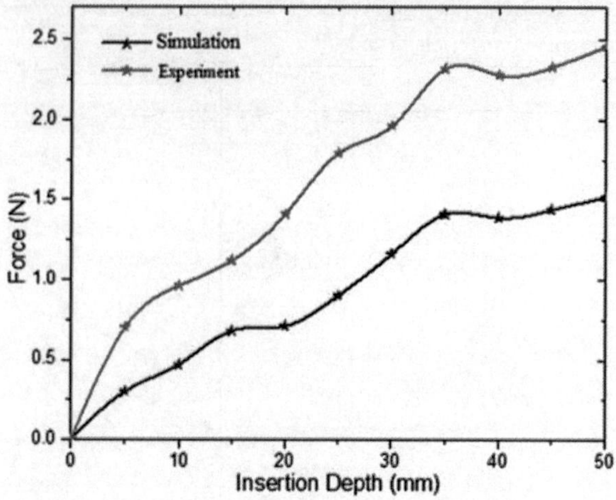

Fig.9 Simulation and experimental force profile

insertion process takes place, dry Coulomb friction will act on the outer surface of the needle. Therefore, the surgical needle needs more force for completion of the insertion process. The maximum deflection was noticed in 0.4 mm diameter needle insertion process. So, to keep the needle track in exact position, needle diameter plays an importance role.

Analysis of simulation and experiment model. In this study, the simulation of surgical needle insertion process was done by Abaqus software by Dassault Systèmes®, and also, we consider the gel object as nonlinear properties because human tissue also contains viscoelastic nonlinear properties. Figure 9 displays that the force summary of both experiment and simulation is increasing with surgical needle penetration depth, but in the event of experimental procedure, the maximum force was observed.

4 Conclusions

Presently, micro-surgery plays an important in modern medical surgery like removal of gall stone, kidney stone, ureteroscopic lithotripsy (URSL). In this study, a robotically controlled surgical needle penetration experiment has been investigated by conducting tests and computational simulation. In this experimentation, two dissimilar speed and vibrational frequencies were used. To get better results, each of the tests was done five times, so that minimum invasive procedures can be analyzed properly. This experimental study creates one thing noticeable that in the travel plan during the micro-surgery process by surgical needle insertion, a number of considerations play an essential character, for example, the velocity parameter of surgical needle insertion, the effect of vibrational characteristics. The experiment indicates that the needle insertion force proportionally rises with the needle vibration and velocity.

In case of stable or const. frequency, the highest surgical needle penetration force is detected at 10 mm/s, and furthermore, at const. speed and const. amplitude, the highest insertion force of surgical needle was observed in 150 Hz.

Acknowledgements The authors would like to express gratitude to all the laboratory mates and laboratory authorities of CHST, Heaton hall laboratory, IIEST, Shibpur, and Department of Urology, R.G. Kar Medical College and Hospital, Kolkata-700004, for their support and encouragement.

References

1. van Gerwen DJ, Dankelman J, van den Dobbelsteen JJ (2012) Needle–tissue interaction forces—a survey of experimental data. Med Eng Phys 34:665–680
2. DiMaio SP, Salcudean SE (2003) Needle insertion modeling and simulation. IEEE Trans Robot Autom 19(5):864–875
3. Barua R, Giria H, Datta S, Roy Chowdhury A, Datta P (2020) Force modeling to develop a novel method for fabrication of hollow channels inside a gel structure. Proc Inst Mech Eng 234(2):223–231. https://doi.org/10.1177/0954411919891654
4. Barua R, Datta S, Datta P, Roy Chowdhury A (2020) Experimental analysis the tissue deformation of needle insertion process in tissue engineering. In: IEEE 1st international conference for convergence in engineering (ICCE). Kolkata, India, pp 83–85.https://doi.org/10.1109/ICCE50343.2020.9290598
5. Abolhassani N, Patel R, Moallem M (2007) Needle insertion into soft tissue:a survey. Med Eng Phys 29:413–431
6. Misra S, Reed KB, Schafer BW, Ramesh KT, Okamura AM (2010) Mechanics of flexible needles robotically steered through soft tissue. The Int J Robot Res 29:1640–1660
7. Oldfield M, Dini D, Giordano G, Rodriguez y Baena F (2013) Detailed finite element modelling of deep needle insertions into a soft tissue phantom using a cohesive approach. Comput Methods Biomech Biomed Eng 16(5):530–543
8. Abayazid M, Roesthuis RJ, Reilink R, Misra S (2012) Integrating deflection models and image feedback for real-time flexible needle steering. IEEE Trans Robot 29(2):542–553
9. Alterovitz R, Branicky M, Goldberg K (2008) Motion planning under uncertainty for image-guided medical needle steering. The Int J Robot Res 27(11–12):1361–1374
10. Glozman D, Shoham M (2006) Flexible needle steering for percutaneous therapies. Comput Aided Surg 11(4):194–201
11. Abolhassani N, Patel RV, Ayazi F (2007) Minimization of needle deflection in robot-assisted percutaneous therapy. Int J Med Robot 3(2):140–148
12. Mallapragada VG, Sarkar N, Podder TK (2009) Robot-assisted real-time tumor manipulation for breast biopsy. IEEE Trans Robot 25(2):316–324
13. Bui HP, Tomar S, Bordas SPA (2019) Corotational cut finite element method for real-time surgical simulation: Application to needle insertion simulation. Comput Methods Appl Mech Eng 345:183–211
14. Li P, Yang Z, Jiang S (2018) Needle-tissue interactive mechanism and steering control in image-guided robot-assisted minimally invasive surgery: a review. Med Biol Eng Comput 56(6):931–949. https://doi.org/10.1007/s11517-018-1825-0 Epub 2018 Apr 21 PMID: 29679255
15. Yang C, Xie Y, Liu S, Sun D (2018) Force modeling, identification, and feedback control of robot-assisted needle insertion: a survey of the literature. Sens (Basel). 18(2):561. https://doi.org/10.3390/s18020561.PMID:29439539;PMCID:PMC5855056
16. De Lorenzo D, Koseki Y, De Momi E, Chinzei K, Okamura AM (2013) Coaxial needle insertion assistant with enhanced force feedback. IEEE Trans Biomed Eng 60(2):379–389. https://doi.org/10.1109/TBME.2012.2227316 Epub 2012 Nov 15 PMID: 23193302

17. Meltsner MA, Ferrier NJ, Thomadsen BR (2007) Observations on rotating needle insertions using a brachytherapy robot. Phys Med Biol 52(19):6027–6037. https://doi.org/10.1088/0031-9155/52/19/021 Epub 2007 Sep 17 PMID: 17881817

A Secured IoT-Based Health Care Monitoring System Using Body Sensor Network

J. Swetha Priyanka, Medamoni Sai Kiran, and Phanidar Nalla

Abstract Nowadays, the advancement in technology is seen replacing the existing methodologies with the intelligent ones in the modern health care system. The main perspective of this proposed work is to monitor the vital parameters of the patient continuously, which is very helpful in controlling chronic diseases. In this paper, an emphasized version of fall recognition is introduced to monitor the stance of a senior citizen or a physically handicapped. Along with this, breathing, heartbeat, and temperature of a person are also monitored to know the patient condition. The sensing elements in this work are temperature sensor (LM35), sound sensor, microelectromechanical system (MEMS) sensor, and pulse sensor, these sensor parameters are given to Raspberry Pi and it will communicate with the cloud, where the monitored data are stored. Whenever an abnormal value is observed, Twilio will send SMS to the mobile of caretaker or doctor.

Keywords Temperature sensor · Sound sensor · Pulse sensor · MEMS · Raspberry Pi · Cloud · Twilio

1 Introduction

At present, the number of doctors is less compared to increased number of patients. As the population in increasing, doctors are not enough to take care about patients. The cost of patient care is also high. People must take care by themselves. They need some technical support to ease their work. Many new devices are replacing older ones. Though they are meant to help people, they are not used by many people like older people, uneducated, etc. This will also help to know the fall detection of the patient. By using these sensors, the sensor information is monitored by Raspberry Pi

J. S. Priyanka · M. S. Kiran (✉) · P. Nalla (✉)
Department of Electronics and Communication Engineering, Vardhaman College of Engineering, Hyderabad, India

J. S. Priyanka
e-mail: swethapriyanka1823@vardhaman.org

N. Marriwala et al. (eds.), *Emergent Converging Technologies and Biomedical Systems*, Lecture Notes in Electrical Engineering 841,
https://doi.org/10.1007/978-981-16-8774-7_39

and sends information to ThingSpeak cloud. This work makes use of communication platform like Twilio. Patient's data can be monitored by the doctor or caretaker when they are connected to the Internet. The emergency alert or message will be sent to the patient caretaker/doctor if the sensor value exceeds given the threshold data. Thus, the doctors can know the symptoms or reactions of a patient for a long amount of time, then it the doctors can treat the patients effectively. So, this helps in speedy recovery of the patients. By this, the cost of patient care can be reduced. This gadget can be further used as medicine reminder also.

2 System Description

In this work, data aggregator is Raspberry Pi, where all the information is collected and it is used as a processor, which performs calculations on the data obtained. All the analog sensors continuously measure temperature, heartbeat, position of patient, etc. These analog signals are given to Raspberry Pi. The sensors include breath sensor, temperature sensor, pulse sensor, and microelectromechanical system (MEMS) sensor. Since Raspberry Pi performs calculations with digital data, an A to D converter is required to convert sensors' analog input data to digital data. Output can be monitored continuously on the monitor while executing. This can be simultaneously recorded on the cloud to store data. We also use Twilio communication platform to send message to caretaker (Fig. 1).

Raspberry Pi 3B+ The Raspberry Pi is a low cost, credit-card sized computer that plugs into a computer monitor or TV using HDMI to VGA converter, and uses a keyboard and mouse to give input to the Raspberry Pi. It is device that enables people of all ages to explore computing and to learn how to do programming in different languages like Scratch and Python. It works on Linux operating system.

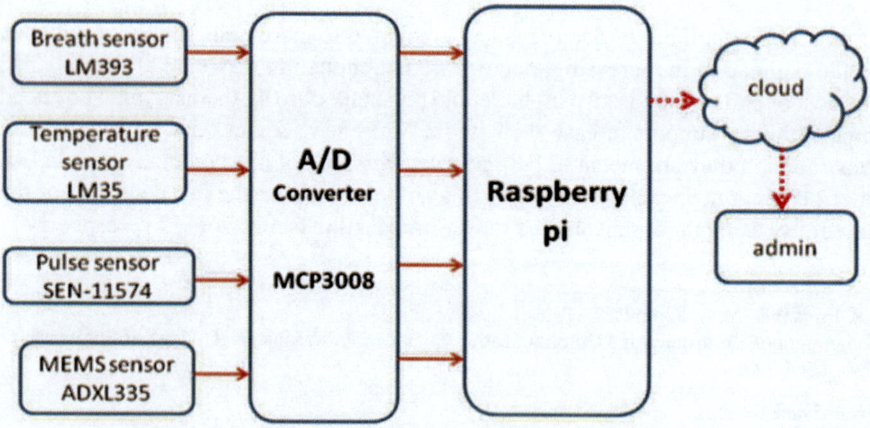

Fig. 1 Block diagram

Raspberry Pi has many features, which are very helpful to build many applications. It is faster than another microcontroller because of its high clock speed, i.e., 1.4 GHz. It can process high-end programs for applications like cloud server, gaming, weather station console, etc.

Analog to Digital Converter (MCP3008) Analog to digital converter MCP3008 uses successive approximation technique having 10-bit resolution. It has sample and hold circuit to get discrete values. It could be programmed for 8 single ended inputs or 4 pseudo input pairs. Integral nonlinearity (INL) and differential nonlinearity (DNL) are specified at ± 1 LSB. It will use the serial peripheral interface bus protocol. Raspberry Pi's GPIO header supports this protocol. It has conversion rate up to 200ksps. Robotics, multichannel data loggers, data acquisition, instrumentation, and measurement are some its applications.

Sound sensor (LM393) A sound sensor (LM393) is used to check whether a person is having any abnormality in breathing. If the person breathes heavily, sound waves are produced from the patient's mouth. If that sound exceeds threshold, it can be detected. The sound sensor module provides an easy way to detect sound and is generally used for detecting sound intensity. This module can be used for security, switch, and monitoring applications.

Temperature sensor (LM35) The LM35 series are exact integrated-circuit temperature devices with an output voltage linearly proportional to the Centigrade temperature. This output voltage can easily be evaluated to obtain a temperature reading in Celsius. The benefit of LM35 over thermistor is external calibration which is not required. The formula for converting the voltage to centigrade temperature for LM35 is temperature (in Centigrade) = voltage read by ADC/10 mV).

Pulse sensor (SEN11574) This sensor is used to offer output digitally of heartbeat at the same time as finger is placed, and this output will connect to microcontroller right now to degree the beats per minute (BPM) rate. While heart is pumping blood through blood vessels, finger becomes more opaque. Because of this, very less amount of light reaches from light emitting diode to the detector. For every pulse, the detector's signal is varied. Electric signal is generated with this varied detector signal by conversion.

MEMS sensor (ADXL335) MEMS is the abbreviation for microelectromechanical systems. The ADXL335 is an accelerometer, which has three axis, i.e., X, Y, Z. Based on the position of axes, signal voltage is conditioned. The output of signal obtained from the extent of diaphragm deformation. It is used to know the position of patient, i.e., standing or sleeping. When the patient fell down suddenly, there will be change in the values of axis. Whenever the value crosses threshold value, it implies that patient has fell down.

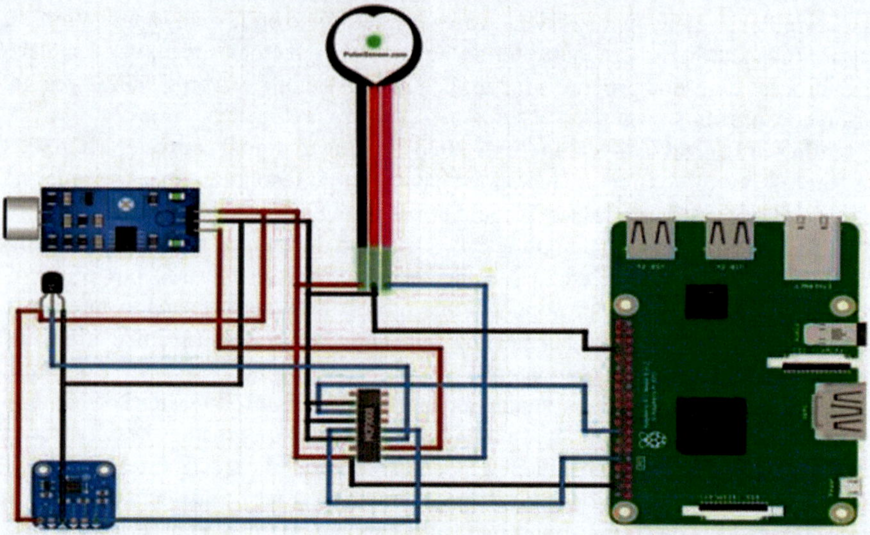

Fig. 2 Schematic diagram

3 System Implementation

The schematic diagram of this device is given below. All the sensors are connected to ADC to convert analog to digital values. The output of ADC is connected to Raspberry Pi. The flow of execution of the implementation is given below (Figs. 2 and 3).

The flow of execution of the proposed implementation is given below:

- Firstly, we convert sensors' analog values to digital values.
- Connect the system to cloud using API key.
- Whenever digital data crosses threshold values, message will be sent to mobile using Twilio.
- If the digital data are less than threshold, the digital values just displayed on the monitor.
- For all the observed data are stored in ThingSpeak cloud simultaneously.

4 Software Implementation

Raspberry Pi is used in this work, and the software required for this work is ThingSpeak cloud and Twilio. In this implementation, Python language is used for software interaction. The Python program is saved in SD card of Raspberry Pi.

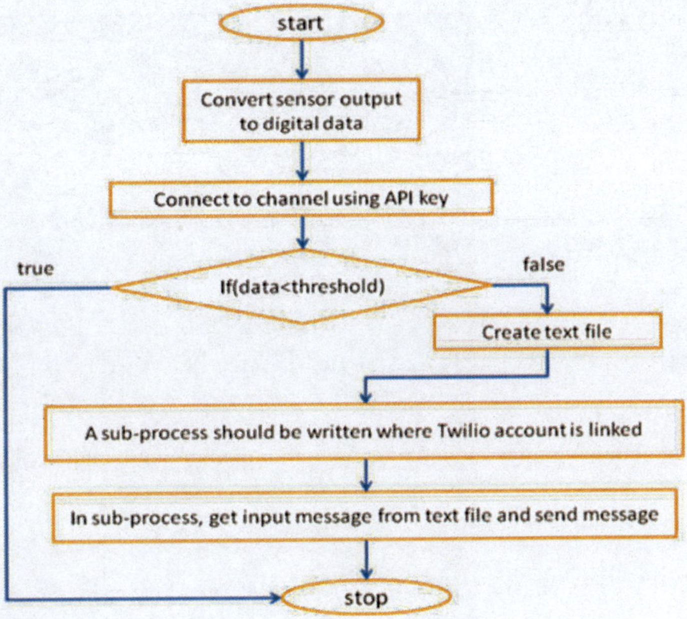

Fig. 3 Flowchart

5 Results

The hardware setup is shown in below Fig. 4.

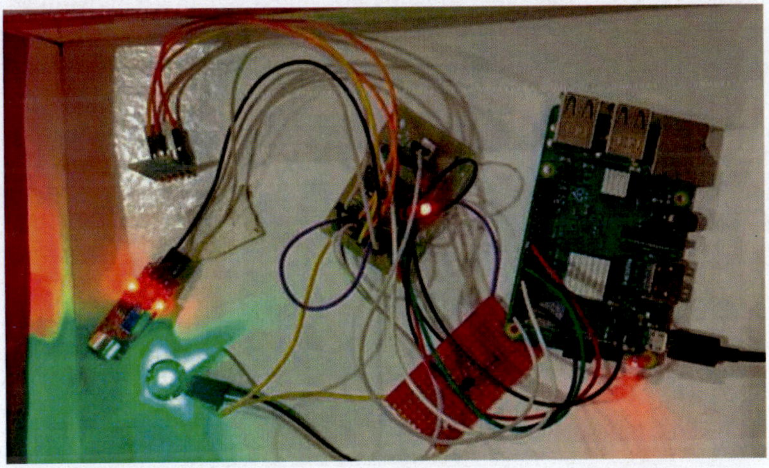

Fig. 4 Hardware setup

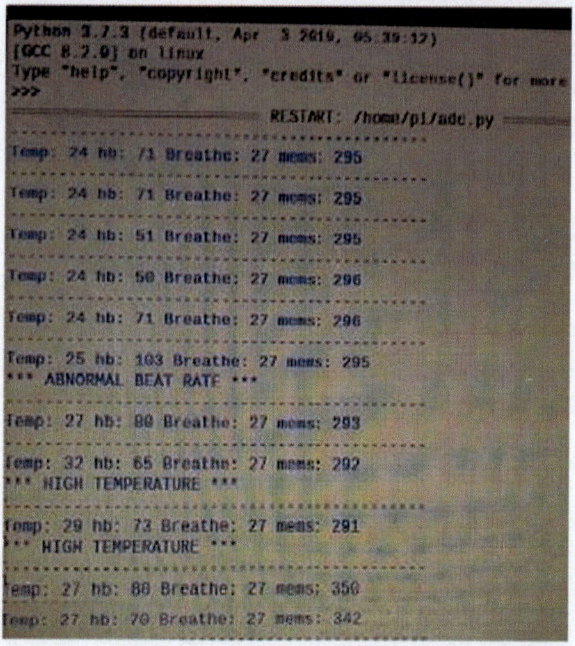

Fig. 5 Output on monitor

The working model for this proposed system is designed and implemented. All the sensors are checked in such a way that their values are below and above the threshold value. Since, the clock speed of Raspberry Pi is high, the calculations performed on digital values are fast enough to get accurate values.

In the Fig. 5, temperature and pulse values have exceeded the threshold values. Then, message is sent to mobile through Twilio. One should have Twilio account to send or receive message. To store data in cloud, a channel must be created. This channel must have fields which contain all the parameters of the patient.

The output on the monitor is observed as shown in the following figures:

While displaying on the monitor, those output on monitor values is simultaneously in the ThingSpeak cloud in the allocated channel. But the only problem with this, user must have connected to Internet to check the recorded data in cloud (Fig. 6).

When an abnormal value is observed, message is sent to mobile as shown in figure (Fig. 7).

6 Conclusions

This system helps to give better health care services to patients in the form of speed and accuracy. The information collected is processed and sent to ThingSpeak cloud. Then, doctors can use this data for analysis of the disease and provide effective solution. This system reduces the cost of patient care by doctors or nurses in hospitals.

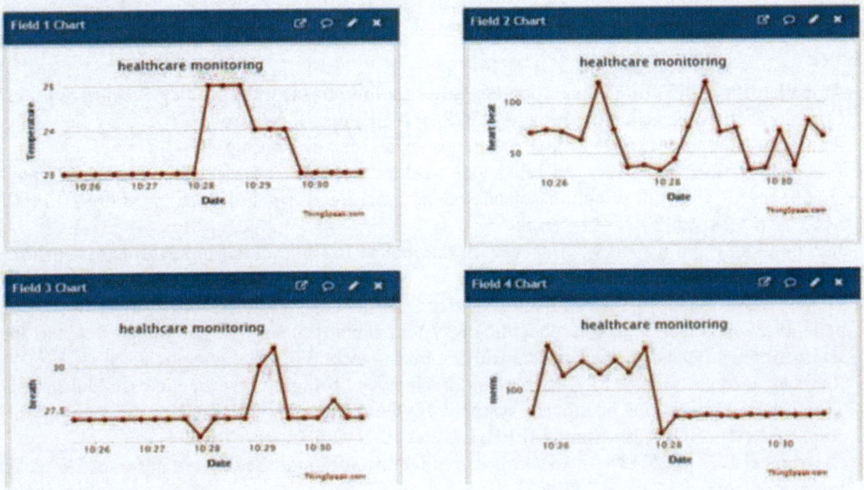

Fig. 6 Data on ThingSpeak

Fig. 7 Received messages

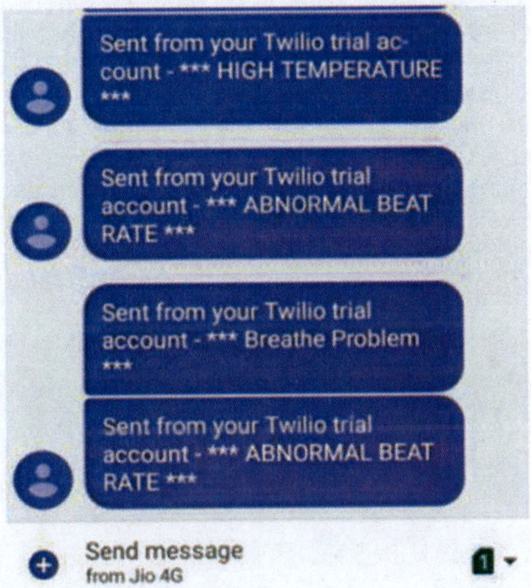

The design and implementation of the work help monitoring the patient's health status from anywhere. Message has been sent using Twilio communication platform. Patient data can be checked at any time. The developed system can be used at home as well as in traveling. This system has special features which involve less need of doctors. This system is easy to operate and can be used for many purposes at a time. This system can be also used medicine reminder, fitness monitoring, chronic disease monitoring, etc.

Bibliography

1. Ambatkar SK (2015) Implementation of healthcare monitoring system using Raspberry Pi. In: Communications & signal processing (ICCSP). IEEE, pp 1083–1086
2. Anuradha Kumari V (2011) Embedded intensive health care unit, pp 169–176
3. Jimenez RT (2015) Building an IoT aware health-care monitoring system. In: International conference of Chilean computer science society. Santiago, pp 1–4. https://doi.org/10.1109/SCCC.2015.7416592
4. Jayashree K, Babu R (2015). A survey on the role of IoT and cloud in health-care. Int J Sci EngTechnol Res 04:2217–2219
5. Jaiswal K, Sobhanayak S, Mohanta B, Jena D (2017) IoT-cloud based framework for patient's data collection in smart healthcare system using raspberry-pi" Computer Science. In: International conference on electrical and computing technologies and applications (ICECTA)
6. Rahmani AM et al (2015) Smart e-health gateway: bringing intelligence to Internet-of-Things based ubiquitous healthcare systems. In: Consumer communications and networking conference (CCNC), 12th Annual IEEE. Las Vegas, NV, 2015, pp 826–834
7. Catarinucci L et al (2015) An IoT-aware architecture for smart healthcare systems. In: IEEE Internet of Things J 2(6):515–526
8. Xu B, Xu L, Cai H, Xie C, Hu J, Bu F (2014) Ubiquitous data accessing method in IoT-based information system for emergency medical services" Computer Science. IEEE Trans Indus Inform
9. Rohokale VM, Prasad NR, Prasad R (2011) A cooperative Internet of Things (IoT) for rural healthcare monitoring and control. In: 2nd international conference on wireless communication, vehicular technology, information theory and aerospace & electronic systems technology (Wireless VITAE). Chennai, pp 1–6
10. Joephine Selvarani S (2011) Online health monitoring system. Int J Comput Sci Eng 3(4)
11. Hartalkar A, Kulkarni V, Nadar A, Johnraj J, Kulkarni RD (2020) Design and development of real time patient health monitoring system using Internet of Things
12. Feng G (2006) A survey on analysis and design of model-based fuzzy control systems. IEEE Trans Fuzzy Syst 14(5):676–697
13. Marci Meingast TR (2006) Security & privacy issues with health care information technology. IEEE

Breast Cancer Patient Classification from Risk Factor Analysis Using Machine Learning Classifiers

Deepti Sharma, Rajneesh Kumar, and Anurag Jain

Abstract Breast cancer-related mortality in females is a rising global health problem. The fact that for the greater duration of its course of spread, it shows no clinical symptoms, further makes it more challenging to control. Earlier diagnosis has deciding role on prognosis of disease. Innovative diagnostic techniques have provided a large database of disease. These databases, with support of machine learning, provide us a framework to arrive at a decision. This paper aims to find machine learning usefulness, its techniques and algorithms for breast cancer prediction. In this work, classifiers such as naïve Bayes, random forest, sequential minimum optimization (SMO) and logistic regression are used for classification of breast cancer patients based on different risk factors. Performance of these machine learning algorithms is analyzed based on accuracy, F-measure, recall and precision using Waikato Environment for Knowledge Analysis (WEKA). Naïve Bayes classifier has given the accurate classification of patients at high risk and low risk of breast cancer.

Keywords Breast cancer · Machine learning · Risk factors · And Risk assessment · Random forest (RF) · Support vector machine (SVM) · Sequential minimum optimization (SMO)

D. Sharma (✉) · R. Kumar
Department of Computer Engineering, MMEC, Maharishi Markandeshwar (Deemed to be University), Mullana, Ambala, Haryana, India

R. Kumar
e-mail: drrajneeshgujral@mmumullana.org

A. Jain
Virtualization Department, School of Computer Science, University of Petroleum and Energy Studies, Dehradun, India
e-mail: anurag.jain@ddn.upes.ac.in

N. Marriwala et al. (eds.), *Emergent Converging Technologies and Biomedical Systems*, Lecture Notes in Electrical Engineering 841,
https://doi.org/10.1007/978-981-16-8774-7_40

1 Introduction

Any tissue growth consisting of mutated cells and which is uncontrolled is known as cancer. It can involve any body part and any type of tissue. Cancer disease can affect both young and old host bodies. In the case of breast cancer, it has been found to have the highest incidence rate in females. It grows much faster in younger females than older ones. It has been found to become double in diameter from within 1.2 months in young females compared to 6.3 years in older females. When it has its origin from cells of the milk duct, it is termed as ductal carcinoma, or in the case of glands, it is termed as glandular carcinoma. It begins as a small tumor mass within breast tissue, which, if having irregular border or speculation, may later become malignant/cancerous [1]. Some of the significant symptoms associated are lumps in the breast with any texture or volume and with hard or soft edges. Another sign is the pain in breast tissue. Also, there may be a change in the nipple region in the form of retraction, ulceration, itching and bleeding [2].

Broadly, breast cancer can be categorized in in situ, i.e., localized breast cancer and invasive breast cancer. In situ carcinoma can further be of two types: ductal carcinoma in situ (DCIS) and lobular carcinoma in situ (LCIS). Out of these two, LCIS is generally believed to be benign and is not having the potential to progress in an invasive variety of cancer. In contrast, invasive cancer variety can develop from DCIS. It grows very slowly and sometimes may not be requiring treatment. Researchers have shown about 20–53% of cases of DCIS get to progress to an invasive type of cancer. Invasive breast cancer constitutes a larger group of breast cancer, making it about 81%. By invasive cancer, it implies that the tumor is infiltrating in nature, and it has broken down the walls of glands and ducts from where it has originated. Initially, breast cancer was considered a single entity, but it has been established that it is having four molecular subtypes and twenty-one histological subtypes. Histology refers to types of tissue from where breast cancer has the origin. Different histologic types have various risk factors, clinical picture, treatment outcome, etc. Histology is classified according to shape, size and arrangements of breast cancer cells [1]. The different types of breast cancers are explained below in Table 1.

The two most common breast cancer risk factors are advanced age and family history of the patient. For estimation of lifetime risk (LTR), many empirical and

Table 1 Classes of breast cancer

1	Invasive breast cancer	• Ductal
		• Lobular
2	In situ	• Ductal carcinoma in situ (DCIS)
		• Lobular carcinoma in situ (LCIS)
3	Other	• Inflammatory • Tubular • Pregnancy-induced

statistical models have been proposed by authors in the past decades. Mostly, models relied on the family history of the patient, but some models relied on other factors as well. These models have a role in patient screening, genetic counseling, testing and research related to breast cancer.

Broadly, these models can be categorized on risk factors they incorporated and the kind of information we get from them. However, they can be classified into three classes: first, which estimates breast cancer risk; second, which determines risk for a genetic mutation in BRCA1 and BRCA2 genes known for increasing breast cancer risk; thirdly, which predicts the risk for both the groups. Based on risk factors, some models incorporated risk factors such as family history, while others were based on hormonal and environmental factors as well. With knowledge, growing, other risk factors have also been added from time to time, like radiographic and histological data. Each model developed is population-specific, for which it has been developed. But, it has to be validated firstly for its implementation. The two most commonly used validation measure techniques are discrimination and calibration [3].

Early-stage breast cancer was usually diagnosed by radiological imaging techniques or molecular. Earlier mammograms by X-ray machines and magnetic resonance imaging (MRI) were methods for more rapid detection of breast cancer. Also, serum micro-RNA and urine DNA damage were seen as initiating lesions for breast cancer. These old techniques are less significant nowadays. American cancer society supports early detection of breast cancer so that it may be identified and cured early. Early diagnosis improves the long-term prognosis of disease as well [4]. Early detection of disease enhances the chances of successful treatment by concentrating on symptomatic patients in an early stage. Late diagnosis of cancer results in the low likelihood of survival, low resource settings, higher costs of care, more significant morbidity of treatment and results in deaths or disability arising from it. Cancer outcome improves from a timely diagnosis and provides better options for the medication to the clinicians. Therefore, the current focus on cancer research is upon etiology and modalities of treatment for cancer prevention and efficient treatment later on, if it arises [2, 3]. The risk factor associated with breast cancer is divided into three main categories like personal or hormonal factors, breast disease-related and hereditary factors [5]. Some classic models like the Gail model, BCRAT model, Claus model, BRCAPRO model, BOADICEA and IBIS Tyrer-Cuzick models are divided according to the risk factors included in them.

This paper is divided into seven sections. The role of machine learning in breast cancer prediction and conventional machine learning techniques have discussed and compared on different parameters is discussed in Sect. 2. Section 3 analyzes performance metrics like accuracy, precision, recall. Methods and materials used and experimental setup are discussed in Sect. 4. Performance evaluation and comparison are in Sect. 5. At last, Sect. 6 gives result and concludes this paper as the scope of future scope of action.

2 Machine Learning in Breast Cancer Prediction

Machine learning is a subdivision of artificial intelligence in which algorithms learn from the data in supervised or unsupervised guidance to classify the data and to provide some valuable predictions. An algorithm in machine learning is designed to accomplish a specific task and trained on data and revised.

Data mining and machine learning techniques have been progressed for the detection and classification of breast cancer [6, 7]. The steps for prediction are divided into pre-processing, feature extraction and classification. The flowchart to construct a machine learning-based model is shown in Fig. 1.

Machine learning is in growing demand day by day because of becoming a service. Expert knowledge is required to understand the concept of machine learning. An expert with the knowledge and skills is needed to understand the concepts of pre-processing, feature selection and classification processes. Applications of machine learning in health care like detection of the type of cancerous cells help doctors in many ways. Techniques of machine learning are very much useful in detecting and classifying the patients in the high category risk of patients and low-risk patients [6]. Scientists have used many screening methods in the early stage of the disease to find the type of cancer before the symptoms arise. New strategies have been developed for detecting cancer at an early stage. A large number of hospitals and cancer research institutes provide cancer patients with data for the community of medical research. Accurate prediction of disease is the ultimate purpose and challenging task for clinicians. Machine learning techniques are commonly used by medical researchers these

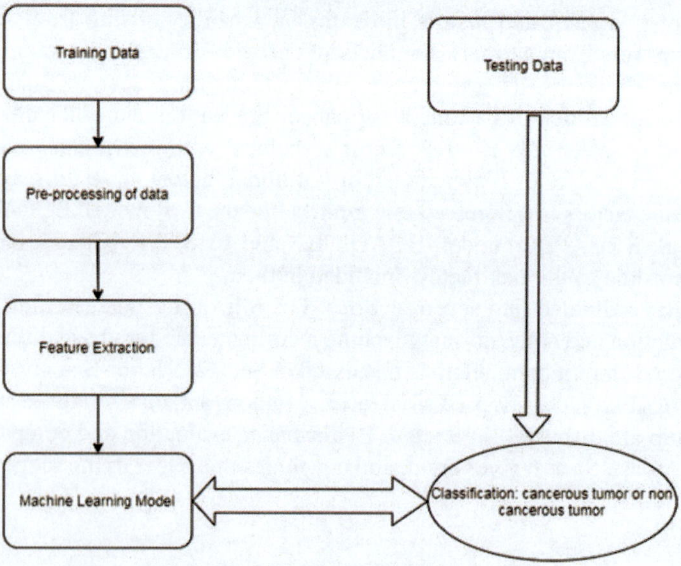

Fig. 1 Flowchart of machine learning-based prediction model

days. These techniques are used to extract patterns and relationships associated with the dataset. The detection and classification of patients are helpful in breast cancer diagnosis.

Screening methods are available and used like mammography, magnetic resonance imaging (MRI), digital breast tomosynthesis (DBT) and ultrasound for the classification of proteomic and genomic malignancies. Machine learning techniques provide identification, classification and detection of tumors and other malignancies [7]. Prediction and prognosis of cancer are different from the purposes of detection and diagnosis. The main concern in prediction or prognosis is with these predictive facts:

(i) The prediction related to the susceptibility of cancer (i.e., risk assessment): Possibility of developing cancer before the recurrence of the disease is formed.
(ii) The prediction of cancer recurrence: Possibility of redeveloping of cancer is formed even after the proper treatment of cancer.
(iii) The prediction of cancer survivability: It is the predictions related to the result or outcome after the diagnosis of the disease. The success depends on the quality of diagnosis in the cases of recurrence and

2.1 *Process of Risk Prediction in Breast Cancer*

The process of risk prediction in breast cancer has been depicted in Fig. 2.

In machine learning or deep learning-based prediction system process, many modules are responsible for the overall correct and accurate prediction. The first step in any prediction is the collection of data like in disease prediction. We need to take electronic health records from any hospital or available online repositories according to our area of research. This process is called capturing of data; after this step, storing and sharing of the data step. Next, the primary phase is to analyze

Fig. 2 Process of disease prediction in breast cancer

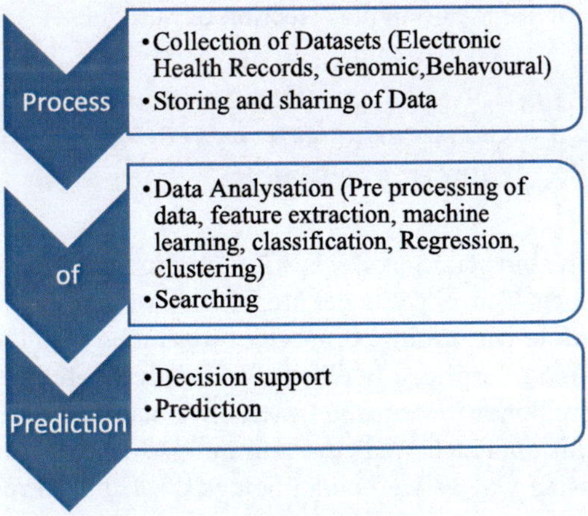

the data by extracting and selection of features and application of machine learning technique and then finally the result in the form of prediction using decision support [8].

2.2 *Machine Learning Techniques in Breast Cancer Prediction*

In machine learning, feature selection is a process in which related attributes of a subset are chosen from various class attributes, and it is essential to build a model. To create a valid predictive model, selection of features is an important task. The choice of features for a model has different methods and advantages. Some advantages of feature selection are:

(i) It makes the machine learning model faster and effective.
(ii) It interprets the results more quickly.
(iii) Reduced the complexity of the model.
(iv) Accuracy of the model is increased if the right features are chosen.
(v) Over-fitting of the model is reduced [9].

The different features for a subset of attributes have interrelationship between them; it is challenging to choose independent and useful features among the subgroup. Many approaches have been proposed in the literature for the feature selection in breast cancer [10]. The main three methods for feature extraction are:

(i) Wrapper Method: The wrapper method chooses the subset that has optimal features. In this, all the best features are guided by the learning process.
(ii) Filter Method: The filter method is a pre-processing step and uses general features. The selection of attributes is not dependent on the learning process in this.
(iii) Embedded Method: This method has the qualities of both the filter and wrapper method in the selection of best subset.

2.3 *Classic Machine Learning Algorithms Related to Breast Cancer Prediction*

Machine learning deals with the programming of machines that learn from experience. Here experiences are for the machines is the kind of data that it has to deal with while performing. It provides machines with the ability to make decisions. It is the kind of artificial intelligence that gives intelligence to machines. In the health care prediction system, the "interactive machine learning" approach is desirable [11], and this approach leads to the improved learning procedure that machines learn in the same way as we human beings do. Humans received knowledge about something

Fig. 3 Training data and testing data

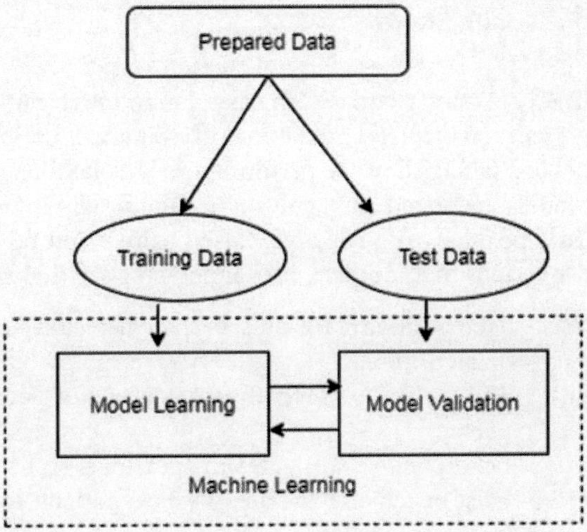

and kept that knowledge in mind and perform the identification of things by using that knowledge experiences from the past to help in making decisions for the future. The human brain trains itself by observing features and patterns available in that knowledge. Machines are also able to learn from data and experience given to them. Data provided to the machines are of two types, as depicted in Fig. 3.

(i) Training data: Machines learn the patterns and features from the training data and trained to make decisions from that data like classification, identification and prediction of new data.
(ii) Test data: Data received from training data are checked with test data to know the accuracy of decisions and predictions of the machines.

3 Performance Metrics

After the process of collecting datasets, pre-processing of data, feature extraction, feature selection, then classification, regression or clustering and getting output as a model, the final step is to check the efficiency of the build model. Various performance evaluation metrics are available for machine learning-based prediction models. The main performance measures are log loss, accuracy, precision, recall, sensitivity, specificity, F-measure, receiver operating characteristic curve (ROC), area under the curve (AUC), etc.

3.1 Confusion Matrix

The confusion matrix is an easy and intuitive outline for prediction. It defines the correct and incorrect predictions of a binary or multiclass classification by each class. Table 2 defines how the performance of a classifier is tested. Many machine learning models are tested and analyzed for the prediction of any disease using this matrix. True positive, true negative, false positive and false negative values are calculated for various matrices that are defined below [12, 13].

(i) True positive (TP): Breast cancer detected, and the patient is identified through an algorithm.
(ii) True negative (TN): Breast cancer not detected, and a patient is a healthy person.
(iii) False positive (FP): Healthy person is identified as a breast cancer patient.
(iv) False negative (FN): Breast cancer patients are identified incorrectly as healthy by the algorithm.

Accuracy (ACC)

It shows that how much the predictions are correct for a classifier, and how many samples are misclassified is also given in this. Accuracy defines the total accurate predictions divided by whole samples. The formula for calculating accuracy is given below:

$$\text{ACC} = \frac{TP + TN}{FP + FN + TP + TN}$$

Sensitivity (recall)

Recall is the no. of true results divided by the finding that has to be returned. It defines all the relevant cases in a database.

$$\text{Recall} = \frac{TP}{TP + FN}$$

Table 2 Confusion matrix

Confusion matrix: Predicted values are denoted by columns, and actual values are indicated by rows		Predicted	
		Breast cancer not detected	Breast cancer detected
Actual	Breast cancer not detected	TN	FP
	Breast cancer detected	FN	TP

Precision

Precision is defined as the no. of true results divided by all returned results. It shows the quality of our prediction.

$$\text{Precision} = \frac{TP}{TP + FP}$$

Specificity

Specificity is defined as the no of True negative values divided by all negative assessments.

$$\text{Specificity} = \frac{TN}{TN + FP}$$

F1-score

The harmonic mean of precision and recall which combines the both is the F1-score measure.

$$\text{F} = 2 * \frac{\text{Precision} * \text{recall}}{\text{Precision} + \text{recall}}$$

In addition to the above metrics, area under curve (AUC) is the measure of threshold settings for the different classification problems. Receiver operator characteristics curve (ROC) plots the positive and negative values to provide information more directly. The shape of the ROC curve contains lots of different values predicted by the confusion matrix. ROC is the probability curve, while AUC is the capability curve [14, 15].

4 Methods and Materials

The data were obtained from the UCI machine learning repository. It includes 286 instances and 10 attributes [16]. The attributes used in the dataset are depicted in Table 3.

4.1 Experimental Setup

To practice the machine learning algorithms, WEKA software has been used. It is an open-source data analysis tool, which takes data in the attribute relation file format (ARFF). It can do the task of pre-processing of data, investigates the behavior and

Table 3 Attributes of the dataset

Number	Attribute
1	Age
2	Menopause
3	Tumor size
4	Inv-nodes
5	Node-caps
6	Degree of malignancy
7	Breast
8	Breast quadrant
9	Irradiation
10	Class: patient at high risk or low risk

finds patterns in the dataset. To test the effectiveness of model, cross-validation (CV) technique is used, which provides performance of any machine learning model.

In a limited data, to evaluate the model, it is a re-sampling procedure. In cross-validation, a sample or portion of data is kept aside on which model is not trained, and this portion or sample is used later for the testing and validation. Patients at low risk and high risk are classified using weighted average in this work [17]. In this work, naïve Bayes, random forest, sequential minimum optimization (SMO) and logistic regression machine learning algorithms are evaluated using Weka software. Classification accuracy of any model is the total number of correct predictions in any dataset divided by the total number of predictions. In classification problems, accuracy is inappropriate for imbalanced data as a performance measure. Accuracy is the combination of F-measure recall and precision; based on these parameters, accuracy can be measured. The accuracy of the predictive model is calculated based on values of F-measure, precision and recall. The performance evaluation of all the four algorithms is shown in Sect. 5, and Figs. 4, 5 and 6 show the comparison of all the various classifiers in the terms of F-measure, recall and precision [18, 19].

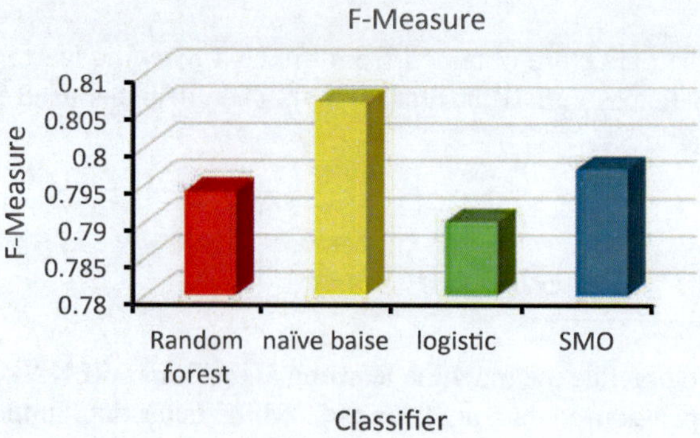

Fig. 4 Comparison of all the four algorithms based on F-measure

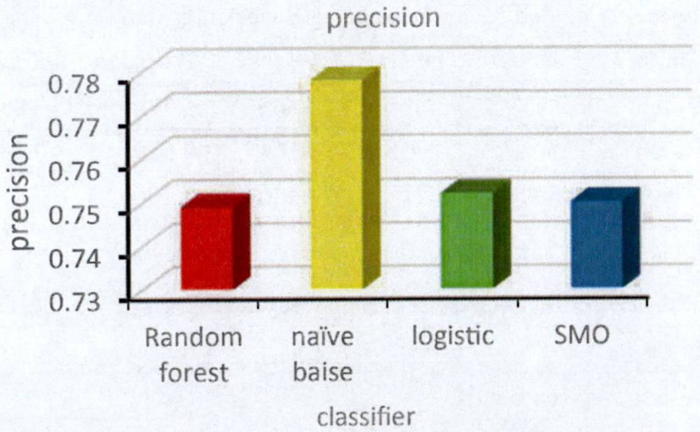

Fig. 5 Comparison of all the four algorithms based on precision

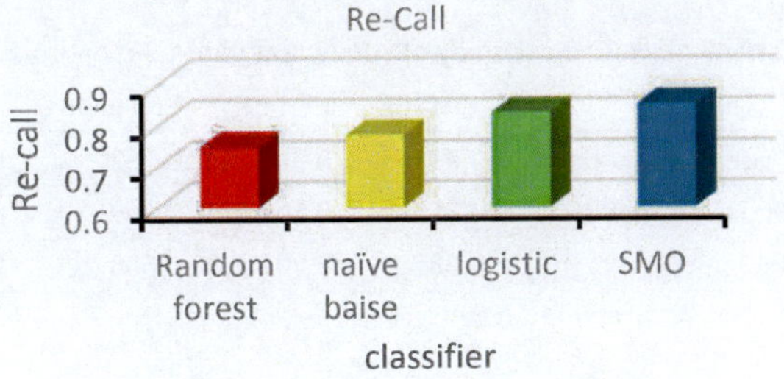

Fig. 6 Comparison of all the four algorithms based on recall

5 Performance Evaluation and Comparison of Classifiers

5.1 Performance Evaluation of Classifiers

Detailed accuracy with random forest algorithm is shown in Table 4, and the confusion matrix corresponding to this is shown in Table 5. Detailed accuracy with naïve Bayes algorithm is shown in Table 6, and confusion matrix of naïve Bayes is shown in Table 7.

Table 4 Detailed accuracy with random forest algorithm

Class	TP rate	FP rate	Precision	Recall	F-measure	ROC area
Patient at low risk	0.846	0.671	0.749	0.846	0.794	0.638
Patient at high risk	0.329	0.154	0.475	0.329	0.389	0.638
Weighted average	0.692	0.517	0.667	0.692	0.674	0.638

Table 5 Confusion matrix of random forest algorithm

Class	A	B
A = low-risk patients	170	31
B = high-risk patients	57	28

Table 6 Detailed accuracy of naive Bayes algorithm

Class	TP rate	FP rate	Precision	Recall	F-measure	ROC area
Patient at low risk	0.836	0.565	0.778	0.836	0.806	0.701
Patient at high risk	0.435	0.164	0.529	0.435	0.477	0.701
Weighted average	0.717	0.446	0.704	0.717	0.708	0.701

Table 7 Confusion matrix of naive Bayes algorithm

Class	A	B
A = low-risk patients	168	33
B = high-risk patients	48	37

Table 8 Detailed accuracy of sequential minimum optimization (SMO)

Class	TP rate	FP rate	Precision	Recall	F-measure	ROC area
Patient at low risk	0.831	0.647	0.752	0.831	0.791	0.646
Patient at high risk	0.353	0.169	0.469	0.353	0.403	0.646
Weighted average	0.689	0.505	0.668	0.689	0.675	0.646

Table 9 Confusion matrix for SMO

Class	A	B
A = low-risk patients	167	34
B = high-risk patients	55	30

Tables 8 and 9 show the accuracy with SMO and its confusion Matrix. Detailed accuracy of logistic regression is in Table 10, and its confusion matrix is in Table 11.

Table 10 Detailed accuracy by class for logistic regression

Class	TP rate	FP rate	Precision	Recall	F-measure	ROC area
Patient at low risk	0.851	0.671	0.752	0.851	0.797	0.59
Patient at high risk	0.329	0.149	0.483	0.329	0.392	0.59
Weighted average	0.696	0.516	0.671	0.696	0.677	0.59

Table 11 Confusion matrix for logistic regression

Class	A	B
A = low-risk patients	171	30
B = high-risk patients	57	28

5.2 *Comparison of Algorithms on the Basis of F-measure, Recall and Precision*

Comparison of F-measure, precision and recall for all the four algorithms on the values in above tables is shown in Figs. 4, 5 and 6, respectively.

6 Result and Conclusion

6.1 *Result*

The nature of training data affects the performance of learning techniques. Confusion matrices have an excellent role for evaluating classifiers. In non-parametric estimation techniques, weighting function is considered as a kernel. In kernel density estimation, it estimates density functions of random variables, and in kernel regression, it estimates the conditional expectation of a random variable. In this, the columns stand for predictions and the rows for the actual class.

A model's performance is measured by the log loss parameter where predicted outcome has its value of probability between 0 and 1. A high log loss is a consequence of probability prediction of 0.101 where true label should be 1. A log loss equation helps in calculating log loss of dataset's each row.

According to the performance of the above observation, naïve Bayes algorithm is higher in terms of classification of patients at the high risk and low risk of breast cancer, and the accuracy of naïve Bayes is 71.6% in prospect to the other classifiers.

6.2 *Conclusion*

Continuously growing electronic health records (EHR) led to a surge of machine learning-based big data prediction models. Conventional methods for database management are incapable of handling big data and of extracting knowledge from this. Real-time analysis and implementation of the machine learning-based model in collaboration with experts to view the effectiveness of these model are essential for any health care decision support system. Timely detection helps doctors in treatment of a patient in an effective manner. In this work, authors have analyzed the existing cancer prediction models, risk factors involved in them, the role of machine learning in prediction, techniques and algorithms used by various researchers. Authors have used the Waikato Environment for Knowledge Analysis (WEKA) for the simulation purpose. On comparing the performance of naïve Bayes, random forest, logistic regression and SMO, it has been found that naïve Bayes algorithm has classified the patient in high-risk and low-risk categories using various risk factors with an accuracy of 71.67%. In the future, authors have planned to propose a new model for detection of breast cancer at early stage.

References

1. Sharma D, Kumar R, Jain A (2021) A systematic review of risk factors and risk assessment models for breast cancer. Mobile Radio Commun 5G Netw 509–519
2. Weedon-Fekjær H, Lindqvist BH, Vatten LJ, Aalen OO, Tretli S (2008) Breast cancer tumor growth estimated through mammography screening data. Breast Cancer Res 10(3):1–13
3. Rakha EA, Reis-Filho JS, Baehner F, Dabbs DJ, Decker T, Eusebi V, Fox SB et al (2010) Breast cancer prognostic classification in the molecular era: the role of histological grade. Breast Cancer Res 12(4):1–12
4. Laurance J (2006) Breast cancer cases rise 80% since the seventies; Breast Cancer. The Independent. London, pp 1–6
5. Cintolo-Gonzalez JA, Braun D, Blackford AL, Mazzola E, Acar A, Plichta JK, Griffin M, Hughes KS (2017) Breast cancer risk models: a comprehensive overview of existing models, validation, and clinical applications. Breast Cancer Res Treatment 164(2):263–284
6. Amir E, Freedman OC, Seruga B, Evans DG (2010) Assessing women at high risk of breast cancer: a review of risk assessment models. JNCI: J Natl Cancer Inst 102(10):680–691
7. Cruz AJ, Wishart DS (2006) Applications of machine learning in cancer prediction and prognosis. Cancer Inform 2:59–77
8. Woolston C (2001) Breast cancer: 4 big questions. Nature 527(7578):120–120
9. Chen M, Hao Y, Hwang K, Wang L, Wang L (2017) Disease prediction by machine learning over big data from healthcare communities. IEEE Access 5:8869–8879
10. Hagerty RG, Butow PN, Ellis PM, Dimitry S, Tattersall MHN (2005) Communicating prognosis in cancer care: a systematic review of the literature. Ann Oncol 16(7):1005–1053
11. Dhahri H, Al Maghayreh E, Mahmood A, Elkilani W, Faisal Nagi M (2019) Automated breast cancer diagnosis based on machine learning algorithms. J Healthc Eng 1–11
12. https://www.cancer.org/content/dam/cance-org/research/cancer-facts-and-statistics/breastcancer-facts-and-figures/breast-cancer-factsand-figures-2019-2020
13. Pilnenskiy N, Smetannikov I (2020) Feature selection algorithms as one of the python data analytical tools. Future Internet 12(3):1–14
14. Akay MF (2009) Support vector machines combined with feature selection for breast cancer diagnosis. Expert Syst Appl 36(2):3240–3247
15. Alghunaim S, Al-Baity HH (2019) On the scalability of machine-learning algorithms for breast cancer prediction in big data context. IEEE Access 7:91535–91546
16. https://archive.ics.uci.edu/ml/datasets.php
17. Chaurasia V, Pal S (2017) A novel approach for breast cancer detection using data mining techniques. Int J Innov Res Comput Commun Eng (An ISO 3297: 2007 Certified Organisation) 2:1–17
18. Li A, Wang R, Liu L, Xu L, Wang F, Chang F, Yu L, Xiang Y, Zhou F, Yu Z (2018) BCRAM: A social-network-inspired breast cancer risk assessment model. IEEE Trans Indus Inform 15(1):366–376
19. Jain A, Tiwari S, Sapra V (2019) Two-phase heart disease diagnosis system using deep learning. Int J Control Autom 12(5):558–573

Designing Deep Learning Architectures for Multiview 3D Shape Estimation Using Image Transformers

Kanika Singla and Parmanand Astya

Abstract The task of 3D shape generation for realistic data is an important challenge that needs to be addressed in the domain of computer vision, robotics, and graphics which serve as a building block for many real-time applications like autonomous driving or 3D modeling, etc. Estimating shapes from a few 2D images are fundamentally ill-posed as numerous 3D shapes can be explained by a few images. In the absence of complete information, recently, deep learning has been used to fill in the gap by leveraging data driven category level priors. In this work, we propose a novel 3D shape estimation network that uses an image transformer to better encode the shape features into a latent representation which is later decoded using a multilayer perceptron. Our experiments show that image transformers are better than convolution-based encoders due to their wide attention capability. We perform both qualitative and quantitative experiments to demonstrate the effect of new architecture on shape quality and detail.

Keywords Computer vision · Multiview shape · 3D reconstruction · Shape estimation · Multiview images · Image transformers

1 Introduction

We are particularly interested in the problem of 3D shape estimation, which involves estimating the complete structure of objects from multiview images of the target. Many relevant real-world applications need this as prerequisite. 3D shape estimation, for example, will help autonomous vehicles track objects [1], and robots find out the best grasping position [2]. Humans can naturally approximate the shapes of objects using only the most basic information. Human eyes can easily perceive the 3D structure from the limited, ambiguous, and even occluded 2D details. However, this task becomes particularly challenging, when this concept is applied to the machines, due to ambiguity generated from single view images, occluded images, and sparse

K. Singla (✉) · P. Astya
Department of Computer Science and Engineering, School of Engineering & Technology, Sharda University, Greater Noida, India

N. Marriwala et al. (eds.), *Emergent Converging Technologies and Biomedical Systems*, Lecture Notes in Electrical Engineering 841,
https://doi.org/10.1007/978-981-16-8774-7_42

point clouds [3]. It is unfair to expect them to predict a deterministic output from an uncertain input [4].

The aim of this paper is to create a geometric representation of the underlying 3D world from a set of images captured from various camera positions. We are estimating the 3D shape of an object using 2D images taken from (digital) cameras by using learned data driven priors of other objects.

With the rising popularity of deep learning, several methods have been proposed to do 3D shape generation from single [5] and multiple images [6]. At the core of this, development is the successes in designing convolutional kernels in 2D/3D space that can learn meaningful features. Frequently, these convolutional neural networks are designed to have several consecutive layers making them "deep" with the objective of increasing their receptive field that is found to aid in learning richer features [6]. Recent research efforts have, however, highlighted the limitations of convolutional neural networks in learning long range relationships in spatial [7] and temporal [7] dimensions. To resolve these limitations, several methods have been investigating transformer networks to learn richer representations that additionally encode long range spatio-temporal dependencies [8].

In this work, we exploit the capability of image transformers to learn such long range dependencies to improve the task of multiimage 3D shape generations. In particular, we show that compared to the popular ResNet-18 [9] encoder, an image transformer such as data efficient transformer (DiT) [7] can capture long range dependencies in the input image and consequently learn richer latent shape representations. We also propose a novel architecture that uses this image transformer and a point-based multilayer perceptron to generate 3D shapes.

While recurrent neural networks (RNNs) have been used in recent approaches to learn object's mapping between distinct views, [10]. These designs are inefficient in terms of computation, and the RNN model's input views are sensitive to the order of permutation [11] which makes it difficult to work with a collection of different unordered acquired views. In contrast, we use Max pooling operation to fuse latent representations from multiple views, thus making our approach permutation invariant.

This paper has been broken down into different sections. The first section of this paper includes the paper's introduction, as well as the problem statement's goal, inspiration, and objectives. Section 2 discusses the literature review of the concepts used in the study. The image transformers' background is detailed in Sect. 3. Section 4 includes qualitative and quantitative experiments analysis. Section 5 covers the interpretation and discussion of the results, as well as the work's contribution to the previous studies. This segment also discusses the potential scope of the work.

2 Related Work

Generating the shape of a 3D object from a few images is an ill-posed problem. We now review the relevant literature in both traditional and learning-based 3D reconstruction. We then briefly review the recent transformer literature as it relates to this work.

A. **Traditional Multiview 3D Reconstruction:** In geometric processing, shape completion has a long history. Many relevant real-world applications need this as a prerequisite such as in tracking objects for autonomous vehicles [1] grasping for autonomous robotic manipulators [2]. For dense point clouds, a common technique to convert them to meshes is Poisson surface reconstruction [12]. Other classical techniques resort to 3D reconstruction from 2D images by leveraging multiview consistency [13]. While more broadly, structure from motion is performed to do large-scale reconstruction with both posed [14] and in the wild images [15], they are often plagued by non-lambertian surfaces, occlusions, small baselines causing degeneracy, and changes in illuminations. Thus, only by collecting millions of images [16] and using hand-crafted edits by artists can such techniques be used reliably. These limitations motivate explorations into data driven methods that do not suffer from such issues.

B. **Deep Learning on 3D Shapes:** Deep learning allows use of data driven priors for resolving shape ambiguities and thus enabling complete shape generation. Broadly, they can be characterized based on the type of 3D representation that is regressed. A mesh-based representation [17] stores the surface information as a list of vertices and faces. Choy et al. [10] put forth a deep generative model for modeling voxelized 3D shapes that leverage 3D convolution kernels for shape generation. To address the drawbacks of the voxel representation, authors argued for generating point clouds [18] instead using a single image. Rich literature on implicit function learning [19, 20] for shape representation and reconstruction tasks has been done by the researchers in the computer vision and graphics community.

C. **Transformers:** Transformer models have excelled at a number of tasks in natural language processing, including computer translation, document classification [21]. The core part of a transformer is its multi-head self-attention mechanism that combines the characteristics of each token pair in the embedding sequence. Transformer has recently been applied to the domain of computer vision with great success [8, 22]. Impactful and promising applications have been shown by [23]. ViT [8] applies transformer to sequences of image-patches for the task of image classification, without using CNN features, when pre-trained on a large-scale dataset, and demonstrates comparable and higher classification accuracy. These have significant advantages over their CNN counterparts when it comes to attending to long range spatio-temporal dependencies. This is key to learning much richer representations opening several avenues for future research not just in 3D reconstruction but also video understanding [24], scene understanding [25].

3 Method, Background, and Notations

We now describe our image transformer-based multiview 3D object reconstruction method, which has been given a set of images (3 in this case) extracts per image latent vectors and fuses them using a Max pooling operation. The pooled representation is permutation invariant and is later used to extract complete 3D shape via a point-based multilayer perceptron network. We will first provide a brief background on the architecture of a vision transformer [8] and then elaborate our proposed pipeline.

3.1 Background on Vision Transformer

Transformers were first introduced in [26] as a two-part architecture (encoder and decoder) that allows you to turn one series into another. However, it differs from existing sequence models like RNN and LSTM in a sense that it does not include recurrent networks. Figure 1 shows the visualization of transformers. The encoder is located on the left, while the decoder is located on the right. Encoder and decoder are both made up of components that can be placed on top of each other several times, as shown by **Nx** in the diagram. As shown in the Fig. 1, the modules are primarily made up of multi-head attention and feedforward layers.

Positional encoding is another crucial component of the model. Since a sequence relies on the order of its components, and we do not have any recurrent networks that can remember how sequences are fed into a model, we need to allocate each component of our sequence a relative place. These coordinates are added to the embedded representation of each letter (n-dimensional vector).

For a sequence of **Y** query vectors (packed into $\mathbf{Z} \in \mathbf{R}^{\mathbf{Y \times d}}$), it produces an output matrix (of size $\mathbf{Y} \times \mathbf{d}$):

$$\mathbf{Attention(Z,\ K,\ V)} = \mathbf{Softmax}\big(\mathbf{ZK^T}/\sqrt{\mathbf{d}}\big)\mathbf{V}, \quad (1)$$

where the Softmax function is applied over each row of the input matrix and the $\sqrt{\mathbf{d}}$ term is used to normalize the result.

3.2 Architecture Details

We now provide details about the network architecture. In the Fig. 2, we show how a set of images (set of 3 in this case) is fed to a ResNet-18 encoder R_ϕ, with shared network weights. This results in view dependent latent vectors L1, L2, L3. In order to fuse them together while maintaining permutation invariance, we use the "Max" operator that takes the max(L1, L2, L3) along the views and results in the global latent code L. This latent code is then decoded via a set of MLP layers Q_θ to generate

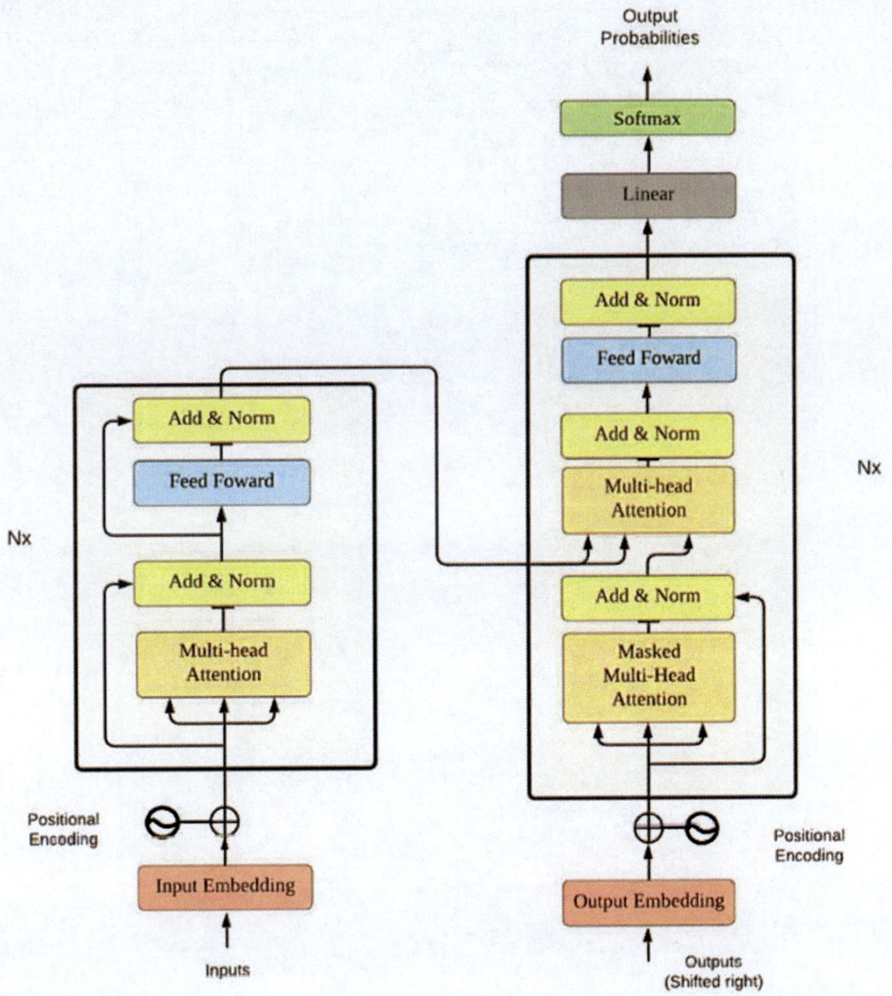

Fig. 1 Transformer model

a point cloud of 1024 points. The MLP being used here has the architecture as [1024, 1000, 1000, 1000, 3072]. While this architecture is plausible and gives us a point cloud based on input views of the object, we propose to further improve the results by means of transformer layers. As discussed above, transformers are able to better capture the long range dependencies in images and as such provide much richer latent codes. Here, the data efficient transformer [8] T_ϕ is used to encode the image set I, which is passed through the max operator to get global latent code L and subsequent point cloud via the decoder Q_θ (same as above). We train both these architectures on

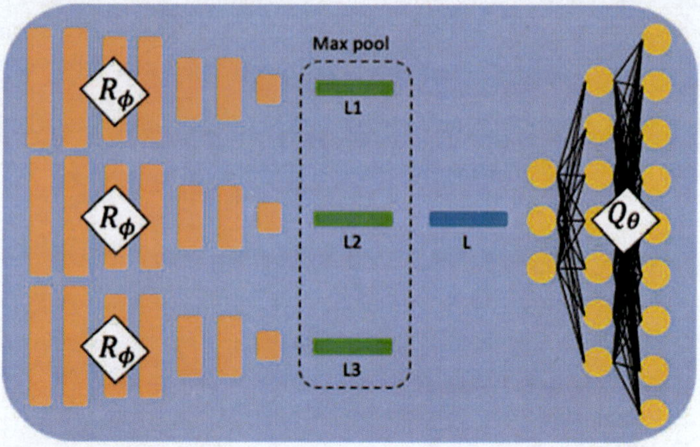

Fig. 2 ResNet-18 as encoder

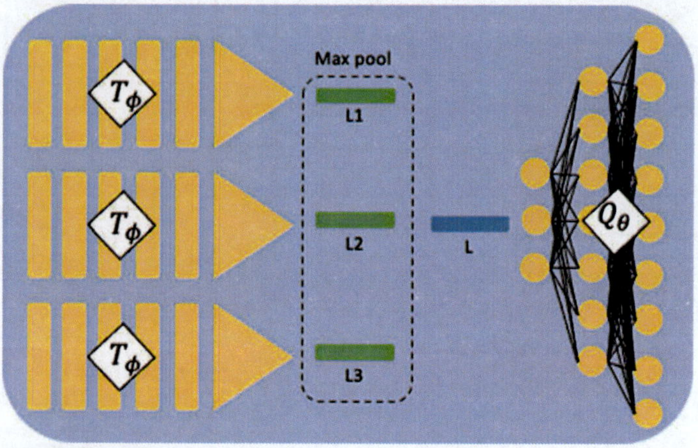

Fig. 3 Image transformer encoding the imageSet

ShapeNet dataset [27] and use the renderings provided by [10] for 120 epochs with a learning rate of 1e-3 and weight decay of 0.98 after every 250 iterations. In total, this takes roughly 30 h on a single NVIDIA 2080Ti GPU (Fig. 3).

4 Experiments and Result Analysis

We now provide some quantitative and qualitative results and comparisons between ResNet-18 encoder and image transformer to highlight benefits of using image transformers for the task of multiview 3D reconstruction.

Table 1 Comparing chamfer distance for multiview reconstruction on resnet-18 and image transformer

Encoder type	Resnet-18	Image transformer (ours)
Chamfer distance	0.83	**0.78**

A. **Quantitative Results**

For quantitative comparisons, we evaluate the bidirectional chamfer distance (Eq. 1) of the generated point clouds. Here, lower values are better. Chamfer distance is a common metric that quantifies distance of two point clouds, from p to q, which is defined as

$$L(\Theta) = \sum \min_{q \in MG} ||p - q||^2 + \sum \min_{p \in MP} ||p - q||^2 \qquad (2)$$

where **MG** and **MP are** ground mesh and predicted mesh, respectively (Table 1).

B. **Qualitative Results**

We now visualize some examples of the reconstructions obtained from ResNet-18 and image transformer encoders, respectively, based on the input image triplets (Table 2).

5 Conclusion and Future Scope

In this work, we presented a novel architecture for 3D shape generation from multiple point clouds and demonstrated that image transformers achieve significantly better performance for this task compared to their ResNet counterparts. We provide both qualitative and quantitative results to establish this claim. In future, we would like to investigate the effects of using a transformer-based decoder (instead of an MLP). I believe that the gains we see by replacing convolutional encoders with transformers will also translate to the decoder side and would hopefully result in much higher fidelity of reconstructions.

Table 2 Qualitative results on 3d reconstruction

Image	ResNet-18	Image transformer (ours)	Ground truth
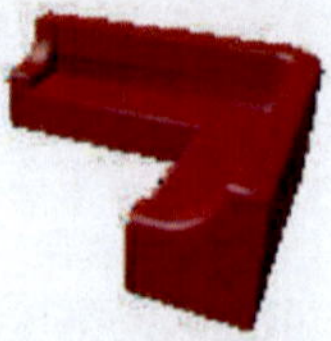	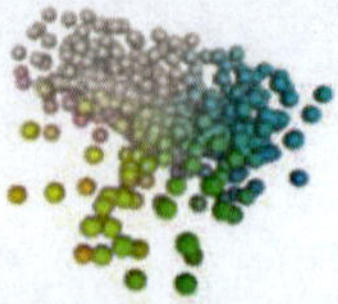	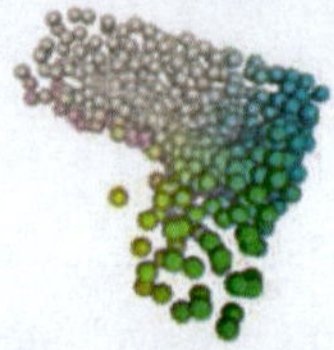	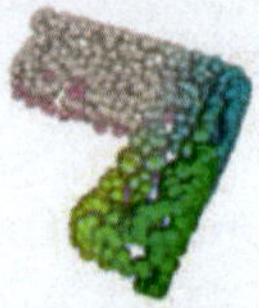
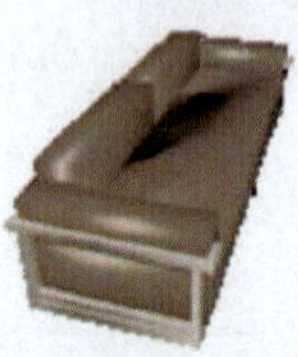	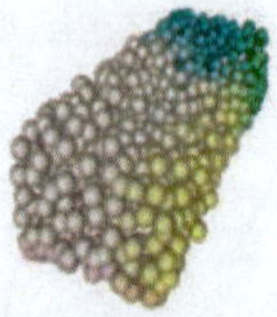	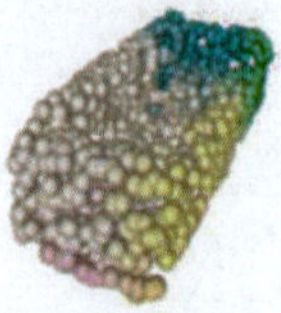	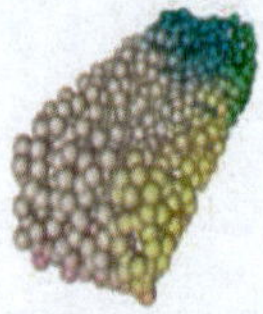
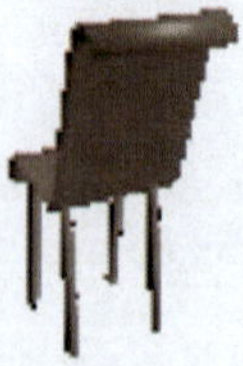	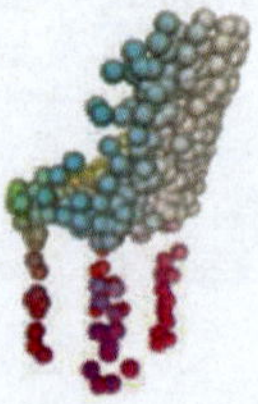	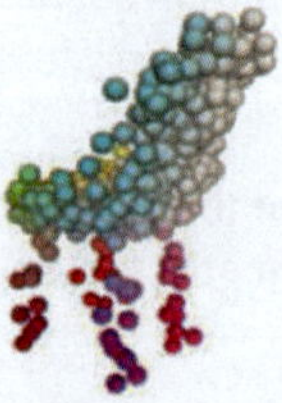	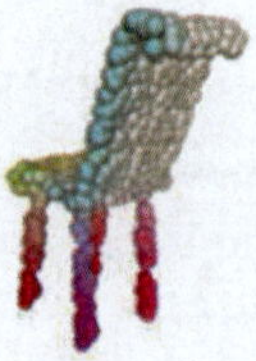
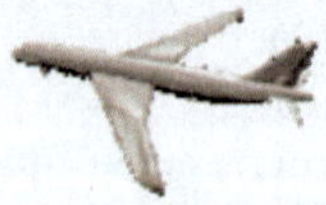	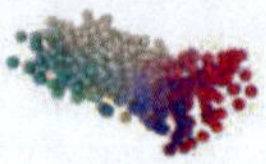	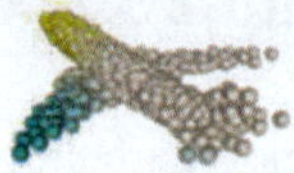	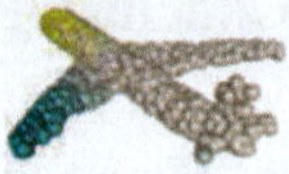

References

1. Giancola S, Zarzar J, Ghanem B (2019) Leveraging shape completion for 3d siamese tracking. In: Proceedings of the IEEE conference on computer vision and pattern recognition, pp 1359–1368
2. Varley J, DeChant C, Richardson A, Ruales J, Allen P (2017) Shape completion enabled robotic grasping. In: 2017 IEEE/RSJ international conference on intelligent robots and systems (IROS), pp 2442–2447. IEEE
3. Qi CR, Su H, Mo K, Guibas LJ (2017) Pointnet: deep learning on point sets for 3d classification and segmentation. In Proc CVPR
4. Mandikal P, Navaneet KL, Agarwal M, Babu RV (2018) 3D-LMNet: latent embedding matching for accurate and diverse 3D point cloud reconstruction from a single image. arXiv preprint arXiv:1807.07796
5. Niu C, Yu Y, Bian Z, Li J, Xu K (2020). Weakly supervised part-wise 3D shape reconstruction from single-view RGB images. In Computer graphics forum, vol 39, No 7, pp 447–457

6. Choy CB, Xu D, Gwak J, Chen K, Savarese S (2016) 3d-r2n2: a unified approach for single and multi-view 3d object reconstruction. In European conference on computer vision (ECCV)
7. Touvron H, Cord M, Douze M, Massa F, Sablayrolles A, Jégou H (2020) Training data-efficient image transformers & distillation through attention. arXiv preprint arXiv:2012.12877
8. Touvron H, Cord M, Douze M, Massa F, Sablayrolles A, J´egou H (2020) Training data-efficient image transformers & distillation through attention. arXiv preprint arXiv:2012.12877
9. Ou X, Yan P, Zhang Y, Tu B, Zhang G, Wu J, Li W (2019) Moving object detection method via ResNet-18 with encoder–decoder structure in complex scenes. IEEE Access 7:108152–108160
10. Choy CB, Xu D, Gwak J, Chen K, Savarese S (2016) 3d-r2n2: a unified approach for single and multi-view 3d object reconstruction. In Proceedings of the European conference on computer vision (ECCV)
11. Vinyals S Bengio, Kudlur M (2016) Order matters: sequence to sequence for sets. In International Conference on Learning Represen-tations (ICLR)
12. Kazhdan M, Bolitho M, Hoppe H (2006) Poisson surface reconstruction. In Proceedings of the fourth Eurographics symposium on Geometry processing, vol 7
13. Hartley R, Zisserman A (2003) Multiple view geometry in computer vision (cambridge university). *C1 C3*, *2*
14. Yingze Bao S, Chandraker M, Lin Y, Savarese S (2013) Dense object reconstruction with semantic priors. In Proceedings of the IEEE conference on computer vision and pattern recognition, pp 1264–1271
15. Wang N, Zhang Y, Li Z, Fu Y, Liu W, Jiang YG (2018) Pixel2mesh: generating 3d mesh models from single rgb images. In Proceedings of the European conference on computer vision (ECCV), pp 52–67
16. Agarwal S, Furukawa Y, Snavely N, Simon I, Curless B, Seitz SM, Szeliski R (2011) Building Rome in a day. Commun ACM 54(10):105–112
17. Achlioptas P, Diamanti O, Mitliagkas I, Guibas L (2018) Learning representations and generative models for 3d point clouds. In International conference on machine learning, pp 40–49. PMLR
18. Liu Y, Fan B, Meng G, Lu J, Xiang S, Pan C (2019) Densepoint: learning densely contextual representation for efficient point cloud processing. In Proceedings of the IEEE/CVF international conference on computer vision, pp 5239–5248
19. Park JJ, Florence P, Straub J, Newcombe R, Lovegrove S (2019) Deepsdf: learning continuous signed distance functions for shape representation. In Proceedings of the IEEE/CVF conference on computer vision and pattern recognition, pp 165–174
20. Michalkiewicz M, Pontes JK, Jack D, Baktashmotlagh M, Eriksson A (2019) Deep level sets: implicit surface representations for 3d shape inference. arXiv preprint arXiv:1901.06802
21. Brown TB, Mann B, Ryder N, Subbiah M, Kaplan J, Dhariwal P, ... Amodei D (2020) Language models are few-shot learners. arXiv preprint arXiv:2005.14165
22. Devlin M-W, Chang K Lee, Toutanova K (2018) Bert: pre-training of deep bidirectional transformers for language understanding. arXivpreprint arXiv:1810.04805
23. Dosovitskiy L, Beyer A, Kolesnikov D, Weissenborn X, Zhai T, Unterthiner M, Dehghani M, Minderer G, Heigold S, Gelly J Uszkoreit, Houlsby N (2021) An image is worth 16 x 16 words: Trans-formers for image recognition at scale. In International Conference on Learning Representations (ICLR)
24. Kwon H, Kim M, Kwak S, Cho M (2020) Motionsqueeze: neural motion feature learning for video understanding. In European conference on computer vision, pp 345–362. Springer, Cham
25. Guo Z, Huang Y, Hu X, Wei H, Zhao B (2021) A survey on deep learning based approaches for scene understanding in autonomous driving. Electronics 10(4):471
26. Vaswani A, Shazeer N, Parmar N, Uszkoreit J, Jones L, Gomez AN, Kaiser LU, Polosukhin I (2017) Attention is all you need. In Guyon I, Luxburg UV, Bengio S, Wallach H, Fergus R, Vishwanathan S, Garnett R (eds) Advances in neural information processing systems, vol 30. Curran Associates, Inc
27. Chang AX, Funkhouser T, Guibas L, Hanrahan P, Huang Q, Li Z, ... Yu F (2015) Shapenet: an information-rich 3d model repository. arXiv preprint arXiv:1512.03012

Comparative Analysis of Term Extraction and Selection Techniques for Query Reformulation Using PRF

Vishal Gupta, Dilip Kumar Sharma, and Ashutosh Dixit

Abstract Query reformulation (QR) is the process to make initial query exact by generating more significant terms. Term extraction and selection are one of the techniques of it. QR eliminates irrelevant and repetitive terms from the top ranked documents and upgrades the effectiveness of IR system. There are various term extraction and selection methods, and each method has its own strength and shortcoming. This paper does comparative analysis of various term extraction and selection techniques for QR using pseudo relevance feedback. Three standard datasets such as CACM, CISI, and Medline are utilized to conduct all the experiments. The outcomes are contrasted with each other in terms of average precision, average recall, and F-measure. It is found that BIM and Okapi BM25 outperform other techniques on both CACM and CISI datasets, while KLD and RSV outperform other techniques on Medline dataset.

Keywords Pseudo relevance feedback (PRF) · Term extraction method · Term selection method · Information retrieval · Query reformulation

1 Introduction

Information retrieval (IR) concerns with the structure, storage, analysis, and access to items of information. This provides the user with easy and efficient access to the relevant information that will satisfy user's information need. To express their information needs, users use unstructured texts called queries. These queries are provided to an information retrieval system which in turn extract relevant resources

V. Gupta (✉) · A. Dixit
J.C. Bose University of Science & Technology, YMCA, Faridabad, Haryana, India

V. Gupta
MMEC, MM(DU), Mullana, Ambala, Haryana, India

D. K. Sharma
GLA University, Mathura, UP, India
e-mail: dilip.sharma@gla.ac.in

N. Marriwala et al. (eds.), *Emergent Converging Technologies and Biomedical Systems*, Lecture Notes in Electrical Engineering 841,
https://doi.org/10.1007/978-981-16-8774-7_43

and presented them to the user. There is a massive difference between the query written by the user to search for the content and the retrieved content that can satisfy the user's intent. One reason for this problem is that the queries written by the user are too small, unstructured, incomplete, or imprecise, which is not enough to explain the user's needs. The average length of the query according to [1] was 2.30 words, which are precisely the same as reported several years before in [2]. So, there is a need for some query representation that can express the user's need for information more efficiently and thoroughly. The major problem faced by the user for efficient information retrieval is vocabulary mismatch according to [3] due to either polysemy (different words with similar meanings) or synonymy (same word having different meanings) which causes retrieval of irrelevant documents. Also, if we retrieve documents that depend only upon the occurrence of query terms inside a document, then we would skip some relevant documents which are more suitable or relevant for the user. To handle this, initial query has been reformulated by adding new terms that help to understand the user's intent and thus generates a more effective query by removing ambiguity. Query reformulation (QR) not only involves adding new query terms to the initial query but also removing irrelevant terms from the query to enhance its formulation. The general process of query reformulation is shown as in Fig. 1.

IR system, according to the user's query, selects terms from document corpus, and these selected terms act as candidate terms for reformulation. These candidate terms along with initial query terms generate a revised query using query reformulation process. The revised query is now applied to the IR system, which in turn generates final ranked documents relevant to the user.

A comparative analysis of various term extraction and selection techniques using pseudo relevance feedback (PRF) is done in this paper. In PRF, firstly, documents are

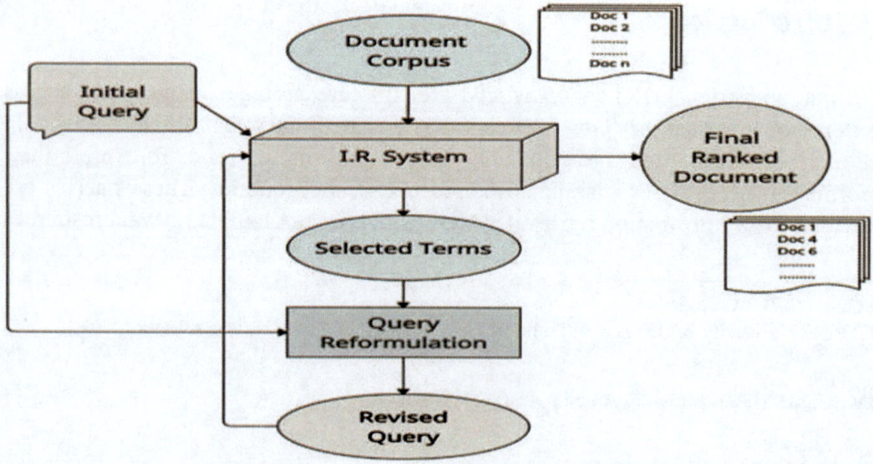

Fig. 1 Query reformulation process

retrieved by executing initial query on a corpus of documents. Then, top retrieved documents are picked as relevant ones for creating a pool of terms. After that by applying various term extraction and selection techniques, candidate terms were generated for query reformulation.

The remaining paper is sorted out as follows. Section 2 presents literature survey. Theoretical foundation of term extraction and selection methods is discussed in Sect. 3. Section 4 presents the experimental study. Finally, Sect. 5 concludes the whole work.

2 Literature Review

This section discusses the state-of-the-art literature related to various query reformulation techniques and highlights the challenges, which still require to be addressed. This section includes various techniques related to indexing, crawling, and ranking of documents for efficient information retrieval that satisfy user's needs.

Authors in [4] presented a review of different query reformulation approaches, along with their advantages and disadvantages. They highlighted the fact that hybrid methods which use both statistical and semantic methods show better performance but retrieving efficient and relevant documents that satisfy user's need is still a challenging task.

Authors in [5] presented a survey on recent automatic query reformulation approaches like query-specific-based, linguistic-based, etc. They also discussed the importance of query reformulation, various steps of automatic query reformulation, different approaches available for query reformulation and their comparison, critical issues faced, and future guidance of automatic query reformulation.

After studying various query optimization techniques, authors selected the pseudo relevance feedback method relevant for efficient retrieval of information, but still, it produces irrelevant results for some queries [6]. To find semantically similar words, authors proposed automated query reformulation technique "Xu" using the concept of high dimensional clustering of word vectors [7]. Researchers in [8] developed divergence from randomness (DFR) model, which assumes that the frequency of informative words is more in relevant documents than in others.

An information-theoretic technique for QR has been presented in [9] which was powerful when used with rocchio's framework for reformulation and weighting of terms. A new automatic query reformulation method (Co) has been introduced in [10] that estimated the correlation between the candidate expansion terms and the query terms. They compared their system (Co) with the Bose–Einstein 2 (Bo2) divergence from randomness (DFR) model. Both Co and Bo2 methods have comparable results, but they found that the success of query reformulation depends upon the type of initial query. An intelligent method via PRF has been proposed in [11] to handle the vocabulary problem, which shows improvements in recall as well as in precision.

In [12], authors summarize various existing soft computing methods that can be employed to increase IR systems efficiency. Majority of the work has been restricted for queries containing only non-numeric terms. Therefore, authors suggested a technique using the fuzzy weighting of query terms that work well for queries containing numerical terms also [13].

A comparative analysis of recent query reformulation approaches based on fuzzy logic was done in [14, 15]. The datasets used for testing performance include TREC-3, CISI, and CACM. The obtained results were compared with approaches given by in [16] and in [17], and performance was validated using a paired t-test analysis.

Authors provided a complete overview of query reformulation techniques from 1960 to 2017 for supporting efficient information retrieval [18]. Authors in [19] used a new scoring technique called in-link score and tf-idf-based score to allocate scores to reformulation terms of Wikipedia and WordNet, respectively, and finally used correlation score to reweigh the selected terms with respect to complete query.

Authors in [20] used multiple methods for selecting terms instead of using individual term selection method for query reformulation. In [21], authors proposed a query reformulation method called maximal marginal relevance-based reformulation (MMRE) which extracts highest MMRE scored top M reformulation terms that match with the user's query but differ from the previously selected reformulation terms by using ConceptNet as dataset.

3 Term Extraction and Selection

As query reformulation is the process of adding new terms and removing irrelevant terms from the query, much focus is on the term extraction and term selection techniques. How new terms are extracted, and out of those extracted terms, how many terms can be added to initial query is an area of research. Various researchers proposed different techniques for term extraction and term selection. It has been found from the survey that query term extraction techniques can be classified into three major categories [22] as co-occurrence information-based [23], class-based [24, 25], and corpus-based [26, 27]. These methods determine the relevance of candidate reformulation terms by calculating similarity scores and ranked them according to their individual score. Some of the popular ones out of them are as follows:

(i) **Cosine:**

The cosine similarity measure between two terms [18] is given as

$$S_{Cosine} = \frac{c_{m_1,m_2}}{\sqrt{\sum_{d_j} w^2_{m_1,m_1} \cdot \sum_{d_j} w^2_{m_2,m_2}}} \tag{1}$$

where $\mathrm{c}_{m_1,m_2} = \sum_{\mathrm{d_k}} \mathrm{w}_{m_1,\mathrm{k}} . \mathrm{w}_{m_2,\mathrm{k}}$ is the correlation value between terms m_1 andm_2, $\mathrm{w}_{m_1,\mathrm{k}}and\mathrm{w}_{m_2,\mathrm{k}}$ represents the weight of m_1 and m_2 in document d, respectively. The $\mathrm{S_{Cosine}}$ measure performs the normalization of correlation value$\mathrm{c}_{\mathrm{m_1,m_2}}$. The cosine measure calculates the co-occurrence of every term presents in the document. This measure does not take into consideration the position of terms w.r.t. each other in a document.

(ii) **Jaccard coefficient:**

The Jaccard similarity score [28] is calculated as

$$S_{Jacard} = \frac{df_{m_1 \cap m_2}}{df_{m_1 \cup m_2}} \tag{2}$$

where $df_{m_1 \cap m_2}$ represents the frequency of documents having both m_1 and m_2, while $df_{m_1 \cup m_2}$ represents the frequency of documents having at least m_1 or m_2.

(iii) **Dice coefficient:**

The Dice similarity score [29] is calculated as

$$S_{Dice} = \frac{2.df_{m_1 \cap m_2}}{df_{m_1} + df_{m_2}} \tag{3}$$

where df_{m_1} and df_{m_2} represent the frequency of documents having terms m_1 and m_2, respectively.

(iv) **Robertson selection value (RSV):**

RSV technique is based on term scoring [30]. It allocates a score to a term based on deviation in term distribution in the top extracted documents. The similarity score of a term is given as

$$RSV_{Score}(m) = \sum_{d \in R} w(m, d).\left[p(m|R_D) - p(m|C_D)\right] \tag{4}$$

where $p(m|C_D)$ represents the probability of candidate term m in corpus C_D and $p(m|R_D)$ represents the probability of candidate term m in relevant documents R_D.

(v) **Kullback–leibler divergence (KLD):**

In [9], authors use the Kullback-Leibler divergence (KLD) that is based on the term distribution differences between top extracted relevant documents and entire document collection. Then, top scored terms are added to reformulate the query. The similarity score of a term is given as

$$KLD_{Score}(m) = \sum_{m \in V} p(m|R_D).\log\frac{p(m|R_D)}{p(m|C_D)} \tag{5}$$

where p(m|C_D) and p(m|R_D) are same as in Eq. (4).

(vi) **Binary independence model (BIM) score:**

The BIM similarity score of query terms for ranking of terms was proposed in [31] and is calculated as follows:

$$\mathrm{BIM}_{\mathrm{Score}}(\mathrm{m}) = \log\frac{\mathrm{p}(\mathrm{m}|\mathrm{R_D})\left[1 - \mathrm{p}(\mathrm{m}|\mathrm{C_D})\right]}{\mathrm{p}(\mathrm{m}|\mathrm{C_D})\left[1 - \mathrm{p}(\mathrm{m}|\mathrm{R_D})\right]} \tag{6}$$

where p(m|C_D) and p(m|R_D) are same as in Eq. (4).

4 Experimental Study

4.1 Methodology

We first retrieve relevant documents against the query using Okapi BM25 ranking function [32, 33]. From the retrieved relevant documents, top "M" documents were used to construct the term pool by collecting all the unique terms from them. The Okapi BM25 similarity score is given [34, 35] as

$$Okapi(Q, C_i) = \sum_{t \in Q \cap C_i} w \frac{(J_1 + 1)tf_t}{J + tf_t} \times \frac{(J_3 + 1)tf_q}{J_3 + tf_q} \tag{7}$$

where initial query consisting of terms is represented by Q, tf_t and tf_q is the term frequency of term t in document C_i and in query Q, respectively. Parameters J_1, α, and J_3 are constants [35] and given as

$$J = J_1 + \left((1 - \alpha) + (\alpha \times \frac{l_d}{l_{ad}})\right) \tag{8}$$

$$w = log\frac{N_d - N_{dt} + 0.5}{N_{dt} + 0.5} \tag{9}$$

where $N_d and N_{dt}$ are total documents and documents having term t, respectively. Parameters l_d and l_{ad} represent document length and average document length. After this, we apply various term extraction and selection techniques to choose expansion terms as discussed above. The selected terms will be added to initial query and finally run the reformulated query again.

4.2 Parameter Selection

To make term pool collection of best candidate expansion terms that may enhance IR system performance, we have used different number (5, 10, 15, 20, 25, 50) of top feedback documents by applying PRF models. We found that 20 top feedback documents give best performance. Secondly, out of generated expansion terms from selected top feedback documents, we select different number (5, 10, 15, 20, 25, 30) of top candidate terms. Out of those, top 10 can be used to reformulate the initial query as they give best performance.

4.3 Datasets

We have used three standard and widely used datasets Medline, CISI, and CACM to perform all the experiments. We have selected all queries from CACM, Medline, and CISI datasets, to test the performance of term extraction and selection approaches and to compare them with each other. The detailed description of these datasets is given in Table 1. First, these datasets were preprocessed, i.e., stop words are removed, and indexing is done.

4.4 Evaluation Parameters

To determine the performance of IR system, we use recall (R), precision (P), and F-measure as evaluation parameters. Recall is defined as.

Recall = Relevant extracted documents (RELEXT)/Relevant documents (REL) and Precision is defined as.

Precision = Relevant extracted documents (RELEXT)/Extracted documents (EXT).

There will, in general, be a trade-off among precision and recall, so naturally, it would be interesting to merge them. Moreover, one method is frequently utilized, called F-measure, which is derived from precision and recall by taking their harmonic mean. Generally, it can be calculated as $F = \left((\partial^2 + 1)P * R\right)/\left(\partial^2 P + R\right)$ where P is precision, R is recall, and ∂ is a parameter usually set to 1. ∂ permits us to choose the relative performance of precision and recall in assessing performance.

Table 1 Summary of datasets

ID	Description	No of documents	No. of queries
CACM	Computer science ACM abstracts	3,204	64
CISI	Information science abstracts	1,460	112
Medline	Biomedicine abstracts	1,033	30

When $\partial = 1$, we refer to the metric as the balanced metric. This puts equal weight on precision and recall. As ∂ drops, more weight is put on precision, and as it rises, more weight is put on recall.

4.5 Comparison of Term Extraction and Selection Techniques

Tables 2, 3, 4 reflect the performance of various term extraction and selection techniques in terms of average precision and average recall on CACM, CISI, and Medline datasets.

Tables 2, 3, 4 show that the performance of BIM and Okapi BM25-based query reformulation term extraction techniques is higher than other term extraction techniques on both CISI and CACM datasets. However, KLD and RSV-based query reformulation term extraction techniques show higher performance on Medline dataset. We also calculate F-measure using precision and recall values as shown in Figs. 2, 3, 4.

Table 2 Average precision and average recall for CACM dataset

Methods	Top 20 retrieved documents	
	Average precision	Average recall
RSV	0.0642	0.1896
KLD	0.0605	0.1843
Jaccard	0.1789	0.2386
Okapi BM25	0.2318	0.1849
Cosine	0.1027	0.3002
Dice	0.1028	0.3004
BIM	0.2319	0.1848

Table 3 Average precision and average recall for CISI dataset

Methods	Top 20 retrieved documents	
	Average precision	Average recall
RSV	0.0591	0.1132
KLD	0.0592	0.1131
Jaccard	0.0592	0.0950
Okapi BM25	0.1162	0.1125
Cosine	0.0813	0.1031
Dice	0.0814	0.1032
BIM	0.1163	0.1124

Table 4 Average precision and average recall for Medline dataset

Methods	Top 20 retrieved documents	
	Average precision	Average recall
RSV	0.1948	0.0905
KLD	0.1949	0.0906
Jaccard	0.0758	0.0433
Okapi BM25	0.1142	0.0914
Cosine	0.1226	0.0405
Dice	0.1227	0.0406
BIM	0.1143	0.0913

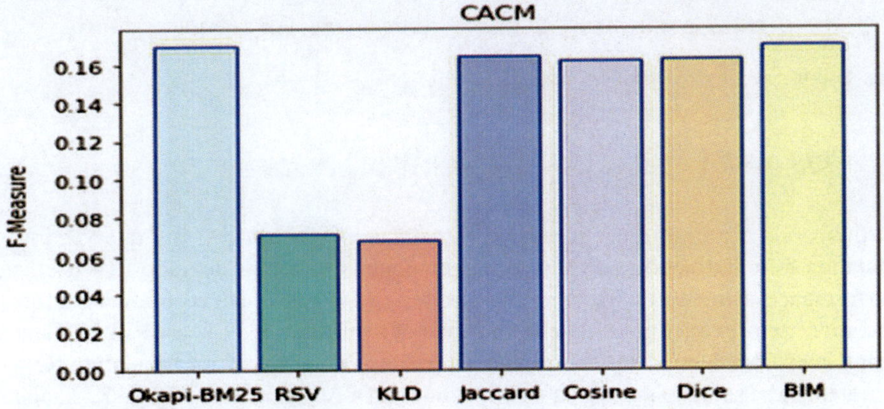

Fig. 2 F-measure for the CACM dataset

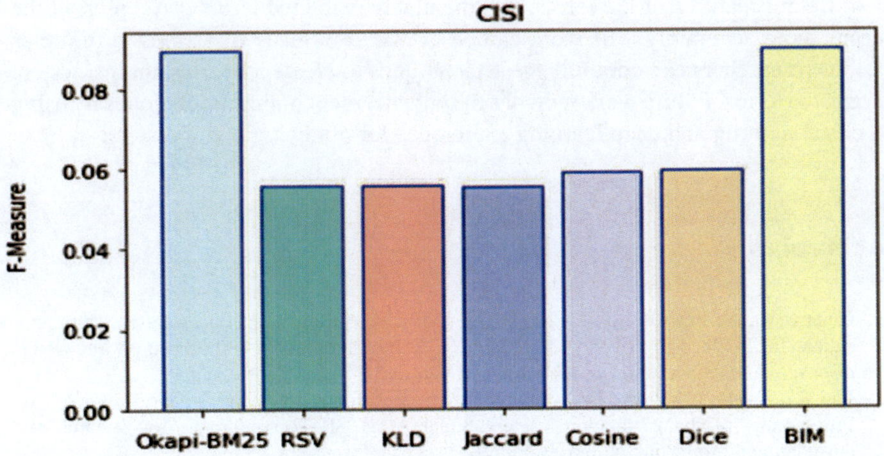

Fig. 3 F-measure for the CISI dataset

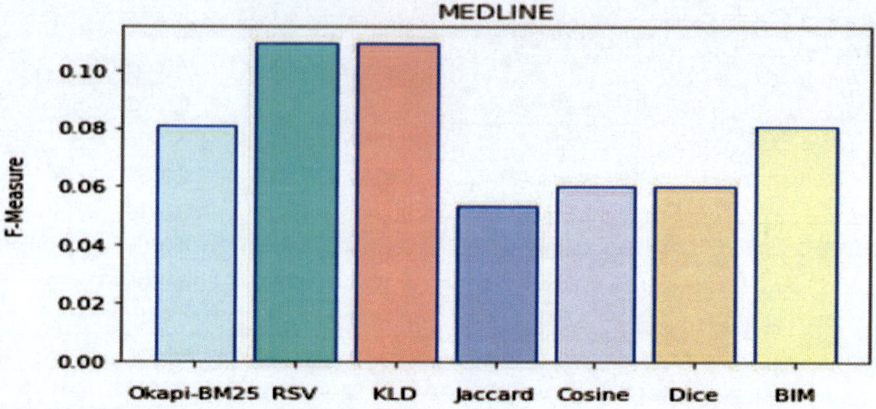

Fig. 4 F-measure for the medline dataset

5 Conclusion

In this work, we have done comparative analysis of various existing query reformulation term extraction and selection techniques utilized to upgrade IR systems performance using PRF. We analyzed and tested the performance of query reformulation term extraction and selection methods on three real datasets. We found that Okapi BM25 and BIM techniques outperform other query reformulation term extraction and selection methods on both CISI and CACM datasets. While KLD and RSV techniques outperform other techniques on Medline dataset. We observed that different query reformulation term extraction and selection techniques can capture the different features of the terms, and the newly extracted terms can represent the corpus more accurately. The work can be extended in many directions in future as various researchers can combine these techniques to create a hybrid ranking system to rank the terms. Future work includes the enhancement of these techniques by using machine learning and deep learning techniques for obtaining better results.

References

1. Crabtree D, Andreae P, Goa X (2007) The vocabulary problem in human-system communication. In: Proceedings of the 13th ACM SIGKDD international conference on knowledge discovery and data mining, pp 191–200. ACM
2. Lau RY, Bruza PD, Song D (2004) Belief revision for adaptive information retrieval. In: Proceedings of the 27th annual international ACM SIGIR conference on research and development in information retrieval, pp 130–137. ACM
3. Gan L, Hong H (2015) Improving query expansion for information retrieval using wikipedia. Int J Database Theory Applic 8(3):27–40
4. Marwi HA, Ghurab M (2018) A review of query expansion approaches. Int J Comput Sci Network 7(4):215

5. Singh J, Sharan A, Siddiqi S (2013) A literature survey on automatic query expansion for effective retrieval task. Int J Adv Comput Res 3(12):170–178
6. Kankaria A (2012) Query expansion techniques. Indian Institute of Technology Bombay, Mumbai
7. Gallant M, Isah H, Zulkernine F, Khan S (2019) Xu: an automated query expansion and optimization tool. In: IEEE 43rd annual computer software and applications conference (COMPSAC), vol 1, pp 443–452. IEEE
8. Ounis I, Amati G, Plachouras V, He B, Macdonald C, Lioma C (2006) A high performance and scalable information retrieval platform. In: SIGR workshop on open source information retrieval
9. Carpineto C, De Mori R, Romano G, Bigi B (2001) An information-theoretic approach to automatic query expansion. ACM Trans Inf Syst (TOIS) 19(1):1–27
10. Ermakova L, Mothe J, Ovchinnikova I (2014) Query expansion in information retrieval: what can we learn from a deep analysis of queries? In: International conference on computational linguistics dialogue, vol 20, pp 162–172
11. Abass OA, Folorunso O, Samuel BO (2017) Automatic query expansion for information retrieval: a survey and problem definition. Am J Comput Sci Inf Eng 4(3):24–30
12. Nagpal N (2018) Applying soft computing techniques in information retrieval. Int J Adv Eng Manag Sci 4(5):386–388
13. Tayal DK, Sabharwal S, Jain A, Mittal K (2012) Intelligent query expansion for the queries including numerical terms. In: Proceedings of International Journal of Computer Applications, pp 35–39
14. Gupta Y, Saini A (2017) A novel Fuzzy-PSO term weighting automatic query expansion approach using combined semantic filtering. Knowl Based Syst, 97–120
15. Singh J, Sharan A (2017) A new fuzzy logic-based query expansion model for efficient information retrieval using relevance feedback approach. Neural Comput Appl 28(9):2557–2580
16. Singh J, Sharan A (2015) Relevance feedback based query expansion model using Borda count and semantic similarity approach. Computational intelligence and neuroscience
17. Gomathi R, Sharmila D (2014) A novel adaptive cuckoo search for optimal query plan generation. Sci World J
18. Azad HK, Deepak A (2019) Query expansion techniques for information retrieval: a survey. Inf Process Manage 56(5):1698–1735
19. Azad HK, Deepak A (2019) A new approach for query expansion using Wikipedia and WordNet. Inf Sci 147–163
20. Singh J, Sharan A (2018) Rank fusion and semantic genetic notion based automatic query expansion model. Swarm and Evolut Comput 295–308
21. Bouchoucha A, He J, Nie JY (2013) Diversified query expansion using conceptnet. In: Proceedings of the 22nd ACM international conference on Information & Knowledge Management, pp 1861–1864
22. Gupta Y, Saini A (2021) A new automatic query expansion approach using term selection and document clustering. In: Innovations in computational intelligence and computer vision, pp 109–121. Springer, Singapore
23. Singh J, Sharan A (2015) Context window based co-occurrence approach for improving feedback based query expansion in information retrieval. Int J Infor Ret 5(4):31–45
24. Li Y, Chung S, Holt J (2008) Text document clustering based on frequent word meaning sequences. Data Knowl Eng 64(1):381–404
25. Aguera J, Araujo L (2008) Comparing and combining methods for automatic query expansion. In: Advances in natural language processing and applications, research in computing science, vol 33, pp 177–188
26. Valdivia M, Galiano M, Raez A, Lopez L (2008) Using information gain to improve multi-modal information retrieval systems. Int J Proc Manag 44(3):1146–1158
27. Carpineto C, Romano G (2012) A survey of automatic query expansion in information retrieval. ACM Comput Survey 44(1):1–50
28. Jaccard P (1912) The distribution of the flora in the alpine zone. New Phytol 11(2):37–50

29. Dice LR (1945) Measures of the amount of ecologic association between species. Ecology 26(3):297–302
30. Robertson SE (1990) On term selection for query expansion. J Document 46(4):359–364
31. Robertson SE, Jones KS (1976) Relevance weighting of search terms. J Am Soc Inform Sci 27(3):129–146
32. Singh J (2017) Ranks aggregation and semantic genetic approach based hybrid model for query expansion. Int J Comput Intell Syst 10(1):34–55
33. Sharma DK, Pamula R, Chauhan DS (2019) A hybrid evolutionary algorithm based automatic query expansion for enhancing document retrieval system. J Amb Intell Human Comp 1–20
34. Singh J, Sharan A (2016) Relevance feedback-based query expansion model using ranks combining and Word2Vec approach. IETE J Res 62(5):591–604
35. Robertson SE, Walker S, Jones S, Beaulieu MMH, Gatford M (1995) Okapi at TREC- 3. In: Proceedings of the third text retrieval conference, pp 109–126
36. Ramalingam G, Dhandapani S (2018) A hybrid batcs algorithm to generate optimal query plan. Int Arab J Inf Technol 15(3):353–359

Enhanced Quality of Service (EQoS)-Enabled Load Balancing Approach for Cloud Environment

Minakshi Sharma, Rajneesh Kumar, and Anurag Jain

Abstract Cloud computing uses the "pay as you go model" to provide on-demand services to its users especially data storage, computing power, network, and others. These services are provided to users without their direct active participation in managing resources. Cloud computing relies upon resource sharing to acquire coherence and economies of scale. Task scheduling in such an environment is used for the task execution on a suitable resource by considering some parameters and constraints to achieve performance. During high demand for these virtualized resources, efficient task scheduling achieves the desired performance criteria by balancing the load in the system. This paper presents a balancing mechanism by practicing task scheduling to increase performance in the cloud environment. It perceives various load balancing approaches based on task scheduling and concludes that their optimization goals are multi-objective. The presented mechanism is an extension of the previous proposed work QoS-enabled JMLQ [1]. This proposed approach has been tested in the CloudSim simulator, and results show that the proposed approach achieves better results in comparison with QoS-enabled JMLQ and its other variants in the cloud environment.

Keywords Cloud computing · Load balancing · JMLQ · CloudSim · Task scheduling

M. Sharma (✉) · R. Kumar
Department of Computer Science and Engineering, MMEC, Maharishi Markandeshwar Deemed to be University, Mullana, Ambala, Haryana 134002, India

R. Kumar
e-mail: drrajneeshgujral@mmumullana.org

A. Jain
School of Computer Science, Univesity of Petroleum and Energy Studies, Dehradun, Uttarakhand 248007, India
e-mail: anurag.jain@ddn.upes.ac.in

N. Marriwala et al. (eds.), *Emergent Converging Technologies and Biomedical Systems*, Lecture Notes in Electrical Engineering 841,
https://doi.org/10.1007/978-981-16-8774-7_44

1 Introduction

The advent of various technologies such as distributed computing, utility computing, autonomic computing, and the unveiling of service-oriented architecture has driven the growth of cloud computing. It points toward the goal to serve the user at a low cost without any expertise or deep knowledge of the system. The services provided by it are software as a service (SaaS), platform as a service (PaaS), and infrastructure as a service(IaaS).

Scheduling of user requests is an important concept in the cloud environment, which includes a mechanism that maps a user request to an appropriate resource for the execution of a task. The performance of the system is directly affected by the efficiency of a scheduling technique. These algorithms are based on the management of physical and virtualized resources in the environment. In this paper, a two-level load balancing mechanism based on task scheduling has been discussed. The research work presented here is a load balancing approach that efficiently schedules tasks to virtual resources to increase the quality of service requirements. It is an incremental approach to our previous proposed work QoS-enabled JMLQ [2, 3]. Enhanced QoS-enabled JMLQ is an improved version of QoS-enabled JMLQ. This proposed algorithm is an attempt to override the random behavior of the algorithm.

2 Related Work

Scheduling of tasks is an important concept in the field of cloud computing, efficient scheduling of tasks not only can meet user requirements but can also improve resource utilization, response time, and other performance parameters, thereby balancing the load on the system [4, 5]. Task allocation is the task assigned to an appropriate resource that suits user requirements while the task scheduling algorithm settles the execution order of each task to be executed on the server [6, 7]. There are different task scheduling algorithm exists in the literature that balances the load on the system and enhances the performance of the system by considering different performance parameter. The following is the research work studied for task scheduling-based load balancing in the cloud environment.

In 2011, Yi Lu et al. proposed a load balancing approach JIQ based on the scheduling of the tasks. The main objective of this proposed approach was to execute the tasks in minimum response time by avoiding extra communication overheads during the process of task assignment. It is a two-fold load balancing mechanism that balances the load for a large system. It uses a data structure, i.e., I-queue that acts as a communication medium during task assignment to the processor. The first level of load balancing works for task assignment by probing the I-queues for idle server, and the load balancing at the second level balances the load by idle processors placement in any random I-queue attached with the dispatchers. The prime consideration factor was response time for this approach [8].

In 2013, X. Wu et al. proposed a QoS-driven task scheduling approach in which tasks were sorted based on the special attribute of tasks to decide precedence among the tasks. Afterward, the completion time of tasks evaluated on different services and the task was scheduled for a service according to the sorted queue based on minimum completion time [9].

In 2015, Babu and Samuel devised a technique to balance the load based on the foraging nature of honey bees. In their proposed technique the task with the lowest priority has the higher chances of being migrated from an overwhelmed virtual machine (VM) to the underwhelm virtual machine. Their algorithm relies on the priority of tasks in a waiting queue for VM. Simulated results demonstrate that for tasks that are limited in number makespan reduces, and there is a reduction in the total number of migrations needed for operation, which shows that the proposed algorithm has low scalability [10].

In 2016, H.E.D. Ali et al. proposed a grouped task scheduling approach for the cloud environment based on QoS parameters. The incoming tasks from the user side were categorized into five groups that depend upon task attributes. The categories are user type, task type, task length, and task latency. The scheduling was carried out in two steps. The first step decides the category to be scheduled based on the high value of the attributes of tasks. The second step was based on tasks within the chosen category to be scheduled first based on the minimum execution time of the tasks. The latency of tasks and execution time considered as a performance parameter [11].

In 2017, Ashish Garg et al. proposed a metaheuristic search technique based on ant colony optimization for solving task scheduling problems. The objective of this algorithm was to balance the load across the system by optimizing the makespan performance parameter. The algorithm attains the local optimal solution by using an ant colony algorithm and at last, a Pareto set of solutions was attained by applying non-domination sorting [12].

In 2018, Chunpu wang et al. devised a load balancing approach for low latency in the cloud environment. The scheduler used a technique to deal with an empty I-queue. The task is allocated to the minimum loaded server after searching for d servers that are randomly chosen. Every dispatcher attached to I-queue implements the same strategy for task allocation when it is met with an empty I-queue. Low latency for service time is considered as a performance parameter. Moreover to avoid the delay in performance, a semiclosed-form expressions were also derived [13].

3 System Model for Enhanced QoS-Enabled JMLQ

The system model for “enhanced QoS-enabled JMLQ” comprises a two-fold load balancing mechanism that consists of n parallel VMs having homogeneous configuration VM (VM_0, VM_1, VM_2, ..., VM_{n-1}) interconnected with some networking components. These VMs join the I-queues of the dispatchers (D_0, D_1, D_2, ..., D_{m-1}) considered in a fixed ratio to the number of VMs, i.e., $r = n/m$ (here, n is the number of VMs, m represents an array of dispatchers, and r represents a ratio that is fixed between n and m). The tasks processed in the system are considered independent, and the rate of task arrival is considered general [14] To represent the current scenario, the G/G/c like queuing model has been considered to represent the large cloud system as there is high variability in the arrival process and service process of the tasks [15, 16]. The system model consists of the following units.

Dispatcher: Every dispatcher is responsible for scheduling tasks and acts as an independent scheduler. Each dispatcher in this proposed approach has its unique id and a specified limit up to which it can possess the VMs in an I-queue.

I-Queue: This is attached to the dispatcher unit and acts as a communication medium for allocating tasks. When a VM completes its task, it joins the I-queue.

Task allocation to VMs: The VMs presented in I-queues are responsible for executing tasks that are removed from I-queues after task allocation. The incoming task is allocated to the first VM present within the I-queue of the first dispatcher with ID D_0 if it is nonempty otherwise, it probes for the other minimum loaded VM in adjacent dispatchers I-queue having dispatcher ID in sequence.

VMs allocation to I-queues using d-limit: This proposed approach place an upper bound on each I-queue set by d-limit. After the task completion, VM is drifted toward the first dispatcher's I-queue having ID D_0, it joins the I-queue if I-queue length is less than d-limit otherwise, it probes for the next dispatcher I-queue in a sequential manner. At a medium load, the I-queues remain well occupied with a large number of VMs and these VMs are equally distributed among all the I-queues using d-limit.

At high load, the VMs present with in these I-queues are very less, most of the I-queues remain empty and the probability of getting an empty I-queue is very high. At this stage, if a VM gets idle, it always joins the first dispatcher I-queue with ID D_0 and the next incoming task allocated to it and task allocation continues for this I-queue until and unless it gets empty. At high load, the algorithm behaves like a centralized policy as an idle VM always join the first dispatcher I-queue with ID $D_{0.}$ This nature of the algorithm helps in a further reduction in response time and to utilize the resource more efficiently. If all the dispatcher I-queues are empty, then the task will be allocated to the minimum loaded VM which is chosen among d random VMs and the algorithm behaves like a randomized algorithm (Table 1).

Table 1 List of variables used in pseudocode

Variable notation	Significance
n	The number of available VMs in the system
m	Represents the number of dispatchers based on a fixed ratio b/w VMs and dispatchers
dl	Represents dispatcher limit, i.e., maximum number of VMs an I-queue can possess
D_0	Represents a dispatcher with dispatcher ID D_0
I-queue Length	Represents the length of dispatcher I-queue that consists of a subset of VMs that are minimum loaded in the system
Waiting task queue length	The no. of tasks in the queue waiting to be allocated to VM
d	Represents any random number from 1 to the total number of VMs (n)
F	Represents a flag value can be 0 or 1
Disipatcher_ID	Represents any dispatcher identity number form 0–999

3.1 Pseudocode for Enhanced Qos-Enabled Join Minimum Loaded Queue (JMLQ)

```
EQoS enabled JMLQ():
  {
      •   n= A set of of available VMs {VM0, VM2, VM3, …..VMn-1}
      •   m= an array of diapatchers {D0, D1, D2, ….Dm-1}
      •   d-limit (dl) = n/m
      •   Make a batch of cloudlets equal to 2n

For (I =0 to n-1)
  {
      •  Allocate 2 cloudlets to I-th VM at one clock_time()
  }
•   Make a procedure call named VM_to_dispatcher_mapping for assigning
    VM to an I-queue of the dispatcher Whenever any VM completes the
    execution of the cloudlet.

While (there is an incoming cloudlet from a consumer in a data center)
{
            For (I = 0 to m-1)
              {
      •   Obtain the Ith dispatcher_ID
      If ( dispatcher D0 I-queue is non-empty)
      {
```

```
                • Allocate cloudlet to the first VM in the I-queue of
                  dispatcher D0
                • After cloudlet allocation remove VM from I-queue of
                  dispatcher D0
                • break;
        }
      Else

        {
                if  dispatcher_ID == Total-no-of-dispatcher -1
                {
                    If the last dispatcher's I-queue length is Nil then
              {
                  • Randomly choose d VMs
                  • Find the one VM having waiting task queue length
                    minimum among the d random VMs.
                  • The task will be allocated to a VM having waiting
                    task queue length is smallest.
                                  }
                                     }
                                  }
                }

   • Make a procedure call named VM_to_dispatcher_mapping for assigning
     VM to an I-queue of the dispatcher Whenever any VM completes the
     execution of the cloudlet.

        }
          }

      VM_to_dispatcher_mapping()
      {
         • dispatcher D0 is selected based on its ID
         If (D0's I-queue length is less than d-limit)
         {
               • VM joins the I-queue of dispatcher D0 which have completed  the
                 cloudlet execution
         }
         Else
         {
           Repeat
           {
                 ▪ Flag = 0
                 ▪ Idle VM searches the adjacent dispatcher ID in a sequence
                   having I-queue length is less than d-limit
                 ▪ On the successful joining of VM in an I-queue set Flag=1
           } until(Flag = 1)
         }
      }
```

4 Experimental Setup and Result

To prove the better optimization effects of performance parameters by practicing "enhanced QoS-enabled JMLQ," the authors selected some load balancing approaches based on task scheduling including the previous versions of the proposed approach JMLQ and QoS-enabled JMLQ [17, 3]. All these selected approaches have been tested and analyzed in the simulated environment. CloudSim (version 3.0.3) has been used for demonstrating the cloud environment. Eclipse IDE is used to

Table 2 Simulation environment configuration

Configuration Details	
Cloudlets of variable length	In-between (600,000–800,000)
Number of hosts	2500, each with four processing elements (Pe)
Number of virtual machines (VMs)	10,000
Different sets of cloudlets	In-between (60,000 – 260,000)
Storage size for each VM	10,000 MB
RAM for each VM	512 MB
Million instructions per second (MIPS)	1000
Bandwidth	1000
Cloudlet scheduler	CloudletSchedulerSpaceShared()
VM scheduler	VmSchedulerTimeShared()

develop and implement the algorithm using JDK 1.8. The following table represents the configuration details used in CloudSim (Table 2).

4.1 Validation of Results for Response Time

Figure 1 represents the comparison of response time for different distributed approaches versus the proposed approach. This proposed approach average response

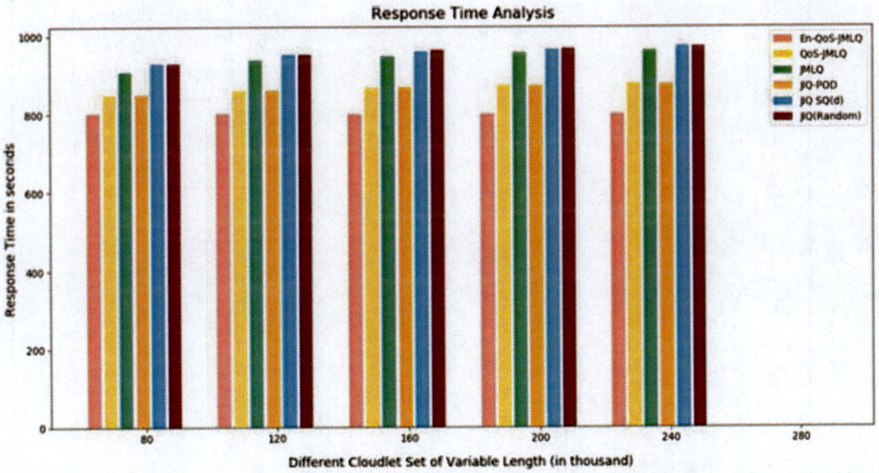

Fig. 1 Comparison of the response time for different distributed approaches with the proposed approach

time is 6.86% less than QoS-enabled JMLQ and JIQ-Pod, 14% less than JMLQ, 15.35% less than JIQ-SQ(d), and 15.53% less than JIQ-Random.

Figure 1 depicts that response time declines with some points as the number of cloudlets increases for the proposed approach, here, cloudlets represent the number of tasks. This proposed approach uses the dispatcher ID for joining a VM in an I-queue, therefore, all the VMs are placed in I-queues in a contiguous form without insertion of empty I-queues, also, these VMs are equally distributed among the I-queues based on d-limit. So an incoming task will always get a VM in an I-queue until these are present in the I-queues. This proposed approach overcomes the random behavior of the previous variants and eliminates the mapping of the incoming tasks with empty I-queues until and unless VMs are not present in the I-queues. After, a set of 160,000 cloudlets response time gets stable.

4.2 Validation of Results for Resource Utilization

Figure 2 represents the percentage of resource utilization for different distributed approaches in comparison with this proposed approach. It depicts from Fig. 2 that the proposed approach utilizes the resource more efficiently in comparison with its variants. The percentage of resource utilization is improved over QoS-enabled JMLQ

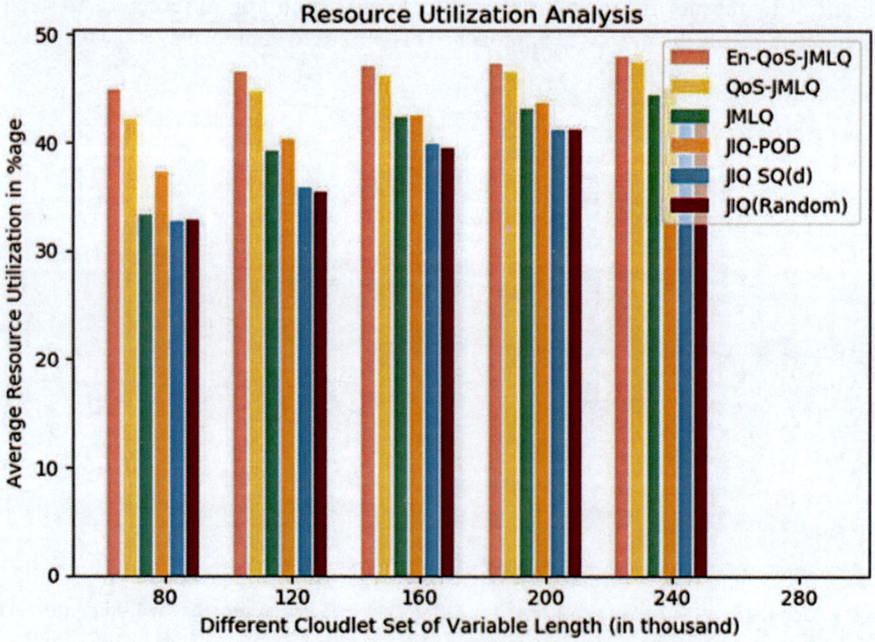

Fig. 2 Number of cloudlets versus percentage of resource utilization

by 2.55%, 16.51% better than JMLQ, 13.14% better than JIQ-Pod, 25.03% improved over JIQ-SQ(d), and 25.88% improved over JIQ-random. It is an important parameter to achieve an efficient load balancing policy that led to a decrease in cost for services from the customer side.

4.3 *Validation of Results for Average Waiting Time*

To determine the optimization of performance parameters for this proposed approach, next, parameter is considered as the average waiting time. The reduction in average waiting time represents a decrease in the waiting period to serve user requests. It can be analyzed from Fig. 3 that an increase in average waiting time with respect to increase in the number of cloudlets is not very significant in comparison with other distributed approaches. The decrease in waiting time observed 0.7% less than QoS-enabled JMLQ, 1.68% less than JMLQ, 15.02% less than JIQ-pod, 16.59% improved over JIQ-SQ(d), and 15.92% less than JIQ-random. These experimental results prove the efficacy of this proposed approach in comparison with other distributed approaches.

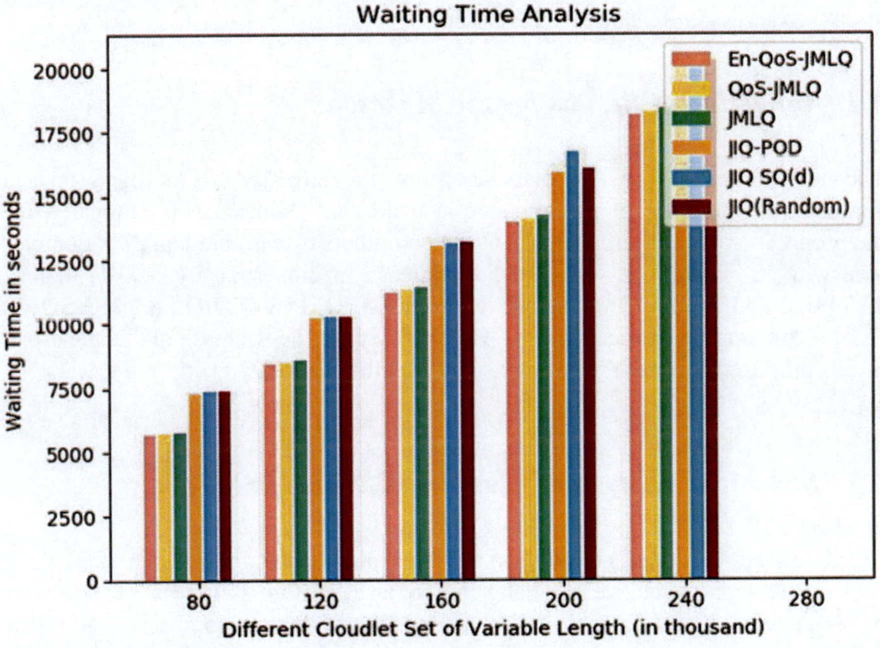

Fig. 3 Average waiting time versus no. of cloudlets

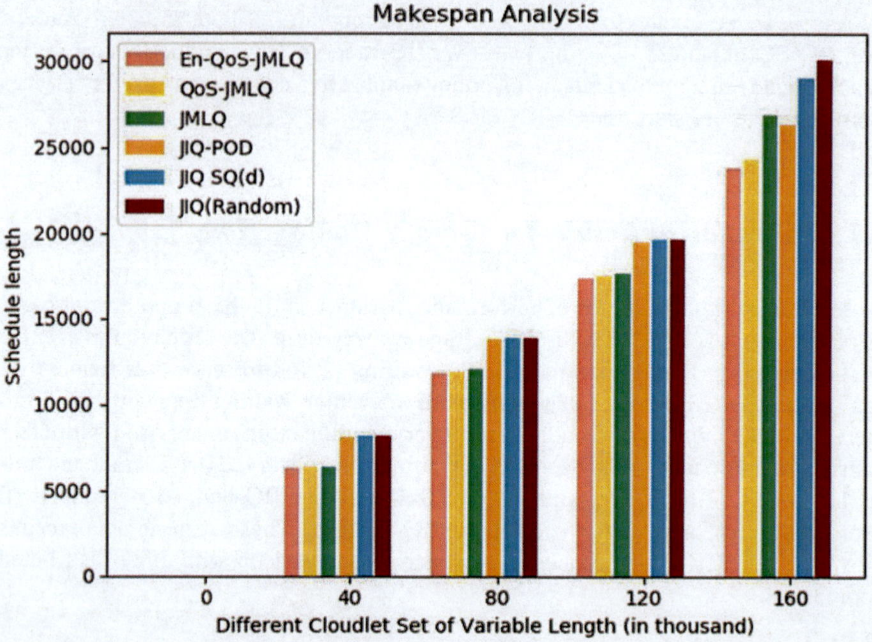

Fig. 4 Makespan versus a different set of cloudlets

4.4 Validation of Results for the Makespan

The next parameter considered to determine the effectiveness of the proposed approach on the scale of performance is makespan. Makespan is compared for the proposed approach for a set of 160,000 cloudlets of variable length in comparison with its variants. It was found a decrease in makespan by 1.04%, 4.56%, 13.74%, 16.55%, 17.47% from QoS-enabled JMLQ, JMLQ, JIQ-pod, JIQ-SQ(d), JIQ-random approaches respectively. Figure 4 depicts the decrease in the makespan of this proposed approach in comparison with other variants.

4.5 Statistical Analysis of Cloudlet Distribution

Equal distribution of tasks (cloudlets) among available resources is one of the most desirable features to achieve load balancing for an algorithm. It increases the stability of the system so cloudlet distribution among the available resources is one of the important parameters to determine the efficiency of an algorithm. Statistical analysis is done to determine the cloudlet distribution. It is based on the standard deviation that determines the variance of cloudlet distribution of the proposed approach in comparison with other distributed approaches. For the proposed approach, the coefficient of

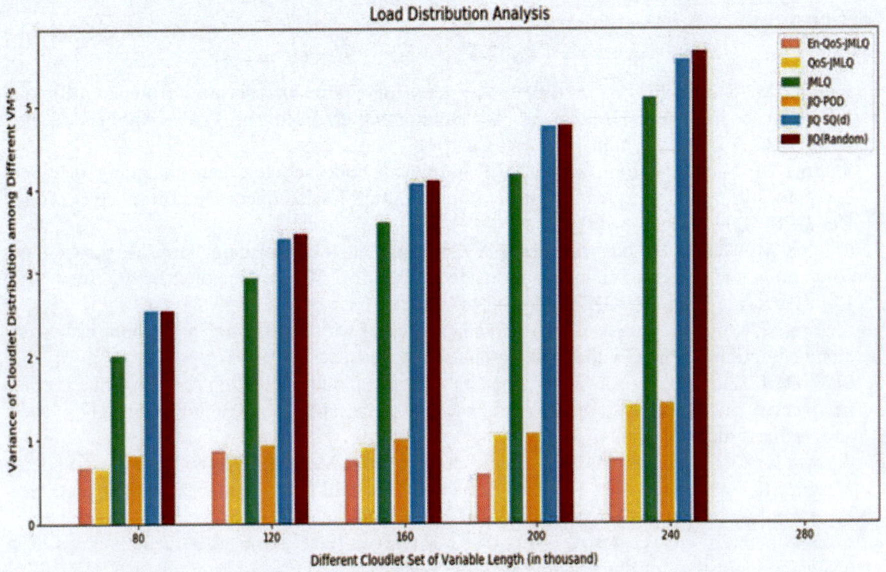

Fig. 5 Number of cloudlets versus the variance of cloudlets distribution

variation has a value less than one, which signifies the distribution of cloudlets with a low variance in comparison with other distributed approaches. Figure 5 represents the variation of the cloudlet distribution of this proposed approach in comparison with others.

5 Conclusion and Future Scope

This research work presented here is a load balancing approach based on task scheduling that efficiently balances the load in a cloud environment by optimizing the performance parameters. The experimental results have been validated and analyzed in a simulation environment developed using CloudSim. The objective of this research work is to achieve multi-dimensional performance parameters. This proposed algorithm minimizes the response time of user requests by utilizing the resource more efficiently by balancing the load in the system. As a future scope, enhanced QoS-enabled JMLQ work can also be extended by developing more hybrid methods during task allocation at high load to minimize response time by invoking intelligence during task allocation based on some intelligent information.

References

1. Sharma M, Kumar R, Jain A (2019) A system of quality of service enabled (QoS) join minimum loaded queue (JMLQ) for cloud computing environment. Patent Application, no. 201911039375, 51328, India
2. Sharma M, Kumar R, Jain A (2020) A proficient approach for load balancing in cloud computing-join minimum loaded queue: join minimum loaded queue. Int J Infor Syst Model Des (IJISMD) 11(1):12–36
3. Sharma M, Kumar R, Jain A (2021) A QoS enabled load balancing approach for cloud computing environment join minimum loaded queue(JMLQ): QoS enabled JMLQ. Int J Grid High-Perform Comput (IJGHPC) 4(14), Article 5
4. Sharma M, Kumar R, Jain A (2019) Implementation of various load-balancing approaches for cloud computing using CloudSim. J Comput Theor Nanosci 16(9):3974–3980
5. Sharma M, Kumar R, Jain A (2021) Load balancing in cloud computing environment: a broad perspective. Intelligent data communication technologies and internet of things. Sringer science and business media, India
6. Åström E (2016) Task scheduling in distributed systems. Model and prototype
7. Mishra SK, Sahoo B, Parida PP (2020) Load balancing in cloud computing: a big picture. J King Saud Univ Comput Inform Sci 32(2):149–158
8. Lu Y, Xie Q, Kliot G, Geller A, Larus JR, Greenberg A (2011) Join-Idle-queue: a novel load balancing algorithm for dynamically scalable web services. Perform Eval 68(11):1056–1071
9. Wu X, Deng M, Zhang R, Zeng B, Zhou S (2013) A task scheduling algorithm based on QoS-driven in cloud computing. Proc Comput Sci 17:1162–1169
10. Babu KR, Samuel P (2015) Enhanced bee colony algorithm for efficient load balancing and scheduling in cloud. Innovat Bio-Insp Comput Applic 424:67–78
11. Ali HGEDH, Saroit IA, Kotb AM (2017) Grouped tasks scheduling algorithm based on QoS in cloud computing network. Egypt Inform J 18(1):11–19
12. Gupta A, Garg R (2017) Load balancing based task scheduling with ACO in cloud computing. In: Proceedings of international conference on computer and applications IEEE (ICCA), pp 174–179
13. Wang C, Feng C, Cheng J (2018) Distributed Join-the-Idle-Queue for low latency cloud services. IEEE/ACM Trans Network 26(5):2309–2319
14. Abraham GT, James A, Yaacob N (2015) Group-based Parallel Multi-scheduler for grid computing. Futur Gener Comput Syst 50:140–153
15. Bramson M, Lu Y, Prabhakar B (2010) Randomized load balancing with general service time distributions. ACM Sigmet Perform Eval Rev 38(1):275–286
16. Atmaca T, Begin T, Brandwajn A, Castel-Taleb H (2015) Performance evaluation of cloud computing centers with general arrivals and service. IEEE Trans Parallel Distrib Syst 27(8):2341–2348
17. Sharma M, Kumar R, Jain A (2019) A system of distributed join minimum loaded queue (JMLQ) for load balancing in cloud environment. Patent Application, no. 201911007589, pp. 12780, India

Classification for Diagnosis of Breast Cancer Using Machine Learning Techniques with Hyperparameter Tuning

K. K. Sreekala and Jayakrushna Sahoo

Abstract Breast cancer mortality has risen dramatically in recent years. However, early diagnosis and treatment may greatly reduce the risk of death. Cancer cells may spread from the breast to other portions of the body over the bloodstream arrangement. They will move early in the process, when the tumour is minor stage, or later in the process, when the tumour will be in major stage. The aim is to propose a method that allows use of supervised machine learning (ML) classifiers such as linear regression, Naive Bayes (NB), support vector machine (SVM) and multilayer perceptron (MLP) that classify the mammogram images as benign or Malignant. The hyperparameters scheme used for the classifiers was manually allocated in order to increase the classifier's accuracy and identify the cancer as benign or Malignant. The results show that by manually tuning the hyperparameters, all of the presented ML algorithms performed well on the classification task. In addition, the Wisconsin breast cancer (WBC) dataset was used in this analysis. The dataset was divided in the following way for the ML algorithms implement to classify the breast cancer: 60% for training and 40% for testing. The main purpose of this work is to compare multiple classifiers to discover the best classifier that provides better accuracy in breast cancer classification. The proposed model's output is evaluated using various parametric values such as precision, recall, sensitivity, and F-measure.

Keywords Machine learning classifier · Breast cancer · Classification · Benign or Malignant and hyperparameters

K. K. Sreekala (✉) · J. Sahoo
Department of Computer Science and Engineering, Indian Institute of Information Technology Kottayam, Kottayam, Kerala 686 635, India
e-mail: sreekalaphd2019@iiitkottayam.ac.in

J. Sahoo
e-mail: jsahoo@iiitkottayam.ac.in

N. Marriwala et al. (eds.), *Emergent Converging Technologies and Biomedical Systems*, Lecture Notes in Electrical Engineering 841,
https://doi.org/10.1007/978-981-16-8774-7_45

1 Introduction

Healthcare is one of the most concerning fields in terms of data collection and processing. With the advent of the digital era and advancement in technology, a large amount of multidimensional data is generated about patients, which include clinical parameters, hospital resources, disease diagnostic details, patients' records and medical devices. The information about vast, voluminous and multidimensional data essentials to be processed and examined for the extraction of knowledge for effective decision-making. Cancer is the Malignant growth of cells, and it can take place in any part of the body. The malignant growth spreads and leads to crowding out of the normal cells and thereby making it difficult for the body to function [1–3]. Malignant growth of cells that is cancer cannot be categorized as a single disease. There are numerous sorts of malignant growth. It is not only one place that gets infected, but malignant growth can also occur in any internal organ and even in the blood cells.

Malignant growths are similar somehow or another, however, they are distinctive in the manners in which they develop and spread [4]. Our body functions with the aid of cells acting like building blocks. Trillions of cells in the body render shape, nutrition and energy to the body. Cells also carry out unique functions like holding on hereditary features and make copies of themselves by dividing itself into two or more cells and those daughter cells further divide into other cells. This process of cell division takes place as a part of a larger cell cycle. Cancer growth happens through the development of tumours or lumps. However, not all irregularities are malignant in nature. Doctors examine a bit of the tumour or lumps and find out whether it is Malignant or not. If it is not a Malignant growth, it is called benign. Apart from the development of tumours, there are a few malignancies, similar to leukaemia (disease of the blood), that develop in the platelets or different cells of the body not as tumours [5].

Data mining progress provides clients with methods to uncover new and unknown instances from large amounts of data. In the healthcare sector, the uncovered knowledge can be used to enhance the precision of diagnosis by medical service administrators and physicians, thus raising and lowering the level of caution. Awareness disclosure of data refers to 'the concealment of data, the retrieval of ambiguous and conceivable useful data' [6]. The aim of hypotheses in knowledge mining is to help people explore designs in data to boost their prosperity [7]. In the healthcare sector, data mining plays an important role in predicting illnesses. A data mining ideal is the forerunner of the forecast. The aftereffects of interventions were discussed in this article, and recommendations for future research were made. A health professional's diagnosis of breast cancer is not 100 per cent correct.

Furthermore, a precise definition of a malignant tumour may prevent patients from receiving appropriate treatment. As a consequence, the proper determination and assignment of breast carcinoma to benign and malignant sets are a widely discussed subject [8, 9]. ML approaches were commonly used in the centuries to identify breast carcinoma and to draw different notions from data patterns. Machine learning is well-known for its use in the classification and simulation of breast cancer. It is a tool for detecting previously unknown regularities and trends in a variety of datasets. It integrates a wide variety of approaches for the revelation of rules, paradigms and relations in classes of data and creates a theory of these relations that can be used to decode new secret data [10]. Various artificial learnings [8–11], deep learning scheme [12, 13] and bio-inspired computation [14] approaches have been used in many medicinal prognoses in recent years. Despite the fact that many modalities have been shown, none of them can produce a 100% right and reliable answer. The doctors must read a vast quantity of imaging data, which limits accuracy. This technique is often time taking, and in particular cases, incorrectly senses the illness.

The remaining of this paper is followed as a literature review of earlier work is focussed in Sect. 2, proposed methodology is offered in Sect. 3, result and discussion of this proposed model are labelled in Sect. 4 and finally, the paper is finished in Sect. 5.

2 Literature Review

In this section, the literature is surveyed to recognize the state of the art and to identify the problem of breast cancer identification. Numerous researches work have been conducted on the identification of breast cancer with machine learning algorithms. But the researchers have applied different ML algorithms on different breast cancer data repositories and the performance of the proposed model with various ML algorithms varies based on the algorithm and the dataset used by different researchers.

The author [11] has projected a duo-phase SVM was showed by combining a duo-phase clustering approach with an operative probabilistic SVM in order to analyze WBC Diagnosis and achieve a classification model accuracy of 99.10%. Unlike other existing schemes, this strategy can identify the figure of the masses and provide efficient analyzes for large bodies.

Kapil and Rana [12] have projected a weight improved DT technique as a modified DT technique and applied it on WBCD dataset obtained from the UCI. Using the Chi-square test, they discovered that they had ranked the each feature and hold the features that were relevant for this classification process. Their proposed technique achieved approximately 99 per cent accuracy on the WBCD dataset, whilst it achieved approximately 85–90% accuracy on the breast cancer dataset.

Banu and Subramanian [13] have emphasized the ML scheme such as NB practises for breast cancer prediction and labelled a comparison study on tree augmented NB, boosted augmented NB and Bayes belief network (BBN). The models were implemented using SAS-EM. In their work, they use the same common WBCD dataset. According to their findings, 91.7 and 94.11% accuracy were achieved using gradient boosting.

Yue et al. [14] have presented complete analyzes on SVM, ANNs, K-NNs and DT machine learning classifier model. By this model for application of medical data diagnosis to classification of breast cancer by evaluate the system to use WBC diagnosis dataset. This study was conducted to combining the two neural network model as ANN architecture (DBNs-ANNs) and deep belief networks (DBNs, in this combination scheme provide the better classification results achieved of 99.68% of accuracy. On other hand, the SVM classification technique achieved a 99.10% of classification accuracy, when combined with the two-step clustering algorithm. They also looked at the ensemble technique, which used to implement SVM, NB and J48. The ensemble method achieved an accuracy of 97.13%.

For the breast cancer diagnosis, a variant of SVM [15] is introduced. There are different types of SVM used for performance evaluation in this article as NSVM, SSVM, LPSVM and LPSVM. The results of typical SVM are compared to those of other types of SVM. For training and testing, four-fold cross-validation is used. In the training phase, St-SVM achieves the highest accuracy, specificity and sensitivity of 97.71, 98.9 and 97.08%, correspondingly. In the testing phase, the highest accuracy of 96.55%, sensitivity of 98.24% and specificity of 96.55% attained by are and 97.14%, respectively.

3 Proposed Methodology

In this section, we discussed the proposed scheme of breast cancer classification and detection by using Wisconsin breast cancer dataset, the proposed scheme is showed in Fig. 1. In primary, the dataset is preprocess to eliminate the noise and irrelevant data from the entire data. Then preprocessed data are given to the feature selection procedure, in this section, we proposed the PCA feature selection model to select the proper feature for better classification result and reduce the computation time. Then, apply different ML model to classify the selected data. The different ML models such as multilayer perceptron, naïve Bayes, SVM and linear regression. In this classifier, we tune the classifier parameter to tune the classifier process to improve the learning rate of the classifier. In classification section, which significantly classify the data as benign or Malignant.

3.1 Dataset Description

In this study, WBC dataset is used for the breast cancer identification process. The dataset is accessible from UCI ML repository website as https://www.kaggle.com/uciml/breast-cancer-wisconsin-data. In the clump depth, benign cells appear to form monolayers, whilst cancerous cells often form multilayers [16]. Cancer cells, on the other hand, differ in size and structure in the standardization of cell size/shape. As a result, these criteria are useful in deciding whether or not the cells are cancerous. Normal cells tend to stay together in the case of marginal adhesion, whilst cancer cells tend to lose this capacity. As a result, lack of adhesion is a symptom of cancer. The scale of a single epithelial cell is linked to the previously described uniformity.

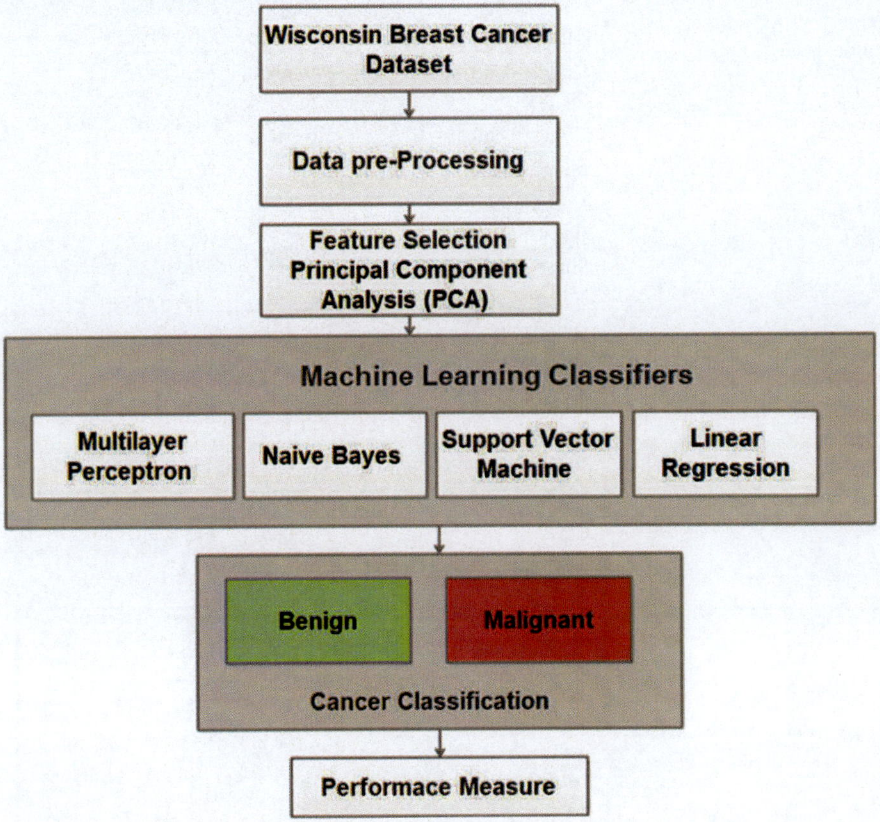

Fig. 1 Proposed method for breast cancer detection

Significantly, swollen epithelial cells may be Malignant cells. The word 'bare nuclei' refer to nuclei that are not enclosed by cytoplasm. These are commonly seen in benign tumours (Table 1).

In benign cells, the bland chromatin represents a 'texture' of the nucleus. The chromatin in cancer cells is coarser. Normal nucleoli are minor size structures that can be found in the nucleus. If the nucleolus is visible in normal cells, it is typically very thin. The nucleoli become more evident in cancer cells, and there are sometimes more of them. As a final stage, Mitoses is known as nuclear division plus cytokines, which result in the development of two identical descendant cells during prophase. It refers to the mechanism by which a cell splits and replicates. By measuring the number of mitoses, pathologists may assess the grade of cancer. Figure 2 depicts an extract from the dataset.

Table 1 WBC dataset attributes [14]

Attribute	Domain
Sample code number (SCN)	Id number
Clump thickness (CT)	1 to 10
Marginal adhesion (MA)	1 to 10
Uniformity of cell shape—(UCSh)	1 to 10
Single epithelial cell size (SECS)	1 to 10
Uniformity of cell size (UCS)	1 to 10
Bare nuclei—(BN) 1–10	1 to 10
Mitoses	1 to 10
Bland chromatin (BC)	1 to 10
Normal nucleoli (NN)	1 to 10
Class	2 as benign, 4 as Malignant

sample code number	clump thickness	uniformity of cell size	uniformity of cell shape	marginal adhesion	single epithelial cell size	bare nuclei	bland chromatin	normal nucleoli	mitoses	class
1000025	5	1	1	1	2	1	3	1	1	benign
1002945	5	4	4	5	7	10	3	2	1	benign
1015425	3	1	1	1	2	2	3	1	1	benign
1016277	6	8	8	1	3	4	3	7	1	benign
1017023	4	1	1	3	2	1	3	1	1	benign
1017122	8	10	10	8	7	10	9	7	1	malignant
1018099	1	1	1	1	2	10	3	1	1	benign
1018561	2	1	2	1	2	1	3	1	1	benign
1033078	2	1	1	1	2	1	1	1	5	benign
1033078	4	2	1	1	2	1	2	1	1	benign
1035283	1	1	1	1	1	1	3	1	1	benign
1036172	2	1	1	1	2	1	2	1	1	benign
1041801	5	3	3	3	2	3	4	4	1	malignant
1043999	1	1	1	1	2	3	3	1	1	benign
1044572	8	7	5	10	7	9	5	5	4	malignant
1047630	7	4	6	4	6	1	4	3	1	malignant
1048672	4	1	1	1	2	1	2	1	1	benign
1049815	4	1	1	1	2	1	3	1	1	benign
1050670	10	7	7	6	4	10	4	1	2	malignant
1050718	6	1	1	1	2	1	3	1	1	benign

Fig. 2 Breast cancer Wisconsin (BCW) dataset

3.2 Dataset Preprocessing

Data preprocessing is a salient step in data mining which deals with the renovation of raw data into a clean, precise and understandable format. Preprocessing activities involve but are not restricted to issues related to cleaning, transformation, mapping, reduction, organization and selection of data. Amongst all the issues, feature selection is of prime importance. To evade inappropriate task of significance, the dataset was uniform using Eq. 1.

$$z = X - \mu\sigma \tag{1}$$

where X is identified as a feature to be standardized, mean value of the feature is specified as μ, and the standard deviation of the feature is represented as σ. The preprocessing process was implemented using the code as below.

- from sklearn.preprocess import StandardScaler
- scaler = Standard Scaler()
- X = scaler.fit_transform(X)

3.3 *Feature Selection*

Choosing features are a significant phase in creating a classification model. To attain the better classification results of the model, it is beneficial to limit the sum of input attributes in a classifier. Instead of using the whole attribute collection, a few dominant features that are good enough to execute the classification task with the same or much better precision is used. Choosing a feature subset not only improves precision, but it also cuts computation time and model complexity [17].

Principal Component Analysis (PCA).

PCA is a technique for evaluating principal components by using them to perform information-based adjustments, often using only the main principal components and skipping the respite. Knowledge may be extracted from a high-dimensional (include) space by predicting it into a low-dimensional subspace. It attempts to preserve the fundamental parts with greater data diversity whilst removing redundant parts with less diversity.

This paper proposes function selection methods based on principal component analysis. The benefits of fit test decides, if an empirical frequency distribution corresponds to a theoretical frequency distribution. PCA is a scientific technique that employs an orthogonal transformation to turn a series of potentially clustered measurements into a set of values of linearly uncorrelated variables known as PCA. The amount of PCA is equal to or less than the number of initial variables.

Cell radius, compactness, concavity, perimeter, area and concave points mean values can be used to define cancer. Higher values of these parameters are associated with Malignant tumours. ii) Mean texture, symmetry, smoothness, or fractal dimension values do not imply a preference for one diagnosis over another. There are no apparent large outliers in any of the histograms that need further cleaning. Table 2 shows the significance of the characteristics in determining whether tumours are malignant or benign.

Table 2 Feature importance

Features importance mean (%)	Importance (%)
Concavity	18.2823
Texture	3.8492
Symmetry	1.6371
Fractal dimension	0.9043
Area	17.3446
Smoothness	1.9023
Radius	11.5543
Perimeter	20.45614
Concave points	19.7067
Compactness	4.3632

3.4 Classification

Classification of diseases is a majorly focussed challenge in medical data mining. When it comes to breast cancer, the main concern is to categorize the occurrences into benign and Malignant cases with high accuracy. Several ML systems for classification of breast cancer data.

3.5 Linear Regression

Despite the fact that, there is an algorithm for the regression problem by using a ML scheme of linear regression classifier in this analysis. This was accomplished by setting a threshold for the contribution of Eq. 2, i.e. subjecting the regress and to Eq. 3.

$$h_\theta(x) = \sum_{i=0}^{n} \theta i \cdot xi + b \tag{2}$$

$$fh_\theta(x) = \begin{cases} 1h_\theta(x) \geq 0.5 \\ 0h_\theta(x) < 0.5 \end{cases} \tag{3}$$

The mean squared error (MSE) was used in Eq. 4 to calculate the loss of the model.

$$L(y, \theta, x) = 1/N \sum_{i=0}^{N} (y_1 - (\theta i \cdot x_i + b))2 \tag{4}$$

where y denotes the real class and (θ x + b) denotes the expected class. The SGD algorithm, which knows the constraints of Eq. 7, is used to minimize this deficit. The same loss minimization approach was used for Softmax regression and MLP.

3.6 Support Vector Machine

The SVM was designed specifically for binary classification. Its main goal is to find the best hyperplane $f(w, x) = w \cdot x + b$ for separating two groups in a given dataset with input features x R p and labels $yi + 1$ by resolving the guarded optimization problem in the SVM is derived below:

$$min 1/p w^T w + \sum_{i=1}^{p} \xi i \tag{5}$$

$$s.t\ y' i\ (w\ \cdot\ x\ +\ b)\ \geq\ 1\ -\ \xi i \tag{6}$$

$$\xi i \geq 0, i = 1, ..., p \tag{7}$$

where w^T w is identified as Manhattan norm, ξ represented as a cost function, its problem of unconstrained optimization is derived in the following as

$$\min\ 1/p\ w^T w\ +\ \sum_{i=1}^{p} \max\ (0, 1 - y' i(w_i x_i\ +\ b)) \tag{8}$$

The predictor function is wx + b. Equation 9's target is known as the primitive form dilemma of L1-SVM with the regular hinge loss. The downside of L1-SVM is that it is not distinguishable, as opposed to its variant, L2-SVM:

$$\min\ 1/p\ ||\ w\ ||_2^2\ +\ C\ \sum_{i=1}^{p} \max(0, 1 - y' i(w_i x_i\ +\ b))^2 \tag{9}$$

The L2-SVM delivers better stable outcomes than its L1 counterpart.

3.7 Multilayer Perceptron

The most commonly used for pattern recognition is MLP, which is known as a feedforward backpropagation neural network system. MLPs are supervised learning classifiers composed compressed a different layers that extract valuable information during learning and allocate modifiable weighting coefficients to input layer components. The preceding words are represented in Fig. 3. Weighted input is allocated to the input units, as well as the nodes in the hidden layer and the output specify the output in the first (forward) pass. The result is compared to the desired result. An

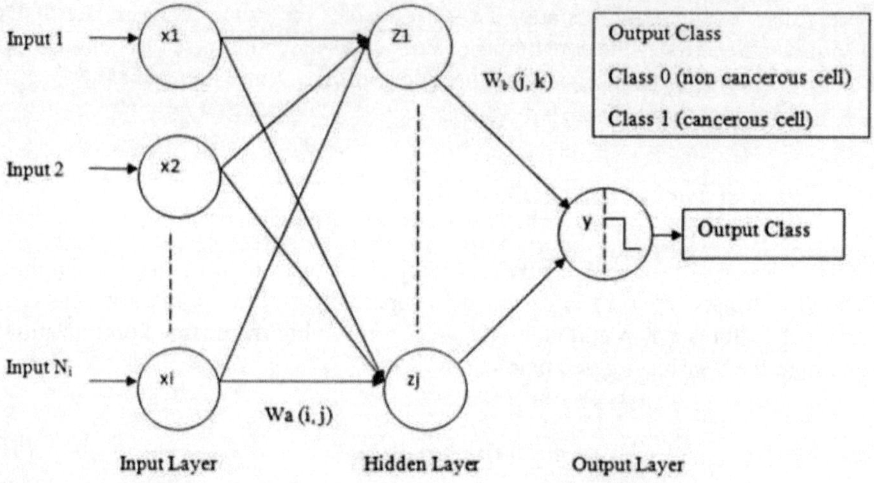

Fig. 3 Architecture of multilayer perception feedforward neural network

error signal is then returned, and the link weights are modified accordingly. During preparation, MLPs create a multidimensional space identified by the activation of secret nodes, in order to separate the three groups (Malignant or benign) as far as possible. The separating surface changes in response to the results.

3.8 Naive Bayes

Bayesian learning methods are important to the ML research for two reasons. First, Bayesian learning algorithms, such as the Naive Bayes classifier, that compute explicit probabilities for hypotheses, are amongst the most effective alternatives to certain kinds of learning problems. The Bayes theorem-based NB classifier is called as a probabilistic classifier. The Nave Bayes classifier provides probability approximations rather than forecasts. They measure the chance that a given example belongs to a given class for each class value. The Naive Bayes classifier has the advantage of having only a limited training data to approximate the parameters used for classification. It is presumed that the influence of an attribute rate on a given class is liberated of the other attributes' values.

4 Simulation Results and Analysis

In this simulation study, we conducted by evaluate the classification and identification of breast cancer by using WBC dataset. The experimentation was compiled by using a Python platform and further materials required as PC with 4 GB RAM Windows

Table 3 Hyperparameter tuning in machine learning model

Hyperparameter	SVM	MLP	NB	Linear regression
Batch size	128	128	128	128
Cell size	128	500	-	500
Dropout rate	1.0	0.5	-	-
Learning rate	0.01	0.001	0.01	0.01
Normal	L2	-	-	L1
Epochs	1500	1500	1500	1500

10. The performance of the machine learning classifier obtained and analysis by using different parameter as accuracy, precision recall and F-measure, which are mathematically expressed in following section. The choice of classifier is based on the percentage of correct prediction. There are at least three machine learning techniques which are generally used to calculate classifier accuracy. First one is to divide the whole dataset in two parts by 60:40 ratio for training and testing dataset. Table 3 demonstrations that the manually allocated the hyperparameters used for the machine learning algorithm.

4.1 Performance Measures

This proposed system in which different classifier performances is measure by using different parametric. The developed system is assessed using evaluation metrics such as TP, FP, TN, FN, sensitivity, precision, specificity, F-measure and accuracy.

- TP—Sum of normal sample is correctly categorized as noncancerous sample.
- TN—Sum of abnormal sample is correctly categorized as cancerous sample.
- FP—Sum of normal sample is wrongly categorized as cancerous sample.
- FN—Sum of abnormal sample is wrongly categorized as noncancerous sample.

Sensitivity

Sensitivity is also called as recall. Sensitivity is distinct as the percentage of sample with abnormal, whose output is positive, and it is calculated using the Eq. 10 as

$$Sensitivity = TP/(TP + FN) \tag{10}$$

Specificity

Specificity is defined as percentage of sample with normal, whose output is negative, and it is calculated using the Eq. 11 as

$$Specificity = TN/(TN + FP) \tag{11}$$

Classification accuracy

Classification accuracy is defined as the sum of correctly classified images, which are separated by the total sum of samples, and then, it is multiplied by 100 to turn it into a percentage. It is calculated using the Eq. 12 as

$$ClassificationAccuracy = (TP + TN)/(TP + FP + TN + FN) \quad (12)$$

Precision

Precision is distinct as the sum of true positives, which is divided by the number of TP and false positives, and it is calculated using the Eq. 13 as

$$Precision = TP/(TP + FP) \quad (13)$$

False positive rate

FPR is distinct as the sum of false positives, which is divided by the sum of false positives and true negative, and it is calculated using the Eq. 14 as

$$FPR = FP/(FP + TN) \quad (14)$$

F-measure

This is the kind of parameter measure, which association of recall and precision. The F-measure is determined by using the Eq. 15 as

$$F - measure = 2 * Recall * Precision/Recall + Precision \quad (15)$$

In Tables 4, 5 and Fig. 4, they show that the performance analysis of different machine learning classifier with and without feature selection method. In SVM classifier, achieved the 97.01% accuracy on with without feature selection and 99.07% of accuracy achieved at combination of feature selection algorithm. Then, MLP achieved 98.89% accuracy and PCA-MLP achieved 99.07% of accuracy. NB classifier achieved the accuracy of 96.13% and PCA-NB achieved 98.00% of accuracy.

Table 4 Comparison analysis of different classifier model without feature selection

Methods	Precession (%)	Recall (%)	F-measure (%)	Accuracy (%)
SVM	97.46	95.32	97.21	97.01
MLP	97.20	96.89	96.45	98.89
Linear regression	94.52	95.99	96.21	96.13
NB	96.33	95.15	94.15	97.33

Table 5 Comparison analysis of different classifier with feature selection technique

Methods	Precession (%)	Recall (%)	F-measure (%)	Accuracy (%)
PCA-SVM	97.99	96.42	98.92	97.92
PCA-MLP	97.85	97.48	97.13	99.07
PCA-linear regression	98.54	97.84	97.88	97.35
PCA-NB	97.82	96.58	98.55	98.00

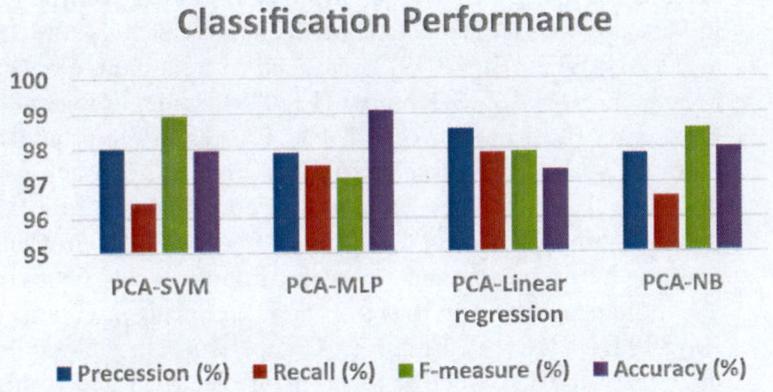

Fig. 4 Graphical representation of classifier performance

PCA-linear regression achieved the accuracy of 97.35% of accuracy. By this comparison, conclude that the PCA-MLP achieved better accuracy than other classifier model.

5 Conclusion

To reduce the mortality rate caused by breast cancer by increasing the accuracy of early detection of breast cancer and achieving effective Remote Diagnosis System through improved Machine Learning and Data Mining Mechanism. In this study, we increased the learning rate of the machine learning classifier by tuning the hyperparameter of the classifier to classify the breast cancer as begin or malignant efficiently. And also, on other hand, we implemented the PCA scheme to select the important feature from the large dataset. By combing the classifier with feature selection algorithm to get better classification result in breast cancer classification and identification. In this experimentation, Wisconsin breast cancer is used to evaluate the performances of the model by obtaining the different parametric values. In testing and training process, by choosing, 60% of data for training process and 40% testing process. And also we set the parameter of each machine learning classifier to train and test the model effectively to get the better result. By this comparative study of different machine learning classifier, principal component analysis with multilayer perceptron achieved the better classification accuracy as 99.07%.

References

1. Ak MF (2020) A comparative analysis of breast cancer detection and diagnosis using data visualization and machine learning applications. In Healthcare Multidisciplinary Digital Publishing Institute 8(2):111–124
2. Rositch, AF., Unger-Saldaña, K., DeBoer, RJ., Ng'ang'a, A., Weiner, BJ.: The role of dissemination and implementation science in global breast cancer control programs: frameworks, methods, and examples. Cancer 126(12), 2394–2404 (2020).
3. Tsang J, Tse GM (2020) Molecular classification of breast cancer. Adv Anat Pathol 27(1):27–35
4. Jenkins C, Ha DT, Lan VT, Van Minh H, Lohfeld L, Murphy P (2020) Breast Cancer messaging in Vietnam: an online media content analysis. BMC Public Health 20(1):1
5. Waks AG, Winer EP (2019) Breast cancer treatment: a review. Jama 321(3):288–300
6. Momenimovahed Z, Salehiniya H (2019) Epidemiological characteristics of and risk factors for breast cancer in the world. Breast Cancer: Targets and Therapy 12(4):141–151
7. Sahu B, Mohanty S, Rout S (2019) A hybrid approach for breast cancer classification and diagnosis. EAI Endorsed Transactions on Scalable Information Systems 6(20):20–31
8. Idri A, Hosni M, Abnane I, de Gea JM, Alemán JL. Impact of parameter tuning on machine learning based breast cancer classification. In World Conference on Information Systems and Technologies 2019 Apr 16 (pp. 115–125). Springer, Cham.
9. Bayrak, EA., Kırcı P., Ensari T.: Comparison of machine learning methods for breast cancer diagnosis. In2019 Scientific Meeting on Electrical-Electronics & Biomedical Engineering and Computer Science (EBBT) 20(12), 1–13 (2019).
10. Bataineh AA (2019) A comparative analysis of nonlinear machine learning algorithms for breast cancer detection. International Journal of Machine Learning and Computing 9(3):248–254
11. Inter Osman, A.H: An enhanced breast cancer diagnosis scheme based on two-step-SVM technique. International Journal of Machine Learning and Computing 9(3), 248–54 (2018).
12. Juneja, K., Rana, C.: An improved weighted decision tree approach for breast cancer prediction. In: International Journal of Information Technology 18(2), 1–8 (2018).
13. Banu AB, Subramanian PT (2018) Comparison of Bayes classifiers for breast cancer classification. Asian Pac J Cancer Prev (APJCP) 19(10):2917–2920
14. Yue L, Tian D, Chen W, Han X, Yin M (2018) Machine learning with applications in breast cancer diagnosis and prognosis. Designs 2(2):13–24
15. Azar AT, El-Said SA (2013) Performance analysis of support vector machines classifiers in breast cancer mammography recognition. Neural Computer Application. 24(5):1163–1177
16. Yadav A, Jamir I, Jain RR, Sohani M (2017) Breast cancer prediction using SVM with PCA feature selection method. International Journal of Scientific Research in Computer Science 5(2):969–978
17. Sahu B, Mohanty S, Rout S (2019) A hybrid approach for breast cancer classification and diagnosis. EAI Endorsed Transactions on Scalable Information Systems 6(20):1–8

An Investigation into the Application of Bidirectional Associative Memory and Pseudorandom Number for Steganography

Garima and Priyanka Dahiya

Abstract Steganography is the craft of concealing the restricted information in the harmless information with the end goal that very presence of the mysterious message is hidden. We propose utilization of bidirectional associative memory alongside pseudorandom number in the field of steganography. Since a message is made out of limited number of ASCII type characters which is powerless against assaults. Hence, we reason to pick a bunch of non-straight codes that has great hamming distance between any two back-to-back codes to supplant the first ASCII type input. This plan will make our framework considerably more shortcoming lenient in correlation with ASCII code-based framework under direct assault. We additionally reason another strategy to shroud the tweaked code in the image utilizing pseudorandom number inclusion method. To recuperate an assaulted code, we utilize bidirectional associative memory to perform vague coordinating. It gives best trial brings about recuperating the information from the mutilated Images.

Keywords Steganography · Bidirectional associative memory · Pseudorandom number · Pattern analysis

1 Introduction

The steganography comprises of techniques to permit the correspondence between two people, concealing the substance as well as the actual presence of the correspondence according to any spectator. So, they should discover some method of concealing their code text in a guiltless looking cover text [1–5].

Associative memory is one of the one of the significant classes of the neural organizations, which are weak impersonation of the human brain's capacity to relate

Garima (✉)
NIT Hamirpur, Himachal Pradesh, India
e-mail: 20bce018@nith.ac.in

P. Dahiya
DIT University, Dehradun, India

N. Marriwala et al. (eds.), *Emergent Converging Technologies and Biomedical Systems*, Lecture Notes in Electrical Engineering 841,
https://doi.org/10.1007/978-981-16-8774-7_46

designs. An associative memory is the storage facility of related examples that are encoded in some structure. At the point when the storage facility is set off with an example, the related example pair is reviewed. The info example could be a precise reproduction of the put away example or contorted one. On the off chance that the related example sets (x, y) are extraordinary and assuming the model reviews y given a x or the other way around, it is named as hetero-associative memory, otherwise if (x, y) refer to the same pattern then the model termed as auto-associative memory. Hetero-associative memories are useful for the association of the pattern and auto-associative memories are useful for image refinement. Auto-associative correlation memories are known as auto-correlators, and hetero-associative correlation memories are known as hetero-correlators. Bidirectional associative memory (BAM) is a two-level nonlinear neural organization dependent on prior examinations and models of cooperative memory [6–8].

This paper is coordinated as follows: In areas II and III, we present an outline of what is bidirectional associative memory and how the steganography works. This is followed NLFFSR in Sects. 4 and 5 describes the generation of the pseudorandom bit sequence using NLFFSR. In Sect. 6, we describe the proposed technique of hiding the data into the image as an application of BAM. The next Sect. 7 describes the method of retrieving the data from the image. In Sect. 8, we discuss Outline and Conclusion is introduced in segment IX which is trailed by the rundown of the referred to references.

2 Bidirectional Associative Memory

Kosko extended the unidirectional auto-associators to bidirectional processes. One of the significant execution credits of BAM is its capacity to review put away combines especially within the sight of noise (Fig. 1).

BAM introduced by Kosko has the following operations:

(2.1) There are N training pairs $\{(A_1, B_1), (A_2, B_2) \ldots (A_n, B_n)\}$ where

$$A_i = (a_{i1},\ a_{i2},\ a_{i3} \ldots\ a_{in})$$

$$B_i = (b_{i1}\text{--},\ b_{i2},\ b_{i3} \ldots\ b_{in})$$

Here, a_{ij} or b_{ij} is either in the ON or OFF state which corresponds to values 1 and 0, respectively, in the binary mode. In the bipolar mode, ON = 1 and OFF = -1.

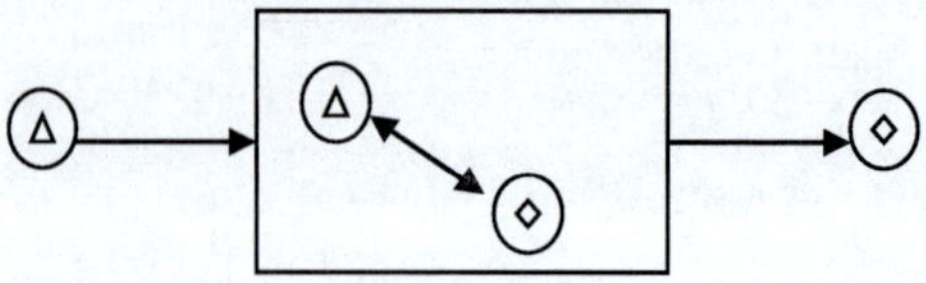

Fig. 1 Basic model of associative memory

(2.2) The corresponding bipolar matrix of the Ai and Bi are Xi and Yi.
We frame the correlation matrix

$$M = \sum_{i=1}^{n} X_i^T Y_i$$

To retrieve the nearest pair (A_i, B_i) given any pair (α, β) we start with (α, β) as the initial condition, we determine a finite sequence (α', β'), (α'', β''), (α''', β''') … until an equilibrium point (α_f, β_f) is reached.

$$\beta' = \phi(\alpha M).$$

$$\alpha' = \phi(\beta' M^T)$$

$$\phi(F) = G = g_1, g_2, g_3 \ldots g_n$$

$$F = (f_1, f_2, f_3 \ldots f_n)$$

$$g_i = 0\,(Binary) f_i < 0 \left\{ \{ {}^{1\,if\ \ f_i > 0}_{-1\,(Bipolar)} \right.$$

Previous g_i, $f_i = 0$.

(2.3) On addition of a new pattern pair (X', Y'), the new correlation matrix M becomes

$$M = X_1^T Y_1 + X_2^T Y_2 + \ldots + X_N^T Y_N + X'^T Y'$$

(2.4) On deletion of a pattern pair (X_j, Y_j), the new correlation matrix M becomes.

$$(New)\ M = M - (X_j^T Y_j)$$

The addition and deletion of the information as pattern pairs resemble the typical human memory exhibiting learning and forgetfulness.

(2.5) Energy function for BAM

An example pair (A, B) characterizes the condition of a BAM. To store an example, the estimation of the energy works for that specific example needs to involve a base point in the energy scene

The stability of a BAM can be identified by an energy function E with each state (A, B). The energy function E is given as

$$E\,(A, B) = -AMB^T$$

for the bidirectional case. However, if the energy E evaluated using the coordinates of the pair (A_i, B_i), i.e.,

$$E = -A_i M B_i^T$$

doesn't establish a neighborhood least, at that point the point can't be reviewed, despite the fact that one beginnings with $\alpha = Ai$. In this viewpoint, Kosko's encoding strategy doesn't guarantee that the put away combines are at neighborhood minima. That is, it cannot guarantee the recall of the pattern pairs even if the pattern pairs are few. But, depending upon the application of the application, it could be essential to ensure the review of a specific example pair, or in reality, all the example sets. Wang presented the "various preparing" idea to guarantee the review of an ideal pair in the arrangement of preparing sets. In this paper, we will utilize this "different preparing" idea to effectively review the example sets. Assume the "numerous preparation" is utilized for every one of the sets in a preparation set; at that point, the connection network becomes

$$M = \sum_{i=1}^{n} q_i X_i^T Y_i$$

where q_i's are positive real numbers. This modified correlation matrix is called the generalized correlation matrix. The necessary and sufficient conditions for the weights q_i, such that all training pairs will be correctly recalled, have been discussed by Wang.

3 How Steganography Work

The plan guideline of steganographic frameworks depends on the reason that most correspondence stations, for example, phone lines and radio stations—send signals joined by some sort of commotion. This commotion can be supplanted by a changed mystery signal unclear from the clamor without the mysterious key. Along these lines, the mysterious sign can be sent undetected. Concealing information in a picture requires two documents. The primary document, called the "cover-picture", will be the guiltless looking picture that holds the secret data. The subsequent document will contain the data to be covered up. At the point when consolidated, the two records will produce a "stego-picture". There exists various approaches to make a stego-picture from the given cover-picture and the information to be covered up. These incorporate LSB (least huge piece) inclusion, veiling and separating, excess example encoding, pseudorandom number generation techniques [3, 9–14].

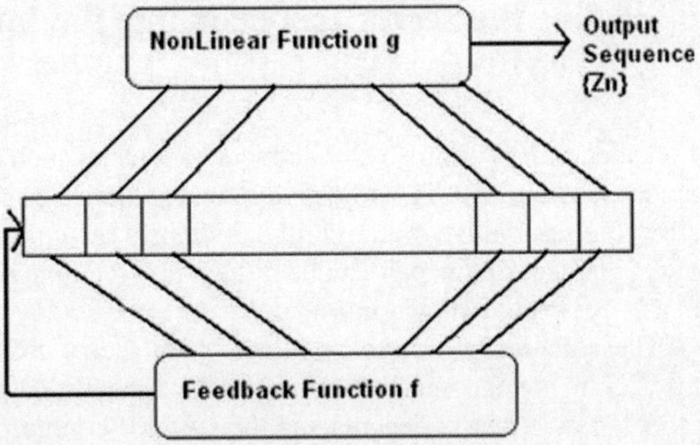

Fig. 2 An n-bit model of NLFFSR

4 What is a Nonlinear Feed Forward Shift Register?

It is a mechanism for generating binary sequences; Fig. 2 shows a general model. It is a linear feed forward shift register with a linear feed forward function f and a nonlinear output function g describing the nonlinear logic (i.e., multiplication of chosen number of bits followed by modulo-2 addition of resultant bits on the contents of the register) giving the output. The output sequence is called nonlinear feed forward sequence. The period of the sequence generated by a n-bit register is 2^{n-1}.

5 Pseudorandom Binary Pattern Generation Using NLFFSR

NLFFSR make amazingly great pseudo-irregular paired example generators. At the point when this register is stacked with some random starting worth (aside from 0 which will create a pseudo-irregular double example of every one of the 0 s). The lone sign fundamental for the age of the twofold example is a clock beat. With each clock heartbeat, a touch of the paired succession is delivered. A model $f = 1 + x + \times 4$ and the non-direct capacity g characterized. Its underlying piece esteems are utilized (1111). The yield succession Zn: 011,111,000,000,001,011,111,000,000,001… generated by period 15, which is equivalent to the time of the grouping produced by NLFFSR of four pieces. The usefulness of the arrangements, for example, determined above depends in enormous part on their having almost haphazardness properties. Subsequently, such groupings are named as pseudo-arbitrary double arrangements. Besides, utilizing fell NLFFSR can give more solidarity to the mysterious keys. The NLFFSR produced arrangements are critical in numerous fields of designing and sciences.

6 Hiding the Secret Text Data into the Image Using NLFFSR

Consider a set of English alphabetical characters such as A, B, C…, which are to be hidden in the image. The objective is to convert these characters into pattern pairs and allow the associative memory model identify the characters presented such that one of the element of this pair can be hidden into the image. The characters are engraved in a 7 × 7 grid as shown in Fig. 3.

These characters are to be related with their ASCII counterparts. Accordingly, the (X, Y) design sets which are to be related utilizing the acquainted memory model are the matrix designs and their ASCII counterparts. The framework designs are addressed as a bipolar vector of the 49 parts. In the event that the pixel in the network is concealed, the vector segment is 1 else it is –1. Additionally, the ASCII quantities of the characters have been addressed utilizing their bipolar counterparts. Figure 4 shows the bipolar coding of the example characters and their ASCII counterparts. We shroud the X of each example pair relating to each character we get in the text that should be covered up. As an illustration to stow away 'A', we conceal the double type of X comparing to 'A' that is 0001000001010001000101000001111111110000011000001 in the image utilizing NLFFSR addition technique. This procedure of NLFFSR addition is utilized to make it more harder for the inceptor to have the option to remove the privileged information. We propose to disperse it in arbitrary bit areas inside a given byte as opposed to restricting ourselves to just the most un-huge bit inside the every bite. For instance, we may shroud the slightest bit of the information at all huge digit of the byte, at that point we may conceal the second cycle of the information in bit number 3 of the subsequent byte, and afterward, we may shroud the third bit of the information in the bit number 6 of the third byte, etc., contingent on the arbitrary grouping produced by a specific NLFFSR utilized by the individual concealing the content. Assume that the double arrangement produced by the NLFFSR is 011111000000001011111000000001… as demonstrated in the segment 5, we set aside three pieces at an effort to build an arbitrary grouping of decimal numbers going from (0–7). The same decimal arrangement gets 3,700,137,001… accordingly the 49 pieces relating to 'A' are covered up as follows the originally cycle '0' is put away in (3 + 1)th bit of the primary byte; the subsequent bit '0' is put away in (7 + 1)th digit of the subsequent byte; the third bit '0' is put away in (0 + 1)th bit of the third byte, etc. We find that there have

Fig. 3 Nonlinear code for ASCII-test

0	0	0	1	0	0	0		1	1	1	0	0	0	0		0	1	1	1	1	0	0
0	0	1	0	1	0	0		1	0	0	1	0	0	0		1	0	0	0	0	0	0
0	1	0	0	0	1	0		1	0	0	1	0	0	0		1	0	0	0	0	0	0
1	0	0	0	0	0	1		1	1	1	0	0	0	0		1	0	0	0	0	0	0
1	1	1	1	1	1	1		1	0	0	1	0	0	0		1	0	0	0	0	0	0
1	0	0	0	0	0	1		1	0	0	1	0	0	0		1	0	0	0	0	0	0
1	0	0	0	0	0	1		1	1	1	0	0	0	0		0	1	1	1	1	0	0

X		**Y**		
Character	Bipolar Equivalent	ASCII	Binary Equivalent	Bipolar Equivalent
0001000	(-1 –1 –1 1 –1 –1 –1)			
0010100	(-1 –1 1 –1 1 –1 –1)			
0100010	(-1 1 –1 –1 –1 1 –1)			
1000001	(1 –1 –1 –1 –1 –1 1)	65	(0 1 0 0 0 0 0 1)	(-1 1 –1 –1 –1 –1 –1 1)
1111111	(1 1 1 1 1 1 1)			
1000001	(1 –1 –1 –1 –1 –1 1)			
1000001	(1 –1 –1 –1 –1 –1 1)			
X		**Y**		
Character	Bipolar Equivalent	ASCII	Binary Equivalent	Bipolar Equivalent
0011100	(-1 –1 1 1 1 –1 –1)			
0100010	(-1 1 –1 –1 –1 1 –1)			
0100000	(-1 1 –1 –1 –1 –1 –1)			
0011100	(-1 –1 1 1 1 –1 –1)	83	(0 1 0 1 0 0 1 1)	(-1 1 –1 1 –1 –1 1 1)
0000010	(-1 –1 –1 –1 –1 1 –1)			
0100010	(-1 1 –1 –1 –1 1 –1)			
0011100	(-1 –1 1 1 1 –1 –1)			

Fig. 4 Sample modulated code for ASCII characters 'A' and 'S'

been not many single piece changes between the raster information subsequent to concealing the data. Utilizing fell NLFFSR, it is feasible to produce more arbitrary piece grouping that would guarantee not very many piece changes.

7 Retrieving the Secret Text Data from the Image Using BAM and NLFFSR

Making use of the Wang associative memory model and choosing q1 = 2 and q2 = 3, we frame the correlation matrix [M] 49 × 8 given by

$$M = 2X_1^T Y_1 + 3X_2^T Y_2$$

We use only training pairs of the two sample characters; we have taken for illustrations and use the weights of 2 and 3, respectively, for the training. When we have obtained the matrix M, we retrieve the X from the image using the same NLFFSR as that was used at the sender side. When we obtain the X of the pattern pair, we calculate the value of corresponding Y as explained in the Sect. 2. We can easily recall the noisy characters using this technique. If the information hidden in the image gets corrupted or distorted, the reconstructed matrix X_{1x49} can get us the right satisfactory results. Thus, it is a major performance attribute of the discrete BAM.

8 Conclusion and Summary

The utilization of BAM assisted us with recovering the information in any event, when it is loud and twisted (Refer Fig. 5). This strategy is extraordinarily helpful in the application where the information should be recovered essentially in any event, when it is altered or contorted; this discovers its application in the field of Copyright Protection of the Images and Fabric Defect Identification. Likewise, we focused on improving the most un-critical piece (LSB) inclusion strategy by joining of the property of arbitrary example succession age showed by nonlinear feed forward shift register. It is accepted that by picking an appropriate NLFFSR or a blend of different NLFFSRs fell together; we can alter the LSB plan so much that the "stego-picture" is a precise copy of the first picture. We are right now arranging an AI-based programming which can get familiar with a ton of examples combines and review

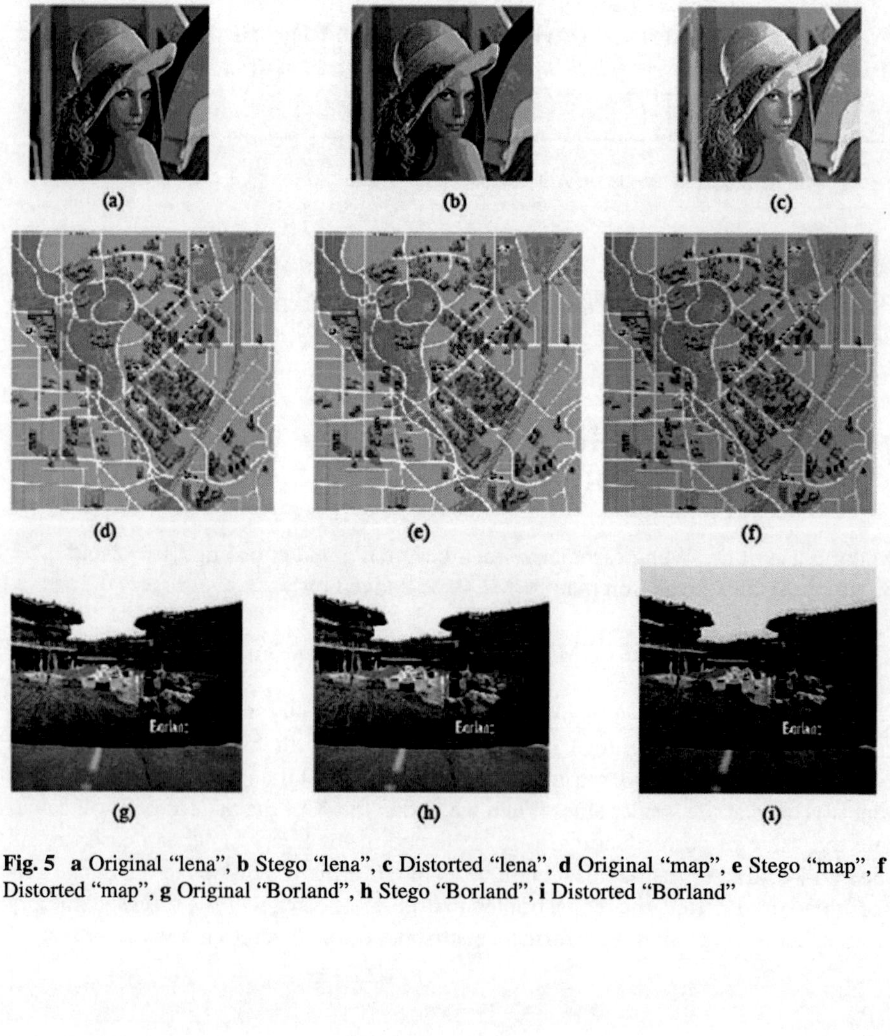

Fig. 5 **a** Original "lena", **b** Stego "lena", **c** Distorted "lena", **d** Original "map", **e** Stego "map", **f** Distorted "map", **g** Original "Borland", **h** Stego "Borland", **i** Distorted "Borland"

them regardless of whether the related pair is boisterous. It will be secure copyright protection programming utilizing BAM strategy.

References

1. Jain M, Kumar A (2017) RGB channel based decision tree grey-alpha medical image steganography with RSA cryptosystem. Int J Mach Learn Cybern 8:1695–1705
2. Jain M, Choudhary RC, Kumar A (2016) Secure medical image steganography with RSA cryptography using decision tree. 2016 2nd Int Conf Contemp Comput Informatics, pp 291–295
3. Kumar A, Ghose MK (2011) Extended substitution–diffusion based image cipher using chaotic standard map. Commun Nonlinear Sci Numer Simul 16:372–382
4. Dahiya P, Nautiyal R, Dahiya A (2019) Application of random block selection and random bit selection in the field of image steganography. J Adv Res Dyn Control Syst 11:335–340
5. Jain M, Kumar A (2017) Secure medical communication using sixteen rectangle substitution cipher and information-location dependent steganography. 2017 Int Conf Intell Commun Comput Tech, pp 189–193
6. Kohonen T (1972) Correlation matrix memories. IEEE Trans Comput 100:353–359
7. Wang Y-F, Cruz JB, Mulligan JH (1989) An enhanced bidirectional associative memory. IJCNN Int Jt Conf Neural Networks 1:105–110
8. Wang Y-F, Cruz JB, Mulligan JH (1990) Two coding strategies for bidirectional associative memory. IEEE Trans Neural Networks 1:81–92
9. Kumar A, Ghose MK (2009) Overview of information security using genetic algorithm and chaos. Inf Secur J A Glob Perspect 18:306–315
10. Kumar A, Ghose SS, Ghose MK (2009) An improved secure data communication using blind source separation and chaos. 2009 11th IEEE Int Symp Multimed, pp 358–362
11. Pandey D, Rawat US, Kumar A (2016) Robust progressive block based visual cryptography with chaotic map. J Discret Math Sci Cryptogr 19:1025–1040
12. Kumar A, Ghose MK (2010) Substitution-diffusion based image cipher using chaotic standard map and 3D cat map. Int Conf Bus Adm Inf Process, pp 34–38
13. Kumar A, Ghose MK (2010) Improved substitution-diffusion based image cipher using chaotic standard map, pp 333–338. https://doi.org/10.1007/978-3-642-12035-0_33
14. Mendiratta A, Dahiya A, De A, Rajpal N (2007) Chaos based audio watermarking. ProcInt Conf Comput Intell Multimed Appl ICCIMA 2008(4):64–69
15. Jain M, Kumar A, Choudhary RC (2017) Improved diagonal queue medical image steganography using Chaos theory, LFSR, and Rabin cryptosystem. Brain Inform 4(2):95–106

Investigations on Motor Imagery in Brain–Computer Interface

Rohtash Dhiman and Pawan

Abstract The authors present an investigation on state of the art of motor imagery (MI) for brain-computer interface (BCI) using electroencephalogram (EEG) in this paper. The EEG-based BCI is the youngest and fastest growing emergent technology that permits encephalic activity alone to computer or artificial system. Motor imagery BCI systems have enticed the great interest ranging from medicine to military points. EEG has been used for medical diagnosis such as seizure detection, brain injury detection, and also used control engineering for object controlling application, object recognition, rehabilitation, and human assistance. The EEG-based BCI system, wavelet transform gives appropriates outputs which enhanced the classification results. The support vector machine (SVM) and deep learning techniques generally used for EEG-based MI-BCI classification tasks. This research shows clear and easy interpretation of each methods used for feature extraction and classification using EEG for motor imagery BCI systems.

Keywords Artifacts · Brain computer interface · Electroencephalogram · Motor imagery

1 Introduction

The electroencephalogram signals are recorded simply by placing electrodes on scalp of subject [1]. EEG brain signals recorded by electrodes placed over the human scalps and are commonly placed as per international 10–20 system, which has been standardized by American Electroencephalographic Society [2, 3]. These electrodes are mostly made of silver chloride and electrodes-scalp contact impendence range varies from 1 kilo-ohm to 10 kilo-ohm during recording being correct biological signal. The human brain without interrupted, generated electrical waves in form of voltage signals from 0.5 to 100 Hz but fundamentally in the range from 0.5 to 50 Hz [4, 5]. This range can further be divided between different frequencies

R. Dhiman · Pawan (✉)
Electrical Engineering Department, Deenbandhu Chottu Ram University of Science and Technology, Murthal, Haryana, India

N. Marriwala et al. (eds.), *Emergent Converging Technologies and Biomedical Systems*, Lecture Notes in Electrical Engineering 841,
https://doi.org/10.1007/978-981-16-8774-7_47

and correlated to various cognitive task or movement. [6]. Electroencephalogram plays a significant role in categorizing brain activity and behavior. EEG-based brain–computer interface (BCI) is direct interface between brain and external device. BCI is also knows as brain machine interface (BHI). There are basically two types of BCI systems, namely invasive BCI and non-Invasive BCI. The non-invasive BCI systems preferred in use due to their affordability and flexibility in capturing the signals from brain. This research study is organized into six sections, Sect. 2, "EEG—the brain signals", Sect. 3, "EEG recorded method and artifacts", Sect. 4, "Signals processing technique for Brain–Computer Interface system", Sect. 5, "Technical challenges for BCI", Sect. 6, " Conclusion".

2 EEG the Brain Signal

First time EEG signal recorded on animal brain by Richard Caton in 1875. Hans Berger was a German psychiatrist first recorded the brain's electrical activity from the scalp in 1924. The electroencephalogram is maximally used signal in BCI due to high temporal resolution, ease of use and safe [7]. It has poor spatial resolution. Electroencephalogram signals are mostly time varying and non-stationary and measured different points of human brain in form of various range of voltage [8]. The EEG has unique property of non-stationary in nature. It is vulnerable to artifacts caused by eye coordination, eye blinks, muscular activities, breathing process, and power line interferences. The classification of electroencephalogram signals based on their frequency band and EEG investigates the events in the form of electrical signals. Using biological signals researcher capable to examine brain illness related with human beings. By evaluating electrical wave variance, capable to discover some of the brain abnormalities like strokes, neurodegenerative diseases. The classification of electroencephalogram signals based on their frequency, amplitude, and shapes is explained below [9].

2.1 Delta Signal

Delta signals represent the gray matter of brain and have highest amplitude and can produce either in cortex or thalamus. These signals are usually associated with all stages of sleep in stage 3 and 4. It is also called as slow-wave sleep (SWS) and aid in characterizing depth of sleep. Its frequency range from 0.5–4.0 Hz and seen normally in adults in slow-wave sleep as well as in infants [10].

2.2 Theta Signal

Theta signals ranges from 4 to 8 Hz. These types of brain signals are observed in meditation and deep relaxation. This signal is show abnormality in adults but in normal for children below age of 13 years. It is responsible for producing of human development hormone and serotonin hormone that rise clam and provides relief from ache.

2.3 Alpha Signal

These are most common in adolescents who are awake, but calm during closed eyes. frequency band range of these from 8 to 13 Hz and are occurs on both side of the head. It acts as a channel between subconscious and conscious brain. Many researchers show that marijuana that initiates a rise in alpha signal power.

2.4 Beta Signal

The frequency band range of this signal is from 13 to 30 Hz. It is seen commonly on both sides of frontal and parietal lobes. These signals are occurring in conscious mind state, judgment, puzzle solving, talking, and decision-making.

2.5 Gamma Signals

These signals have frequency band between 30 to 100 Hz and related with consciousness and perception [11]. These waves accurately combine memory and sense together for ideal experience.

3 EEG Recording Method and Artifacts

3.1 EEG Recording Method

The neurons of cerebral cortex generated various electrical fields on surface of skull that can be captured and recoded with appropriate electrodes. During EEG biological signal recording, electrodes are located discretely on scalp by 10–20% international standards of the human head [12]. Every silver chloride electrode connected to an amplifier for recording EEG. After captured EEG signals from the electrode, it

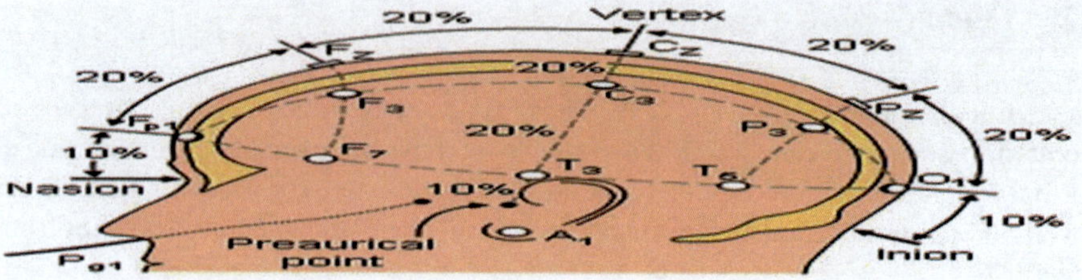

Fig. 1 Side view of 10–20 electrode system [14]

reaches an amplifier or differential amplifier. The filtering processes are performed inside the amplifier for both highpass as well as lowpass filter. Each and every electrode positioned in 10/20 system is marked by a number and a letter [13]. The number recognized the hemisphere and letter identified lobes of brain. The right part of hemisphere electrodes is positioned by even numbers, while left hemisphere is positioned by odd numbers. The English alphabets letter F stands for frontal, and T, C, P, O, A are stands for temporal, central, parietals, occipital, and auricular, respectively, while "Z" is used to refer to electrodes positioned on midline (Fig. 1).

3.2 *Artifacts*

It contaminates the original signal giving noisy signals. The signal artifacts are more substantial while collecting EEG data from recording systems. Usually, EEG artifacts can be broadly classified into two categories termed as physiological and non-physiological artifacts [15]. During recording and signal processing, some physiologic and non non-physiologic artifacts are added with EEG signals are giving below Table 1.

Table 1 Type of artifacts

S.No	Physiological Artifacts	Non-Physiological Artifacts
1	Eye blink and movements	Electrodes impedance
2	Muscular movements	Electrical power line interference 50 to 60 Hz
3	Cardiac muscle movement	Bad of electrodes position
4	Pulsation of blood vessel	Low battery of signal processing devices
5	Skin sweating	Dry scalp-electrodes contact

4 Signals Processing Technique for Brain–Computer Interface System

The brain–computer interface system involved the mainly four stage of data acquisition, data preprocessing, feature extraction, classification, and command translation [16–18]. Brain–computer interface also called NCI mean neural control interface. The BCI techniques should be capable of classifying mental tasks as precisely from EEG signals. It has become a collaborative mixture of computational neuroscience, engineering, signal processing, computer science, and many other types of research. The operation of brain–computer interface commonly involves several steps as shown in below Fig. 2.

4.1 Data Acquisition Process

For data acquisition 10–20 international system is used with electrodes having 8 mm. The data acquisition unit is accountable for capturing electrophysiological waves that deliver input to brain–computer interface. These waves are recorded from surface of subject's brain for checking neuronal activity and amplifying the signal. Brain–computer interface use invasive or non-invasive technique for signal recording. The invasive technique has enhanced wave's quality as compared to non-invasive techniques. Non-invasive techniques for acquiring biological signals are EEG, magnetoencephalogram, near-infrared spectroscopy and functional magnetic resonance imaging. The recorded biological signal is amplified for heighten the power then digitized before they are used by any of the artificial devices.

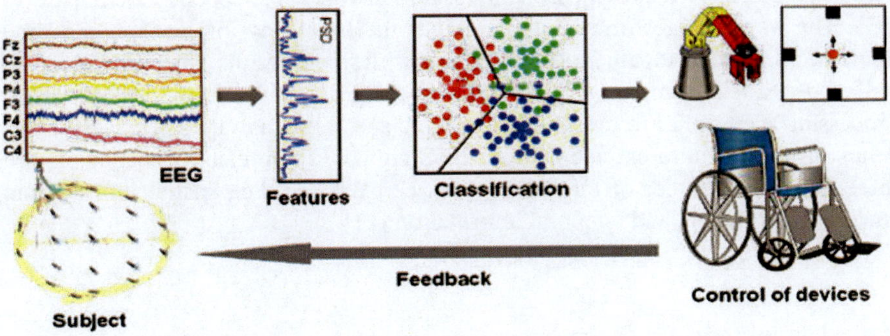

Fig. 2 Brain–computer interface system [19]

4.2 Signal Processing

The signal processing techniques are heart of current medical instrumentation, and main goal of preprocessing is to prepare recorded signals for processing by increasing signal-to-noise ratio. The SNR is measure of relative strength of valuable information in a signal capture by noise vs. overall strength of signal, involved noise. Notch filter having null frequency of 50 Hz is preferred to use for removal of artifacts as well as noise. The signals having large frequency noisy components are eliminated with help of LPF having cut of frequency 40–70 Hz [20]. However, the recorded electrical signal always be dirtied with artifacts and then affect the analysis of EEG signal. Hence, it is important to develop techniques to efficiently detect and extract the clean electroencephalogram data during EEG recordings. The numerous approaches have been proposed to eliminate artifacts, but the research on artifact elimination still to be an open problem.

4.3 Feature Extraction

The most crucial step in signal processing of EEG is stage of feature extraction which provides greatest possible success of classification stage, and it reduces the dimensions of data without loss of signal information through classification stage in real-time operation. There are many feature extraction methods and some are as follows: The FFT calculates relative strength of EEG signal by decomposes biological signal into frequency components. It does not examine non-stationary electrical signal. For investigating such signal used short-term Fourier transform (STFT). The autoregression model is calculating power spectrum density of EEG signal for brain–computer interface. It provided better resolution fort short epochs as compare to FFT. The wavelet transform (WT) combines the frequency information and time domain information together so that WT provides best results when compared to FFT and AR. The common spatial pattern is commonly used for multiple channel processing and applies to tune subject specific spectral band range. The CSP algorithms used to feature extraction from EEG signals. From electroencephalogram, three important sources of information can be extracted, i.e., spatial information, spectral information, and temporal information [21].

4.4 Classification Techniques

After feature extraction and selection, biological signal should be classified using classification methods to get accurate control signal for desired actions. The various classification techniques have been used for identifying biological signals. Basically, linear and nonlinear two type of classier used in brain–computer interface systems

Table 2 Classification techniques

S.No	Technique	Advantages	Disadvantages
1	LDA [24]	- It is linear classifier and closely related to ANOVA - It is very simple to apply and has less computational work	- It will not give satisfactory results if discriminatory information is not in mean but in variance of data - It is not fit for nonlinear dataset
2	SVM [25]	- It constructs a set of hyper-planes in an infinites dimensional region - It is linear and supervised learning methods	- To obtain best results, SVM algorithms have many key parameters that required set correctly
3	ANN [26]	- It is a nonlinear classifier and example of supervised learning technique - Remove artifacts in best manners	- Approximate results are obtained trail and error methods - It requires more is a time for computational task
4	NBC [27]	- It is based on Bayes theorem - It is fast to implement any given problem	- It is very sensitive for input dataset - There is possibility an error during classification
5	K-NN[28, 29]	- It is non-parametric technique apply for classification or regression - K-NN is simplest classifier, and it is an instance-based learning technique	- It has slow learning process - It ignores attributes importance during computation

for classification task [22, 23]. Some important classifier used in signal process to get desired action descried in Table 2 and the latest literature of various MI-brain computer interface system in Table 3.

5 Technical Challenges for BCI

5.1 Nonlinearity

The human brain is an extremely complex nonlinear arrangement in which show very chaotic behavior. EEG biological signals can be well categorized by nonlinear dynamic techniques than linear approaches [43].

5.2 Maximum Error Rate

Brain–computer interface system use noninvasive method to capture biological signal which have artifacts. The noise and artifacts make the EEG signal erroneous.

Table 3 Comparison table of various MI-brain–computer interface applications

Aim of the research work	Preprocessing techniques	Feature extraction	Classification methods	Accuracy
MI classification (right and left hand) [30]	Band pass filter	CSP	CCA	87.09 ± 2.28%
MI classification (right and left hand) [31]	Spatial filter	CSP	KSVM	60%
MI classification(right side, left side and right-side limb) [32]	Spatial filter	PCA, FLD	ELM	96.44%
Classification (fingers movements included right hand) [33]	Band pass filters	QFTD	Multi-class SVM	77.1%
MI classification(right and left hand) [34]	Band pass filters	CSP	LDA,SVM	82%
MI classification(right and left hand) [35]	Band pass filters	AAR	SVM	76.82%
MI classification (lower limbs) [36]	Band pass filter	CSP and Open ViBe software		Good
MI classification(left hand, right hand, foot, or tongue) [37]	Spatial filter	CSP	SVM	73.37%
MI classification(right and left limbs) [38]	Spatial filter	CSP	SVM (Dataset with two classes)	86.49%
MI classification (right and left limbs and tongue) [39]	Spatial filter	CNN	LSTM	87.31%
MI classification(left hand, right hand) [40]	Spatial filter	CSP	FBCSP algorithm	79.80%
MI classification [41]	Band pass filter	CFS algorithm	SVM	80%
MI classification right hand) [42]	Band pass filter	Morlet wavelet approach	M-D-based classifier	80%

5.3 *Training Process*

MI-brain–computer interface systems have training process little time consuming [44]. During training, it should be guided by user.

5.4 *Low Signal Strength*

EEG signal is not easy to capture from human brain due to weak signal strength [45]. The good strength signal getting process is very challenging task. To overcome this, problem amplifier is used.

6 Conclusion

This research paper has surveyed a large variation of literature on motor imagery BCI using EEG which helps and motivates the researchers who don't have wide experience in MI-brain–computer interface research. We investigated that MI-BCI systems basically have four main parts: EEG signal types, signal acquisition, feature extraction and selection, and classification. The wavelet transform approach better choice for feature extraction and provide better accuracy for classification process. For this study, it can conclude that SVM and deep learning techniques deliver the better classification results for EEG-based MI-BCI systems. The BCI applications are not limited. It is used into many areas such as communication, motor re-establishment, ecological control, locomotion, and entertainment. This literature survey is intended to give the readers a fast overview of MI-brain–computer interface systems.

References

1. Kumar JS, Bhuvaneswari P (2012) Analysis of electroencephalography (EEG) signals and its categorization—a study. Procedia Eng 38:2525–2536
2. Dvorak D, Shang A, Abdel-Baki S, Suzuki W, Fenton AA (2018) Cognitive behavior classification from scalp EEG signals. IEEE Trans Neural Syst Rehabil Eng 26(4):729–739
3. Donoghue JP (2002) Connecting cortex to machines: Recent advances in brain interfaces. Nat Neurosci 5(11s):1085–1088
4. Muangjaroen P, Wongsawat Y (2012) Real-time index for predicting successful golf putting motion using multichannel EEG. Proc Annu Int Conf IEEE Eng Med Biol Soc EMBS, pp 4796–4799
5. Lu N, Yin T, Jing X (2020) Deep learning solutions for motor imagery classification: a comparison study. 8th Int Winter Conf Brain-Computer Interface, BCI 2020, vol. c, pp 628–637
6. Wan X et al (2019) A review on electroencephalogram based brain computer interface for elderly disabled. IEEE Access 7(c):36380–36387

7. Wolpaw JR, Birbaumer N, McFarland DJ, Pfurtscheller G, Vaughan TM (2002) Brain-computer interfaces for communication and control 113(6):767–791
8. Dhiman R, Saini JS, Priyanka (2014) Genetic algorithms tuned expert model for detection of epileptic seizures from EEG signatures. Appl Soft Comput J 19:8–17
9. Abo-Zahhad M, Ahmed SM, Abbas SN (2015) A new EEG acquisition protocol for biometric identification using eye blinking signals. Int J Intell Syst Appl 7(6):48–54
10. Nawrocka A, Kot A (2011) Methods for EEG signal analysis. Proc 2011 12th Int Carpathian Control Conf ICCC'2011, pp 266–269
11. Mahdi SS, Al-Hajaj MR (2012) Design and implementation of EEG measuring system. 2012 1st Natl Conf Eng Sci FNCES-2012, pp 7–9
12. Padmasai Y, Subba Rao K, Raghavendra Rao C, Sita Jayalakshmi S, Koteshwar Rao MD (2008) EEG analysis using chi-square association metric. IETJE Res 54(1):74–80
13. Abdulkader SN, Atia A, Mostafa MM (2015) Brain computer interfacing: applications and challenges, pp 213–230
14. Alotaiby T, El-samie FEA, Alshebeili SA, Ahmad I (2015) A review of channel selection algorithms for EEG signal processing. EURASIP J Adv Signal Process, pp 352–362
15. Schalk G, Leuthardt EC (2011) Brain-computer interfaces using electrocorticographic signals. IEEE Rev Biomed Eng 4:140–154
16. Aggarwal S, Chugh N (2019) Signal processing techniques for motor imagery brain computer interface: a review. Array 1–2(January):100003
17. Bularka S, Gontean A (2016) Brain-computer interface review. 2016 12th Int Symp Electron Telecommun ISETC 2016 - Conf Proc, pp 219–222
18. Zhang W, Tan C, Sun F, Wu H, Zhang B (2018) A review of EEG-based brain-computer interface systems design. Brain Sci Adv 4(2):156–167
19. Iftikhar M, Khan SA, Hassan A (2019) A survey of deep learning and traditional approaches for EEG signal processing and classification. 2018 IEEE 9th Annu Inf Technol Electron Mob Commun Conf IEMCON 2018, pp 395–400
20. Francisco S (1987) Element of the signal processing. Int J Clin Monit Comput, 85–98
21. Al-Fahoum AS, Al-Fraihat AA (2014) Methods of EEG signal features extraction using linear analysis in frequency and time-frequency domains. ISRN Neurosci 2014:1–7
22. Sreeja SR, Rabha J, Nagarjuna KY, Samanta D, Mitra P, Sarma M (2017) Motor imagery EEG signal processing and classification using machine learning approach. Proc - 2017 Int Conf New Trends Comput Sci ICTCS 2017 2018-Janua:61–66
23. Oikonomou VP, Georgiadis K, Liaros G, Nikolopoulos S, Kompatsiaris I (2017) A comparison study on EEG signal processing techniques using motor imagery EEG data. Proc - IEEE Symp Comput Med Syst 2017-June(1):781–786
24. Preethi J, Science C (2014) A survey on EEG based emotion analysis using various feature extraction techniques. Int J Sci Eng Technol Res 3(11):3113–3120
25. KavitaMahajan M, Rajput M (2012) A comparative study of ANN and SVM for EEG classification. Int J Eng 1(6):1–6
26. Abinaya A, B. T, E. T, and M. M, "EEG Signal Classification Using Principal Feature Analysis and Artificial Neural Network for Brain Disease Diagnosis," Int. J. Adv. Res. Sci. Eng., vol. 4, no. 1, pp. 802–813, 2015.
27. Szuflitowska B, Orlowski P (2017) Comparison of EEG signal classifier LDA, NBC and GNBC based on time frequency features. Promiary Automatyka Robotyka, ISSN 1427–9126(R21):39–45
28. Mohanchandra K, Saha S, Murthy KS, Lingaraju GM (2015) Distinct adoption of k-nearest neighbour and support vector machine in classifying EEG signals of mental tasks. Int J Intell Eng Inform 3(4):313
29. Harikumar R, Narayanan BS (2003) Fuzzy techniques for classification of epilepsy risk level from EEG signals. IEEE Reg 10 Annu Int Conf Proceedings/TENCON 1:209–213
30. Yan N et al (2020) Quadcopter control system using a hybrid BCI based on off-line optimization and enhanced human-machine interaction. IEEE Access 8:1160–1172

31. Lee SB, Kim HJ, Kim H, Jeong JH, Lee SW, Kim DJ (2019) Comparative analysis of features extracted from EEG spatial, spectral and temporal domains for binary and multiclass motor imagery classification. Inf Sci (Ny) 502:190–200
32. Venkatachalam K, Devipriya A, Maniraj J, Sivaram M, Ambikapathy A, Iraj SA (2020) A novel method of motor imagery classification using eeg signal. Artif Intell Med 103:101787
33. Alazrai R, Alwanni H, Daoud MI (2019) EEG-based BCI system for decoding finger movements within the same hand. Neurosci Lett 698(September 2018):113–120
34. Belwafi K, Gannouni S, Aboalsamh H, Mathkour H, Belghith A (2019) A dynamic and self-adaptive classification algorithm for motor imagery EEG signals. J Neurosci Methods 327(July, 2019)
35. Chatterjee R, Maitra T, Hafizul Islam SK, Hassan MM, Alamri A, Fortino G (2019) A novel machine learning based feature selection for motor imagery EEG signal classification in Internet of medical things environment. Futur Gener Comput Syst 98:419–434
36. Tariq M, Trivailo PM, Simic M (2018) Motor imagery based EEG features visualization for BCI applications. Procedia Comput Sci 126:1936–1944
37. Sun L, Feng Z, Chen B, Lu N (2018) A contralateral channel guided model for EEG based motor imagery classification. Biomed Signal Process Control 41:1–9
38. Dose H, Møller JS, Iversen HK, Puthusserypady S (2018) An end-to-end deep learning approach to MI-EEG signal classification for BCIs. Expert Syst Appl 114:532–542
39. Yang J, Yao S, Wang J (2018) Deep fusion feature learning network for MI-EEG classification. IEEE Access 6(c):79050–79059
40. Ang KK, Guan C (2017) EEG-based strategies to detect motor imagery for control and rehabilitation. IEEE Trans Neural Syst Rehabil Eng 25(4):392–401
41. Bhattacharyya S, Konar A, Tibarewala DN (2017) Motor imagery and error related potential induced position control of a robotic arm. IEEE/CAA J Autom Sin 4(4):639–650
42. Edelman BJ, Baxter B, He B (2016) Nickerson - knowing & misjudging what others know.pdf. 63(1):4–14
43. Hassani M, Karami MR (2018) Improved EEG segmentation using non-linear volterra model in bayesian method. IETE J Res 64(6):832–842
44. Jain VK, Agarwal A (1976) Spectrum analyser for EEG signals. J Inst Electron Telecommun Eng 22(12):797–802
45. Singh G, Gupta V, Singh D (2010) Coherence analysis between ECG signal and EEG signal. Control 7109:25–28

Texture Analysis of Liver Ultrasound Images

Niranjan Yadav, Rajeshwar Dass, and Jitendra Virmani

Abstract The main goal of this work is to classify liver ultrasound images based on texture features for the early detection of liver abnormalities. A total of 60 liver ultrasound (30 benign and 30 malignant) images have been used for the analysis. A total of 302 texture features have been extracted, namely histogram, co-occurrence matrix, run-length matrix, absolute gradient, autoregression, and wavelet-based by using MaZda. In this work, most uncorrelated features are selected using principal component analysis (PCA), and three classifiers, namely (a) probabilistic-neural network (PNN), (b) K-nearest neighbors (K-NN), and (c) support vector machine (SVM) has been used to classify liver abnormities. A total of 20 statistical features have been selected using PCA and SVM yields optimal accuracy as 95%. It is observed that texture analysis using the MaZda package has been a more feasible and convenient method for analysis of abnormalities of the soft tissue.

Keywords Texture analysis · MaZda · PCA · SVM · GLCM · GLDS · GLRLM

1 Introduction

Various medical imaging modalities are widely used for characterization of soft tissue as x-ray, ultrasound, MRI, PET CT scan. Sonography has been widely used for analysis of soft tissue due to (a) low cost, (b) radiation free, (c) easy availability [1, 2]. The sonography reveals the texture of the soft tissue includes appearances, position, and structure of lesion. The texture features of an image are computed using several mathematical process by evaluation of grayscale intensity and position of pixel [3, 4]. Texture analysis provides intra-lesion heterogeneity and relationship among, the gray-level values in the image [5]. The histogram-based texture features mean, variance, skewness, and kurtosis attains uniformity, histogram as asymmetry,

N. Yadav (✉)
DCRUST Murthal, Sonipat, India

R. Dass · J. Virmani
CSIR-CSIO, Chandigarh, India

N. Marriwala et al. (eds.), *Emergent Converging Technologies and Biomedical Systems*, Lecture Notes in Electrical Engineering 841,
https://doi.org/10.1007/978-981-16-8774-7_48

irregularity, histogram flatness, and dispersion, respectively [6]. The texture feature based on first and second order are the important diagnostic information used in prediction [7]. Texture analysis employs a models to achieve an accurate assessment of lesion heterogeneity, spatial relationship, and dissimilarity [5–7]. Texture feature extraction remains a challenging task in the medical imaging due to complex computation [7]. The statistical modeling involved three orders of parameters named as first, second, and higher order. First order explores the distribution of frequency using histogram and measures intensity, standard deviation, etc. Second order explores co-occurrence and run-length matrix assessing a length of pixels based on gray-level intensity. High-order statistical parameters explore the overall differences between pixels via gray-tone difference matrix [8].

MaZda is a software package used for medical image texture examination. It is widely used in the medical imaging modality due to free of cost, reliability, and accurate. It was developed by IET University, Poland in 1996 for texture analysis of medical application [9]. MaZda provides much quantitative information about pixel, neighboring pixels, and spatial gray-level intensity within the image. In this work, texture analysis has also been explored to better characterize hepatic fibrosis, emphysema, and liver cirrhosis as benign and malignant using MaZda software package [8, 9]. Brief description of related study as shown in Table 1.

From Table 1, it is concluded that texture feature extraction becomes a difficult task in machine learning. It is very difficult to train the model with a large number of feature sets and less the features, the performance of the model improved. Feature extraction was computed in two ways (a) subset of features are combined in two or more approach (b) overall features extraction in one approach. Matlab extracts the subset of features and combined the all subset using a fusion approach. It is time-consuming and always chances of redundancy. MaZda is a tool that extracts all texture feature using one approach and very less of redundancy in the features set. The performance of the train network depends upon the number of features

Table 1 Brief description of related study

Investigator(s)	Feature extractor tool	Classifier
Ali Abbasian Ardakani et al. [8]	MaZda	1-NN and A-NN
Xiaowei Huang et al. [11]	MaZda	KNN
Tommaso Banzato et al. [13]	MaZda	1-NN and A-NN
Soo-Yeon Kim et al.	Matlab	t or chi-square test
Ganesh et al. [14]	Matlab	BPN
Salih et al. [15]	Matlab	Texture variation analysis
Neofytou et al. [16]	Matlab	PNN and KNN
Hui Mai et al. [17]	MaZda	KNN

selected from the features set. PCA, LDA GA, etc., are used for the reduction of the features set in the machine learning. PCA is the most common feature reduction method by combining multiple features into the new one. It works on the variance and correlation pattern in the database so that significantly reduced the dimensionality without any loss of important diagnostic information from the medical images. The main challenges in the feature extraction are human readability and scalability. In this work, the MaZda software package is used as a feature extractor due to overcomes all the challenges, and the PCA is used as a feature selection method.

2 Method and Material

The workflow adopted for characterization of liver ultrasound images as benign and malignant using MaZda software are shown in Fig. 1.

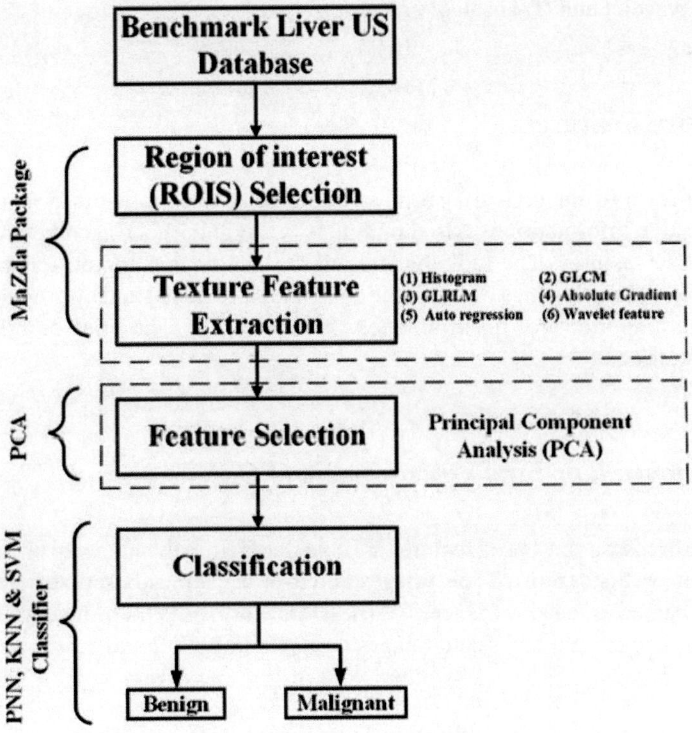

Fig. 1 Workflow adopted for the characterization of liver ultrasound images

2.1 Liver Database and Bifurcation

The liver US images have been taken from the standard benchmark database available at [10]. A total of 60 liver US (30 benign and 30 malignant) images have been used for the analysis. For training (20 benign and 20 malignant), liver US images are considered and for testing (10 benign and 10 malignant) are considered for analysis.

2.2 Texture Analysis

The texture analysis involved three orders of parameters named first, second, and higher. The first and second order explore the distribution of frequency and length of pixels based on gray-level intensity. High-order statistical parameters explore the overall differences between pixels via gray tone difference matrix. The texture features named as (a) Histogram based (b) Co-occurrence (c) run length (d) difference matrix (e) wavelet and (f) absolute gradient [8–12].

3 Texture Features

The visual form of image is transformed into precise descriptive information, and this descriptive information is based on intensity, neighborhood, and heterogeneity called texture features. The radiologist considers the texture region for the visual appearance of abnormalities of the tissue so that texture inside and outside the tumor boundary is important for discrimination of cancer [11]. The brief description of texture features as follow.

3.1 Histogram or First-Order Statics (FOS)

First-order or histogram-based features are calculated from the intensity of frequency distribution or histogram of the images. First-order statics-based features using histogram named as mean, variance, skewness, and kurtosis [9]. The histogram-based analysis for benign and malignant images is shown in Figs. 2 and 3, respectively.

3.2 GLCM Features

The spatial relationship is computed using the angular relationship θ and the distance d between the neighboring pixels [6]. Texture analysis is based on the co-occurrence

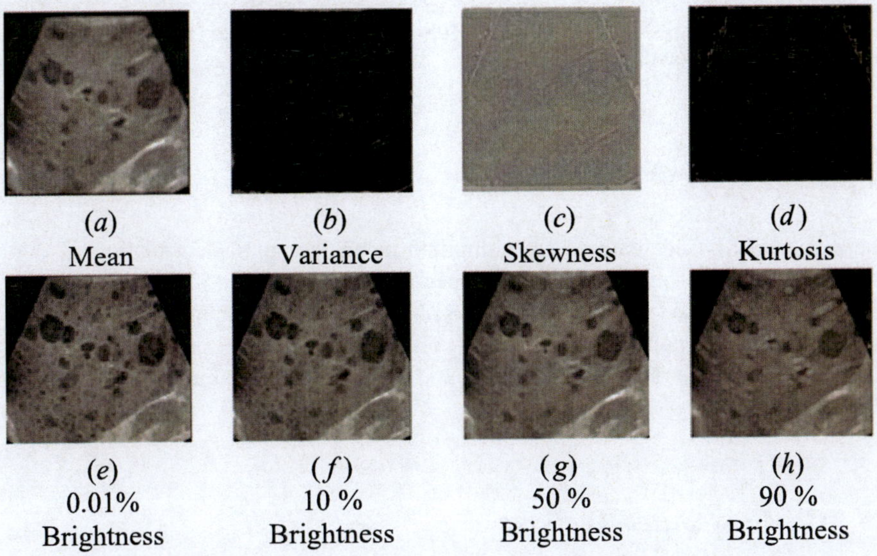

Fig. 2 Histogram-based features images

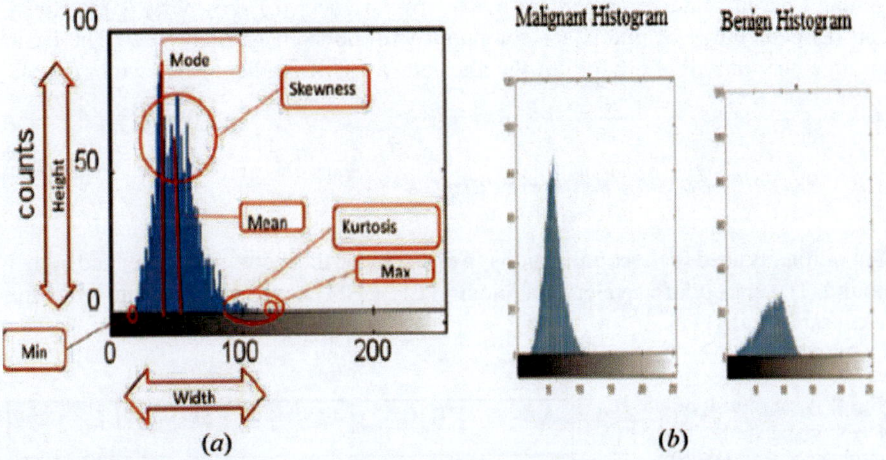

Fig. 3 **a** Histogram analysis and histogram-based features **b** Histogram of the benign and malignant liver ultrasound image

matrix, i.e., relationship of two pixels in the spatial domain. There are eleven GLCM features named as (a) entropy, (b) sum of entropy, (c) difference entropy, (d) sum average, (e) inverse difference moment, (f) sum of square, (g) difference variance, (h) correlation, (i) sum variance, (j) contrast, (k) angular 2nd moment computes for 4 direction and 5 distances [9, 10]. It measures angular relationship and pixel distance in the direction (0°, 45°, 90°, and 135°), pixel distance d = 1, 2, 3, 4 & 5. P (i, j) is the probability of gray-level combination, and P (i, j, θ, d) is representing some pixels pair at distance d and direction θ.

3.3 GLRLM Features

The run-length based features are computed using the spatial correlation of two or more pixels. It is measured using a specific direction (0°, 45°, 90°, and 135°). Gray-level variation is measure using GLRLM features in the images. There are five run-length features named as (a) "RL-uniformity (b) gray-level non-uniformity (c) long-run emphasis (d) short-run emphasis and (e) fraction computing in second-order category [9].

3.4 Gradient-Based Features

Gradient features are computed using the neighborhood of image pixel X (i, j) and the neighborhood absolute value of the gradient for each pixel [6]. There are five gradient-based features named (a) mean, (b) variance, (c) skewness, (d) kurtosis, and (e) percentage of pixels are computed with nonzero gradient [11]. The basic arrangement of neighborhood for the absolute value of gradient is shown in Fig. 4.

3.5 Wavelet-based Texture Features

Gabor filter is used for decompositions so that achieve the theoretical lower and higher bound. The energy of wavelet coefficient in LL, LH, HL, and HH is computed at the successive scale [11].

Fig. 4 Arrangement of neighborhood for the absolute value of gradient

A	B	C	D	E
F	G	H	I	J
K	L	X(i, j)	N	O
P	Q	R	S	T
U	V	W	X	Y

4 Analysis of Liver Ultrasound Images

Tissue characterization remains challenging for all scenarios. Texture analysis is much accurate, reliable, and implements for both homogenous as well as non-homogeneous tissues. It gives better results than the spectral parameter analysis. MaZda is a computer-based program that serves to calculate texture features for medical images. It has been developed by IET University, Poland in 1996 for texture analysis, and it has been under research and development since 1998 to fulfil the requirements and the used for quantitative analysis of MRI, Ultrasound and mammograms [9]. The program MaZda package used C++-based programming and complied through window7/8/10 operating system [9–11]. In this work, MaZda is used for discrimination of liver tissues in ultrasound images and provides support to the radiologist for early detection of cancer as benign or malignant. In MaZda, ROIs can be drawn in different shapes and colors. The basic layout of MaZda and histogram of the region of interest is shown in Figs. 5 and 6, respectively.

4.1 Feature Selection

A total of 302 texture features are combining as set (TFS) from training and testing images. Some features are interrelated to each other's so that these redundant features

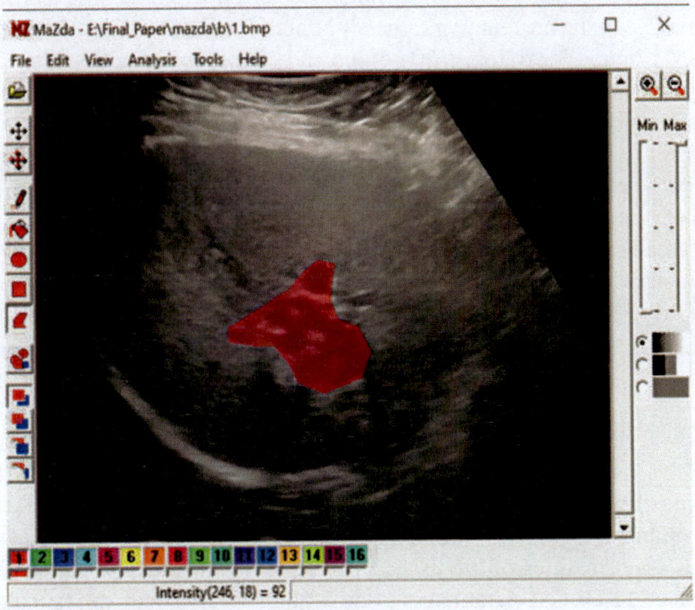

Fig. 5 MaZda software with the region of interest (ROI)

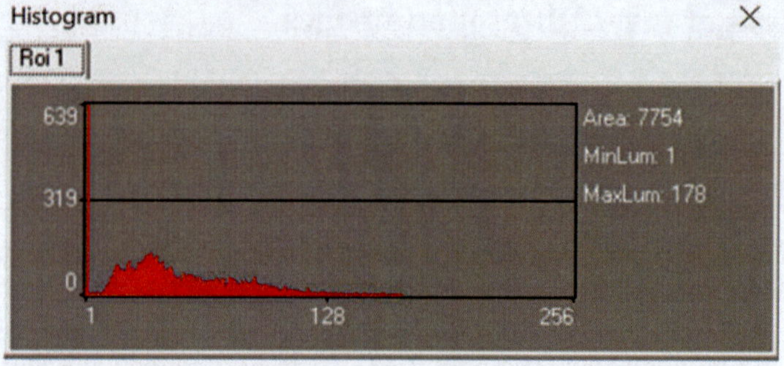

Fig. 6 Histogram of the region of interest

are not useful information for differentiating abnormalities. These texture feature sets are converted into optimal uncorrelated feature set (OFS) using principal component analysis (PCA) method. The number of PCs in the range of 2–20 for optimizing the features set.

5 Result and Discussion

The k-nearest neighbor (K-NN), probabilistic neural networks (PNN), and support vector machine (SVM) classifier are strong popular tools for machine learning in the medical images. In the present work, the SVM classifier has been implemented using the LibSVM library. For training, 20 benign and 20 malignant are selected, whereas for testing, 10 benign and 10 malignant are used. A receiver operating characteristic (ROC) analysis curve for the PCA-PNN, PCA-KNN, and PCA-SVM classifier is shown in Fig. 7. The network has been trained with an optimal feature set, the area under the curve expressively higher as 0.95 with PCA-SVM. The results of the three classifiers are shown in Table 2.

From Table 1, it is obtained that texture feature extracted using the MaZda package yields optimal results using principal component analysis selection method and SVM classifier (Table 3).

6 Conclusion and Future Work

The MaZda software package is the most reliable and efficient tool for texture analysis. It is computed better correlation parameters from the image and used a new tool for analysis abnormalities of the tissue. MaZda software package extracts valuable information as 11 GLCM parameters (4 direction and distances varies from 1 to 5), 5 GLRLM parameters with 4 direction resulting 20 features, gradient features with

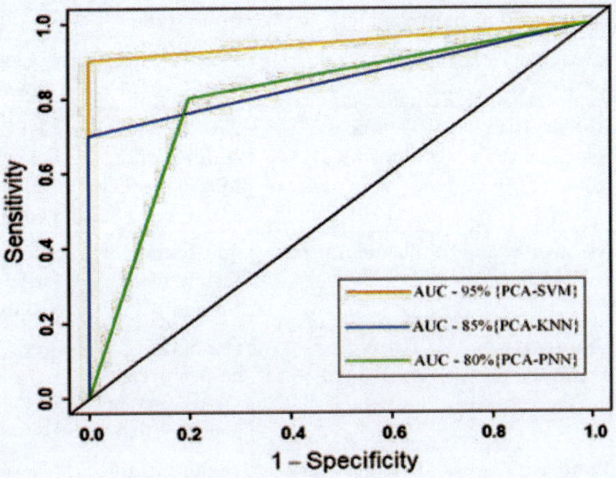

Fig. 7 Receiver operating characteristics curve

Table 2 Classifier results

Classifier	Confusion matrix			Accuracy (%)	Sensitivity (%)	Specificity (%)	ICAB (%)	ICAM (%)
PCA-PNN		B	M	80	80	80	80	80
	B	8	2					
	M	2	8					
PCA-KNN	B	10	0	85	100	70	100	70
	M	3	7					
PCA-SVM	B	10	0	95	100	90	100	90
	M	1	9					

Note B-Benign, M-Malignant, ICAB- Individual Class Accuracy for Benign, ICAM- Individual Class Accuracy for malignant

a mask size 3 × 3, and wavelet feature with (LL, LH, HL and HH partitioning). The most common type of abnormalities in the liver is hepatocellular carcinoma and other types of hepatoblastoma, cholangiocarcinoma. Tissue characterization of the human liver using ultrasound is the most challenging task. In this work, the MaZda package has been used for feature extraction from the liver ultrasound images, and these extracted features are selected using feature selection method principal component analysis. These selected features are classified using PNN, KNN, and SVM classifiers. It is observed that the PCA-SVM classifier yields optimal classification accuracy as 95%. In the future, morphological features are combined with texture feature, and more classifiers will be used in the model.

Table 3 Comparative analysis with existing studies

Investigator(s)	Tissue	Feature extraction	Feature selection	Classifier
Ali Abbasian Ardakani et al. [8]	Thyroid ultrasound	270 Texture feature using MaZda package	Fisher and average correlation coefficients	1-NN and A-NN
Xiaowei Huang et al. [11]	Plaque images	300 Texture feature using MaZda	Linear discriminant analysis	KNN
Soo-Yeon Kim et al.	Thyroid ultrasound	Histogram, co-occurrence matrix features using Matlab	–	t or chi-square test
Tommaso Banzato et al. [13]	B-mode ultrasound images	Texture feature using MaZda package	Correlation coefficients	1-NN and A-NN
Ganesh et al. [14]	Skin disease images	GLCM features using Matlab	–	BPN
Salih et al. [15]	Chest muscle Ultrasound	FOS, GLCM features using Matlab	–	Texture variation analysis
Neofytou et al. [16]	Hysteroscopy images	Dependence and difference matrices using Matlab	–	PNN and KNN
Present study	Liver ultrasound images	302 texture feature using MaZda	Principal component analysis	PNN, KNN, and SVM

References

1. https://www.radiologyinfo.org. Accessed July 2020
2. https://en.wikipedia.org/wiki/Ultrasound. Accessed July 2020
3. Kriti JV, Agarwal R (2019) Effect of despeckle filtering on classification of breast tumors using Ultrasound images. Biocybern Biomed Eng 39(2):536–560. https://doi.org/10.1016/j.bbe.2019.02.004
4. Flores WilfridoGómez, Coelho W, de AlbuquerquePereira A, CatelliInfantosi F (2014) Breast Ultrasound despeckling using anisotropic diffusion guided by texture descriptors. Ultras Med Biol 40(11):2609–2621. https://doi.org/10.1016/j.ultrasmedbio.2014.06.005
5. Snekhalatha U, Gomathy V (2018) Ultrasound thyroid image segmentation, feature extraction, and classification of disease using feed-forward backpropagation network. Progr Adv Comput Intell Eng 563:89–98. https://doi.org/10.1007/978-981-10-6872-0_9
6. Song G, Xue F, Zhang C (2015) A model using texture features to differentiate the nature of thyroid nodules on sonography. J Ultrasound Med 34(10):1753–1760. https://doi.org/10.7863/ultra.15.14.10045
7. Jitendra V, Kumar V, Kalra N, Khandelwal N (2014) Neural network ensemble based CAD system for focal liver lesions from B-Mode ultrasound. J Digit Imaging 27(4):520–537. https://doi.org/10.1007/s10278-014-9685-0

8. Ardakani AA, Mohammadi AGA (2015) Application of texture analysis method for classification of benign and malignant thyroid nodules in ultrasound image. Iranian J Cancer Prev 8(2):116–124
9. Szczypiński PM, Strzelecki M, Materka A, Klepaczko A (2009) MaZda—a software package for image texture analysis. Comput Methods Programs Biomed 94(1):66–76. https://doi.org/10.1016/j.cmpb.2008.08.005
10. https://www.ultrasoundcases.info/cases/abdomen-and-retroperitoneum/liver/. Accessed July 2020
11. Huang X, Zhang Y, Qian M, Meng L, Xiao Y, Niu L, Zheng R, Zheng H (2015) Classification of carotid plaque echogenicity by combining texture features and morphologic characteristics. J Ultrasound Med 35:2253–2261. https://doi.org/10.7863/ultra.15.09002
12. Virmani J, Kumar V, Kalra N, Khandelwal N (2013) SVM based Characterization of liver cirrhosis by single value decomposition of GLCM matrix. Int J Artif Intell Soft Comput 3(3):276–296. https://doi.org/10.1504/IJAI
13. Tommaso Banzato, Enrico Fiore, Massimo Morgante, Elisabetta Manuali, Alessandro Zotti (2016)Texture analysis of B-mode ultrasound images to stage hepatic lipidosis in the dairy cow: a methodological study. Res Veterin Sci 108:71–75. https://doi.org/10.1016/j.rvsc.2016.08.007
14. Ganesh VN, Vibha, Prajwitha J Puthran, Fidelia Chaitra Siri, Varnasri Jain M (2019) Skin disease recognition using texture analysis. Intern J Eng Res Technol (IJERT) 8(6):410–413
15. Salih NM, Dewi DEO, Yusof NSM, Noor NM, Yahya A, Mohamed F (2016) Ultrasound chest muscle characterization using 2D texture analysis. IEEE EMBS Conf Biomed Eng Sci (IECBES) 30–34. https://doi.org/10.1109/IECBES.2016.7843409
16. Neofytou MS, Pattichis MS, Pattichis CS, Tanos V, Kyriacou EC, Koutsouris DD (2006) Texture-based classification of hysteroscopy images of the endometrium. Annual international conference of the IEEE engineering in medicine and biology society. IEEE Eng Med Biol Soc 3005:3008. https://doi.org/10.1109/IEMBS.2006.259811
17. Mai H, Mao Y, Dong T, Tan Y, Huang X, Wu S, Huang S, Zhong X, Qiu Y, Luo L, Jiang K (2019) The utility of texture analysis based on breast magnetic resonance imaging in differentiating phyllodes tumors from fibroadenomas. Front Oncol 9:1021. https://doi.org/10.3389/fonc.2019.01021

Recent Advancements on Recommendation Systems in Healthcare-Assisted System

Gauri Sood and Neeraj Raheja

Abstract Present recommendation schemes such as content grounded filtering and collaborative filtering practice dissimilar databases to create references. Content-based filtering creates recommendations built on customer favorites for product types. Collaborative filtering mimics user-to-user recommendations. Both approaches have limits. Content-based filtering recommends a new item but requests more data of customer preference to include the finest match. Like, collaborative filtering wants a huge dataset with lively customers who valued a product before to create precise predictions. The arrangement of these dissimilar recommendation schemes is named hybrid systems. These schemes can blend the topographies of the item itself and the favorites of other customers. This paper reviews recent advances in recommendation approaches and their findings.

Keywords Recommender system · Convolutional neural network · Deep neural network · Deep Boltzmann

1 Introduction

The explosive progress in the work of digital data and the large count of people on the Internet has produced an impending task of data burden that obstructs the well-timed entrance to things of importance on the Internet. Recommender schemes are facts purifying arrangements that contract with the difficulty of data excess by clarifying vibrant evidence portion out of the huge volume of vigorously produced data allowing to customer's favorites, awareness, or practical activities around point [1]. For the healthcare field machine learning and its subfield, i.e., deep learning is useful and the fastest developing technologies. Machine learning offers superior assistances in better disease analyses, investigations, and avoidance. Lots of

G. Sood (✉) · N. Raheja
CSE Department, Maharishi Markandeshwar (Deemed to be University), Mullana 133207, India

N. Raheja
e-mail: neeraj_raheja2003@mmumullana.org

N. Marriwala et al. (eds.), *Emergent Converging Technologies and Biomedical Systems*, Lecture Notes in Electrical Engineering 841,
https://doi.org/10.1007/978-981-16-8774-7_49

machine learning-based classifications have been considered to deliver adapted daily life recommendations/mediation (Fig. 1).

Recommender schemes create recommendations and references to help their customers in various supervisory practices. Customers are further expected to access suitable produces and facilities using the recommender classifications (Fig. 2).

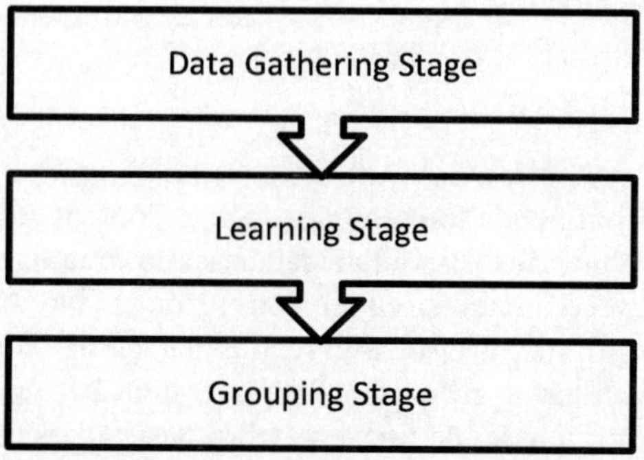

Fig. 1 Recommendation system process [1]

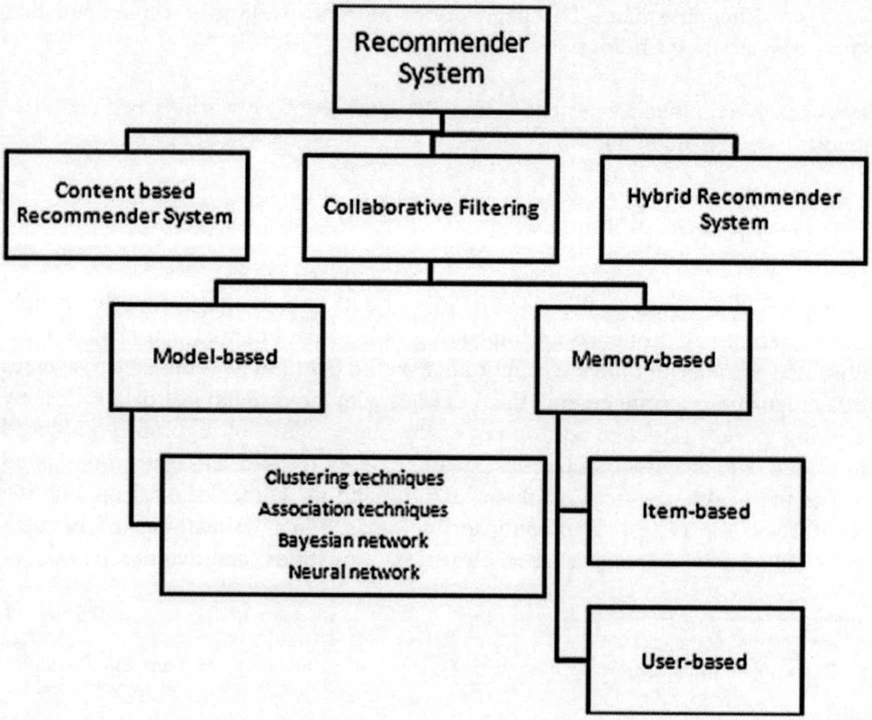

Fig. 2 Recommendation techniques [1]

According to Adomavicius and Tuzhilin 2005 recommender, schemes can be categorized into three main types.

1.1 Collaborative Filtering Recommender

CF recommender schemes create suggestions to its customers built on the likings of other consumers with comparable perceptions. It is an area self-governing expectation procedure for content that cannot simply and effectively be designated by metadata such as pictures and composition. This method works by the construction of a catalog (user-item matrix) of inclinations for things by customers. Collaborative filtering then contests customers with related importance and inclinations through scheming resemblances among their profiles to create references [2] (Fig. 3).

1.2 Content-Based Recommender System

Content-based recommender schemes create suggestions founded on resemblances of fresh articles to those that the customer be fond of in the previous by manipulating the imaginative features of objects. It is an area-reliant procedure and highlights further the examination of the characteristics of objects in direction to make guesses, where official forms such as network sheets, newspapers, and newsflash are to be suggested, a contented-created filtering system is best effective [3].

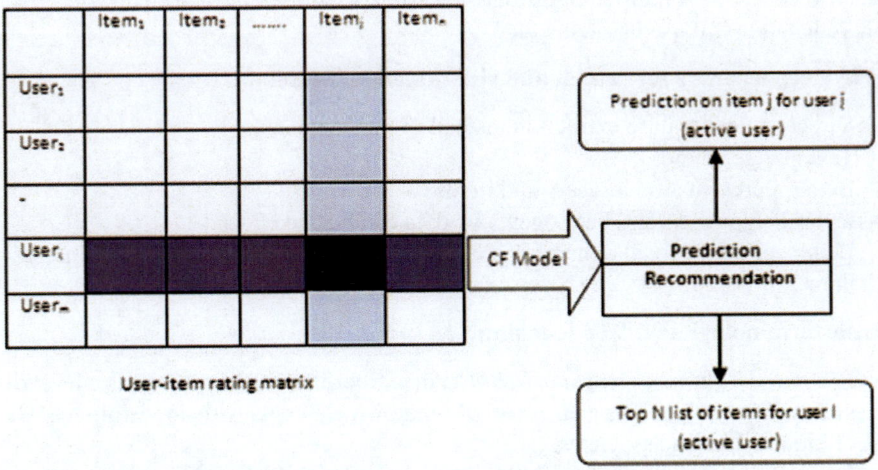

Fig. 3 Collaborative filtering

1.3 Hybrid Recommender System

Hybrid recommender schemes employ several methodologies together, and they overwhelmed the drawbacks of certain methods by manipulating the recompenses of the other. Hybrid filtering system pools dissimilar recommendation procedures in direction to advance improved classification optimization to evade certain limits and difficulties of clean reference schemes.

1.4 What is Deep Learning?

- It comes underclass of machine learning systems
- It uses the hierarchy of nonlinear processing layers and complex model structure
- Layers learn to represent different representation of facts
- Advanced stage features are constructed from minor stage abstract features
- Trendy name for "Neural Networks with deep layers".

Deep learning has become increasingly more famous all through subfields of software engineering, for example, natural language preparing, picture and video handling, PC visualization, and information withdrawal because there has not been such a typical way to deal with taking care of various types of figuring issues previously. With such part of profound learning systems, they are not just exceptionally equipped for helping complex issues in numerous fields; however, they additionally structure a mutual terminology and shared view for these exploration grounds. Deep learning strategies also assist these subfields to team up with one another, wherever this was somewhat questionable earlier because of the assorted variety and unpredictability of used systems [4, 5].

Why deep learning for search and recommender system?

- Direct content feature extraction instead of metadata
- Text, image, audio
- Better representation of users and items
- Hybrid algorithms and heterogeneous data can be used
- Better suited to model dynamic behavioral patterns and complex feature interactions.

Basic terminologies of deep learning

- *Restricted Boltzmann machine (RBM)*: An extraordinary BM containing a level of perceptible components and a level of unknown elements with no visible–visible or hidden–hidden associates.
- *Deep Boltzmann machine (DBM)*: An exceptional BM in which the unseen modules are structured in a deeply layered fashion, simply neighboring covers are joined, and the identical layer has no visible-visible or hidden-hidden contacts.

- *Deep neural network (DNN)*: It is a system with several unseen layers and loads that are completely coupled and pre-taught using fixed restricted Boltzmann machine (RBM) or deep Boltzmann machine DBM [2].

Deep Learning Techniques

Deep learning can in general deliberated as a subfield of artificial intelligence. The characteristic central principle of deep learning is to acquire profound exemplifications, i.e., knowledge of many stages of depictions as well as thoughts from statistics. In real-world explanations, any neural network design can be considered as deep knowledge as extended as it improves a defined independent purpose using a variety of stochastic grade backgrounds (SGB). Neural designs have established incredible achievement in equally controlled and unproven learning tasks. In this section, we explain various architectural prototypes [6].

- *Multilayer Perceptron (MLP)*

It is a type of feed-frontward neural system having many (more than one) hidden layers connecting the input and output layer. The perceptron can service random initiation tasks and does not certainly signify a firmly twofold classifier. MLP can be taken like weighted covers of nonlinear alterations, knowledge graded feature depictions. MLPs are also recognized to be general estimates. Both common sigmoidal activation function used for multiperceptron is described as:

$$x(y_i) = \tanh(y_i) \text{ and } x(y_i) = (1 + e^{-vi})^{-1}$$

- *Recurrent Neural Network (RNN)*

It is appropriate for demonstrating consecutive statistics. The contrasting feed-forward neural system, RNN to recollect previous calculations has rounds and recollections. Two variations long short-term memory (LSTM) and gated recurrent unit (GRU) systems are frequently installed now to overwhelm the threatened gradient difficulty. The recursive formula could be given as:

$$Z_t = R_w(Z_{t-1}, Y_t)$$

Here, Z_t is the state at time step t; Y_t is the input at time step t, and R_W is the recursive function.

- *Convolutional Neural Network (CNN)*

It is a distinctive kind of feedstuff frontward neural network including density layers and merging processes. CNN is clever to capture the comprehensive and native sorts and expressively improves the effectiveness and correctness. CNN achieves sound in handing out statistics with a grid-like structure. An asteris $k*$ symbol is commonly used to describe convolution in mathematics. If an input image is represented by $Y(x)$ and a filter is represented by h, the expression is:

$$X = Y * h$$

- *Neural Autoregressive Distribution Estimation (NADE)*

It is an unsubstantiated neural net constructed above autoregressive prototypical and feedstuff frontward neural systems. NADE is a controllable and well-organized estimator for demonstrating statistics delivery and bulks. Collaborative filtering replicates the division of ratings by the user. Suppose, if we have different ratings for different movies then, CF-NADE uses the chain rule given by:

$$S(x) = \pi_{j-1}^{F} S(x_{nbj} | x_{nb<j})$$

where F is the total number of items rated by the user; n_j is the jth rated item's index, and x_{nbj} is the user rating given to item n_{bj} [5, 7, 8].

2 Literature Work

See Table 1.

3 Accuracy Comparison of Various Classifiers Used in Existing Healthcare Recommender System

With massive amounts of unprocessed data and information overload, recommender systems are becoming increasingly common as a means of filtering large datasets and information. There is a need for a new HRS that will strengthen the healthcare system and deal with a patient that is plagued with diseases. Below is the Table 2 demonstrating the existing classifiers used in the healthcare recommendation system.

A brief explanation of the above table is as follows:

(i) As shown in the table, for the diet recommendation system, various classifiers of deep as well as machine learning are applied for the medical dataset, which was gathered from the Internet and hospitals, consists of 30 patients' data, 13 disease features, and 1000 items. Out of all the classifiers (MLP, RNN, GRU, LSTM, Naive Bayes, and logistic regression), LSTM provides the maximum accuracy of 96.5% [37].

(ii) As shown in the table, for cancer diagnosis, ANN and GLM show better accuracy as compare to SVM methodology, i.e., 95% and 96%, respectively, as both are deep learning techniques, and they produce better results when trained for a large amount of data as opposed to machine learning techniques [36].

Table 1 Findings of various recommendation systems

Author(s)	Year	Approach	Findings	Limitations/Future Scope
Joseph A. Konsta John Riedl	2012	Enhancing user experience by including algorithm in recommender system [4]	• Reported advances in collaborative filtering recommender systems, progression from research concentrating on the ironic set of queries concerning the consumer involvement with the recommender	• The amalgamation of collaborative, content-based, and contextual approaches into realistic recommender systems
Kulev, Igor Vlahu-Gjorgievska	2013	To use collaborative filtering in a physical activity recommendation scheme [9]	• Collaborative filtering to classify similar users and learn their physical activity habits to improve their health and make suggestions based on that information	• Accuracy can be improved further
Kim, J., Lee, D., and Chung, K. Y.	2014	In a collaborative filtering method, a context-aware collaborative model uses context knowledge to fill in the missing values [10]	• The hybrid recommender integrates content-based, utility-based, and demographic filtering to tailor health recommendation messages	• The most significant flaw in current collaborative filtering is the failure to address missing values for user preferences which can be improved further
Xun Zhoua, Jing Heb, Guangyan Huang, Yanchun Zhang	2015	Proposal of singular value decomposition-based incremental algorithm [11]	• Error analysis for demonstrating the efficiency of the performance of incremental Appro SVD algorithm	• Accuracy can be improved further

(continued)

Table 1 (continued)

Author(s)	Year	Approach	Findings	Limitations/Future Scope
Ashwin Belle, Raghuram Thiagarajan	2015	Three encouraging and impending capacities of medicinal investigation: image, genomics, and gesture-centered Big Data analytics in Healthcare [12]	• The enormous capacity of medicinal statistics directed can be developed by joining multimodal records from distinct foundations	• Areasof data aggregation, wrangling, and harmonizing discrete and continuous medical data formats need to be explored further • A novel approach for signal processing toward physiological signals needs to be developed
Lidong Wang and Cheryl Ann Alexander	2015	Conversion of innovative analyses for big data [13]	• Big data has unlimited prospective to develop medicine; monitor clinicians in supplying value-based carefulness	• Issues in data storage, retrieval, and visualization because of the large volume and variety of big data • Challenges in consolidating and processing segmented data, and analyzing unstructured data • Issues like information security and privacy need to be resolved
Carlos Luis Sánchez Bocanegra	2015	Used SNOMED-CT and Bio-ontology semantic skills to endorse healthiness Web sites [14]	• Mostly all Web sites recommending health videos were relevant provided through semantic skills	• For enhancing recommendation quality, experiments with health consumers need to be performed • Video dataset needs to be generalized

(continued)

Table 1 (continued)

Author(s)	Year	Approach	Findings	Limitations/Future Scope
Hors-Fraile, S., Benjumea, F. J. N., Hernández	2016	To help people quit smoking, two collaborative filtering-based recommendation systems have been developed [15]	• To customize health recommendation messages, the hybrid recommender incorporates content-based, utility-based, and demographic filtering	• Other weighting formulas for the hybrid algorithm, as well as the demographic similarity function—including the attributes—should be tested in the future study
Alejandro Baldominos Fernando De Rada, Yago Sae	2017	Apache Spark, an open-source collection workout structure [16]	• The proposed framework is intelligent to recover facts from devices that are set up in the healthcare center places and form appropriate info	• The system is not able to identify the healthcare personnel attending the patients • Limited information of planned tours and that is also limited to visit times and visited rooms
Mohamed Hussein Abdi	2017	A Study on Context-Aware Healthcare Recommender System points out that a socio-technical issue of privacy, security, and trust is emerging [17]	• The incorporation of contextual information is limited even though it is suggested as a key ingredient to improving the quality of the recommendations and the accuracy of the predictions	• Security and trust issues that are inherent in the traditional recommender systems need to be resolved
Hanna Schafer	2017	Personalization of recommender systems based on customers trust and evaluation approaches and actions (consumer fulfillment) in HRS [18]	• Helping users with customized, complex medical support, or interventions with precautionary healthcare measures	• Issues such as ethics, domain modeling, user interaction, and privacy need to be addressed

(continued)

Table 1 (continued)

Author(s)	Year	Approach	Findings	Limitations/Future Scope
J. Archenaa, Dr E. A. Mary Anita	2017	Big data for developing effective health recommendation engine [2, 19– 21]	• On multi-structured healthcare data on lifestyle, mental health factors, physical health factors, and their social network behaviors, the proposed solution used a Bayesian network	• To boost the accuracy of recommendations, further research into the collaborative filtering-social profile enhanced recommendation methodology will be considered
Weiwei Yuan, Chenliang Li Donghai Guan, Guangjie Han Asad Masood Khattak	2018	Deep learning-based socialized healthcare service recommendation [22]	• A new deep learning-driven socialized healthcare service recommender prototypical that proposes services based on suggestions from recommenders who have both confidence and mistrust relationships with active users	• Potential research will primarily concentrate on the development of new high-performance recommendation algorithms that take advantage of trust and distrust data
Gourav Bathla, Himanshu Aggarwal	2018	Recommendation approach centered on deep knowledge and outsized scale graph splitting [23]	• Deep knowledge and outsized scale graph splitting approaches provide better recommendation accuracy for large-scale social data	• Accuracy can be improved further
Jun Yi LIU	2018	A recommendation approach to extract customers and objects topographies centered on deep learning neural system [24]	• The proposed recommendation approach focuses on real-world situations for better accuracy, cost competence, and low resource depletion in real-world use	• Practical implementation of more real-world situations for accurate real-time prediction

(continued)

Table 1 (continued)

Author(s)	Year	Approach	Findings	Limitations/Future Scope
Hanafi, Nanna Suryana	2018	A recommendation approach centered on application field Arrangement using deep learning [25]	• Provides enhanced performance to capture appropriate consciousness concerning examination, feedback, theoretical, and product description	• More research is needed in recommender systems adopting deep learning
K. U. Kala, M. Nandhini	2018	Applicability of deep knowledge practices in recommender schemes [26]	• Deep learning practices are very effective in the area of recommendation schemes	• For improving scalability, a multi-view environment needs to be developed
Shadi Alian, Juan Li	2018	Personalized recommendation system for diabetic American Indians [27]	• Provides tailored guidelines for AI patients, such as dietary consumption and physical activity, based on their specific socioeconomic, educational, and environmental circumstances	• Evaluation with real-tribe user's needs to be done
Zeynep-Batmaz, Ali Yurekli	2018	An approach to examine the relation among deep knowledge classifications and purposive things of recommendation schemes [28]	• Efficiently categorizes the journals into the conforming recommender arrangement category	• Scalability and accuracy can be improved further
Riccardo Miotto, FeiWang, Shuang Wang, Xiaoqian Jiang, and Joel T. Dudley	2018	Examination, opportunities, and challenges in deep learning for health care[29]	• Deep learning approaches may be the key to turning large amounts of biomedical data into better human health	• Enrichment of features and how to interpret the implications of these models and how to make them more understandable to create trustworthy and effective systems

(continued)

Table 1 (continued)

Author(s)	Year	Approach	Findings	Limitations/Future Scope
Liao Liang Jiang	2018	A reliance constructed ecommerce recommendation scheme using collaborative filtering scheme [30]	• Deployment of slope one algorithm in various recommender systems based on the combination of user similarity and trusted data	• More research needs to be done to tackle the problem of cold-start
Oleg Rybakov, Vijai Mohan	2018	Formulating recommendation problems to predict the future behavior by encoding historical behavior using soft data split, combining predictor and autoencoder models [31]	• Learning the significance (time decay) of the purchases depending on the purchase date by introducing a convolutional layer and indicating that the shape of the time decay function can be approximated by a parametrical function	• Accuracy can be improved further
Georgia Koutrika	2018	Focus on multi-armed bandits, matrix factorization, and methods for amalgamation of recommendation [32]	• Matrix factorization provides good performance in terms of recommendation excellence and scalability	• Problems such as data exploration, query optimization, and data integration need to be worked upon
Ahmed Fadhil, Yunlong Wang	2018	To propose a supervised machine learning algorithm to classify users and help caregivers to personalize their intervention feedback[33]	• CoachMe, a prototype procedure, was present, to encourage a healthier lifestyle and activities while lowering the risk of chronic diseases	• The solution should be tested and validated with actual users in the future

(continued)

Table 1 (continued)

Author(s)	Year	Approach	Findings	Limitations/Future Scope
Sahoo, A. K., Pradhan, C., Barik, R. K., and Dubey, H.	2019	A collaborative filtering-based deep learning-based health recommender system [34]	• Proposed an intelligent HRS using a deep learning system based on CNN and RBM	• Develop an algorithm to provide better accuracy while preserving a high degree of privacy
Qiwei Han	2019	Temporal dynamics of patient–doctor relationships using consultation histories [35]	• The proposed model displays greater extrapolative accurateness than both a collaborative filtering method and a heuristic model	• Transforming service provision into a more person-centered primary care is still an issue of concern
Jenni A. M. Sidey Gibbons, Chris J. Sidey Gibbons	2019	Use of machine learning techniques for cancer detection [36]	• Other dynamic functions, such as natural language processing and image recognition, can easily be applied to the principles illustrated	• A drawback of this approach is that several of the nuances and complexities of ML analyses, such as high dimensionality or sparsity, are not properly represented in the results
Iwendi, C., Khan, S., Anajemba, J. H., Bashir, A. K., and Noor, F.	2020	Diet recommendation framework for patients using deep learning and machine learning model [37]	• LSTM provides maximum accuracy as opposed to other classifiers mentioned in the paper	• The patient–dietician justification for the recommender method is also a mystery to medical professionals
Farman Ali, Shaker El-Sappagh, S. M. Riazul Islam	2020	Based on feature fusion and ensemble deep learning, a smart healthcare monitoring system for heart disease prediction [38]	• This recent structure not only finds the finest selection of features, but in addition measures their unique importance in the datasets, enhancing prediction precision	• To achieve effective performance, a more advanced approach for eliminating irrelevant features and handling missing values and noise will be investigated

(continued)

Table 1 (continued)

Author(s)	Year	Approach	Findings	Limitations/Future Scope
Ponselvakumar, A. P., Anandamurugan, S., Logeswaran, K., Nivashini, S., Showentharya, S. K., and Jayashree, S. S.	2021	Deep learning methods advance precision medicine and recommendation system for clinical trials [39]	• The use of a recommendation framework in conjunction with deep learning and big data could lead to high-quality results in personalized medicine	• To achieve better outcomes, concentrate on demographic-based patient data collection, interpretation, and healthcare mechanisms

Table 2 Accuracy of various classifiers

Author	Year	Approach	Dataset	Classifier	Accuracy
Celestine Iwendi, Suleman Khan, Joseph Henry Anajemba	2020	Diet Recommendation framework for patients using deep learning and machine learning model [37]	Internet and hospitals	MLP RNN GRU LSTM Naive Bayes	92.91% 94.5% 95.29% 96.5% 92.81% 92.79%
Jenni A. M. Sidey Gibbons, Chris J. Sidey Gibbons	2019	Use of machine learning techniques by developing three predictive models for cancer diagnosis [36]	breast cancer Wisconsin Diagnostic dataset	ANN SVM GLM	95% 94% 96%
Varun Gulshan, Lily Peng, Marc Coram	2016	Automated detection of diabetic retinopathy [40]	EyePACS-1 and Messidor-2 dataset (retinal images)	DCNN	94% 96%
John A. Quinn Nakasi	2016	Histological and microscopical elements detection [41]	microscopic image	DCNN and shaped features like the moment and morphological	100% for Malaria; 99% for tuberculosis and hookworm
Korsuk	2016	Features extraction and detection of abnormalities [42]	ADNI dataset Alzheimer disease using the dataset of PET, MRI, combination of PET and MRI	DBM	92.38% 92.20% 95.35%
Sarraf	2016	Alzheimer's and Parkinson's diseases detection [43]	fMRI and MRI images	CNN	97.77% and 100% for fMRI and MRI subjects
Iidaka T	2015	Functional connectivity and classification of brain disorders [44]	fMRI data	Deep learning classifiers	90%

(iii) For automated diabetic retinopathy, DCNN gives an accuracy of 94% for the EyePACS-1 dataset which consists of 9963 images from 4997 patients, and 96% accuracy for the Messidor-2 dataset which contains 1748 images from 874 patients. DCNN, i.e., deep convolution neural network is used as a dataset consist of retinal images [40].

(iv) Similarly, DCNN produces 100% and 99% accuracy when used for malaria as well as tuberculosis detection, respectively. The dataset again consists of microscopic images DCNN is more appropriate. The task of detecting malaria had the highest accuracy—possibly because it had the largest training collection [41].

(v) DBM is used for the detection of abnormalities using three different datasets, i.e., PET, MRI, and a combination of both yielding accuracies of 92.38%, 92.20%, and 95.35%, respectively [42].

(vi) For Alzheimer's and Parkinson's disease detection, CNN is used giving an accuracy of 97.77% for fMRI and 100% for MRI subjects [43].

(vii) Lastly, when deep learning classifiers are used for the classification of brain disorders, it yields an accuracy of 90%. The multi-center research project provided imaging data from 328 subjects with typical growth and 312 subjects with ASD. In this study, only subjects under the age of 20 were included [44].

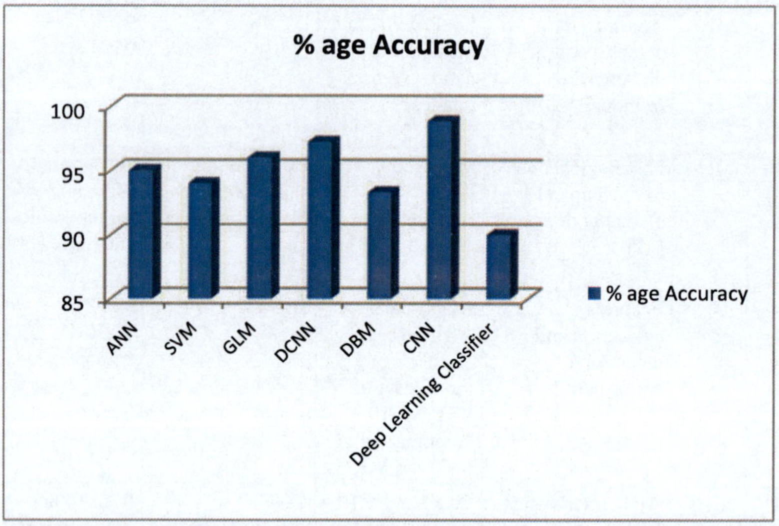

As shown in the graph, CNN and DCNN (kind of CNN but with more layers as compared to CNN) yield improved accuracy as compared to the rest of the classifiers, i.e., SVM, ANN, GLM, etc. Hence, it is concluded that as compared to machine learning techniques deep learning techniques provide better accuracy because the more the number of layers, the more is accuracy obtained.

4 Conclusion

Collaborative filtering is reflected as more superior to other tree approaches (contents centered, knowledge centered, and demographic filtering). A deep learning methodology for collaborative and content-centered methods will permit the traditional model to acquire dissimilar topographies of customers and things routinely to progress the accuracy of recommendations. Collaborative filtering recommendation procedure with deep learning technology provides good accuracy. This model uses a feature extraction scheme built on a quadric polynomial regression model, which gets the hidden topographies further precisely by the old-style matrix factorization procedure. Then, these hidden features are considered as the input of the deep neural system.

References

1. Adomavicius G, Tuzhilin A (2005) Toward the next generation of recommender systems: a survey of the state-of-the-art and possible extensions. IEEE Trans Knowl Data Eng 17(6):734–749
2. mySugr Bolus Calculator (2018) Available in diabetes healthcare. https://mysugr.com/mysugr-boluscalculator/
3. Vlahu-Gjorgievska E, Trajkovik V (2011) Personal healthcare system model using collaborative filtering techniques
4. Konstan JA, Riedl J (2012) Recommender systems: from algorithms to user experience. User Model User-Adap Inter 22(1):101–123
5. Sahu SP, Nautiyal A, Prasad M (2017) Machine learning algorithms for recommender system–a comparative analysis. Int J Comput Appl Technol Res 6(2):97–100
6. Betru BT, Onana CA, Batchakui B (2017) Deep learning methods on recommender system: a survey of the state-of-the-art. Int J Comput Appl 162(10):17–22
7. Zhang L, Luo T, Zhang F, Wu Y (2018) A recommendation model based on a deep neural network. IEEE Access 6:9454–9463
8. Wang D, Liang Y, Xu D, Feng X, Guan R (2018) A content-based recommender system for computer science publications. Knowl-Based Syst 157:1–9
9. Kulev I, Trajkovik V, Koceski S, Vlahu-Gjorgievska E (2013) Recommendation algorithms based on collaborative filleting and their application in health care. In: Proceedings of the 10th conferences on informatics and information technology (CIIT), pp 34–38
10. Kim J, Lee D, Chung KY (2014) Item recommendation based on a context-aware model for personalized u-healthcare service. Multimed Tools Appl 71(2):855–872
11. Zhou X, He J, Huang G, Zhang Y (2015) SVD-based incremental approaches for recommender systems. J Comput Syst Sci 81(4):717–733
12. Belle A, Thiagarajan R, Soroushmehr SM, Navidi F, Beard DA, Najarian K (2015) Big data analytics in healthcare. BioMed Res Int
13. Wang L, Alexander CA (2015) Big data in medical applications and health care. Am Med J 6(1):1
14. Bocanegra CLS, Ramos JLS, Rizo C, Civit A, Fernandez-Luque L (2017) HealthRecSys: a semantic content-based recommender system to complement health videos. BMC Med Inform Decis Mak 17(1):1–10
15. Hors-Fraile S, Benjumea FJN, Hernández LC, Ruiz FO, Fernandez-Luque L (2016) Design of two combined health recommender systems for tailoring messages in a smoking cessation app. arXiv:1608.07192
16. Baldominos A, De Rada F, Saez Y (2018) DataCare: big data analytics solution for intelligent healthcare management. Int J Interact Multimed Artif Intell 4(7)
17. Mohamed HA, George OO, Ronald WM (2017) A survey of context-aware healthcare recommender systems. Int J Sci Res (IJSR) 962–967
18. Schäfer H, Hors-Fraile S, Karumur RP, Calero Valdez A, Said A, Torkamaan H, Trattner C et al (2017) Towards health (aware) recommender systems. In: Proceedings of the 2017 international conference on digital health, pp 157–161

19. Archenaa J, Anita EM (2017) Health recommender system using big data analytics. J Manag Sci Bus Intell 2(2)
20. glaucoma (2018). https://www.glucomen.co.uk/rapidcalc/
21. Diabetes (2018) M-your diabetes management app-keep diabetes under control. https://www.diabetes-m.com/
22. Yuan W, Li C, Guan D, Han G, Khattak AM (2018) Socialized healthcare service recommendation using deep learning. Neural Comput Appl 30(7):2071–2082
23. Bathla G, Aggarwal H, Rani R (2018) Improving recommendation techniques by deep learning and large-scale graph partitioning. Int J Adv Comput Sci Appl 9:403–409
24. Liu JY (2018) A survey of deep learning approaches for recommendation systems. J Phys Conf Ser (IOP Publishing) 1087(6):062022
25. Suryana N, Basari ASBH (2018) Deep learning for recommender system based on application domain classification perspective: a review. J Theor Appl Inf Technol 96(14)
26. Kala KU, Nandhini M (2018) Applicability of deep learning techniques in recommender systems. IIOABJ 10(1):11–20
27. Alian S, Li J, Pandey V (2018) A personalized recommendation system to support diabetes self-management for American Indians. IEEE Access 6:73041–73051
28. Batmaz Z, Yurekli A, Bilge A, Kaleli C (2019) A review on deep learning for recommender systems: challenges and remedies. Artif Intell Rev 52(1):1–37
29. Miotto R, Wang F, Wang S, Jiang X, Dudley JT (2018) Deep learning for healthcare: review, opportunities, and challenges. Brief Bioinform 19(6):1236–1246
30. Jiang L, Cheng Y, Yang L, Li J, Yan H, Wang X (2019) A trust-based collaborative filtering algorithm for an E-commerce recommendation system. J Ambient Intell Humaniz Comput 10(8):3023–3034
31. Rybakov O, Mohan V, Misra A, LeGrand S, Joseph R, Chung K, Luo R et al (2018) The effectiveness of a two-layer neural network for recommendations
32. Koutrika G (2018) Recent advances in recommender systems: matrices, bandits, and blenders. In: EDBT, pp 517–519
33. Fadhil A (2018) Towards automatic and personalised mobile health interventions: an interactive machine learning perspective. arXiv:1803.01842
34. Sahoo AK, Pradhan C, Barik RK, Dubey H (2019) DeepReco: deep learning-based health recommender system using collaborative filtering. Computation 7(2):25
35. Han Q (2019) A hybrid recommender system for patient-doctor matchmaking in primary care
36. Sidey-Gibbons JA, Sidey-Gibbons CJ (2019) Machine learning in medicine: a practical introduction. BMC Med Res Methodol 19(1):1–18
37. Iwendi C, Khan S, Anajemba JH, Bashir AK, Noor F (2020) Realizing an efficient IoMT-assisted patient diet recommendation system through machine learning model. IEEE Access 8:28462–28474
38. Ali F, El-Sappagh S, Islam SR, Kwak D, Ali A, Imran M, Kwak KS (2020) A smart healthcare monitoring system for heart disease prediction based on ensemble deep learning and feature fusion. Inf Fusion 63:208–222
39. Ponselvakumar AP, Anandamurugan S, Logeswaran K, Nivashini S, Showentharya SK, Jayashree SS (2021) Advancement in precision medicine and recommendation system for clinical trials using deep learning methods. In: IOP conference series: materials science and engineering, vol 1055, No 1, IOP Publishing, p 012110
40. Gulshan V, Peng L, Coram M, Stumpe MC, Wu D, Narayanaswamy A, Webster DR et al (2016) Development and validation of a deep learning algorithm for detection of diabetic retinopathy in retinal fundus photographs. JAMA 316(22):2402–2410
41. Quinn JA, Nakasi R, Mugagga PK, Byanyima P, Lubega W, Andama A (2016) Deep convolutional neural networks for microscopy-based point of care diagnostics. In: Machine learning for healthcare conference. PMLR, pp 271–281
42. Sirinukunwattana K, Raza SEA, Tsang YW, Snead DR, Cree IA, Rajpoot NM (2016) Locality sensitive deep learning for detection and classification of nuclei in routine colon cancer histology images. IEEE Trans Med Imaging 35(5):1196–1206

43. Sarraf S, Tofighi G, Alzheimer's Disease Neuroimaging Initiative (2016) Deep AD: Alzheimer's disease classification via deep convolutional neural networks using MRI and fMRI. BioRxiv, 070441
44. Iidaka T (2015) Resting-state functional magnetic resonance imaging and neural network classified autism and control. Cortex 63:55–67

Assessment of De-noising Filters for Brain MRI T1-Weighted Contrast-Enhanced Images

Sarita, Rajeshwar Dass, and Jitender Saini

Abstract Noise in the medical images is always of great concern because it can lead to misinterpretation for advance process. With advancements in technology, the quality of image capturing through MRI improved, but noise is still present; therefore, noise present in the MRI images should be removed to get the good quality of images for accurate diseases detection and its diagnosing. In this work, five different filtering algorithms, named as non-local mean (NLM) filter, anisotropic filter, Weiner filter, bilateral filter, and Gaussian filter, used to eradicate the different types of noise named (salt and pepper, speckle, and Gaussian) through brain MRI images. PSNR, SSIM, and MSE are statistical parameters used for analyzing the performance of the filters. The study shows that for Gaussian noise, Weiner filter is considered the most efficient filter. For salt and pepper noise, Gaussian filter work better than other filters. In the case of speckle noise, anisotropic works better on low noise density, whereas for high noise density, Gaussian filter works better.

Keywords NLM · Anisotropic filter · Weiner filter · Bilateral filter · Noises · SSIM · PSNR · MSE

1 Introduction

In the medical field, image quality is vital for the detection of diseases. MRI provides a highly detailed image of human tissue and organs, and it also does not use radiations; therefore, it is a frequently used examination method to find brain diseases. Despite good MRI scanner technology, MRI quality is affected by the noise that occurs during acquisition. The noise in MRI image limits further analysis processes like feature

Sarita (✉)
ECED, D.C.R. University of Science and Technology, Murthal, Sonipat, Haryana, India

R. Dass
D.C.R. University of Science and Technology, Murthal, Sonipat, Haryana, India

J. Saini
Department of Neuroimaging & Intervention Radiology, NIMHANS, Bengaluru, India

N. Marriwala et al. (eds.), *Emergent Converging Technologies and Biomedical Systems*, Lecture Notes in Electrical Engineering 841,
https://doi.org/10.1007/978-981-16-8774-7_50

extraction, segmentation, and classification. To improve MRI images' quality, noise should be removed while retaining the image features before subsequent analysis [1]. MRI images are prone to salt and pepper, Gaussian, and speckle noise [2]. In brain MR images, Gaussian is the most common noise [3], also known as electronic noise, which arises in the MRI machine's detector and amplifier. Salt and pepper noise have black and white pixels, and it is also known as impulse noise [4]. Speckle noise occurs due to the environmental effect on the sensor of an image-capturing device.

This paper's primary purpose is to evaluate different filters' performance in removal of types of noise through brain MRI images. PSNR, MSE, and SSIM parameters are used for assessing the noise filtering quality of these filters.

Paper's organization is as follows: research background in first segment. In segment 2, we discussed the previous work done by the researchers. Segment 3 describes the material and method used in the work. Results are discussed in segment 4, and the outcome of the study is concluded in segment 5.

2 Literature Review

In past few years, many researchers worked on removing noise from the MRI images with preserving the optimum information. Chandrashekar et al. [5] explained the noise model and nonlinear de-noising algorithm such as anisotropic, bilateral, and nonlocal mean (NLM) filter. They found that NLM filter works better than the other two filters in terms of the high value of parameters like PSNR and SSIM, but the execution time of NLM is 200 s which is higher than the anisotropic and bilateral filter. Riji et al. [6] proposed an iterative bilateral algorithm for removing Gaussian noise from the MRI images and compared the results with the NLM, UNLM, and LMMSE de-noising algorithms in terms of statistical parameters such as mean SSIM and PSNR; results confirmed that the proposed filtering algorithm by them has better noise removing quality than the other filters. Nagarjan et al. [7] performed de-noising of the MR images having Gaussian noise with block division-based filtering algorithm. Compared the result with median, bilateral, anisotropic, NLM, IBLF and WBNLM, SANLM algorithm in term of PSNR, SSIM, RMSE and execution time. They found that prosed technique works better than all other algorithms with less execution time, i.e., 26.28 s for T1 weighted, 9.945 s for T2 weighted, and 9.366 s PD-weighted images, respectively. Anitha et al. [8] applied the median and Weiner filter for removing the noise and found that the median filter works better than Weiner filter. Zeng et al. [9] performed the de-noising of brain MR images by hybridizing the Weiner filter, wavelet soft threshold, and wavelet hard threshold and found that hybrid algorithm works better than each method alone. Saladi et al. [10] compared the performance of PCA, NLM, bilateral, and SANLM de-noising algorithm by statistical parameters and found that SANLM works better than other filters. Mundada et al. [11] investigated the noise parameter's effect on the image restoration of brain MRI images and found that change in standard deviation of noise results in change of noise distribution also. For a lower range of standard deviation, i.e., Gaussian distribution for noise range 1–4.27, and for standard deviation 4.51 or greater than this, noise is Rician noise. They found that for de-noising brain MRI images, the Gaussian filter works better for Gaussian noise distribution, whereas for Rician distribution, the hybrid filter works better. Isa et al. [12] evaluated three de-noising algorithms named median, adaptive, and average filter for Gaussian, speckle, and salt and pepper noise. Their work proves that the median filter works better for Gaussian and salt and pepper noises with PSNR value 38.3 dB, whereas the average filter do filtering better for speckle noise with PSNR of 56.2 dB. Rai et al. [13] proposed hybrid algorithm ICA-DWT for removing noise like Gaussian, speckle, and Salt and Pepper with noise variance of 0.1–0.9 and compared this with the traditional algorithms such as ICA, DWT, and UDWT. They found that proposed technique works better for high noise variance levels and preserves the structure of MRI.

3 Methodology

3.1 DataSet

For this work, brain MRI dataset of T1-weighted contrast-enhanced images (3064) are used, which were downloaded from [14]. This dataset contains 3064 MRI images from 233 patients, in axial, sagittal, and coronal view. We have taken 10 images for our work.

3.2 Filters

Non-local mean (NLM) filter performs the mean of all neighboring pixels and put weight to these by the similarity of pixels to the center pixel. Weights are used to determine the closeness of the pixel from the target pixels. Common weighting functions are Gaussian and discrete algorithms. NLM is a powerful method for noise removal, but it is limited by the high execution time [15].

Wiener filter is used to de-noising the image, whose quality is decreased by additive noise and blurring. For calculating assumption requires that the noise and signal both processes are of second order. Zero mean noise is considered [16].

Wiener filters generally apply in the frequency domain [17]. Take a corrupted image, $i(n, m)$, takes DFT to get $I(k, l)$. To estimate the original image spectrum, multiplication of $I(n, m)$ and Weiner filter $W(n, m)$ is taken:

The Wiener filter is as follows:

$$W(k,l) = \frac{H^*(k,l)P_s(k,l)}{|H(k,l)|^2 P_s(k,l) + P_n(k,l)} \tag{1}$$

Bilateral filter is an algorithm for removing noise while protecting the edges. In this, each pixel is replaced by average of the neighboring pixels, so the formulation is easy. It depends on the size and contrast of the feature to protect. Computational speed is high; therefore, it can be used at iterative speed for large size image [18].

Gaussian filter is a linear filter used to reduce noise and blurring from the image. It takes the weighted average of the neighboring pixels. It uses zero mean Gaussian distribution.

Anisotropic diffusion filter is also called Perona–Malik diffusion filter because Peeerona and Malik introduced it in 1987. It removes the noise from the image without distorting the image details like edges. The diffusion process of the filter is space invariant and linear of the original image.

4 Result and Discussion

Performances of the filters are measured using the statistical parameter PSNR, SSIM, and MSE.

Mean square error (MSE) is computed by doing an average of the square of the difference in the input image's intensity and the output image's intensity [19]:

$$MSE = \frac{1}{mn} \sum_{i=0}^{mn-1} \left(d(i) - \hat{d}(i) \right)^2 \tag{2}$$

Peak signal-to-noise ratio (PSNR), and is calculated by [20]:

$$PSNR = 10 \log 10 \left(\frac{255^2}{MSE} \right) \tag{3}$$

PSNR value must be greater or near 48 dB for better performance of the filter. SSIM stands for the structure similarity index, and it is calculated by as [21]:

$$SSIM = \frac{(2\mu_x \mu_y + C_1)(2\sigma_{xy} C_2)}{(\mu_x^2 \mu_y^2 C_1)(\sigma_x^2 \sigma_y^2 + C_2)} \tag{4}$$

Filter having SSIM value near to1 is considered as the most effective filter.

Qualitatively analysis of the different filters using the statistical parameters like MSE, PSNR, and SSIM is shown in Tables 1, 2 and 3, respectively.

Table 1 MSE of different filters

Noise variance	0.05	0.1	0.5	0.9
Gaussian noise				
NLM	1999.0894	3742.1724	11487.058	14643.792
Anisotropic diffusion	500.2552	1059.066	4176.353	5782.596
Weiner	**399.9964**	**790.1641**	**3214.55**	**4508.743**
Bilateral	527.1559	1103.33	4231.541	5868.273
Gaussian	609.7047	1067.795	3611.562	4910.483
Salt and pepper noise				
NLM	1389.8414	2753.3822	13740.169	24635.022
Anisotropic diffusion	249.9103	522.4391	4522.417	11365.16
Weiner	146.6004	286.7802	3177.689	9312.235
Bilateral	242.037	550.3864	4530.614	11483.2
Gaussian	**97.3878**	**219.3397**	**3079.496**	**3104.496**
Speckle noise				
NLM	114.4543	281.9931	1403.0609	2007.9464
Anisotropic diffusion	**18.7696**	34.1259	205.7021	319.7328
Weiner	18.9268	36.3139	159.5432	232.757
Bilateral	21.854	46.5252	236.3332	346.2618
Gaussian	26.2175	**32.9796**	**82.2954**	**117.219**

Table 2 PSNR of different filters

Noise variance	0.05	0.1	0.5	0.9
Gaussian noise				
NLM	15.1225	12.3996	7.5287	6.4743
Anisotropic diffusion	21.1389	17.8816	11.9228	10.5096
Weiner	**22.1102**	**19.1536**	**13.0596**	**11.5902**
Bilateral	20.9114	17.7037	11.8658	10.4457
Gaussian	20.2796	17.8459	12.5497	11.2196
Salt and pepper noise				
NLM	16.7012	13.7321	6.7509	4.2153
Anisotropic diffusion	24.153	20.9504	11.5771	7.575
Weiner	26.4695	23.5553	13.1097	8.4403
Bilateral	24.292	20.7241	11.5692	7.5302
Gaussian	**28.2458**	**24.7196**	**13.246**	**13.2103**

(continued)

Table 2 (continued)

Noise variance	0.05	0.1	0.5	0.9
Speckle noise				
NLM	27.5445	23.6284	16.66	15.1033
Anisotropic diffusion	**35.3963**	32.8	24.9984	23.0829
Weiner	35.36	32.5301	26.102	24.6474
Bilateral	34.7355	31.4539	24.3956	22.7368
Gaussian	33.9449	**32.9484**	**28.977**	**27.4408**

Table 3 SSIM of different filter

Noise variance	0.05	0.1	0.5	0.9
Gaussian noise				
NLM	0.0628	0.0377	0.0119	0.0087
Anisotropic diffusion	0.2663	0.1885	0.0828	0.0593
Weiner	0.333	0.2655	0.1486	0.1171
Bilateral	0.2478	0.1769	0.0795	0.0581
Gaussian	**0.3402**	**0.2812**	**0.1595**	**0.1267**
Salt and pepper noise				
NLM	0.285	0.1225	0.0132	0.0028
Anisotropic diffusion	0.3638	0.2508	0.078	0.0182
Weiner	0.4692	0.3701	0.163	0.0556
Bilateral	0.3797	0.2565	0.0803	0.0169
Gaussian	**0.5352**	**0.402**	**0.1683**	**0.1611**
Speckle noise				
NLM	0.8513	0.7734	0.6656	0.646
Anisotropic diffusion	**0.966**	0.9423	0.82	0.7853
Weiner	0.1025	0.0857	0.0509	0.0448
Bilateral	0.9505	0.9157	0.8058	0.7752
Gaussian	0.9619	**0.9501**	**0.8912**	**0.8626**

5 Conclusion

In this paper, the performance of de-noising filters evaluated for three different types of noise on brain MRI images. Performance is evaluated on the basis of statistical parameters such as PSNR, MSE, and SSIM. From results, it is observed that for Gaussian noise, Weiner filter works more prominent than other filters. In case of salt and pepper noise, Gaussian filter works better. For speckle noise, anisotropic diffusion filter works better on low noise density with MSE 18.7696 at 5% noise density, whereas for high noise density, Gaussian filter works better with MSE value 117.219 at 90% noise density.

References

1. Lakshmi Devasena C, Hemalatha M (2011) Noise removal in magnetic resonance images using hybrid KSL filtering technique. Int J Comput Appl 27(8):1–4. https://doi.org/10.5120/3324-4571
2. Sivasundari MKS, Siva Kumar R (2014) Performance analysis of image filtering algorithms for MRI images. Int J Res Eng Technol 03(05):438–440. https://doi.org/10.15623/ijret.2014.0305080
3. Gudbjartsson H, Patz S (1996) The Rician distribution of noisy MRI data. Magn Reson Med 36(2):332; 34:910 (1995)
4. Gonzalez RC, Woods RE (2007) Digital image processing, 3rd ed. Prentice Hall
5. Chandrashekar L (2017) Assessment of non-linear filters for MRI images, 2
6. Jeny RR, Jan R, Madhu S (2015) Iterative bilateral filter for Rician noise reduction in MR images. Signal Image Video Process 1543–1548. https://doi.org/10.1007/s11760-013-0611-6
7. Priya INGGL (2019) Removal of noise in MRI images using a block difference-based filtering approach. June:1–13. https://doi.org/10.1002/ima.22361
8. Anitha S, Kola L, Sushma P, Archana S (2018) Analysis of filtering and novel technique for noise removal in MRI and CT images. In: International conference on electrical, electronics, communication computer technologies and optimization techniques, ICEECCOT 2017, vol 2018-Janua, pp 825–827. https://doi.org/10.1109/ICEECCOT.2017.8284618
9. Zeng Y et al (2020) Magnetic resonance image denoising algorithm based on cartoon, texture, and residual parts. Comput Math Methods Med 2020. https://doi.org/10.1155/2020/1405647
10. Saladi S, Amutha Prabha N (2017) Analysis of de-noising filters on MRI brain images. Int J Imaging Syst Technol 27(3):201–208. https://doi.org/10.1002/ima.22225
11. Mundada K (2019) Investigation of effect of noise parameter on brain MR image restoration. In: 2019 IEEE 5th international conference on convergence technology, pp 1–5
12. Isa IS, Sulaiman SN, Mustapha M, Darus S (2015) Evaluating de-noising performances of fundamental filters for T2-weighted MRI images. Proc Comput Sci 60(1):760–768. https://doi.org/10.1016/j.procs.2015.08.231
13. Rai HM, Chatterjee K (2019) Hybrid adaptive algorithm based on wavelet transform and independent component analysis for de-noising of MRI images. Meas J Int Meas Confed 144:72–82. https://doi.org/10.1016/j.measurement.2019.05.028
14. https://figshare.com/articles/dataset/brain_tumor_dataset/1512427. Accessed 12 April 2021
15. Buades A, Coll B, Morel J (2005) A non-local algorithm for image de-noising. In: 2005 IEEE computer society conference on computer vision and pattern recognition (CVPR'05), San Diego, CA, USA, vol 2, pp 60–65. https://doi.org/10.1109/CVPR.2005.38
16. Dass R, Devi S (2012) Effect of wiener - H elstrom filtering cascaded with bacterial foraging optimization to despeckle the images ultrasound images. 9(4):372–380
17. Dass R (2018) Speckle noise reduction of ultrasound images using BFO cascaded with wiener filter and discrete wavelet transform in homomorphic region. Procedia Comput Sci 132:1543–1551. https://doi.org/10.1016/j.procs.2018.05.118
18. Kumar N, Nachamai M (2017) Noise removal and filtering techniques used in medical images. Orient J Comput Sci Technol 10(1):103–113. https://doi.org/10.13005/ojcst/10.01.14
19. Rajeesh T, Moni J, Palanikumar RS, Gopalakrishnan S (2010) Noise reduction in magnetic resonance images using wave atom shrinkage. Int J Image Process 4(2):131–141
20. Shreyamsha Kumar BK (2013) Image denoising based on non-local means filter and its method noise thresholding. Signal Image Video Process 7(6):1211–1227. https://doi.org/10.1007/s11760-012-0389-y
21. Ai D, Yang J, Fan J, Cong W, Wang X (2015) Denoising filters evaluation for magnetic resonance images. Optik (Stuttg) 126(23):3844–3850. https://doi.org/10.1016/j.ijleo.2015.07.155

Consensus-Based Distributed Control in Microgrid Under Switching Topology

Rinku Kumar, Pankaj Mukhija, and Manish Kumar Saini

Abstract Microgrids are an emerging source for emergency as well as remote load centers power supply. It provides power security with generation from the locally available resources. The most probably the resources used for power generation are renewable sources. Where at certain time of a day power production of renewable dependent source may reduce to zero. A centralized controller may handle such problems. However, distributed control under plug and play of DG units is very difficult task in renewable dependent microgrid. In this paper, a consensus-based distributed secondary controller adaptive to switching communication topology is designed for enhanced performance and reliable power supply. The load requirements along with the local load are met satisfactorily by the distributed control strategy devised in this paper. The simulation results show the efficacy of the proposed control strategy to achieve global voltage regulation and proportional load sharing when there is frequent change in the number of DGs operating in a microgrid.

Keywords Microgrid · Renewable integration · Switching topology · Consensus · Distributed control

1 Introduction

Microgrids are new and fast developing entity in power supply sector for delivering power to the locality where typically it is very difficult to supply power from the utility grid or for the critical loads. The microgrids are good supplement to the power grid for mitigating the power quality issues arising from switching of heavy loads and faults in the supply system, etc. For ancillary service supports, power generation industries have developed their own microgrids at different locations. Due to

R. Kumar · M. K. Saini (✉)
Deenbandhu Chhotu Ram University of Science and Technology, Sonipat, Haryana, India
e-mail: manishkumar.ee@dcrustm.org

P. Mukhija
National Institute of Technology, Delhi, India

N. Marriwala et al. (eds.), *Emergent Converging Technologies and Biomedical Systems*, Lecture Notes in Electrical Engineering 841,
https://doi.org/10.1007/978-981-16-8774-7_51

capability of microgrids to operate in grid connected as well as islanded mode, microgrids are the first choice for critical loads. Moreover, technical advancements, green energy production, depleting fossil fuels, environmental pollution, reliable power supply, etc., are the major factors for development and installation of renewable-based distributed power generation units [1]. Microgrid gives added features like improved reliability, better power quality, fault resiliency, ancillary services and support to meet the increasing power demands to utility grid in grid connected mode [2].

For satisfactory operation of microgrid, hierarchical control scheme is adopted. The hierarchical control structure has three different layers (primary, secondary and tertiary control) of implementation to track the references [2–4] required for the controller to achieve the desired output from the distributed generating units (DGs) connected to microgrid. Microgrid central control (MGCC), is the conventional scheme to control the microgrid [5–7] in which, all data for various DGs is collected to a common point to generate the control action for every DG's controller corresponding to the required set points [8, 9]. As the system size increases, the MGCC becomes sluggish due to increase in data dimensions. In addition to that, requirement of huge communication network, high bandwidth, system global knowledge, privacy concerns and presence of single point of failure, etc., are the major problems with centralized control of microgrid. To overcome these problems, the researchers have developed number of distributed control schemes [10–12]. The distributed control schemes are almost fully resilient to system faults and instability caused from overloads, system expansions, etc., [9, 13–15]. In distributed control, each DG is capable to take action without affecting the nearby units. The control hierarchy is implemented in distributed fashion. This paper aims to design a consensus-based distributed control scheme in which multiple agents agreed upon a certain quantity of interest to reach the desired objective. The stability analysis is of consensus scheme depends upon the communication tree among the agents, which describes the adjacency of all agents with respect to each other.

The designed controller is able to regulate the DC bus voltage and achieves proportional loading of the participating DGs in microgrid. The consensus-based cooperative control is a two-level control algorithm [13]. The top or secondary level replaces the MGCC by collecting information from the neighboring units only. The primary controller is augmented with two correction terms arising from voltage agreement and proportional load sharing between the generating units. To address flexibility of plug and play of DERs allowing space for some units to come in and go out in microgrid there is not much literature available [14, 16, 17]. Also, there is always variation in communication topology after addition and removal of DERs from microgrid which complicates the monitor and control of microgrid due to its random nature. When renewable-based DER such as PV unit is operating then either due to change in weather or change in solar irradiations the output power is not fixed. Such units cannot be considered as connected or disconnected at these instants of time until it is not generating any power. No major studies have been done to focus this point of renewable-based generation in proportional loading of DGs. The objective of this paper is to design a consensus-based distributed controller adaptive to plug and play of DERs and capable to handle the power demand of renewable-based DER microgrid. Rest of the paper is organized as follows: The communication graph adjacency and Laplacian matrix design are discussed in Sect. 2. Consensus protocol adopted and implementation scheme is given in Sect. 3. Section 4 contains the simulation and results of the proposed control strategy. Finally, the conclusion and future possibilities are discussed in Sect. 5.

2 Communication Graph Preliminaries

The communication graph indicates the flow of information (i.e., states of DERs) between the agents. Communication graph also known as weighted diagraph when certain weight is assigned to edges. Let $G = (V, E, A)$, is weighted diagraph with nodes $V = (V_i \in N)$, $N = (1, 2, 3, \ldots, n)$, the set of edges, $E \subseteq V \times V$, $A = [a_{ij}]$ is the adjacency matrix. Each entry of adjacency matrix indicates the connection between DERs, if ith DER is connected to jth DER then $[a_{ij} = 1]$ otherwise 0, also $[a_{ii}] = 0$. The elements of the graph Laplacian matrix $L = [l_{ij}]$, $l_{ij} = \sum_{k=1}^{n} a_{ik}$ for $i = j$ and $l_{ij} = -a_{ij}$ for $i \neq j$. For detailed study on graphs and related terminology readers can refer [18, 19].

3 Consensus in Microgrid Under Switching Topology

The renewable based DGs such as wind, tidal or PV generator do not generate constant power for a full day. Also, some active consumers do not have enough power to feed the microgrid every time. Such incidents cause change in number of DGs sharing the load at common bus. Centralized/non centralized control microgrid control strategies evaluate reference values for individual DG, on the basis of total available power and load demand by collecting state information. This requires a communication link between the control center and DG controller. In distributed control schemes a spars communication network is enough to achieve the desired objective. The DGs connected via communication channel and capable to share information among them are known as neighbors of each other. The addition and removal of DGs indirectly emphasize that the microgrid should operate generously to facilitate the plug and play feature and allowing space for some units to come in and go out.

The poor communication among the DGs can also cause certain DGs to disappears/appears from/in the network. The distributed control scheme based on consensus theory is incorporated with switching communication topology is designed in this paper. When a new unit is to be connected to the existing structure, it only needs global parameters for synchronization. In AC microgrid frequency, phase and voltage are needed for synchronization while in case of DC microgrid the bus voltage is global parameter for synchronization [20]. Then depending on the available surplus power, the controller takes action and accordingly the converter's output is controlled.

The consensus protocol makes an agreement on certain quantity of interest among the interconnected agents by sharing the state information of neighboring units only. In mathematical form, the consensus protocol is given by Eq. (1), as follows:

$$\dot{\hat{x}}_i(t) = \dot{x}_i(t) + \sum_{j \in Ni} a_{ij}\left(\hat{x}_j(t) - \hat{x}_i(t)\right) \tag{1}$$

where $\hat{x}_i$ is aggregated state (voltage or current in case of microgrid control objectives) of ith DER. N_i—is the neighbors of the ith DER in fixed communication topology. If communication topology is varying, the neighbors of DGs becomes a variable quantity and (1) is modified as:

$$\dot{\hat{x}}_i(t) = \dot{x}_i(t) + \sum_{j \in Ni(t)} a_{ij}\left(\hat{x}_j(t) - \hat{x}_i(t)\right) \tag{2}$$

where $N_i(t)$—is the neighbors of the ith DER at time "t".

The convergence of above protocol relies on the formation of spanning tree between all agents and the graph must be balanced [21]. In balanced graphs, the sum of incoming and outgoing channels is equal. A communication tree is said to be spanning tree if each node is accessible from any node in the direction of information flow without encountering any node twice. A bidirectional graph is always balanced [10] as sum of incoming and outgoing channels is always equal so, the communication channels which can carry information in both directions are considered in this investigation. To investigate the switching topology operation, a set with finite collection of all possible spanning tree topology is designed in advance [21, 22]. Further, before adding a new unit to the microgrid, the output voltage of new DG is synchronized with DC bus voltage. The newly added unit after integration to microgrid will share the load proportional to its own power rating. The rated capacity of individual DG itself is taken as the base unit to determine the percentage loading of respective DG. The communicated states of DG's are processed by the controller of individual DG, for reference update for the droop controller to take action for proportional load sharing.

Droop controller takes action for the change in the load demand, low gain of droop controller causes the DG to aggressively change its output while high gain makes it sluggish. The droop gain of adaptive virtual droop controller is calculated as per the capability of the DG without adversely affecting its performance [16]. The droop gain is calculated as:

$$r_d = \Delta V_{\max}/I_{\max} \tag{3}$$

where $\Delta V_{\max}$ is maximum allowable change in voltage and $I_{\max}$ is maximum current rating. To incorporate intermittent generation, the droop gain of the adaptive droop controller is given by:

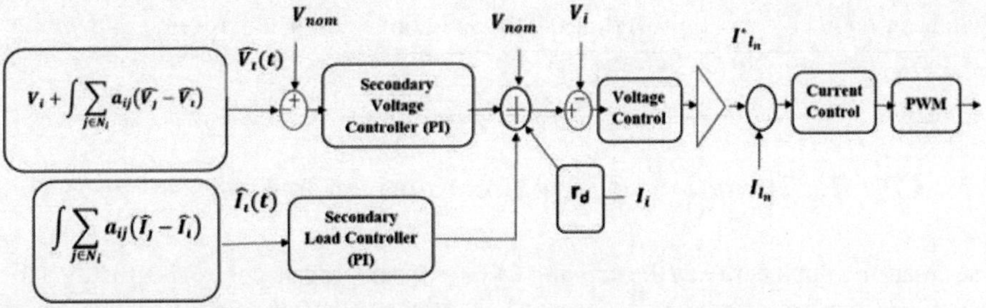

Fig. 1 Proposed consensus-based distributed control scheme of *i*th DG

$$r_{d\max} = \Delta V_{\max}/I_{\max} \tag{4}$$

where $r_{d\max}$ is the droop resistance used when DG is operating at its maximum rated capacity.

The reference current is fed to the inner current controller extracted from "*G*" block as shown in Fig. 1, and given to a PI controller to adjust the output. Figure 1 shows the complete distributed control strategy of distributed consensus-based secondary controller.

4 Results and Discussion

The test bed microgrid is simulated in MATLAB. The DC bus voltage is taken as 380 V. Four DG sources of capacity DG1 = DG2 = DG3 = DG4 = 7.6 kW with respective local loads L1 = L2 = L3 = L4 = 2.4 kW are connected to DC bus as shown in Fig. 2. Load connected to DC bus is 12 kW and a switching load of 2.4 kW,

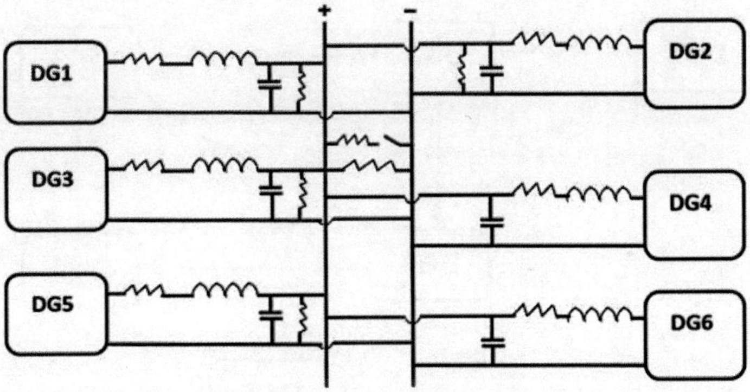

Fig. 2 Electrical connection of all DERs with microgrid bus

switching on at 3 s and removed at 6 s is also connected to microgrid. The whole strategy is divided into four cases.

4.1 Case 1: Formation of New Communication Link

The creation of link between the existing DG's in the microgrid control is investigated to analyze the performance of proposed distributed control scheme in this case. Keeping the configuration same explained above the communication topology is varied. In this case, at t = 4 s, a link between the DG3 and DG4 were established as indicated by blue dotted line in Fig. 3. This new link has no effect on the output of any DG as both units were already the part of the communication tree. Yet, this may cause high convergence rate to achieve consensus. The change visible at t = 3 s, is because connection of 2.4 kW switching load connected to the microgrid bus (Fig. 4). No visible traces can be seen for this change in communication graph, see Fig. 5 as system has already reached consensus.

4.2 Case 2: Addition/ Plug and Play of DG's

Two new DG units named as DG5 and DG6 are added to the microgrid as shown in Fig. 2. The communication topology for newly connected DGs is shown in Fig. 3. Before synchronization, the DG output voltage is brought up to the DC bus voltage. These DG units are connected to DC bus at t = 2 and t = 3, respectively, the output voltage of new plugged DGs is highlighted in black and sky blue colors in Fig. 6. The new units share load corresponding to their rated capacity and voltage drops slightly from no load to loaded condition. Figure 7 shows the current supplied by the each

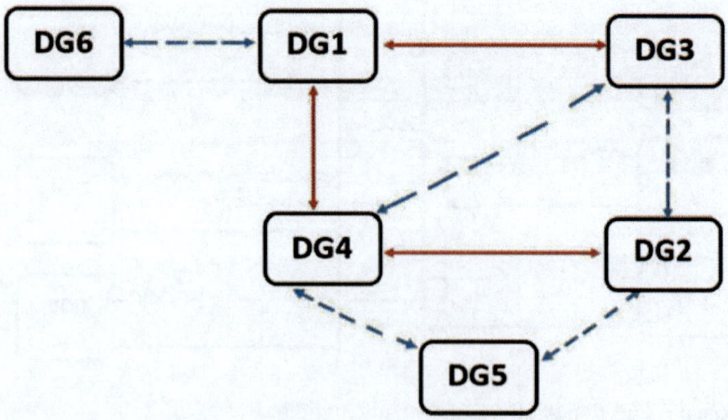

Fig. 3 Communication topology between the microgrid DGs

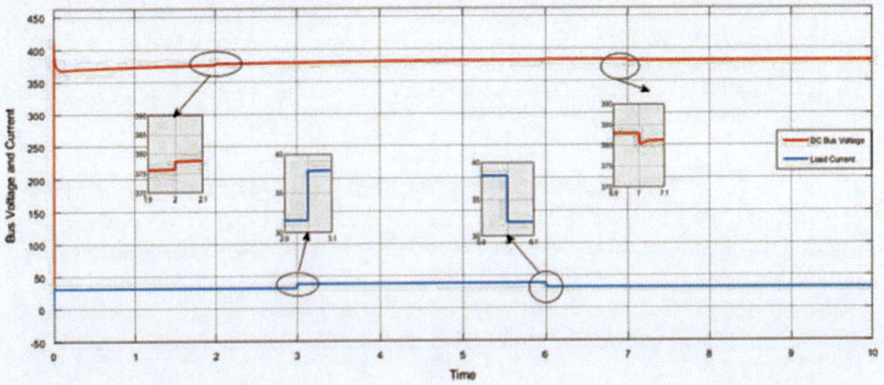

Fig. 4 DC bus voltage and current

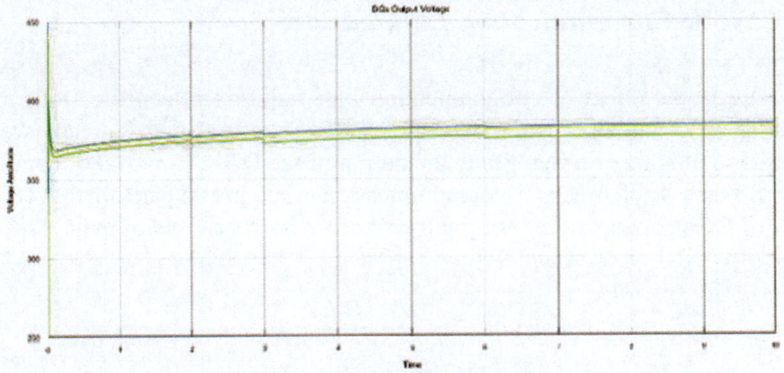

Fig. 5 DERs voltages without plug in of 5th and 6th DGs

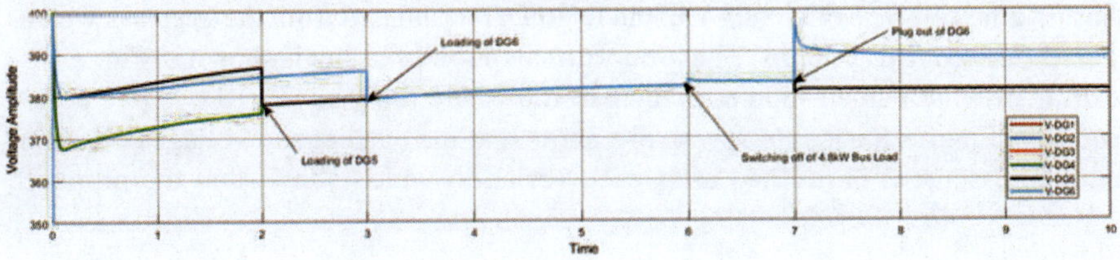

Fig. 6 DERs voltages with additional DG unit

DG to the microgrid common load. The amount of load shared by new DGs reduces the current loading of all other DG's correspondingly.

No local is connected to the new units, emulating units like fuel cell, electric vehicle or battery storage power supply. The rating of new unit is taken same as that of other DGs.

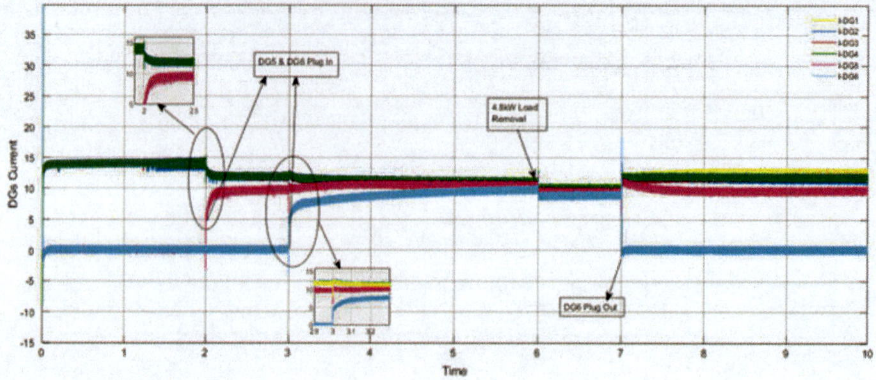

Fig. 7 DERs load sharing

4.3 Case 3: Communication Link Failure

To investigate the effect of communication link failure between the DG's a link connecting DG3 and DG2 is removed at t = 8 s. But, as all units already were in consensus so, it makes no changes in the output of the DG's. Removal of communication link such that it breaks the communication graph in two parts, in that case the two set of DGs corresponding to graph will reach to consensus in their respective set.

4.4 Case 4: Removal of a DG from the Microgrid

To investigate the performance of the designed controller for proportional load sharing after removal of certain DG the DG6 DG is isolated from the graph as well as form the microgrid at t = 7 s. The proportional of load sharing is shown in Fig. 7. The loading of all remained sources is increased to share the load shared by DG6 before isolation. Figures 8 and 9, respectively, show that the current and voltage consensus among all sources is reached after each variation which shows that the proposed

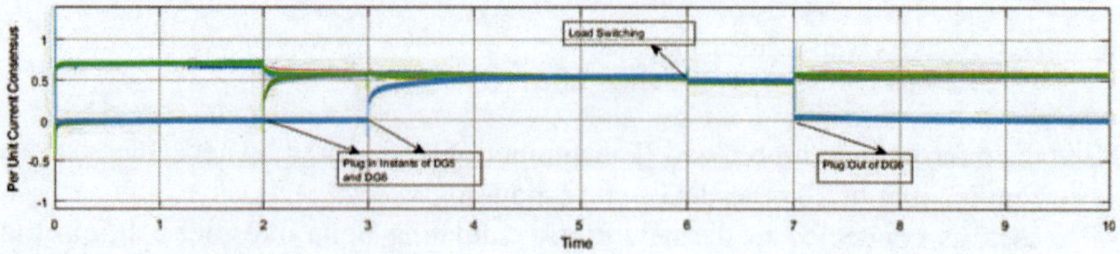

Fig. 8 DERs current consensus after each disturbance

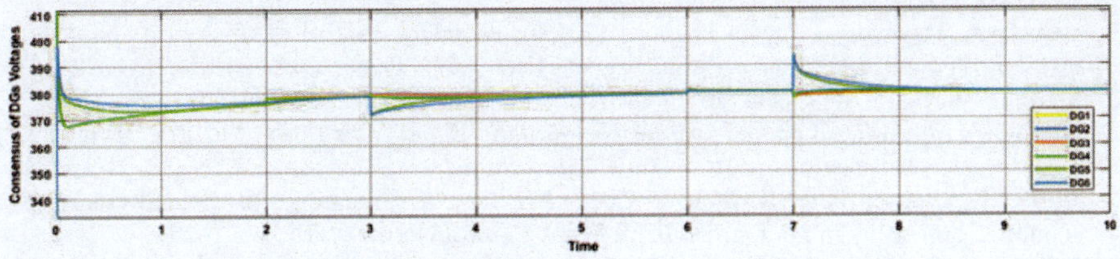

Fig. 9 DERs voltage consensus after each disturbance

controller is working effectively under variable communication topology and plug and play of DG's. The DC bus voltage is regulated within acceptable tolerance shown in Fig. 4.

5 Conclusion

The proposed consensus-based distributed secondary controller is effective to restore the microgrid voltage within acceptable deviations under switching topology of sources. The proportional load sharing between sources respective to their rating is successfully achieved even when certain DG unit either fails to communicate with neighbors or removed from the microgrid without affecting the performance of the other DGs of the microgrid. The proposed strategy can be extended for discontinuous data communication to reduce the communication cost. To have fast response characteristics, finite time consensus solutions can be adopted.

References

1. Green M (2016) Community power. Nat Energy 1:16014
2. Gumerman E, Bharvirkar, La Commare R, LaCommare KH, Marnay C (2003) Evaluation framework and tools for distributed energy resources. Lawrence Berkeley Natl Lab 1(1):1–59
3. Ahmadi S, Shokoohi S, Bevrani H (2015) A fuzzy logic-based droop control for simultaneous voltage and frequency regulation in an AC microgrid. Int J Electr Power Energy Syst 64(1):148–155
4. Unamuno E, Barrena JA (2015) Hybrid AC/DC microgrids - Part I: review and classification of topologies. Renew Sustain Energy Revolut 52(1):1251–1259
5. Xiao J, Weng P, Setyawan L et al (2015) Hierarchical control of hybrid energy storage system in DC microgrids. IEEE Trans Ind Electron 62(8):4915–4924
6. Micallef A, Apap M, Spiteri-Staines C, Guerrero JM, Vasquez JC (2014) Reactive power sharing and voltage harmonic distortion compensation of droop controlled single phase islanded microgrids. IEEE Trans Smart Grid 5(3):1149–1158
7. Palizban O, Kauhaniemi K (2015) Hierarchical control structure in microgrids with distributed generation: island and grid-connected mode. Renew Sustain Energy Rev 1(44):797–813
8. Guo F, Wen C (2014) Distributed control subject to constraints on control inputs: a case study on secondary control of droop-controlled inverter-based microgrids. In: Conference 2014, industrial electronics and applications, vol 1. IEEE Hangzhou, China, pp 1119–1124

9. Bidram A, Davoudi A, Lewis FL et al (2013) Secondary control of microgrids based on distributed cooperative control of multi-agent systems. IET Gener Trans Distrib 7(8):822–831
10. Meng L, Zhao X, Tang F et al (2016) Distributed voltage unbalance compensation in islanded microgrids by using a dynamic consensus algorithm. IEEE Trans Power Electron 31(1):827–838
11. Dorfler F, Simpson-Porco J, Bullo F (2016) Breaking the hierarchy: distributed control & economic optimality in microgrids. IEEE Trans Control Netw Syst 3(3):241–253
12. Pullaguram D, Mishra S, Senroy N (2018) Event-triggered communication based distributed control scheme for DC microgrid. IEEE Trans Power Syst 33(5):5583–5593
13. Xin H, Qu Z, Seuss J et al (2011) A self-organizing strategy for power flow control of photovoltaic generators in a distribution network. IEEE Trans Power Syst 26(3):1462–1473
14. Katiraei F, Iravani MR (2006) Power management strategies for a microgrid with multiple distributed generation units. IEEE Trans Power Syst 21(4):1821–1831
15. Simpson-Porco JW, Dorfler F, Bullo F (2013) Sychronization and power sharing for droop-controlled inverters in islanded microgrids. Automatica 49(9):2603–2611
16. Meng L, Shafiee Q et al (2017) Review on control of DC microgrids and multiple microgrid clusters. IEEE J Emerg Select Top Power Electron 5(3):928–948
17. Shafiee Q, Guerrero JM, Vasquez JC (2014) Distributed secondary control for islanded microgrids—a novel approach. IEEE Trans Power Electron 29(2):1018–1031
18. Godsil C, Royle G (2001) Algebraic graph theory, 1st edn. Springer-Verlag, New York
19. Diestel R (2000) Graph theory, 1st edn. Springer-Verlag, New York
20. Stefano R, Fabio S, Giancarlo FT (2015) Plug-and-play voltage and frequency control of islanded microgrids with meshed topology. IEEE Trans Smart Grid 6(3):1176–1184
21. Olfati-Saber R, Murray RM (2004) Consensus problems in networks of agents with switching topology and time-delays. IEEE Trans Autom Control 49(9):1520–1533
22. Ren W, Beard RW (2005) Consensus seeking in multi-agent systems under dynamically changing interaction topologies. IEEE Trans Autom Control 50(5):655–661

Ice Berg Detection in SAR Images Using Mask R-CNN

M. S. Sivapriya and P. Mohamed Fathimal

Abstract Ice berg is large piece of water which could be in different size and in different length. These ice bergs is formed on land and starts to float on water bodies like river lake and ocean. These ice bergs are the main threat for fatal ship sinking. So many tools and techniques have been developed for ice berg detection. Recent trends in image capturing and image processing can be used to locate ice berg in ocean. Synthetic Aperture Radar image is one of the imaging which can be used to detect iceberg. Nowadays CNN is largely used for image classification. Mask-R-CNN is a type of CNN and also hot deep learning algorithm in recent days for image classification, object detection, object localization due to its high accuracy level. In this proposed system, Mask Region based CNN architecture is going to be used for ice berg detection in Synthetics Aperture Radar image.

Keywords Synthetic aperture radar · CNN · Mask region-based CNN

1 Introduction

Ice berg is a kind of mass that floats on water bodies such as sea or ocean which could be broken off from glacier and looks like ice mountain. It dynamically change on its scale depends on the climatic change in glacier around it. Ice bergs can be in the height varies from starting size of 16 feet above sea level and wideness can be up to 164 feet. It can be widely seen in Antarctic and Arctic Ocean. We have a list of sunk ship due to hits with ice berg, in which the flag ship Titanic places important role. This ship lost 1522 passengers life in 1912.

From there, ice berg monitoring is facing big challenges due to dynamic change in size. Even though it is easily visible for human eyes since it is large in size, the

M. S. Sivapriya (✉) · P. Mohamed Fathimal
SRM Institute of Science and Technology, Vadapalani Campus, Chennai, Tamil Nadu, India
e-mail: sivapris@srmist.edu.in

P. Mohamed Fathimal
e-mail: fathimap@srmist.edu.in

N. Marriwala et al. (eds.), *Emergent Converging Technologies and Biomedical Systems*,
Lecture Notes in Electrical Engineering 841,
https://doi.org/10.1007/978-981-16-8774-7_52

human is not able to find its depth in underwater. So, we are in need of science to calculate its in depth information. The ice berg can be detected and calculated by Radar or sonar. Now it is most common to use satellite imaging technology for iceberg discovery.

Radar satellite imagery is a famous imagery which is mainly useful for ice berg monitoring. Radar satellite has a capability of capturing image in day and night in any climate. Due to this, talent Radar satellite imagery is very much useful for all type of natural environment monitoring. One of the important Radar satellite imagery is Synthetic Aperture Radar which has acronym as SAR.

Synthetic Aperture Radar is a type of Radar which can be used to produce two dimensional image and can be reconstructed to three dimensional image also. This Synthetic Aperture Radar can be mounted to any moving platform and it can move around target location. The microwave can be transmitted from Radar and further it will be reflected to construct image at receiving end. While returning back from the target, the reflected signal usually contains speckle noise which should be despeckled for post processing operation. This despeckled image can be used for all type of environment monitoring.

This SAR image can be used in ice berg discovery also. So many researches had undergone for ice berg detection using SAR imagery.

1.1 Related Work

Kelley has validated [1] the performance of Radar for ice berg detection who has used RADARSAT–1 Synthetic Aperture Radar and ENISAT Advanced Synthetic Aperture Radar. Here, they have calculated the size, age, type of ice by getting back scatter value of Radar and also calculated the probability of detection of Radar.

Mazur proposed [2] ice berg detection algorithm which is based on spatial values of Advanced Synthetic Aperture Radar images and this object-based detection algorithm is applied on the SAR images of Amundsen Sea. In this system, segmentation started at single pixel value and merged with another in each iteration with the condition of shape and brightness. Here still false alarm exist when extremely misshapen ice bergs are existent.

Qian implemented Mask R-CNN to detect objects in multitemporal SAR images. In this system, transfer learning was used for weight initialization trained by ImageNet [3]. Both single mask and multiple mask have been created during mask development stage. They increased speed of algorithm without disturbing accuracy by reducing proposed region size.

Ma suggested a system for ocean surveillance through high resolution SAR imageries produced by GF3 [4] satellite. This team used CNN which contains six convolution layer, three pooling layers and two fully connected layer. To extract more features single shot multi-box detector along with multi resolution input is implemented.

Gallego has done automatic classification of ships in optical aerial images by using CNN. Here, the classification done on optical aerial imagery for small unidentified objects and ships [5]. Finally this system concluded whether there is a presence of ships or not in given image. This is done by diving neural nodes produced from CNN to KNN for classification.

Zhan used data augmentation and stacking of multiple outputs which results in significant improved accuracy [6]. This system achieved accuracy by using transfer learning a convolutional neural network.

Su came with new object detection and segmentation technique using MASK R-CNN for remote sensing imagery [7]. This method consists of two stage which are region proposal network and Fast R-CNN classifier. To avoid quantization of coordinates due to continuous gradient precise ROI pooling was implemented.

Soldal [8] used Sentinel-1 Extra Wide Swath (EWS) SAR images to discover ice berg in the area of Barents Sea. They have used HV polarized intensity for improving the contrast between after that they have applied combination filter for blob discovery. But the responses from low HV polarized cannot be detected and also the highly strong scattering responses from hard ice berg may cause false alarms.

Bailey [9] has taken scattering properties of Synthetic Aperture Radar microwave pulses. With scattering properties they have also clubbed polarimetirc behavior of SAR of ice berg. Specifically, they dealt with quad-pol polarimetry for ice berg classification. After evaluating polSAR parmeters they used multi scale analysis for ice berg discovery with different window size 5×5 and 11×11. This system faced struggle for identifying accurate scaling parameters of ice berg.

Hass proposed deep learning approach to discriminate icebergs and ships. They mapped ocean objects by using YOLOV3 which is a kind of convolutional network [10]. They used YOLO with 53 layer deep convolutional neural network with residual connections.

Stofa detected ships in harbor area using DenseNet architecture with various fine tuning [11]. They take advantage of DenseNet which reduces vanishing gradient problem. They also addressed over fitting problem reduction by using transfer learning. Here, adam optimizer is used for updating the parameters for loss function.

Heiselberg dealt classification of ship and ice berg using neural network in SAR and multi spectral satellite images with neural network [12]. They also compared the result with support vector machine algorithm and proved convolutional neural network gives better result than SVM. Here two CNN network was used which are CNN1 (562,241 parameters) and CNN2 (1,134,081 parameters). It was found that deeper network gives better accuracy at the same time increases cost due to longer computation.

1.2 Convolutional Neural Network

Deep learning is a subset of machine learning which applies neural networks with several layer. It creates multi-level representations of input image. These representations is fed to the very first layer to implement the transformations and forward the resultant to the next layer [13]. This process is continued till the last layer where it achieves the final output. Low level features can be acquired at initial transformation like edges and corners. But when it jumps to next level layers these transformation fine tune the representations which helps to identify the object with in an image with high accuracy.

Convolutional neural network is one of the deep learning architecture which makes image classification with the help of assigning measurable weights and biases to the objects in the image. CNN has convolution layer which is followed by pooling layer. This pooling layers may or may not have fully connected layer as a follower. In recent days, CNN came up with different flavor like Googlenet, Alexnet, Resnet for classification of images.

Nowadays, CNN has been used for remote sensing data for variety of purposes. These architectures have been used for classification or identification of object in remote sensing imagery [14].

1.3 Preliminaries

Region-based convolutional neural network (R-CNN) is a kind of CNN which implements selective search technique that extracts region of interest. This region of interest is represented by rectangle box which is boundary of the respective object at most of the time. This boundary box helps to recognize the object. This R-CNN now came in four different extension like Fast R-CNN, Faster R-CNN, Mask R-CNN and Mesh R-CNN.

Mask R-CNN:

Mask R-CNN is an extended version of Faster R-CNN. For each object in addition to class label and boundary box, it also returns mask of the object which is called as segmentation mask. Mask R-CNN uses residual neural network as a backbone model for feature extraction.

2 Proposed System

The proposed system takes Synthetic Aperture Radar image as an input which is undergone preprocessing steps like logarithmic transformation for despeckling. Then the despeckled image is given to feature extraction part where ResNet101 architecture is used. This extracted feature acts as input to the next layer.

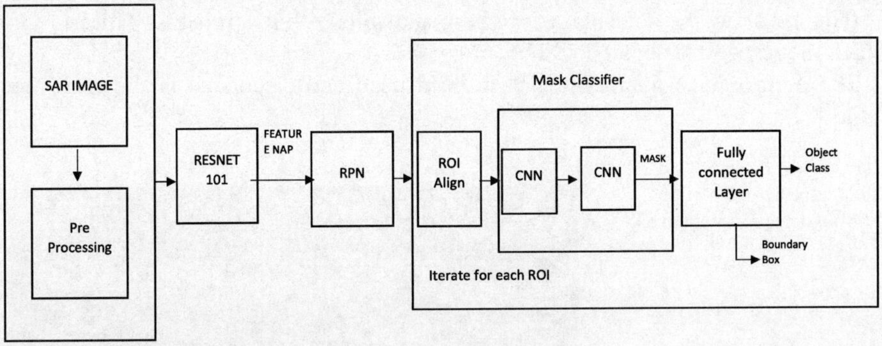

Fig. 1 Mask R-CNN for SAR

The next step is application of region proposal network. The purpose of this step is to find the presence of object in that region and to map the feature as feature maps. The problem of this RPN is, it gives regions in different sizes. So to solve this problem application of pooling layer is needed. This pooling layer transfers all the regions in same shape and size. The next step is prediction of class label and bounding boxes. For this fully connected network is applied on the regions and bounding boxes with class labels are predicted.

Mask R-CNN's main feature is generation of segmentation mask which needs the calculation of Intersection over Union (IoU). IoU can using following formula be calculated

$$\text{IoU} = \text{Intersection Area}/\text{Union Area} \tag{1}$$

If this IoU value is larger than 0.5 then that region will be considered as Region of Interest (RoI) else the respective region will be discarded. After calculating RoI and IoU mask branch has to be added which yields segmentation mask. This segmentation mask will be in size of 28 $\times$ 28. Now all the masks that contains objects can be predicted for ice berg and ship.

The architecture diagram shows the function flow of proposed system (see Fig. 1).

2.1 *Experiments and Results*

For this proposed system sentinel 1 images over Greenland was used since Greenland has abundant ice bergs. The algorithm has been implemented by using python with keras 2.0.8 and tensorflow 1.3.0, opencv, etc. ResNet101 is used as backbone architecture. This model gives mask with size of 28 $\times$ 28. System learnt with learning rate of 0.001. ROI positive ratio as 0.003 and mask size as [28 $\cdot$ 28]. 1000 steps per epoch has been taken.

Figure 2 show the detection of ice berg and ship with its probability measure in which the respective object could be.

The performance metrics that have been used and calculated is shown in the Table 1.

Fig. 2 Ice berg detection and ship detection with mask

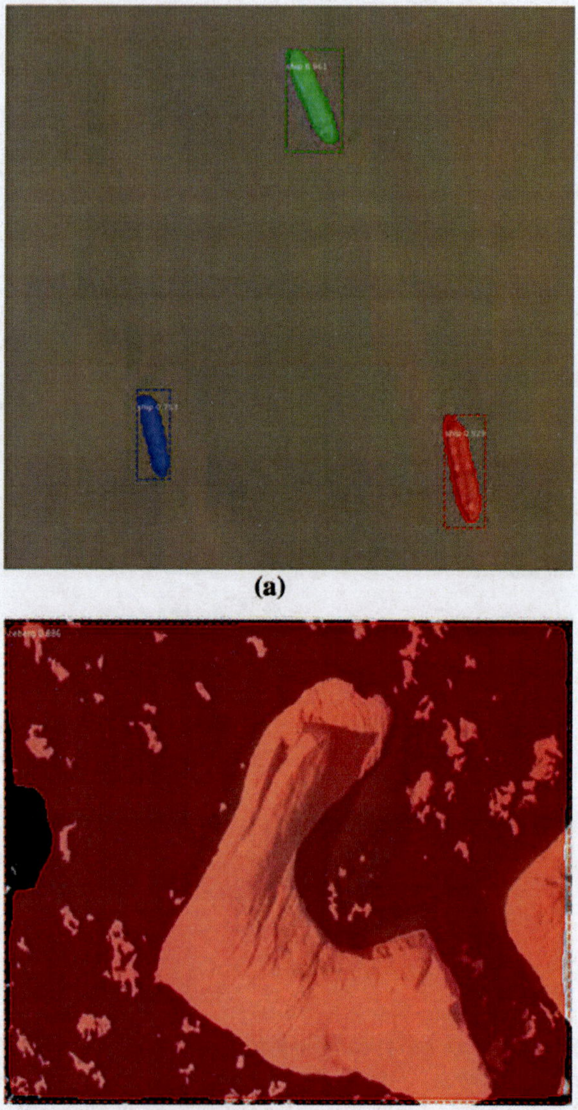

(a)

(b)

Fig. 2 (continued)

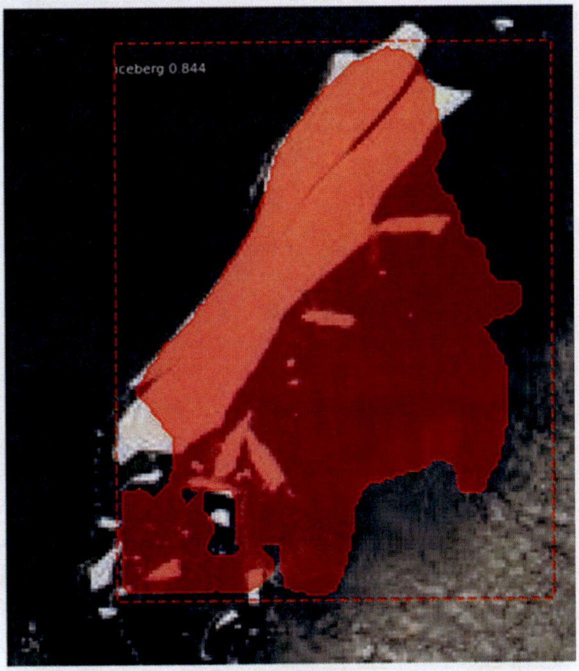

(c)

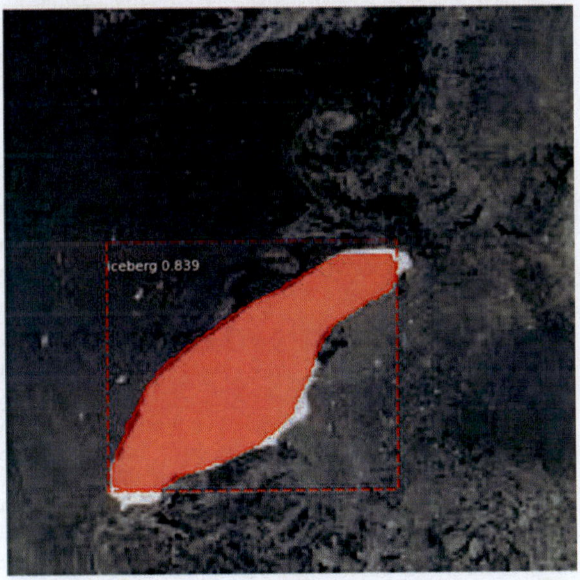

(d)

Table 1 Performance metrics comparison of Mask R-CNN with CNN and Fast R-CNN

Metric	CNN	Fast R-CNN	Mask R-CNN
Precision	0.842105	0.894737	0.947368421
Accuracy	0.8	0.866667	0.933333333
Misclassification rate	0.2	0.133333	0.066666667
TPR	0.842105	0.894737	0.947368421
FPR	0.272727	0.181818	0.090909091
TNR	0.727273	0.818182	0.909091

2.2 Conclusion

Ice berg detection for marine life is a vital and difficult task. This can be assisted with the help of Radar imaging and recent techniques of deep learning. This system used both concepts to give accurate model to detect iceberg. Mask R-CNN is a recent technique which gives upright metrics. So the system uses Mask R-CNN for iceberg detection and the result shows success of the model proposed.

References

1. Lane K, Power D, Youden J, Randell C (2004) Validation of synthetic aperture radar for iceberg detection in sea ice. IEEE, 0-7803-8742-2/04
2. Mazur AK, Wahlin AK, Kerezel A (2016) An object-based SAR image iceberg detection algorithm applied to the Amundsen Sea. Remote Sens Environ 0034-4257
3. Qian Y, Liu Q, Zhu H, Fan H, Du B, Liu S (2018) Mask R-CNN for object detection in multitemporal SAR images
4. Ma M, Chen J, Liu W, Yang W (2018) Ship classification and detection based on CNN using GF-3 SAR images. Remote Sens. https://doi.org/10.3390/rs10122043
5. Gallego A-J, Pertusa A, Gil P (2018) Automatic ship classification from optical aerial images with convolutional neural networks. Remote Sens. https://doi.org/10.3390/rs10040511
6. Zhan C, Zhang L, Zhong Z, Didi-Ooi S (2018) Deep learning approach in automatic iceberg – ship detection with SAR remote sensing data. In: The society of exploration geophysicists and the Chinese petroleum society
7. Su H, We S, Yan M, Wang C, Shi J, Zhang X (2019) Object detection and instance segmentation in remote sensing imagery based on precise mask R-CNN. IEEE, 978-1-5386-9154-0
8. Soldal IH, Dierking W, Korosov A, Marino A (2019) Automatic detection of small icebergs in fast ice using satellite wide-swath SAR images. Remote Sens 11:806. https://doi.org/10.3390/rs11070806
9. Bailey J, Marino A (2020) Quad-polarimetric multi-scale analysis of icebergs in ALOS-2 SAR data: a comparison between icebergs in west and east Greenland. Remote Sens 12:1864
10. Hass FS, Arsanjani JJ (2020) Deep learning for detecting and classifying ocean objects: application of YoloV3 for iceberg–ship discrimination. Int J Geo Inf. https://doi.org/10.3390/ijgi9120758
11. Stofa MM, Zulkifley MA, Zaki SZM (2020) A deep learning approach to ship detection using satellite imagery. IOP Conf Ser Earth Environ Sci 540:012049
12. Heiselberg H (2020) Ship-iceberg classification in SAR and multispectral satellite images with neural networks. Remote Sens. https://doi.org/10.3390/rs12152353

13. Gua J, Wangb Z, Kuenb J, Mab L (2017) Recent advances in convolutional neural networks. Remote Sens
14. Heiselberg H (2019) Ship-iceberg detection & classification in sentinel-1 SAR images. In: Marine navigation and safety of sea transportation

Augmentation Techniques on Mammogram Images for CNN Based Breast Cancer Classification

P. Pratheep Kumar, V. Mary Amala Bai, and Geetha G. Nair

Abstract Deep learning is now the fastest expanding area of several medical image classification and identification. Convolutional neural networks (CNN) are the primary method used for classification across many deep neural networks (DNN). In breast cancer, classification using mammogram image has several challenges such as small dataset size and class imbalance issues. Small dataset issue is a major challenge while performing classification of medical images. Large set of training data is required to build a reliably performing machine learning model for classification. Practically, it is very difficult to generate a bench marked, pathologically tested, large set of medical images. To overcome this problem by proposed and implemented the image data augmentation is a method that can be used. We choose 115 breast mammography photographs with masses from the INbreast database for this study. The amount of breast mammography images was increased to 7732 image data by data augmentation. We utilize the preprocessing process to the breast mammography images, and then apply the CNN ideal is used to classify the images as benign or malignant. In this comparison, the quantitative analysis of classification performance between two processes such as before augmentation technique achieved 94.56% and after augmentation technique achieved better classification accuracy of 98.91%, respectively.

Keywords Breast cancer · Neural network · Convolutional neural network · Augmentation technique · INbreast database · And benign or malignant.

P. Pratheep Kumar (✉)
Department of Computer Science and Engineering, Noorul Islam Centre for Higher Education, Kumaracoil, Tamil Nadu, India

V. Mary Amala Bai
Department of Information Technology, Noorul Islam Centre For Higher Education, Kumaracoil, Tamil Nadu, India

G. G. Nair
Consultant in Obstetrics and Gynaecology, Women and Children Hospital, Thycaud, Thampanoor, Kerala, India

N. Marriwala et al. (eds.), *Emergent Converging Technologies and Biomedical Systems*, Lecture Notes in Electrical Engineering 841,
https://doi.org/10.1007/978-981-16-8774-7_53

1 Introduction

Breast cancer is a severe public health issue globally. It causes more than 1500 deaths in Switzerland alone annually. It is also the typical cancer mortality cause among women. Experts can prevent and cure breast cancer no matter at what stage it is discovered. However, earlier detection is presently the only effective choice available to reduce the illness's related physiological and psychological burden [1–3]. Mammography is the utmost sensitive method available for earlier detection of breast cancer. A discussion into mammography's efficiency to detect breast cancer early is a closed topic. Systematic mammography screening of women between 50 and 60 years is necessary to lower breast cancer mortality. Mammographic density, a robust breast cancer risk factor is increasingly being used to tailor preventive, and screening schemes. It is a primary determinant of mammography screening sensitivity and thereby of interval cancer rates. Mammography is the most important of all imaging methods to examine breast tissue, as it is efficient and accepted [4, 5]. Many computer-aided diagnosis (CAD) techniques were suggested to facilitate discovery of masses in mammograms, an important breast cancer display. The classification of tumour as benign or malignant, the features of these tumours are specified in Table 1.

CNNs produce an outcomes in a number of classification activities, but they still have a number of obstacles to face amid broad perspectives. They have problems both with over-setting and generalisation due to the vast scale of the networks touching millions of limits as well as the absence of sound workout data sets. Finally, the averting of the adversarial attacks [6] that could mislead the DNNs is a rising concern for researchers.

The researchers are battling to resolve these issues and to produce better outcomes by amending the design of the networks, designing and acquiring new learning algorithms. Lack of quality data in sufficient numbers, or an unequal level of class balance within the datasets is the most common issue [2]. The most efficient DNNs today are very large, so that a lot of data is required, which is often difficult to deliver. The famous CNN VGG16 architecture, for instance, consists of a total of 16 neuron layers with a total parameter of 138 million [7]. Moreover, ImageNet, the data set which

Table 1 Differences between benign and malignant mass tumour

Benign mass tumour	Malignant mass tumour
Benign mass are moving in nature	Malignant mass are fixed mass
Soft and clear round with besetment fibrous capsule	Irregular shaped with no capsule
Easy to remove the benign mass and does not recur again	Problematic to remove the malignant mass and may recur again
Tumour cells multiply slowly	Tumour cells multiply rapidly
The growing tumour by expanding and pushing away and against nearby tissue	The tumour growth by invading and destroying nearby tissue

holds more than 1 million pictures from 1000 non-overlapping categories, generally tests the efficiency of new architectures [8]. Data increase by data synthesis is one way of tackling this problem. The interest in multiplied data and the popularity of CNNs have been rapidly increased. The traditional and affinity-orientated transformations: creating new images through a rotation of the original image, zooming in and out, moving, applying distortions, changing the colour palette are the maximum standard and recognised operative practice for data extension. Although, advantages in some cases are not enough for simple classical operations to substantially improve the accuracy of the neural network or overawed the overfitting problem [9]. Furthermore, the current study of so-called CNN attacks has shown that deep neural networks can be easily misclassified by only limited rotations and image translations, addition of noise to images [10], or even altering a pixel in the image [11].

An algorithm presented for automated breast cancer segmentation in mammographic images scheme [12] resulted in a better classification performance. Application of thresholding technology and morphological preprocessing was the principal contribution to this algorithm in order to remove radiopaque products and labels and to separate the background area from the breast profile. The MIAS database for all mammographic images was extensively tested to show the validity of the proposed segmentation system. This database included 322 images with rectangular labels of high intensity. Bright scanning artefacts have been found in most database images. Achieved the detection accuracy about 99.06% using the high intensity square labelling. In the qualitative assessment, the method was precisely segmented throughout the breast region by covering all density classes in a large variety of digitized mammograms.

Currently developed methods for image enhancement are not only traditional methods and CNN methods. An interesting approach is a random technique proposed in [13], which can be quickly and relatively easily implemented but which gives good results in CNN generalization capacity. A noise-filled rectangle is painted randomly in a picture with the method, which leads to changes in the original pixels. As authors said it lessens the hazard of overpassing and makes the model additional robust by extending the data set to different levels of occlusion.

2 Proposed Methodology

The breast cancer classification and identification by using mammogram image proposed architecture is shown in Fig. 1. Initially we take the small breast cancer Mammography images of INbreast dataset, which has small amount of image data. As we have seen, small dataset cannot provide better classification rate. By this problem, we introduced the data augmentation technique to create the several images from small number of images by using different image augmentation scheme as flipping, cropping, noise injection, rotate, and random brightness augmentation. Primarily, we choose only 115 breast mammography images with masses and enhance the image quality by using CLAHE technique. After the data augmentation technique applied

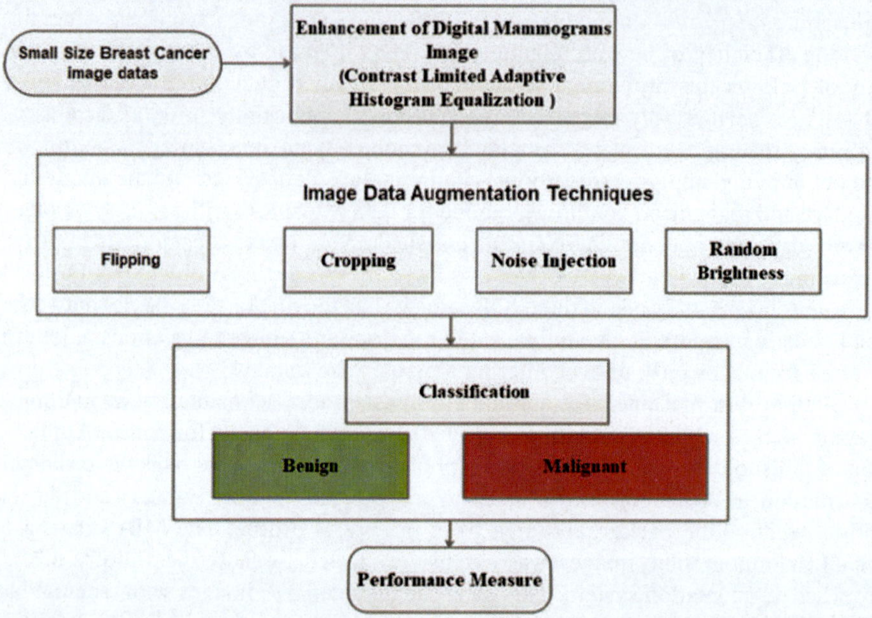

Fig. 1 Flow diagram of proposed method

to increase the image data to increase the learning rate. Further, the increased image data that is given as training and test data to a deep learning-based CNN classifier is ideal to classify the image a benign or malignant.

2.1 Data Description

Originally collected from the Centro Hospitalar S. Joao [SJSB] mammograms from the INbreast database that contain 115 cases with 410 images in total [14]. Of these, 90 were women with both breasts disease. There are four types, including the mass, calcification, asymmetry, and deformation of breast diseases detailed in the database. The images of this database contain Craniocaudal (CC) and Mediolateral oblique (MLO) views, and the breast density according to BI-RADS standards is divided into four categories, which are described in following Table 2 and also dataset sample is showed in Fig. 2.

Table 2 The benign and malignant class labels for breast density

Category	Number
Density-1 with Benign	12
Density-1 with Malignant	30
Density-2 with Benign	4
Density-2 with Malignant	32
Density-3 with Benign 1	13
Density-3 with Malignant	8
Density-4 with Benign	6
Total	115

Fig. 2 Dataset sample image

3 Data Augmentation Process

Data augmentation is a vital measure of training discriminative CNNs. A variety of augmentation strategies, including flipping, cropping, noise injection, rotate, and random brightness augmentation are implemented.

3.1 Cropping

Cropping method may be used by cutting a central patch of the image in a practical manner for image with a diverse height and width. Random crops can also be used for the effect of translations very similar. In contrast, the size of the input is reduced by cutting, as a pixel ratio of (256, 256) to (126, 126) whereas translations maintain the spatial dimensions of the image. This may not be a label-preserving conversion according to the reduction threshold chosen for crops.

3.2 Noise Injection

A random value matrix generally from the Gaussian distribution consists of the injection of noise. Adding image noise can help to make CNNs more robust. Geometric changes are excellent solutions for the location differences found in training results. The distribution of training data from test data can be separated from a wide range of potential sources of bias. If there are positional distortions, such as the fact that every face is effortlessly focused in the frame, geometric changes can be a great solution. Besides great aptitude to overcome positional biases, geometric changes are beneficial, since they are simply carried out. The noise injected images is showed as in Fig. 3.

In order to start operations like horizontal flipping and rotation, many imaging processing libraries are available. Geometric transformations have the difficulties that include additional memory requirement, computer transformation, and extra training time. Some geometric transformations must be observed manually, such as reduction or random cropping, to ensure that the image label is not altered. Finally, the distances between training data and the test data are additional complex than the positional and translation variances in several application fields covered, such as medical image investigation. The scope of the application of geometric changes is therefore relatively limited.

Fig. 3 Noise injected image

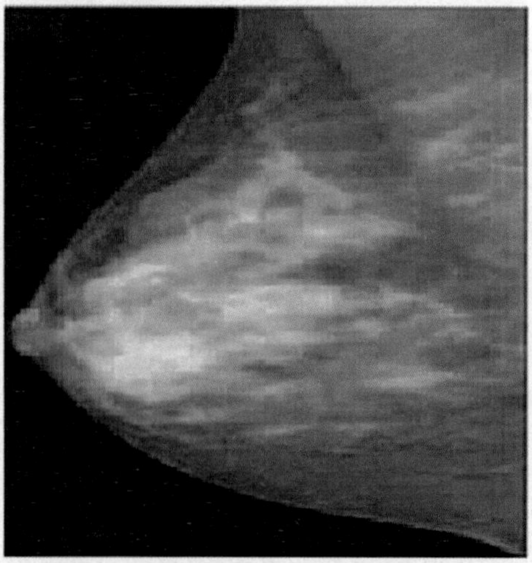

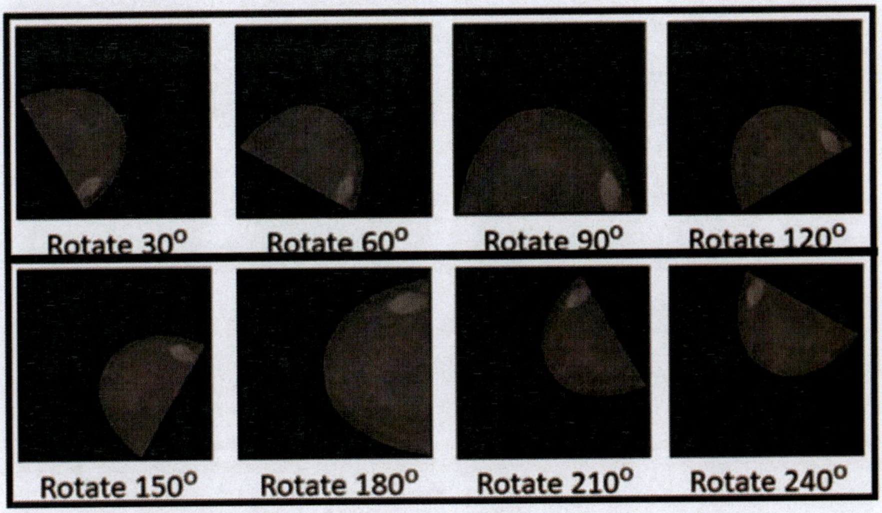

Fig. 4 Rotation of different angle image [14]

3.3 Rotation

In multi-angle-rotation data increase (modify = 30, 60, 90, 120, 150, 180, 210, 240, 270, 300, 330°), and then horizontally and vertically rotate the original image and the 11-angle-rotation images. Not only does the process increase the number of samples, it also avoids overfitting. The different rotation of breast images is exposed in Fig. 4.

3.4 Flipping

In case of a vertical or horizontal breast image flip, an image flip means to reverse rows or columns of pixels. Vertical flips, we assume, capture a special medical image property, that is to say, invariance in vertical reflection. Normally only horizontal flips are used for natural pictures because vertical flips do often not represent natural pictures. However, a vertical flip of a mass would still result in a realistic mass (Fig. 5).

3.5 Random Brightness Augmentation

This is the important augmentation techniques, the brightness is randomly given to the image to create various random brightness image, which is showed in Fig. 6 (Table 3).

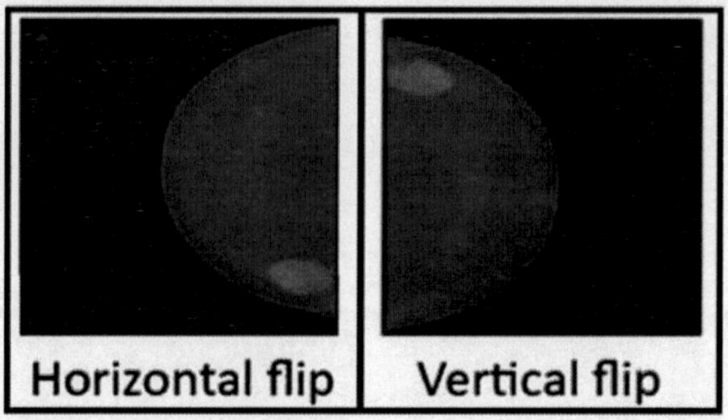

Fig. 5 Flipping breast cancer image [14]

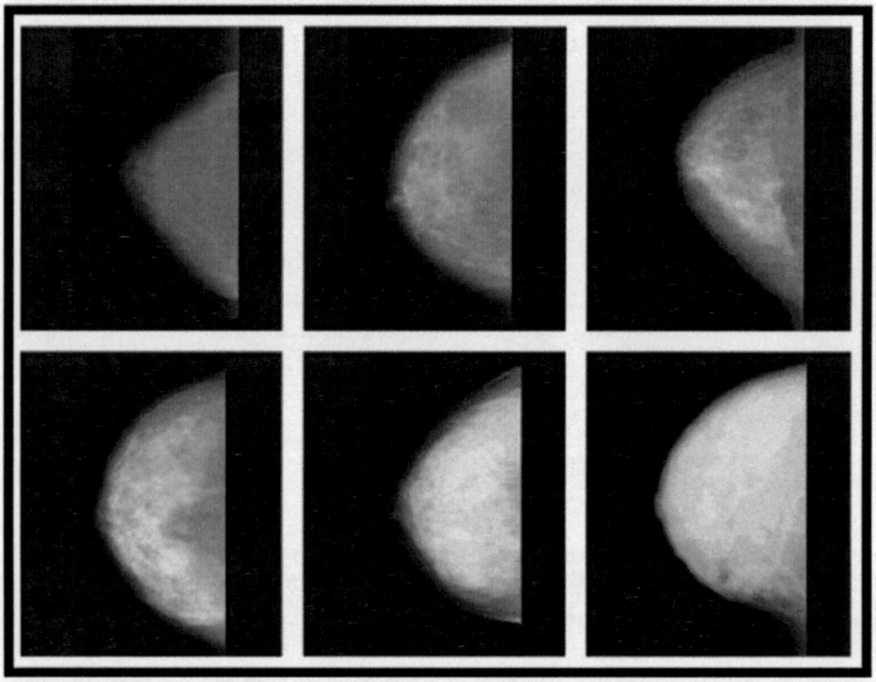

Fig. 6 Brightness augmentation images [14]

3.6 Digital Mammograms Enhancement

The CLAHE approach [15] is used to improve the contrast that some mammograms include, sometimes degraded, in some pictures. In proportion to the pixel intensity in the local intensity histogram, the intensity of a pixel converts into value within the display range. CLAHE is a case of adaptive histogram equalization (AHE) in which

Table 3 Dataset images after image augmentation [14]

Category number	All image	Training data	Testing data
Density-1 with Benign	874	701	173
Density-1 with Malignant	2170	1738	432
Density-2 with Benign	298	230	68
Density-2 with Malignant	2314	1843	471
Density-3 with Benign 1	946	739	207
Density-3 with Malignant	586	461	125
Density-4 with Benign	442	356	86
Density-1 with Benign	102	68	34
Total	7732	6136	1596

the images are improved to the highest contrast enhancement factor by the level of a consumer film. In this technique, improvements are made in small areas so that the over-improvement is very low compared with AHE due to noise or the effect of edge shadows.

Initially, the CLAHE method was established to decrease the shade and sound emitted by medical images in homogeneous areas [16]. The approach was used to develop digital mammograms and has shown good improvements in visual efficiency mammograms.

A small block input image I with M * N dimensions is separated. CLAHE is then used to increase each block's contrast. Bilinear interpolation is finally used to reconnect the next blocks to whole pictures. The steps mentioned in CLAHE are as follows.

(1) Patches of the images shall be divided into blocks of 8 * 8 size which are non-overlapping.
(2) Calculation of the histogram of any block.
(3) A histogram clip limit, t = 0.001, is set for enhancing patches in comparison.
(4) The histogram is redistributed after clipping the threshold value.
(5) The following transformation function modifies each block histogram:

$$\sum_{i=0}^{t} p_t(A_i) \tag{1}$$

where $p_t(A_i)$ is represent as the input patch image greyscale probability density function value and $p_t(A_i)$ is describe as

$$p_t(A_i) = \frac{m_i}{m} \tag{2}$$

where m_i is represent as the grey scale value of input pixel I and m is represent as the total sum of pixels in a block.

(6) Bilinear interpolation is used in any patch to association the next blocks. In the new histogram, the grey scale value of the patch is also modified.

We used the block size of 8 * 8 for our experiment, and the histogram clip limit is set to 0.001.

4 Convolution Neural Network for Classification Task

The relevance of CNN's findings has been shown in the classification of photographs. CNN has an architecture of multi-layered layer shadowed by a maximum layer of pooling. The sum of layers varies with the designer. A fully connected layer like MLP is fed the final maximum pooling layer output and then forwarded to Softmax.

The pooling layer is used to reduce the convolution layer's dimensionality. Average pooling, mean pooling, and full pooling are the most commonly used pooling layer algorithms. During preparation, a random disabling of the neurons is used for the discontinuation algorithm, usually with a 0.3–0.6 dropout ratio. The last layer of CNN is a soft max layer, which includes the output neuron by the sum of classes of the problem and is given a trust score.

The kernel sizes of 7 * 7 are used in both conv and max pooling layers. There are 16 kernels in the convolution layers, and 5 * 5 kernels in the second layer are included. Then the neural layer is completely linked. In the experiment the dropout ratio is 0.55. The layer of Softmax is used for classification CNN preparation. Figure 7 presents the complete network architecture of CNN.

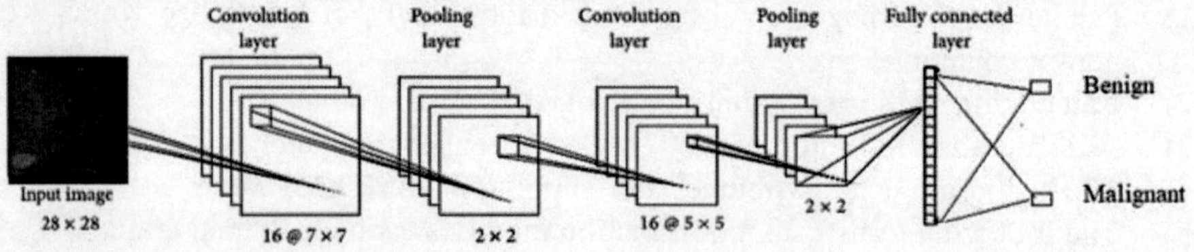

Fig. 7 Convolution neural network model

5 Simulation and Results

In this section, we discussed the performance of the CNN classifier by increase the input data set image by using data augmentation technique. In this simulation, experiment conducted by using software tool as python with system requirement of 4 GB RAM with 2 GHZ Intel i3 core processor. The validation of testing and training the data by using the breast cancer dataset image. The proposed system performance is estimated by using the different parametric metrics, which are explained in following section.

5.1 Performance Measures

The proposed system, in which different classifier performances is measure by using different parametric. The developed system is assessed using evaluation metrics such as TP, FP, TN, FN, sensitivity, precision, specificity, F-measure, and accuracy.

- TP—Sum of benign image is correctly categorized as noncancerous image.
- TN—Sum of malignant image is correctly categorized as cancerous image.
- FP—Sum of benign image is wrongly categorized as cancerous image.
- FN—Sum of malignant image is wrongly categorized as noncancerous image.

Sensitivity

Sensitivity is also called as recall. Sensitivity is distinct as the percentage of image with abnormal, whose output is positive and it is calculated using the Eq. 3 as

$$Sensitivity = TP/(TP + FN) \tag{3}$$

Specificity

Specificity, is defined as percentage of image with normal, whose output is negative and it is calculated using the Eq. 4 as

$$Specificity = TN/(TN + FP) \tag{4}$$

Classification Accuracy

Classification accuracy is defined as the sum of correctly classified images, which is separated by the total sum of images and then it is multiplied by 100 to turn it into a percentage. It is calculated using the Eq. 5 as

$$Classification\ Accuracy = (TP + TN)/(TP + FP + TN + FN) \times 100 \tag{5}$$

Precision

Precision is distinct as the sum of true positives, which is divided by the number of TP and false positives and it is calculated using the Eq. 6 as

$$Precision = TP/(TP + FP) \quad (6)$$

False Positive Rate

FPR is distinct as the sum of false positives, which is divided by the sum of false positives and true negative and it is calculated using the Eq. 7 as

$$FPR = FP/(FP + TN) \quad (7)$$

F-Measure

This is the kind of parameter measure, which association of recall and precision. The F-measure is determined by using the Eq. 8 as

$$F\text{-}measure = 2 * Recall * Precision/Recall + Precision \quad (8)$$

Mean Square Error (MSE)

Measure of fidelity of image. The parameter used to compare between the two images by providing quantitative or similarity rate. MSE calculation formula is expressed Eq. 9 as

$$MSE = \frac{1}{PQ} \sum \sum (f(i, j) - f^R(i, j))^2 \quad (9)$$

In Table 4, it represents that the performance of different augmentation technique with different parameter measures. In this analysis, the combination of entire augmentation technique achieved better performance than separate technique performance.

Table 4 Comparison analysis of different data augmentation technique with classification

Data augmentation methods	Precession (%)	Recall (%)	F-measure (%)	MSE (%)
Flipping	97.46	95.32	97.21	6.48
Cropping	96.40	95.59	96.44	5.67
Rotation	94.52	95.09	96.21	6.97
Noise injection	93.58	94.68	95.22	6.49
Random brightness	96.33	95.17	94.45	5.84
Combination of entire augmentation	98.49	97.92	98.64	4.63

Table 5 Comparison of classification accuracy with augmentation

Data augmentation methods	Accuracy (%)
Flipping	96.46
Cropping	95.21
Rotation	97.36
Noise injection	94.56
Random brightness	95.32
Combination of entire augmentation	98.91

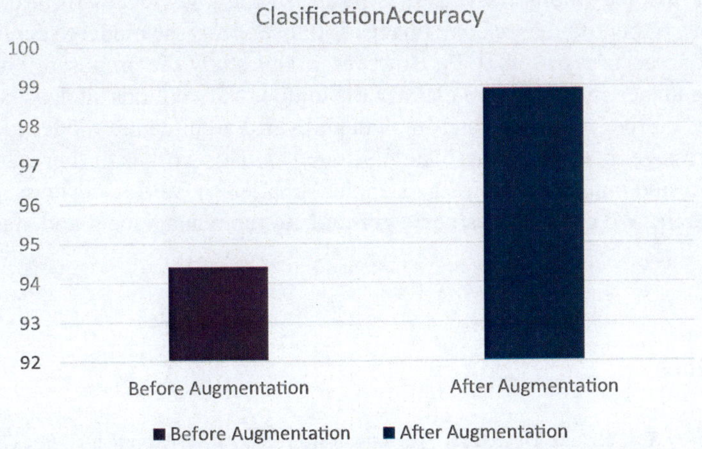

Fig. 8 Comparison of classification accuracy before and after augmentation

Table 5 represents that the accuracy performance of different augmentation technique; in flipping technique it reached 96.46%, cropping technique achieved 95.21% and rotation method reached 97.36% by the noise injection scheme it achieved the 94.565, which is the least value than other models. However, the combination of entire augmentation achieved the better classification accuracy of 98.91%, which is better accuracy performance than the other individual methods.

In Fig. 8, it shows the graphical representation of performance before and after augmentation. In without augmentation data technique, it achieved the least classification accuracy of 94.56%. Whereas, after the image data augmentation technique, the model achieved the better classification accuracy of 98.91%, respectively.

6 Conclusion

In this study, we did the analysis of learning ability of the training model. Using a small dataset, it may be poor due to the lack of potential useful learning information. Data augmentation techniques are implemented to increase the size of image data. In this augmentation technique, we included some methods as flipping, cropping, noise injection, rotate, and random brightness augmentation. In every technique, we separately analysed the classification accuracy by CNN classifier with different parametric measures. In CNN architecture, we implemented the proper kernel filter to achieve the maximum classification result. In this, we successfully create the maximum number of breast cancer images to train and test the model to achieve high classification accuracy as 98.91%. However, in this study the proposed model is to create or enhance image data to classify the tumour as two kinds such as benign or malignant. Further we design and implement hybrid architecture model to classify the breast images at various classification strategies. This work is further extended to clinically tested mammogram image samples supplied by VPS Lakeshore Hospital, Kochi, Kerala. We extend our sincere gratitude to the management and staff of the hospital.

References

1. McKinney SM, Sieniek M, Godbole V, Godwin J, Antropova N, Ashrafian H, Back T, Chesus M, Corrado GS, Darzi A, Etemadi M (2020) International evaluation of an AI system for breast cancer screening. Nature 577(7788):89–94
2. Pratheep Kumar P, Mary Amala Bai V, Geetha GN (2021) Challenges and solutions in CNN based diagnostic techniques on breast mammographic images: a survey. Int J Pharm Res 13(2)
3. Bahl M, Mercaldo S, Dang PA, McCarthy AM, Lowry KP, Lehman CD (2020) Breast cancer screening with digital breast tomosynthesis: are initial benefits sustained. Radiology 295(3):529–539
4. Shaikh TA, Ali R, Beg MS (2020) Transfer learning privileged information fuels CAD diagnosis of breast cancer. Mach Vis Appl 31(1):1–23
5. Karale VA, Singh T, Sadhu A, Khandelwal N, Mukhopadhyay S (2020) Reduction of false positives in the screening CAD tool for microcalcification detection. Sādhanā 45(1):1–12
6. Engstrom L, Tsipras D, Schmidt L, Madry A (2017) A rotation and a translation suffice: fooling CNNs with simple transformations. arXiv:171202779
7. Simonyan K, Zisserman A (2014) Very deep convolutional networks for large-scale image recognition. arXiv:14091556
8. ImageNet (2018). http://image-net.org/. Accessed 05 Feb 2018
9. Wang J, Perez L (2017) The effectiveness of data augmentation in image classification using deep learning. Tech Rep 11(2):112–124
10. Jin J, Dundar A, Culurciello E (2015) Robust convolutional neural networks under adversarial noise. arXiv:151106306
11. Su J, Vargas DV, Kouichi S (2017) One pixel attack for fooling deep neural networks. arXiv:171008864
12. Mahmood M, Isa M, Ashidi (2015) A fully automated breast separation for mammographic images. In: 2015 IEEE international conference on biosignal analysis, processing and systems (ICBAPS), vol 12, no 3, pp 37–41

13. Zhong Z, Zheng L, Kang G, Li S, Yang Y (2017) Random erasing data augmentation. arXiv: 170804896
14. Huang ML, Lin TY (2020) Dataset of breast mammography images with masses. Data Brief 1(31):105–128
15. Khan SA, Hussain S, Yang S (2020) Contrast enhancement of low-contrast medical images using modified contrast limited adaptive histogram equalization. J Med Imaging Health Inf 10(8):1795–1803
16. Farhan AH, Kamil MY (2020) Texture analysis of mammogram using histogram of oriented gradients method. In: IOP conference series: materials science and engineering, vol 881, no 1. IOP Publishing, pp 21–49

Automated Diagnosis of COVID-19 Using Squeeze Net Architecture Based on Deep Learning

J. Syed Nizamudeen Ahmed, M. Mohamed Sathik, Krishnan Nallaperumal, Senthamarai Kannan Kaliaperumal, and Kumar Parasuraman

Abstract Coronavirus infection (COVID-19) is an extremely contagious infection produced by severe acute respiratory coronavirus syndrome 2. The infection started in Wuhan, China, in December 2019, and has extended worldwide to more than 200 countries since then. The effect is such that the World Health Organization (WHO) has announced a Global Health Emergency of International Significance on the present pandemic of COVID-19. As many countries gets affected by this rampant virus, it is important for the healthcare workers to keenly observe every patient and give the accurate results like if they been affected or not. As we know healthcare worker are the real worriers as they sacrifice their lives to save others, so helping them with advance technologies will be a big deal. So, in this paper a CNN model is been used for precisely classify patients as they are affected or not. Experimentation results depicts that the proposed model attains an accuracy of 93.9%.

Keywords Convolutional neural networks · COVID-19 · COVID-19 diagnosis · World health organization · X-ray images

1 Introduction

The new Corona virus (COVID-19) is a basic lethal disease that started in the area of Wuhan, China, in December 2019 and reached out over the world. The pandemic of COVID-19 was significant trouble to the well-being service as no fruitful treatment has been identified [1, 2]. The common arrangement of COVID-19 includes

J. Syed Nizamudeen Ahmed (✉) · K. Nallaperumal · K. Parasuraman
Centre for Information Technology and Engineering, Manonmaniam Sundaranar University, Abishekapatti, Tirunelveli 627012, Tamil Nadu, India

M. Mohamed Sathik
Department of Computer Science, Sadakathullah Appa College, Tirunelveli 627011, Tamil Nadu, India

S. K. Kaliaperumal
Department of Statistics, Manonmaniam Sundaranar University, Abishekapatti, Tirunelveli 627012, Tamil Nadu, India

N. Marriwala et al. (eds.), *Emergent Converging Technologies and Biomedical Systems*, Lecture Notes in Electrical Engineering 841,
https://doi.org/10.1007/978-981-16-8774-7_54

a positive-based single-fiber RNA-type and it is attempting to fix the infection in light of its changing credits. Clinical specialists overall are experiencing extreme exploration to make a proficient treatment for the contamination. Today, COVID-19 is the main wellspring of lakhs of fatalities around the world, with huge occurrences in the Blocked States, France, Italy, Japan, the Blocked Kingdom, India, and so forth there are a few types of COVID-19, and the infections are generally found in untamed life. COVID-19 is found in individuals, bats, pigs, cats, canines, rodents and poultry. Signs of COVID-19 are sore throat, nausea, runny nose, and hacking. The infection will cause the casualty of people with traded off safe models [3, 4]. Corona virus is essentially spread by actual contact starting with one human then onto the next. Generally, stable individuals may be compromised through interaction with breathing, hand touching, or mucous touch with humans having COVID-19 [5]. The respiratory exchange of the contamination from one human to another has set off a snappy reached out of the flare-up [6]. Although COVID-19 induces small indications in around 82% of persons, the others are serious or dangerous [7]. Coronavirus cases count averagely 335,403 of which 14,611 died and 97,636 were improved. The quantity of humans actually diagnosed is 223,156. Around 95% of the affected persons survive the infection marginally, 5% of the infected affected persons have a severe or critical condition [8]. SARS-CoV-2 causes various difficulties for high-salaries and low-salaries or middle-salaries countries (LMICs). A main concern about spreading worldwide is because of the poor health systems. Few countries, such as Nigeria, have been active in handling individual cases so far. However, colossal outbreaks can inadvertently beat LMIC's healthcare administrations. The brutal truth is that nations in quite a bit of sub-Saharan Africa do not know about the COVID-19 flare-up. Also, there are not various nations in Latin America and the Middle East. Environmental safety interventions, as like monitoring, systematic touch tracking, social distancing, travel bans, public health awareness, the availability of medicine for vulnerable and resistant humans, and delaying non-essential procedures and facilities would both play a role in slowing the extended of illness and disbanding strain on hospitals. Private governments will have to determine where to create a line on the implementation of these process. Ethical, social and economic risks will have to be weighed against proven health benefits. Indication definitely means that elected officials will push quickly and forcefully. The fatality of affected persons with SARS-CoV-2 pneumonia is high. As stated by the Lancet Respiratory Medicine recently, "The seriousness of SARS-CoV-2 pneumonia is a major burden on significant care resources in hospitals, specifically if it does not have sufficient staff." This corona virus is destroying the humans. The political reaction to the outbreak will consequently represent the national health danger raised by SARS-CoV-2. Environmental safety interventions, as like monitoring, systematic touch tracking, social distancing, travel bans, public health awareness, the availability of medicines for vulnerable and resistant humans, and delaying non-essential procedures and facilities would both play a role in slowing the extended of illness and disbanding strain on hospitals. Private governments will have to determine where to create a line on the implementation of these process. Ethical, social and economic risks will have to be weighed against proven health benefits. National administrations have also made recommendations to healthcare practitioners, but written suggestion alone is inadequate. Guidance on how to handle the affected persons with COVID-19 must be given as a matter of urgency to health workers and evaluation kits will be made accessible and supply chains reinforced. The medical committee advises that hospitals build up a central committee, comprising medical administrators, an infection reaction staff leader, an infectious infection consultant, and professionals from the Intensive Care Block, incident and emergency departments.

2 Related Works

Castiglioni et al. [9] also suggested a slightly various method, utilizing a set of data which they have compiled and which is not present. Two hundred and fifty COVID-19 and 250 visuals of healthy ones were utilized for planning and a free test set of 74 positive and 36 negative models was utilized. They prepared a social event of 10 Res Nets and accomplished a ROC-AUC of 0.80 for the limit of assortment. Its introduction is a ton of more deplorable than those uncovered in the writing, yet they have utilized both anterior posterior and poster anterior projections and do not encounter the evil impacts of the issue of set of data affirmation that we include in this paper.

In ongoing exploration, Maguolo and Nanni [10] differentiated and examined different test techniques used for the computerized assessment of COVID-19 X-ray pictures. We demonstrate that indistinguishable results can be achieved by using X-ray images that do not cover any of the lungs. We will avoid the lungs from the photographs by changing the center of the X-ray output to dark and rehearsing our classifiers just on the external piece of the images. We consequently accept that some exploration rules for acknowledgment are not fitting and that neural organizations are learning measures in the arrangement of information that are not predictable with the presence of COVID-19. In future exploration, we propose to check the decency of the test convention using our devices and urge analysts to search for preferred strategies over those that we propose.

Toğaçar et al. [11] reconfigured the information clusters utilizing the Fuzzy Color strategy as a preprocessing method and stacked the visuals that are designed with the first visuals. The stacked informational assortment was set up with significant learning models (MobileNetV2, Squeeze Net) on the accompanying stage and the modules accomplished from the models were realized through the Social Mimic headway strategy. Incredible limits were then united and explored using SVM. The typical characterization rate came to by the suggested procedure was 99.27%. It is apparent from the suggested method in this analysis that the system will make an important contribution to the diagnosis of COVID-19 infection.

3 Methodology

3.1 Set of Data

In the theoretical study, we utilize three types of sets of data that are openly accessible. Such groups are common, with pneumonia and COVID-19 photos of the lung (Fig. 1).

Two arrangements of information are X-beam records, and all the document is meant JPG. As COVID-19 is another illness, the quantity of visuals related with this contamination is limited. We joined two openly present sets of data made up of COVID-19 visuals. The first set of data of COVID-19 was distributed on the website. After the verification of the visuals, they were made present to the public. For this study, 76 visuals named with COVID-19 were selected [2]. The second set of data of COVID-19 comprises of visuals provided through a team of researchers. The second set of data of COVID-19 is present on the Kaggle website. Two sets of data comprising COVID-19 visuals were joined for this study and a new set of data comprising of 295 visuals was made. In this examination, the second arrangement of information is fundamental for contrasting COVID-19 breast visuals using DL models. The second arrangement of information involves typical visuals of the chest and visuals of the chest pneumonia. Pneumonia chest visuals comprises the viruses and bacteria, and the visuals are obtained from 53 affected persons. The photographs were made by specialists and circulated openly. The data set comprises of three groups. Details regarding the groups of set of data and the quantity of visuals in the groups are as follows (Figs. 2 and 3).

A check of 295 visuals were gathered in the COVID-19 set. Standard social event X-ray visuals are 65 under control, and pneumonia bunch of X-ray visuals are 98 in count. The total number of visuals in the data combination is 458. In the test examination, 70% of the plan of data was utilized as preparing information and 30% as test data. In the last development of the examination, the k-crease cross-endorsement procedure was utilized for stacked visuals. Test set of data visuals are showed up in

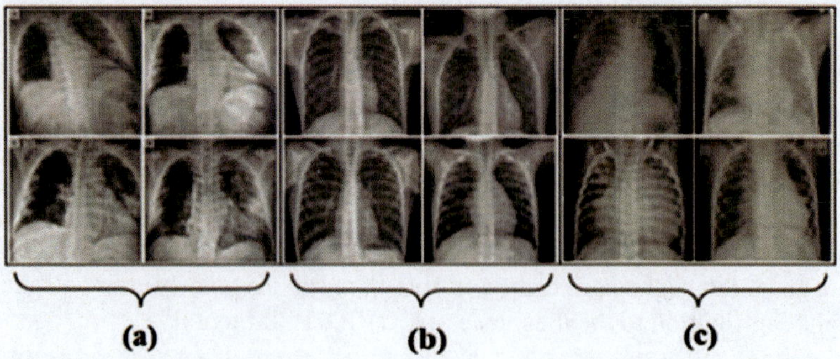

Fig. 1 **a** Visuals of COVID-19 affected lung images, **b** visual of normal image of lung, **c** pneumonia chest visuals

Fig. 1. The input images undergo a preprocessing stage. Contrast enhancement techniques are applied to increase the contrast of the image. Morphological operations are applied on the image to segment the required area. Desired features are extracted from the segmented area and passed over to the neural network which finally analyses the stages of the image as abnormal or normal.

3.2 Deep Learning System

Squeeze Net is an DL learning framework with an info size of 224 × 224 pixels, contained convolutionary levels, pooling levels, ReLU, and Fire levels. Complex and easy bypass interfaces have also culminated in an increase in precision over the Squeeze Net vanilla design. Ironically, the easy bypass allowed it possible to increase precision better than the complicated bypass.

Figure 4 presents the plan of stage. Squeeze Net system produced more Fig. 5 UMAP of the pre-trained network feature space profitable results, with roughly 50 times less features than the Alex Net system, reduce the price of the system [11]. While the layer nuances are referred to in the Squeeze Net structure, the fire (Fl2, Fl3, Fl9) levels seems like another layer containing two divisions, explicitly the compression and expansion parts. This framework uses just a 1 × 1 convolution channel in the fire layer compression part of the info visual. In the expansion parcel, the information visual utilizations both 1 × 1 and 3 × 3 convolution channels.

Fig. 2 Block diagram of the proposed system

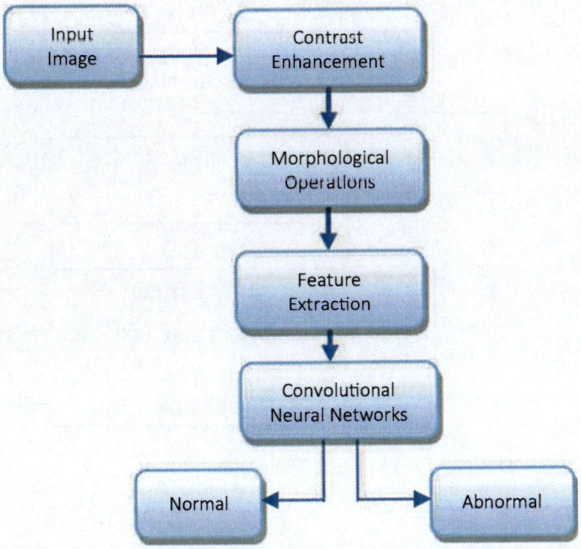

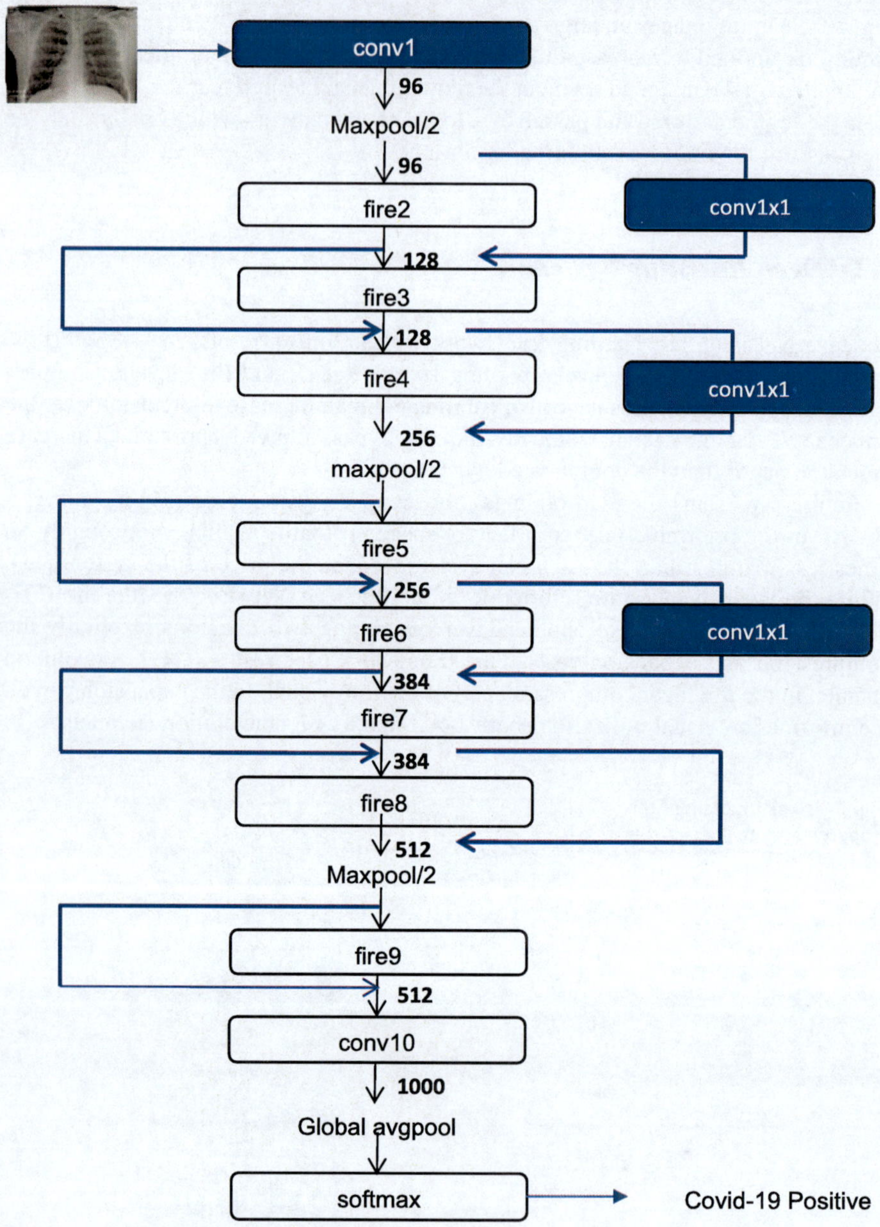

Fig. 3 Design of the Squeeze Net system

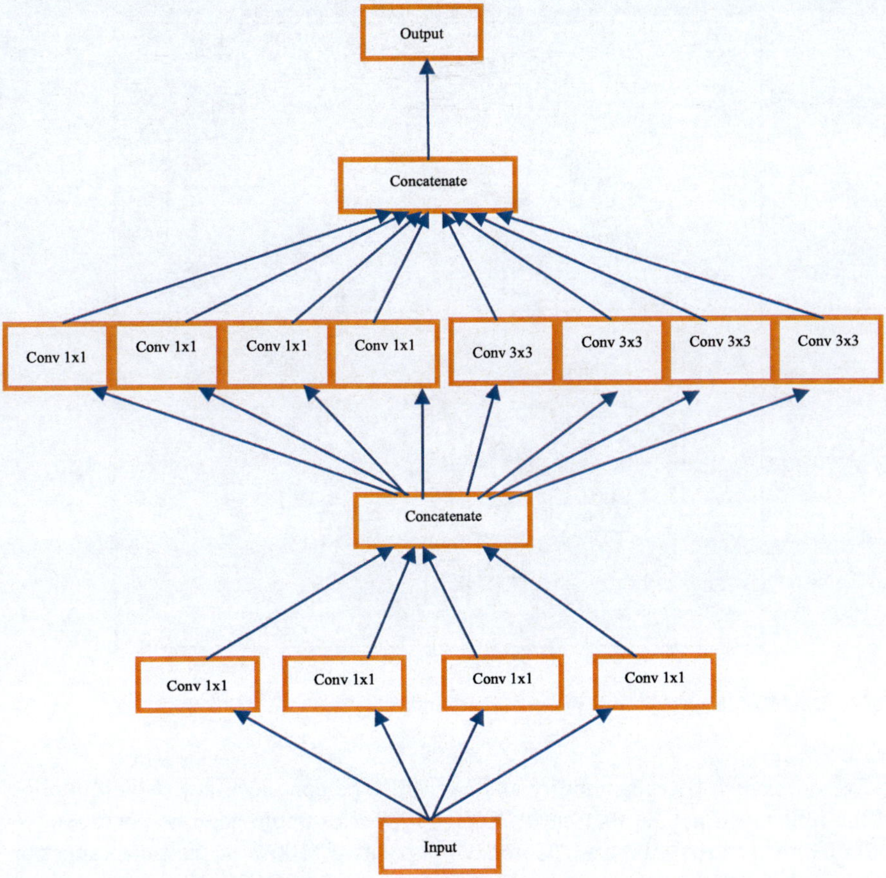

Fig. 4 Fire levels of Squeeze Net

4 Results and Discussion

Here this area will discuss brief about the experimental analysis of Squeeze Net. When an X-ray image is given as input, these are converted into greyscale and filters are used enhance, contrast of the image. Thereby improving several features of images. Then these are segmented by performing morphological operation over CT images. While preprocessing an image a small matrix called kernel convolutional matrix is used for blurring, sharpening, edge detection, and more. Here after all the process is done, they are given to CNN model, here to be specific its Squeeze Net which classifies as normal or affected tissue. These estimations uncovers that the programmed COVID-19 identifier acquires ~90–92% exactness of our information assortment dependent on X-ray visuals—no additional data, tallying actual position, populace thickness, and so forth, have been utilized to prepare this gadget.

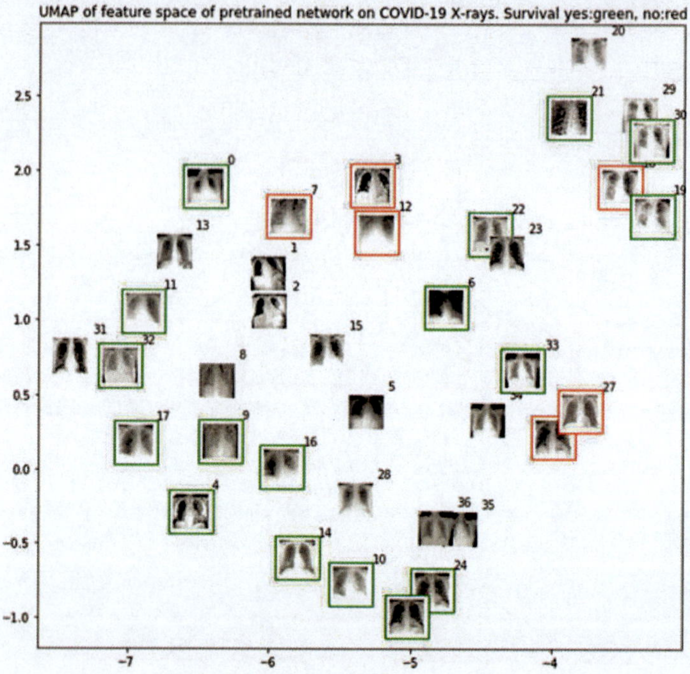

Fig. 5 UMAP of feature space of pre-trained network

We do have 100% adaptability and over 90% percent accuracy, which implies of the influenced people that have COVID-19 (for example genuine positive), we will effectively group them as "Coronavirus positive" 100% of the time using our framework. For affected persons who may not contain COVID-19 (i.e., real negatives), about 80 per cent of the time using our system may be precisely grouped as "COVID-19 negative." As the training history plot reveals that the network is not over-equipped, even though it has restricted training data (Fig. 6).

Being able to precisely identify COVID-19 with 100% precision is good; in reality, the affected persons should be assured that they are COVID-19 negative, and then make them go to their house and get in touch with their families and friends, so that the infection can be extended further. The false positive rate should be handled carefully. A healthy individual not be recognized as "Coronavirus positive," detach them with other positive COVID-19 influenced people, and afterward communicate an illness to somebody who did not really have the infection. Affectability and explicitness adjusting is testing especially infectious diseases that can be immediately spread, for example, COVID-19.

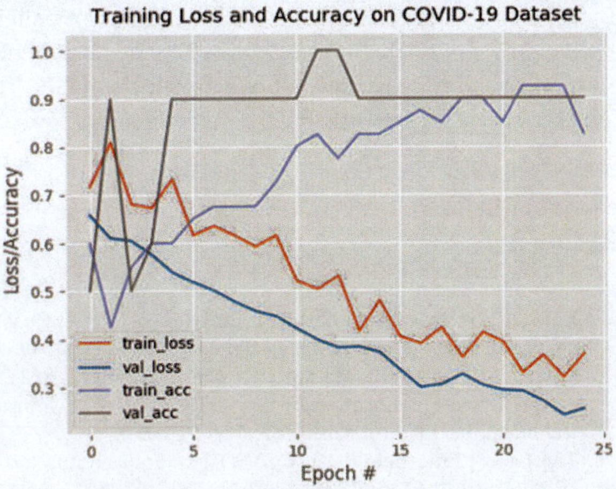

Fig. 6 Precision and loss curves

5 Limitations, Improvements, and Future Work

Clinics needs more rooms to treat the quantity of COVID-19 cases and, given influenced people rights and secrecy, it is much harder to gather quality clinical visual informational collections in an ideal way. I envision we will have greater COVID-19 visual informational collections in the following 12-year and a half; yet until further notice, we can just do what we have. It is plausible that our framework comprises of learning styles that are not related COVID-19, and they are only contrasts among the two information parts. A trained medical professional and through checking would be required to verify the results of the COVID-19 detector. At last, future COVID-19 detectors are going to be multimodal. For now, we are just utilizing visual evidence better automated COVID-19 detectors can exploit several non-visual data streams, including affected person vitals, population level, geographic position, etc. In fact, visual data of its own is not appropriate for this form of use.

6 Conclusion

This article uses an effective network architecture to detect any abnormality produced by COVID-19 by means of chest X-ray visuals. Experiments were conducted to evaluate the performance of the neural network in the COVID-19 set of data utilizing two approaches flat group and hierarchical group. While sets of data are still incipient and thus restricted in the amount of visuals applicable to COVID-19, efficient research on deep neural networks has been rendered possible by the use of transfer learning and data optimization techniques. With regard to the evaluation, the suggested method brought improvements compared to baseline work with a precision of 93.9%, COVID-19 sensitivity of 96.8% and positive prediction of 100% with a computational efficiency of more than 30%. We believe that the present proposal is a promising candidate for integration into medical devices or even mobile phones for physicians and for assistance in the diagnosis of COVID-19, given that more mature COVID-19 visual sets of data are made present.

References

1. Rothe C, Schunk M (2020) Transmission of 2019-nCoV infection from an asymptomatic contact in Gerseveral N. Engl J Med 382:970–971. https://doi.org/10.1056/nejmc2001468
2. Aswathy SU, Jarin T, Mathews R, Nair LM, Rroan M (2020) CAD systems for automatic detection and classification of Covid-19 in nano CT lung image by using machine learning technique. Int J Pharm Res. ISSN: 0975-2366
3. The Lancet Editorial (2020) COVID-19: too little, too late? Lancet 395:755. https://doi.org/10.1016/S0140-6736(20)30522-5
4. Razai MS, Doerholt K, Ladhani S, Oakeshott P (2020) Coronavirus infection 2019 (Covid-19): a guide for UK GPs, vol 800, pp 1–5
5. Peng X, Xu X, Li Y, Cheng L, Zhou X, Ren B (2020) Transmission routes of 2019-nCoV and controls in dental practice
6. Huang C, Jin Q, Wang J, Cao B (2020) Clinical features of affected persons infected with 2019 novel coronavirus in Wuhan, China. The Lancet 395(10223):497–506
7. https://www.nationalgeographic.com/science/2020/02/here-is-what-coronavirus-does-tothe-body/ 20.03.2020
8. https://www.worldometers.info/coronavirus/
9. Castiglioni I, Ippolito D, Interlenghi M, Monti CB, Salvatore C, Schiaffino S, Polidori A, Gandola D, Messa C, Sardanelli F (2020) Artificial intelligence applied on chest X-ray can aid in the diagnosis of COVID-19 infection: a first experience from Lombardy, Italy. MedRxiv
10. Maguolo G, Nanni L (2004) A critic evaluation of methods for COVID-19 automatic recognition from X-ray visuals. arXiv:2004.12823
11. Toğaçar M, Ergen B, Cömert Z (2020) COVID-19 recognition utilizing deep learning models to exploit social mimic optimization and configuration chest X-ray visuals utilizing fuzzy color and stacking approaches. Comput Biol Med

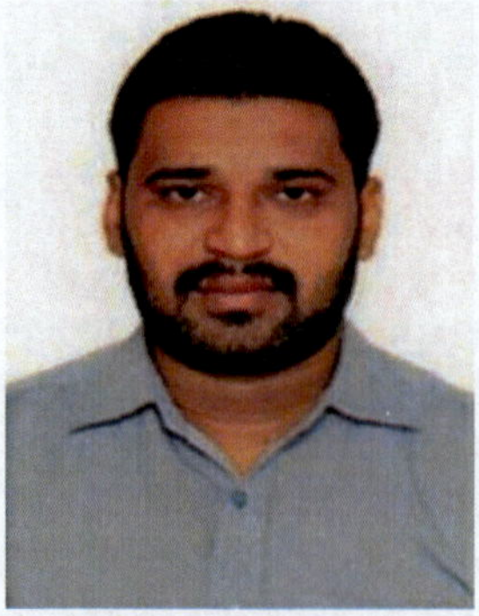

J. Syed Nizamudeen Ahmed received the Bachelor of Technology in Information and Communication Technologies in 2015, Master of Technology in Information and Communication Technologies in 2017 and pursuing Doctor of Philosophy degree in Information Technology and Engineering under regular mode in the department of Centre for Information Technology and Engineering, Manonmaniam Sundaranar University, Tirunelveli, Tamil Nadu, India. His research interests include Image Processing, Computer Vision, Data Analytics, Digital and Signal Image Processing.

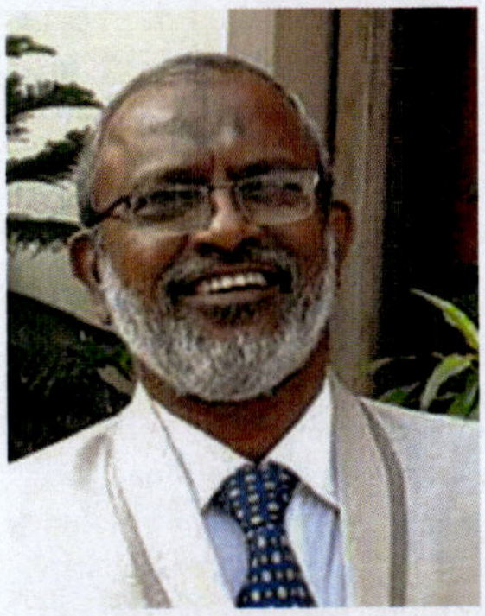

Dr. M. Mohamed Sathik M.Tech., M.Phil., M.Sc., M.B.A., M.S., Ph.D. (CS)., Ph.D. (C&IT) from Manonmaniam Sundaranar University, Tirunelveli, Tamil Nadu, India has so far guided more than 35 research scholars. He has published more than 150 papers in International Journals/proceedings and also two books. Currently he is the Principal, Sadakathullah Appa College, Rahmath Nagar, and Tirunelveli. He is a member of curriculum development committee of various universities and autonomous colleges of Tamil Nadu. His specializations are VRML, Image Processing and Sensor Networks.

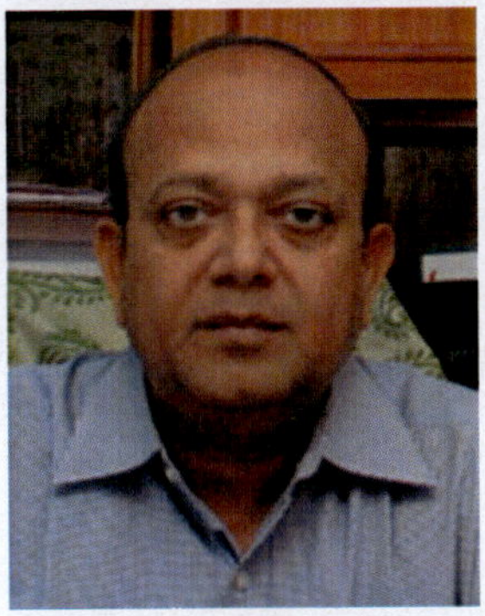

Krishnan Nallaperumal received M.Sc. degree in Mathematics from Madurai Kamaraj University, Madurai, India in 1985, M.Tech degree in Computer and Information Sciences from Cochin University of Science and Technology, Kochi, India in 1988 and Ph.D. degree in Computer Science and Engineering from Manonmaniam Sundaranar University, Tirunelveli. Currently, he is the Professor and Head of Center for Information Technology and Engineering of Manonmaniam Sundaranar University. His research interests include Signal and Image Processing, Remote Sensing, Visual Perception, and mathematical morphology fuzzy logic and pattern recognition. He has authored three books, edited 18 volumes and published 150 scientific papers in Journals/proceedings/books and has produced 35 Ph.D. Scholars. He is a Senior Member of the IEEE and chair of IEEE Madras Section Signal Processing/Computational Intelligence/Computer Joint Societies Chapter.

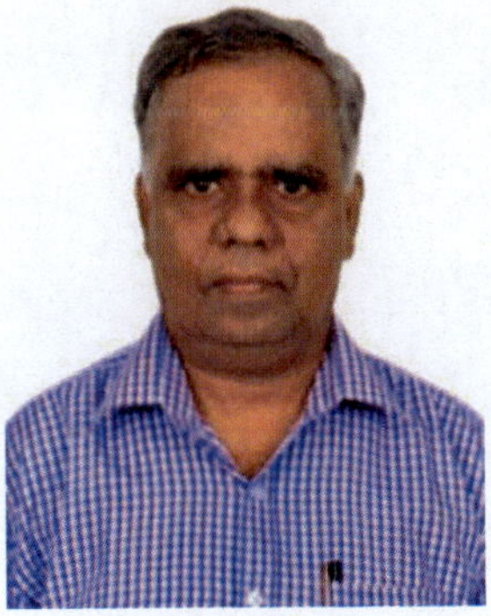

Dr. Senthamarai Kannan Kaliaperumal received the M.Sc, M.Phil., Ph.D., (Statistics) degree from Annamalai University, Tamil Nadu, India and M.Tech. Ph.D., (C&IT) degree from Manonmaniam Sundaranar University, Tamil Nadu, India. He is currently as Senior Professor and Head, Department of Statistics, Dean of Science, Manonmaniam Sundaranar University, India. He has published more than 200 research papers in International/National journals/proceedings/books and has produced 45 Ph.D. Scholars also received prestigious honors/awards from UGC-BSR, Academic Excellence Awards, UGC-SAP DRS, DST-FIST, UGC Innovative Proramme etc. His current research \interests include Stochastic Processes, Queuing Theory, Time Series, Outliers, Data Mining and Image Processing.

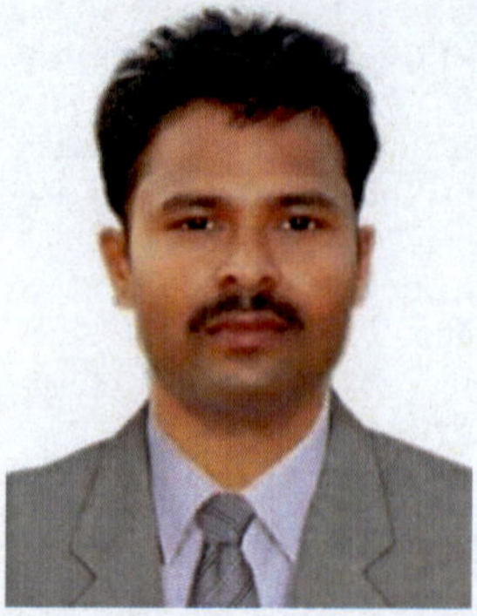

Dr. Kumar Parasuraman received the M.Tech. degree in Information Technology in 2008 and the Doctor of Philosophy in Information Technology-Computer Science and Engineering in 2012 from ManonmaniamSundaranar University, Abishekapatti, Tirunelveli, Tamil Nadu, India and M.B.A.degree in Systems from Alagappa University, Karaikudi, Tamil Nadu, India in 2018. He is currently an Assistant Professor (Stage III) in the department of the Centre for Information Technology and Engineering, ManonmaniamSundaranar University, Abishekapatti, Tirunelveli, Tamil Nadu, India. He has published more than 100 research papers in International/National journals/proceedings/books. His current research interests include signal and image processing, visual perception, Cyber Security, Computer Networks, Pattern Recognition, and Data Analytics.

Voting Classification Approach for Breast Cancer Detection

Ravi Kumar Barwal, Neeraj Raheja, and Pankaj Kumar

Abstract The cancer of breast is the most frequent type of cancer among ladies worldwide following by the lung cancer. A cycle of regeneration procedures in body is maintained with the cells. In general, the natural functioning of the body is maintained by balancing the development and death rate of cells. The pipeline of breast cancer detection includes many tasks such as preprocessing, segmentation, feature extraction and classification. In this research work, voting classification approach is applied for the breast cancer detection. The proposed approach improve performance in comparison to existing models in compliance with precision, recall and accuracy.

Keywords Breast cancer · GLCM · Threshold segmentation · Voting classification

1 Introduction

The technique of image processing is becoming progressively advanced and the trend is to develop more and more automation. The technology of image processing aims to improve crude imagery got from various sources or images clicked in typical day-to-day life to serve different purposes. Digital Image Processing (DIP) is an area of special importance in CSE and has its roots to the multiple areas as well. The significance of image processing technology in the healthcare sector is not hidden from anyone. This technology process images in digital manner using artificial intelligence algorithms. The effect of digitized pictures on present day culture is so incredible, and is a crucial part of science and technology. As of now, the sample of bloods are taken to laboratory and prepared with different substrates to generate outcomes. Image indexing and extraction based on content- has been a significant exploration zone in software engineering throughout the previous few years. Numerous digitized images are usually clicked and stored in different databases in different formats. Thus,

R. K. Barwal (✉) · N. Raheja
CSE Department, Maharishi Markandeshwar (Deemed to be University), Mullana 133207, India

P. Kumar
CSE Department, Government College for Women, Shahzadpur, Ambala, India

N. Marriwala et al. (eds.), *Emergent Converging Technologies and Biomedical Systems*, Lecture Notes in Electrical Engineering 841,
https://doi.org/10.1007/978-981-16-8774-7_55

enormous datasets containing images are being made and utilized in numerous applications [1]. The cancer of breast is the most frequent type of cancer among ladies worldwide following by the lung cancer. A cycle of regeneration procedures in body is maintained with the cells. In general, the natural functioning of the body is maintained by balancing the development and death rate of cells. In any case, this is not generally the situation. Once in a while, an unusual circumstance takes place which leads to abnormal growth in some cells. Consequently, cancer occurs in a specific area of the body and spreads to other areas [2]. Distinct kinds of cancer may occur in individual's body and the cancer of breast is one that is considered as a serious health concern. Women have more susceptibility against breast cancer as compared to men because of the anatomy of the human body. Several reasons may cause breast cancer such as age, medical history, fatness and drinking, etc. The breast of a woman is made up of nipples, ducts and fatty tissues and lobules. In general, epithelial tumors are developed inside the lobules and ducts which cause tumor in the breast later on. The cancer after its initiation disseminates to the other areas of the body.

Breast cancers generally are of two types: Benign and Malignant. The first case has non-cancerous cells that do not cause death. However, in some scenarios, these cells could turn into cancerous cells. The defense system of body referred to as "sac" normally is useful in segregating the benign tumors from harmful cells and expels them from the body. The second type of cancer initiates when cells are growing abnormally and quickly. These cells can spread to the neighboring tissues [3]. The malignant tissue's nuclei is often larger than the regular tissue and can be life threatening [4]. Breast cancer is considered as the heterogeneous disease whose formation is done with different entities such as distinctive biological, histological and clinical attributes. The radiology images are deployed to carry out the clinical screening such as mammography, ultrasound imaging and MRI.

The preprocessing aids the localization of region for irregularity detection. The major concern in mammogram preprocessing faces is to outline the Pectoral Muscle (PM) boundary from the remaining breast area. The PMs generally occur in MLO views of the mammograms. The occurrence of PMs in the MLO view may disturb automated recognition of lesions and can intensify the false positive (FP) alarms. Most of the studies backed the elimination of PMs for making the diagnostic accuracy of the CAD system better. Therefore, it is highly important to successfully remove PMs for preventing false detection [5]. Additionally, it not only decreases the time complexity but also improves the accuracy besides preventing the intra-observation inconsistencies.

Mammograms do not deliver good contrast between healthy glandular breast tissues and cancerous tissues and between the malignant lesions and the background particularly in dense breasts. Poor contrast is inherent to mammography images. The Beer-Lambert equation states that the thicker the tissue is, the rarer the photons go through it. This implies that the X-ray beam goes through malignant breast tissues and normal glandular tissues [6] in dense breast tissue will not create attenuation with huge difference between the two tissues, and therefore less contrast between the healthy glandular and cancerous tissues will occur. Noise is the other common issue in mammograms. The non-uniform image brightness in the parts representing the same tissues causes noise in mammograms [7]. The non-uniform distribution of photons may be the reason of noise. This is known as quantum noise. This noise degrades the quality of images particularly in small objects with low contrast, for example, a mini tumor in a dense breast. Increase in exposure time may reduce quantum noise. The occurrence of noise in a mammogram makes it grainy. The grainy appearance decreases the discernibility of some features in the image specifically for small objects with low contrast representing the scenario for a mini tumor in a dense breast.

2 Literature Review

Wang et al. [8] projected a densely deep supervision technique for increasing the detection sensitivity in efficient manner. To achieve this, multi-layer attributes were employed. In addition, a threshold loss was put forward for presenting voxel-level adaptive threshold to determine the image as discerning cancerous or non-cancerous. Consequently, great sensitivity with was attained with less false positives (FPs). A dataset gathered from 219 patients that comprised 745 cancer regions were executed to calculate the accuracy of projected technique. The outcomes of experiment proved that the sensitivity provided through the projected technique was counted 95% with 0.84 false positives. An effectual cancer detection system was obtained from the projected technique to analyze the breast with the help of ABUS.

Khasana et al. [9] intended to implement watershed transform (WT) approach during segmentation procedure for creating the position of the tumor and distinguishing the matters on the basis of background. Afterward, the thresholding binaries were employed for splitting the tumor image in the form of an object. In the last stage, the area of cancer was computed. The outcomes indicated that the intended algorithm had provided the accuracy and error rate of around 88.65 and 11.35% of the overall tested data. The testing results showed that the intended algorithm was useful to detect the breast cancer with the help of ultrasound image.

Kavya et al. [10] put forward a strategy to detect the breast cancer in which imaging schemes namely, mammography and thermography were implemented. The computer aided diagnosis (CAD) tool was deployed as an effective technique for segmenting and classifying the digital images. The data taken from hospital was analyzed using this technique. The Cyber-physical system (CPS) was exploited to collect the data and share the details to particular systems. Furthermore, the network was integrated, human was interacted with system and system was made flexible, scalable and optimized with the help of CPS. The suggested approach was capable of detecting the breast cancer and providing high safety for the patients for which errors rates were mitigated and the data was monitored.

Varma et al. [11] introduced an approach for analyzing the digital mammograms. For this purpose, texture segmentation was employed for visualizing and detecting the images. Afterward, the attributes were extracted effectively due to which enhanced detection was obtained and proper action was taken for diminishing the risks related to breast cancer. Moreover, the introduced approach was adaptable to alleviate the processing time and enhance the processing speed. The final output images demonstrated that the introduced approach was efficient to outline the anomalies in the breast tissue and successfully detected the breast cancer.

Soliman et al. [12] designed an effective system for detecting the breast cancer with image processing methods. The significant attributes of the breast were extracted from the region of interest (ROI) whose segmentation was done from the thermal input image. Afterward, a neural network (NN) classification algorithm was utilized to categorize the image as cancerous or normal on the basis of these features. A benchmark dataset was applied to quantify the designed system and a success rate was obtained around 96.51%. The outcomes revealed that the designed system was efficient.

Liu et al. [13] presented two diverse microwave imaging techniques for detecting the breast cancer. In the initial technique, SAR an high-quality imagery technique was utilized and the second technique was planned on the basis of inverse scattering quantitative imaging technique for reconstructing the relative permittivity for the breast cancer. The presented techniques were tested on 2D simplified breast phantom. The outcomes of testing depicted the efficiency of presented techniques for detecting the breast cancer cell with good resolution.

Razavi et al. [14] recommended a computer aided diagnosis (CAD) method in which preprocessing median and Gaussian filters were deployed first of all. The cells of interest areas were segmented using an adaptive thresholding technique and watershed algorithm. Thereafter, the recommended technique was utilized to compute the ratio amid green and red FISH signals of all decomposable cells. Enormous Fluorescence in situ hybridization (FISH) images were deployed for presenting the automatic gene expression of epidemic growing feature receptors-2 (HER2) status. The outcomes exhibited the effectiveness of the recommended method to specify the HER2 state of probable patients.

Sangeetha et al. [15] established a new mechanism for detecting the breast asymmetry and micro calcification cancer cells in which various methods of digital image processing (DIP) were integrated that had not utilized in this research area. The established mechanism assisted in detecting the breast cancer in initial phase. An end to end (E2E) solution was acquired from this mechanism. The outcomes generated through the established mechanism were highly accurate in terms of true positive (TP) and true negative (TN).

Yin et al. [16] developed a new RAR algorithmic approach that planned a neighborhood pair-wise correlation-based weighting for dealing with the negative impacts of both artifact and glandular tissues. The maximum combination of these coefficients was applied to weight, sum and time-shift the backscattered signals. The three-dimensional finite-difference-time-domain models were exploited to evaluate the developed algorithm in anatomic and dielectric manner. The developed RAR algorithm had potential to recognize and detect the cancer under various scenarios. The outcomes validated that the developed algorithm was applicable for breast cancer screening.

3 Research Methodology

This noise degrades the quality of images particularly in small objects with low contrast, for example, a mini tumor in a dense breast. Increase in exposure time may reduce quantum noise. The occurrence of noise in a mammogram makes it grainy. The grainy appearance decreases the discernibility of some features in the image specifically for small objects with low contrast representing the scenario for a mini tumor in a dense breast.

Various phases are executed to predict the breast cancer and these phases are defined as.

3.1 *Data Acquisition*

This phase includes the collection of data from distinct clinical organizations to conduct tests.

3.2 *Data Preprocessing*

The entirety is accomplished and the data is analyzed to deploy the machine learning methods and the preprocessing is performed on the data. The redundant attributes are removed from the dataset in order to transmit the clean and de-noised data for enhancing the efficacy of training framework.

3.3 *Feature Selection*

The GLCM algorithm is applied in this phase for the feature extraction. This algorithm can be used for extracting multiple texture features. For this purpose, the considered metrics are as follows:

G denotes applied no. of Gray levels.

μ indicates the mean of P.

μ_x, μ_y represent the means while σ_x, σ_y denote standard deviation P_x, and P_y, respectively. $P_x(i)$ Signifies the ith entry in the marginal-probability matrix achieved after adding the rows of $P(i, j)$.

Contrast: This metric measure the local variations of an image.

$$CONTRAST = \sum_{n=0}^{G-1} n^2 \left\{ \sum_{i=1}^{G} \sum_{j=1}^{G} P(i, j) \right\}, \quad |i - j| = n \tag{1}$$

This metric that computes variance in contrast or local intensity favors aids from $P(i, j)$ outside the diagonal: $i \neq j$.

Homogeneity: This metric measures the nearness of the spreading of components in the GLCM to the diagonal of GLCM.

$$\sum_i \sum_j \frac{P_d[i, j]}{1 + |i - j|} \tag{2}$$

Local Homogeneity, Inverse Difference Moment (IDM):

$$IDM = \sum_{i=0}^{G-1} \sum_{j=0}^{G-1} \frac{1}{1 + (i - j)^2} P(i, j) \tag{3}$$

The image homogeneity also affects IDM. IDM gets mini support from inhomogeneous regions $(i \neq j)$ as a result of the weighting factor $\left(1 + (i - j)^2\right)^{-1}$.

The low value of IDM for inhomogeneous images, and a comparatively greater value for homogeneous image is obtained as the result.

Entropy: This metric measures the content of the information. It is a measure of the unpredictability of distributed intensity. Inhomogeneous images have low 1st order entropy. A homogeneous image. On the other hand, has a great entropy.

$$-\sum_{i=0}^{G-1} \sum_{j=0}^{G-1} P(i, j) \times \log(P(i, j)) \tag{4}$$

Correlation: This metric measures the gray level linear dependency amongst the pixels at the definite positions regarding each other.

$$\sum_{i=0}^{G-1} \sum_{j=0}^{G-1} \frac{\{i \times j\} \times P(i, j) - \{\mu_x \times \mu_y\}}{\sigma_x \times \sigma_y} \tag{5}$$

Sum of Squares, Variance:

$$VARIANCE = \sum_{i=0}^{G-1} \sum_{j=0}^{G-1} (1 - \mu)^2 P(i, j) \tag{6}$$

This attribute lays comparatively high weights on the components different from the average rate of $P(i, j)$.

4 Voting Classifier

The voting classifier is a machine learning model that trains the integration of multiple models and predicts the output (class) according to their higher chances for the selected class as a result.

It simply summarizes the findings of each classifier transmitted to the voting classifier and predicts the output phase according to the number of votes. The idea is that instead of building separate dedicated models and obtaining each of them, we create a single model that trains these types and predicts the output according to their combined votes for each output phase (Fig. 1).

Voting Classifier supports two types of votings.

4.1 *Hard Voting*

In hard voting, the predicted output class is a class with the highest majority of votes, i.e., the class which had the highest probability of being predicted by each of the classifiers.

In this case, the class that received the highest number of votes $N_c(y^t)$ will be chosen. Here, we predict the class label $\hat{y}$ via majority voting of each classifier.

$$\hat{y} = \arg\max(N_c(y_t^1), N_c(y_t^2), \ldots, N_c(y_t^n)) \tag{7}$$

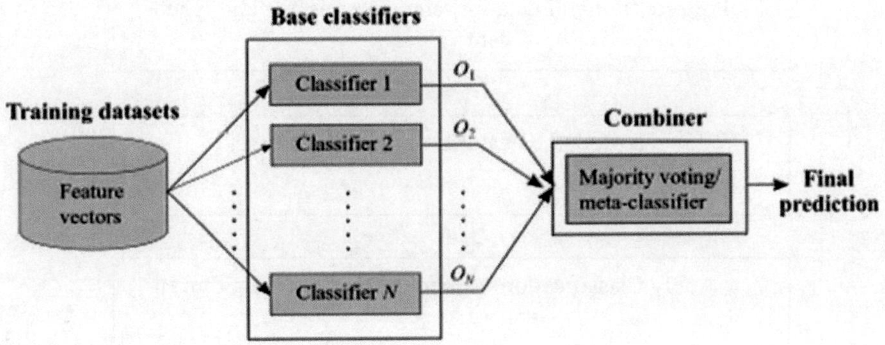

Fig. 1 Voting classifier

4.2 Soft Voting

For soft voting, the withdrawal phase is a prediction based on the proportion of opportunities given to that class.

$$\hat{y} = \arg\max \frac{1}{NClassifiers} \sum\nolimits_{Classifiers} (p1, p2, p3, \ldots pn) \tag{8}$$

This algorithm employs the input from the extracted features. Two classes are defined in this research work. The microarray cancer denotes that the person has probability of occurrence of microarray cancer. The normal is utilized for the person without any possibility of microarray cancer (Fig. 2).

5 Result and Discussion

The dataset is collected from the kaggle. The dataset is generally categorized into two labels. The anaconda is the tool of python which is used for the implementation of the

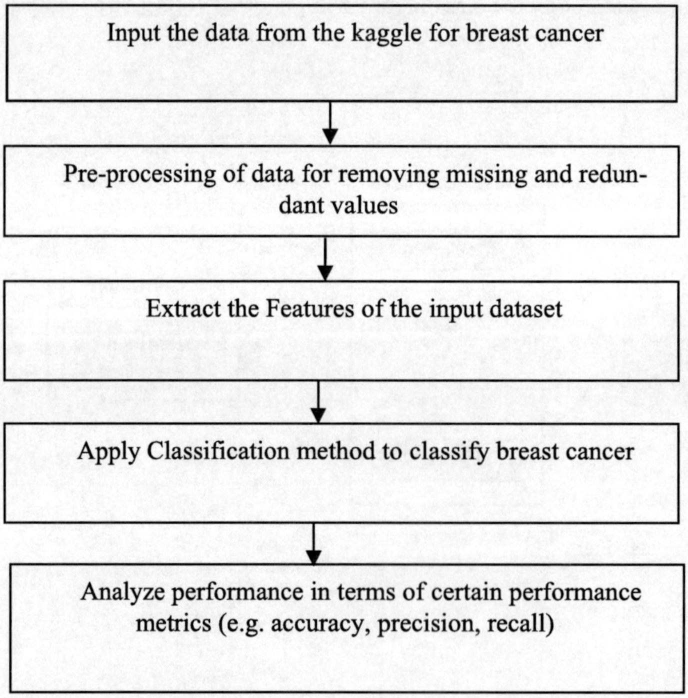

Fig. 2 Proposed methodology

proposed methodology. The various performance analysis parameters like accuracy, precision and recall.

Various presentation metrics are used to calculate the system performance of the classification system (existing and proposed system). These are described below:

$$Accuracy = \frac{Tp + Tn}{Tp + Fp + Tn + Fn} \tag{9}$$

The precision main motive is to calculate the true +ive (TP) units relative to false +ive (FP) units.

$$Precision = \frac{Tp}{Tp + Fp} \tag{10}$$

The main motive of recall is to calculate true +ive (TP) units in relation to false –ive (FN) units that are not at all classes. The arithmetic performance or expression form of recall parameter is declared in:

$$Recall = \frac{Tp}{Tp + Fn} \tag{11}$$

As shown in Fig. 3, the performance of random forest is compared with voting classification for the breast cancer prediction. It is analyzed that accuracy of voting classification is 96%, precision value is 76% and recall value is 78% which improve performance up to 5% (Table 1).

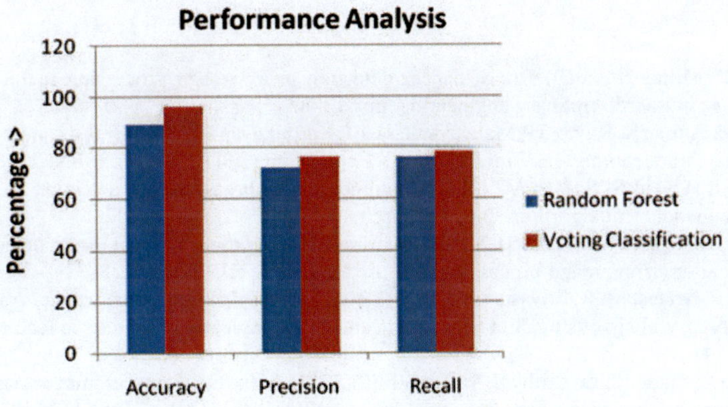

Fig. 3 Performance analysis

Table 1 Performance analysis

Performance parameter	Random forest (%)	Voting classification (%)
Accuracy	89	96
Precision	72	76
Recall	76	78

6 Conclusion

The survival rate of breast cancer has expanded, and a significant fall in the number of deaths due to these diseases has been noticed in the last few years. There are several factors behind this. One of the most considerable factors is the detection of this disorder in the early stage. The timely detection of this disease contributes significantly in the disease healing. It also offers deep insight of the disorder which further leads to the conclusion. The breast cancer detection has various phases which include preprocessing, segmentation, feature extraction and classification. The threshold-based strategy is applied for the segmentation. The textural feature extraction algorithm called GLCM is applied for the feature extraction and in the last voting classification method is applied for classifying the cancer of breast. The performance of the developed model is compared with standard models in the context of accuracy, precision and recall. It is been analyzed that results are optimized up to 7% for the breast cancer detection.

References

1. Sahni P, Mittal N (2019) Breast cancer detection using image processing techniques. In: Advances in interdisciplinary engineering, pp 813–823
2. Chtihrakkannan R, Kavitha P, Mangayar karasi T, Karthikeyan R (2019) Breast cancer detection using machine learning. Int J Innov Technol Explor Eng (IJITEE) 8(11). ISSN: 2278-3075
3. Patel VK, Uvaid S, Suthar AC (2012) Mammogram of breast cancer detection based using image enhancement algorithm. Int J Eng Technol Adv Eng 2(8):143–147
4. Yadav BK, Panse MS (2018) Virtual instrumentation based breast cancer detection and classification using image-processing. Int J Res Sci Innov (IJRSI) 5(4):25–31
5. Kumar R, Srivastava R, Srivastava S (2015) Detection and classification of cancer from microscopic biopsy images using clinically significant and biologically interpretable features. J Med Eng 1–14
6. Ramani R, Suthanthiravanithy S, Valarmathy S (2012) A survey of current image segmentation techniques for detection of breast cancer. Int J Eng Res Appl (IJERA) 2(5):1124–1129
7. Radha M, Adaekalavan S (2016) Mammogram of breast cancer detection based using image enhancement algorithm. Int J Adv Res Comput Commun Eng 5(7):218–221
8. Wang Y, Wang N, Xu M, Yu J, Qin C, Luo X, Yang X, Wang T, Li A, Ni D (2020) Deeply-supervised networks with threshold loss for cancer detection in automated breast ultrasound. IEEE Trans Med Imaging 866–876
9. Khasana U, Sigit R, Yuniarti H (2020) Segmentation of breast using ultrasound image for detection breast cancer. In: International electronics symposium (IES)

10. Kavya N, Usha N, Sriraam N, Sharath D, Ravi P (2018) Breast cancer detection using non-invasive imaging and cyber physical system. In: 3rd international conference on circuits, control, communication and computing (I4C), pp 1–4
11. Varma C, Sawant O (2018) An alternative approach to detect breast cancer using digital image processing techniques. In: International conference on communication and signal processing (ICCSP), pp 0134–0137
12. Soliman OO, Sweilam NH, Shawky DM (2018) Automatic breast cancer detection using digital thermal images. In: 9th Cairo international biomedical engineering conference (CIBEC), pp 110–113
13. Liu H, Shang X, Ye X (2018) Breast cancer detection using synthetic aperture radar imaging and distorted born iterative method. In: International applied computational electromagnetics society symposium - China (ACES), pp 1–2
14. Razavi S, Hatipoğlu G, Yalçın H (2017) Automatically diagnosing HER2 amplification status for breast cancer patients using large FISH images. In: 25th signal processing and communications applications conference (SIU), pp 1–4
15. Sangeetha R, Murthy K (2017) A novel approach for detection of breast cancer at an early stage by identification of breast asymmetry and microcalcification cancer cells using digital image processing techniques. In: 2nd international conference for convergence in technology (I2CT), pp 593–596
16. Yin T, Ali FH, Reyes-Aldasoro CC (2015) A robust and artifact resistant algorithm of ultrawideband imaging system for breast cancer detection. IEEE Trans Biomed Eng 62(6):1514–1525

Design and Development of Smart Bed to Monitor Infants

Vinayak Sharma, Rohan Mittal, and Ashwani Kumar Dubey

Abstract Presently, due to the increase in the number of working mothers in the world, caretaking of babies and monitoring have become a quotidian obstacle for many households as well as parents. Most of the functioning guardians send their youngsters to their grandparent's homes or to the infant care houses. Notwithstanding, the guardians cannot persistently watch their children all the time either in ordinary or unusual conditions. Parents in the present world have always been busy with their work in their vocational life hereby not getting abundant time to take care of their babies. It is widely a great problem for parents to constantly keep an eye on their newborn baby and its conditions while doing their work. In this paper, a smart bed is proposed to monitor the baby all time and take care of them via the mode of automation and sensing. In this, we monitor the baby's body temperature, pulse, crying, motion and bed-wetting through sensors. These boundaries are critical in deciding baby's conditions because they cannot tell anything or explain anything about any surrounding or environment. The estimation of the temperature and pulse gives a quick sign of whether a child is in any pain, while the estimation of bed-wetting can be utilized to decide if the infant is in proper solace. Ceaseless checking of crucial signs requires connection of sensors to the body that should be possible in several ways.

Keywords Bed-wetting · Body temperature · Cry detection · Infant · Heartbeat · Smart bed

1 Introduction

In this paper, we have targeted to build up an instrumented smart bed with sensors to differently screen extremely youthful age newborn children. It will be finished with the assistance of sensors that can recognize temperature variety and certain physiological states, for example, breathing rate and pulse, without the need to connect

V. Sharma · R. Mittal · A. K. Dubey (✉)
Department of Electronics and Communication Engineering, Amity School of Engineering and Technology, Amity University Uttar Pradesh, Noida, Uttar Pradesh, India

N. Marriwala et al. (eds.), *Emergent Converging Technologies and Biomedical Systems*, Lecture Notes in Electrical Engineering 841,
https://doi.org/10.1007/978-981-16-8774-7_56

wired sensors to the individual's body. The sensor yields will, at that point, be corresponded with normal breath rate and pulse. This will help in the automation in the medical industry that will solve many problems for the hospitals and medical institutions and will help working parents to constantly watch their children for effective treatment and on time medication. In most of the nations worldwide, male workers are favored to have high hold on jobs in the industry market more extensively than female workers. All over the globe, the industry force partaking of the female workers of substantial serviceable age has markedly seen an increase in the past gone years of the current generation.

In certain territories of the world, the normal expansion in female workforce cooperation has dropped down or even eased back marginally lately. The number of ladies having infants has prompted the precarious development in the deals of observing gadgets including infant screens. Therefore, people tend to spend money on the automation industry that is helpful for them to monitor their children.

2 Related Work

In certain territories of the world, the normal expansion in female workforce cooperation has dropped down or even eased back marginally lately. Due to this, newborn babies do not get the perfect care from the parents that are very much required for them and is of utmost priority for the parents also. To understand the existing infrastructure related to monitoring and care of the infants, an exhaustive review has been performed.

Lourino [1] has discussed in his paper the sleep disorders and have implemented a smart sensing bed to improve sleep time. Similarly, Gracia [2] has discussed and used big data analytics to stimulate sleep movements. Yousefi [3] has published a paper based on treatment of acute diseases related to bed sores and ulcers. Shivanantham [4] has published a paper on breathing pattern monitoring and detecting heartbeat. Many engineers and scientists have tried to develop smart beds for diversified applications. Brush [5] has also discussed the prevention of ulcers and bed sores in his paper. Symon et al. [6] have done research on smart baby monitoring systems using microcontroller Raspberry Pi. Dubey and Damke [7] have proposed image processing and IoT-based systems for baby monitoring. In a diversified work, Rajesh [8] implemented a baby monitoring system using wireless sensor networks. In [9], the authors have developed a smart baby monitoring cradle system consisting detection of movement, cry and temperature. In [10], the authors have developed a system to monitor the elderly people or paralyzed people.

Fisher [11] discussed the urinary incontinence and developed a sensor material. Similar work on smart bed monitoring is also done by various researchers in [12] using various technologies like IoT and other computing techniques. Gaddam [13] has created a smart digital home care for elder people. Some researchers have done work in the field of improving respiration rate and rehabilitation also to improve the patient's life [14, 15]. An innovative research is done by J. Kim to implement self-tracking device that will track our activities like sleep and dieting [16].

In the literature, there is no complete solution for the monitoring of infants. Therefore, it is highly needed to develop a smart bed which itself takes care of infant's position, bed-wetting, crying, movements, temperature monitoring, etc., and update the situation of the infant with the parents and caretakers.

3 Methodology

Based on the exhaustive literature review, it has been found that a lot more work needs to be done to make bed even smarter.

3.1 Proposed Design of Smart Bed

The proposed design of smart bed is shown through block diagrams in Figs. 1, 2, 3, 4 and 5. In the proposed smart bed, there are primarily five sensing modules such as (i) bed-wetting sensors and alarm module; (ii) cry sensing and alarm module; (iii) temperature sensing and display module; (iv) heartbeat sensing and display module; and (v) IR sensor module for position monitoring.

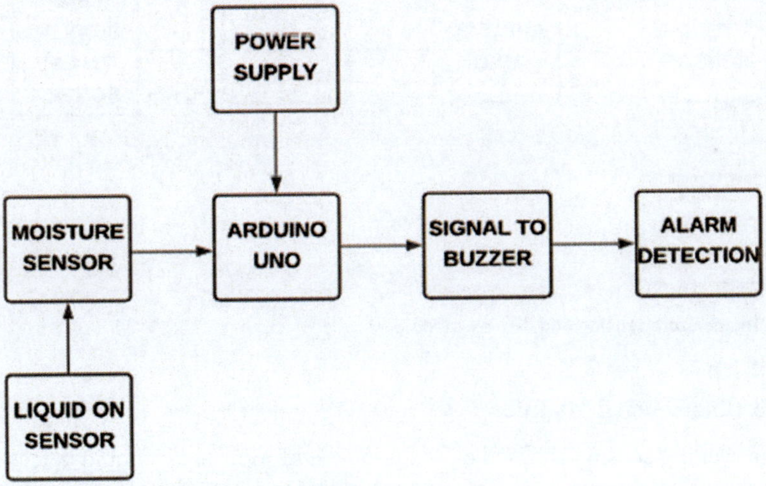

Fig. 1 Bed-wetting sensing and alarm module

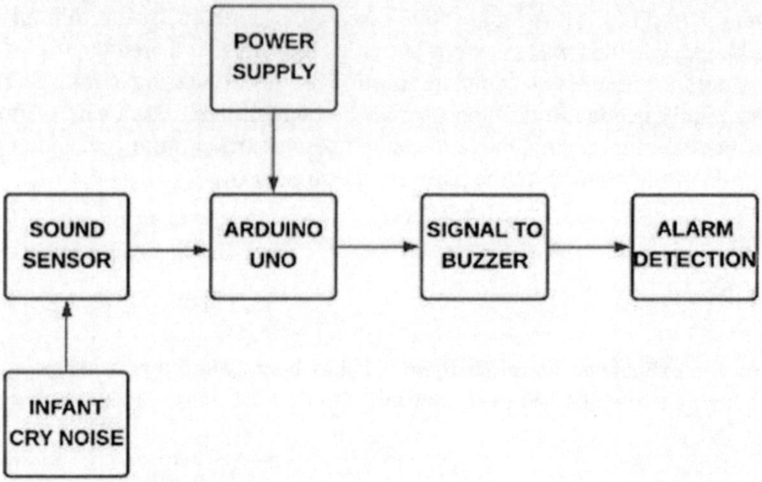

Fig. 2 Cry sensing and alarm module

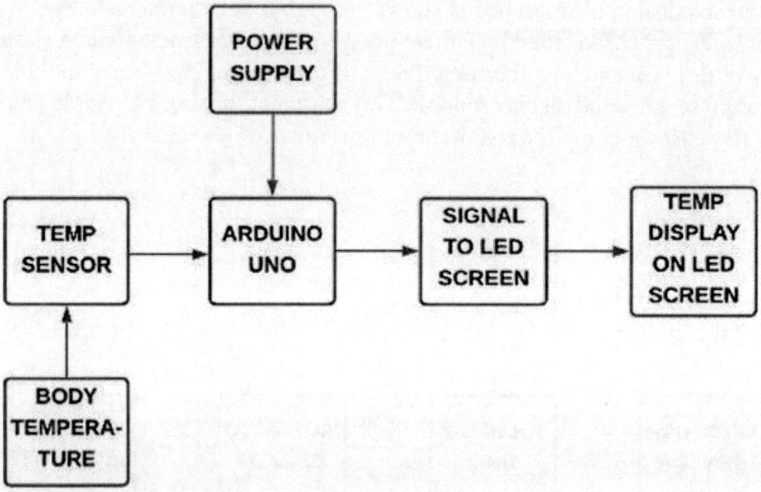

Fig. 3 Temperature sensing and display module

Bed-Wetting Sensing Module

The bed-wetting sensing is based on the principle of moisture or liquid detection. It detects the dielectric permittivity of the surrounding medium that is water or urination of the infant in this scenario. This sensor creates a voltage change that is proportional to the water content present in the surrounding. It will send the signal or will indicate that the circuit is completed responding to the buzzer to ring the alarm. This will give response to the user that the bed is wet, and some liquid is detected. The complete

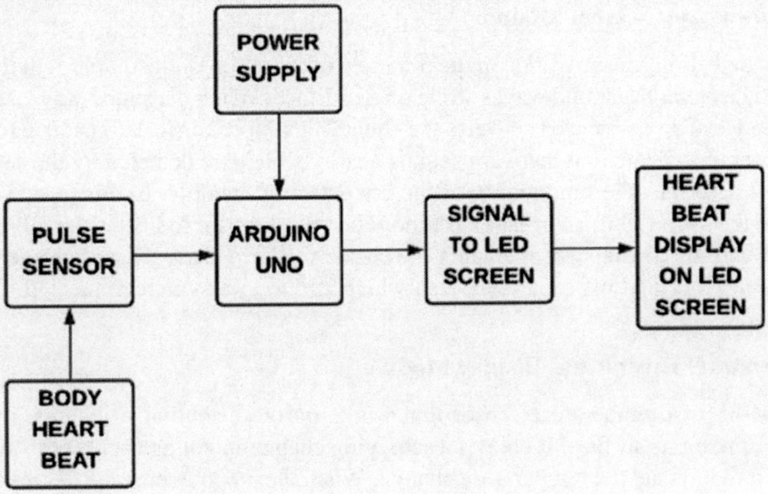

Fig. 4 Heartbeat sensing and display module

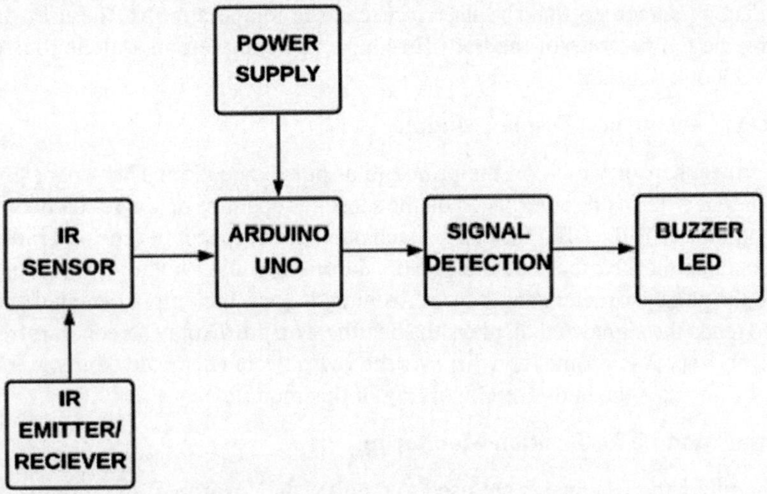

Fig. 5 IR sensor module for position monitoring

bed-wetting system is shown in Fig. 1. In this system, a supply is given to the moisture sensor with the help of Arduino while the buzzer is connected to the moisture sensor. Whenever the circuit is completed from the sensor side, it will make the buzzer to ring the alarm.

Cry Sensing and Alarm Module

The cry detection sensor works on the principle of vibration of the diaphragm that is caused whenever the sound waves strike on its surface. When the sound waves touch the sound sensor, the sensor converts the sound signal to electrical signal triggering the buzzer to indicate that there are sounds nearby which are detected by the sensor. Figure 2 describes the functioning of the cry detection module. In this, a supply is given to the sound sensor through Arduino. The sound sensor indicates the falling of sound waves on its diaphragm leading the buzzer to alarm. This sensor has a feature that it can be turned off separately also which is due to a switch connected to the circuit.

Temperature Sensing and Display Module

The LM-35 is a temperature sensor that works on the detection of change in the temperature on its surface. It creates a satisfying change in voltage across the terminals of it to indicate the temperature change. When the 5 V power supply is given to this sensor through Arduino, it indicates the change in temperature and notifies the value to display the temperature that is detected by the sensor. The sensor refreshes itself in every 2 s to get the newest value of temperature, and the Arduino sends it to the display screen so that the user can read the temperature of the user that is checking the temperature of the body. In Fig. 3, the complete module is illustrated through a block diagram.

Heartbeat Sensing and Display Module

The heartbeat sensor works on the principle of pulse detection. The sensor gives a digital output when a finger is placed on the sensor. It operates on the fundamentals of light modulation as the LED flashes on each pulse with respect to time and indicates and calculates the heartbeat of the person. In this module, when power supply is given to the pulse oximeter sensor from Arduino, it gives the output detected and the Arduino reads the signal and displays the heartbeat on the display screen. It refreshes at a rate of every 2 s gap and then displays the newest value detected from the sensor. Figure 4 illustrates the end-to-end working of this module.

IR Sensor Module for Position Monitoring

In this module, the IR sensors are used to monitor the position of the infants in real time. The IR sensors detect the presence of IR rays on the photodiode and indicate the results. In this system, we try to determine whether the infant is in the correct position or not. That is when the infant comes between the path of the IR receiver and transmitter, the sensor will give us a buzz output to know that the infant is not in the correct place. This situation will only take place when the infant is at the edge of the bed which will help us to alarm that the child may fall from the bed. Also, as the models have LEDs as alarms for IR sensors, it can also be used as a foot light so that the person does not fall due to less vision at night. In Fig. 5, the working of IR sensors is explained in a much simpler way.

The process flowcharts of the proposed smart bed are shown in Fig. 6.

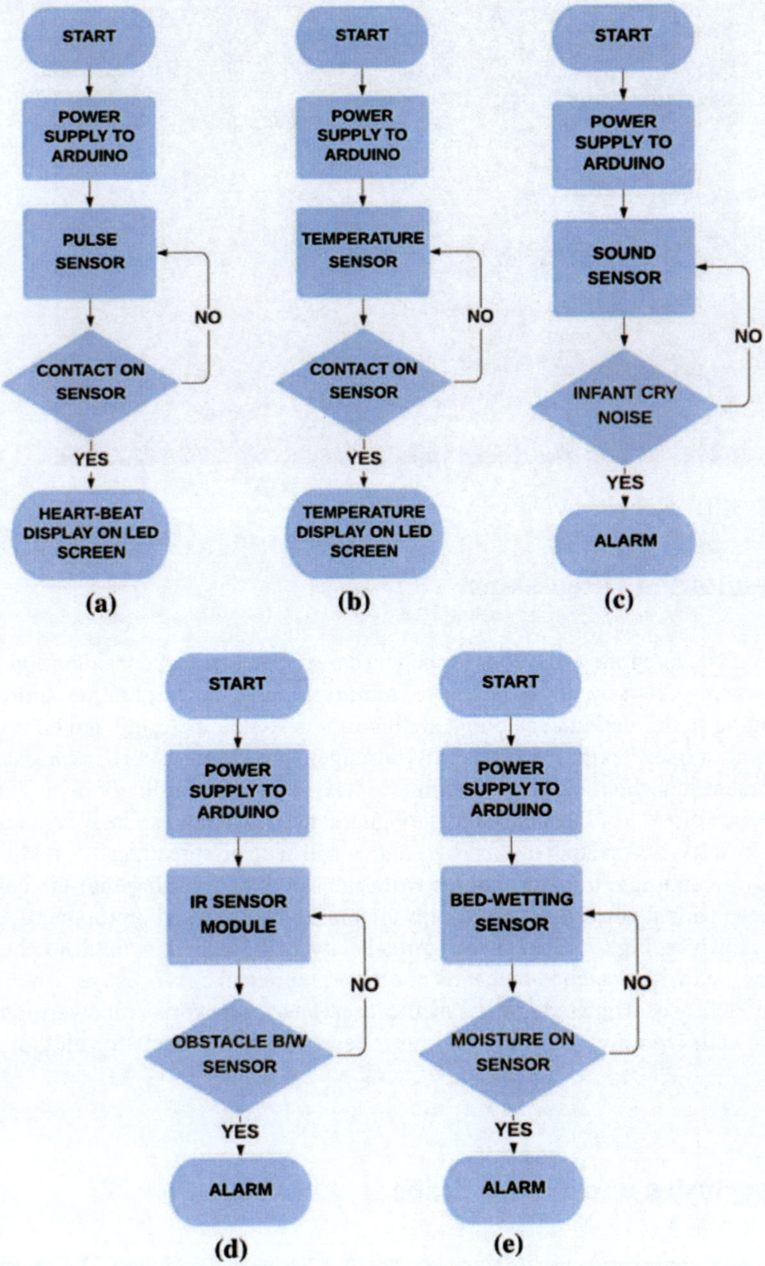

Fig. 6 Process flowcharts of the different modules of proposed smart bed

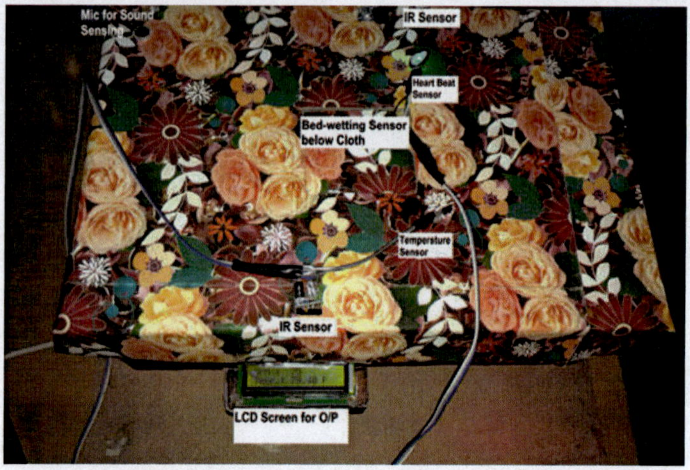

Fig. 7 Prototype of smart bed

4 Results and Discussions

Smart beds are integrated solutions for patient care understanding, consideration, help and observing, in view of an extensive, multidisciplinary configuration approach. Exploration in this field is basic in a setting of worldwide maturing and controlled by a flood in open doors for availability arrangements. Medical beds, consistently incorporated into the medical care framework, have an extraordinary open door in empowering more proficient endeavors for guardians and more responsive conditions for patients. It is normal that these progressions will keep on spreading into additional robotization and plan transformations, with the savvy bed turning into the core of the shrewd patient care climate of things to come. The proposed prototype of smart bed is shown in Fig. 7. The maximum capacity of keen beds would not just be accomplished with detached mechanical or morphological advances, yet when they are consistently coordinated into the medical services framework, empowering more effective endeavors for guardians and more responsive conditions for mothers and infants.

5 Conclusion and Future Scope

In this paper, noninvasive sensors-based smart bed has been developed. The prototype of smart bed is working as per the design specifications. All modules have been tested and found perfectly responding up to the specified range. This smart bed is further being integrated with IoT-based system to monitor the infants in real time through smart phones. In addition, we are developing computer vision-based monitoring of infants and protecting the infants falling from the bed. The module is in the testing phase. The proposed smart bed is cost effective. As we are using low-voltage sensors, hence, chances of getting shock are negligible. We are further extending our work toward the power optimization of the sensors.

References

1. Laurino M et al (2020) A smart bed for non-obtrusive sleep analysis in real world context. IEEE Access 8:45664–45673. https://doi.org/10.1109/ACCESS.2020.2976194
2. García-Magariño I et al (2018) Agent-based simulation of smart beds with internet-of-things for exploring big data analytics. IEEE Access 6:366–379. https://doi.org/10.1109/ACCESS.2017.2764467
3. Yousefi R et al (2011) A smart bed platform for monitoring & ulcer prevention. In: 2011 4th international conference on biomedical engineering and informatics (BMEI), Shanghai, China, pp 1362–1366. https://doi.org/10.1109/BMEI.2011.6098589
4. Sivanantham A (2015) Measurement of heartbeat, respiration and movements detection using smart bed. In: 2015 IEEE recent advances in intelligent computational systems (RAICS), Trivandrum, India, pp 105–109. https://doi.org/10.1109/RAICS.2015.7488397
5. Brush Z et al (2013) Design and control of a smart bed for pressure ulcer prevention. In: 2013 IEEE/ASME international conference on advanced intelligent mechatronics, Wollongong, NSW, Australia, pp 1033–1038. https://doi.org/10.1109/AIM.2013.6584230
6. Symon F (2017) Design and development of a smart baby monitoring system based on Raspberry Pi and Pi camera. In: 2017 4th international conference on advances in electrical engineering (ICAEE), Dhaka, pp 117–122. https://doi.org/10.1109/ICAEE.2017.8255338
7. Dubey YK, Damke S (2019) Baby monitoring system using image processing and IoT. Int J Eng Adv Technol 8(6):2225–2229. https://doi.org/10.35940/ijeat.F9254.088619
8. Rajesh G (2014) Baby monitoring system using wireless sensor networks. ICTACT J Commun Technol 5(3):963–969. https://doi.org/10.21917/IJCT.2014.0138
9. Jabbar WA et al (2019) IoT-BBMS: internet of things-based baby monitoring system for smart cradle. IEEE Access 7:93791–93805. https://doi.org/10.1109/ACCESS.2019.2928481
10. Hong YS (2018) Smart care beds for elderly patients with impaired mobility. Wirel Commun Mobile Comput 2018:1–13. https://doi.org/10.1155/2018/1780904
11. Fischer M (2019) Development of a smart bed insert for detection of incontinence and occupation in elder care. IEEE Access 7:118498–118508. https://doi.org/10.1109/ACCESS.2019.2931041
12. Elsokah MM, Zerek AR (2019) Next generation of medical care bed with internet of things solutions. In: 2019 19th international conference on sciences and techniques of automatic control and computer engineering (STA), Sousse, Tunisia, pp 84–89. https://doi.org/10.1109/STA.2019.8717204
13. Gaddam A et al (2008) Necessity of a bed-sensor in a smart digital home to care for elder-people. Sensors 2008, IEEE, Lecce, Italy, pp 1340–1343. https://doi.org/10.1109/ICSENS.2008.4716693
14. Azimi H (2017) Breathing signal combining for respiration rate estimation in smart beds. In: 2017 IEEE international symposium on medical measurements and applications (MeMeA), Rochester, MN, USA, pp 303–307. https://doi.org/10.1109/MeMeA.2017.7985893
15. Onchi E et al (2016) Design and implementation of a mechatronic smart bed for improved rehabilitation. In: 2016 IEEE international conference on industrial technology (ICIT), Taipei, Taiwan, pp 1482–1487. https://doi.org/10.1109/ICIT.2016.7474978
16. Kim J (2014) Analysis of health consumers' behavior using self-tracker for activity, sleep, and diet. Telemed J E Health 20(6):552–558. https://doi.org/10.1089/tmj.2013.0282

Smart Mask for COVID-19 E-wear

R. Subhash, C. Gnana Kousalya, G. Rohini, and Nikhil Madhavan

Abstract COVID-19 has been one of the most disastrous pandemics of the decade which has impacted several human lives and global economy. It is really difficult to control this kind of problem in a developing country like India where we have huge population. It is also difficult to maintain social distancing in such places. So, we have come up with an idea for the people to self-monitor and protect themselves from the spread of the virus. This paper aims to implement a smart mask which uses digital technology, for detection, prevention and precaution from this deadly virus. This virus is bound to spread in the event of interaction with other people, and we use technology to detect and prevent the virus by forming a personalized mask, which is capable of monitoring your vitals and indicating if the patient is infected by the virus. We are integrating the heart rate pulse sensor, infrared thermometer—MLX90614, respiratory sensor and Dht11 sensor which are used to monitor the inner temperature and humidity present inside the mask. This sensor is mounted on the mask which helps us to monitor the person who is wearing it 24/7. The overall equipment is less bulky with all the required features, rechargeable and replaceable filter. The vitals are monitored through personalized cloud using ThinkSpeak and mobile-based monitoring with alert system. The mask has an OLED display for real-time monitoring.

Keywords Smart mask · Heart rate pulse sensor · Infrared thermometer · Respiratory sensor · Dht1

1 Introduction

The coronavirus pandemic had caused a havoc and had disrupted health and economies of several nations, at the wake of 2019. It has been one of the most disastrous pandemics of the decade which has impacted several human lives. E-wear mask is a special mask which is used to monitor people to prevent them from the

R. Subhash (✉) · C. G. Kousalya · G. Rohini · N. Madhavan
Department of Electronics and Communication Engineering, St. Joseph's Institute of Technology, Chennai 600119, Tamil Nadu, India

N. Marriwala et al. (eds.), *Emergent Converging Technologies and Biomedical Systems*, Lecture Notes in Electrical Engineering 841,
https://doi.org/10.1007/978-981-16-8774-7_57

disease, and this mask has important features like heart rate monitoring sensor along with temperature sensor with the help of which we can measure heart pulse and temperature of the patient wearing the mask. We also have curated design features like air purifier filters which are placed at the front part of the mask. It has two chambers: an inlet and an outlet; by this we can easily inhale and exhale the air; we have decomposable filtrates (any porous material which is biodegradable). Once the sensors measure the value, the data is sent to the controller. Since the microcontroller we use has both analog and digital ports through which the values are recorded. A threshold limit is fixed in the controller; once the threshold limit is reached, the recorded data will be transferred wirelessly using Bluetooth module to the paired mobile phone, which can then be used to intimate the nearby hospital in case of an emergency. There are several challenges that the various industries are currently facing under this pandemic; this includes complete shutdown of factories and slowing down of production and manufacturing. This causes loss of income and growth. This paper focuses on creating a product that will serve the purpose of a secure mask as well as a personal digitalized vital monitoring system. What follows is a discussion on how the latest technological trend can be adopted to eliminate the effect of the virus.

1.1 Literature Survey and Related Work

In the meantime, many systems have been developed for COVID-19 in terms of sophisticated protective gear. In 2020, Atif et al. [1] proposed a system where all protective personal wear was digitally transformed through various concepts in IOT which enables us with a framework for a most sophisticated approach toward health monitoring. These devices have already been applied in COVID-19 conditions, not only to gather digital health data, but also to ensure that people obey certain lockdown and quarantine regulations. Valsalan et al. [2] had a similar framework where they integrated sensor fields to make a smart patient monitoring system. These sensors are embedded on the patient body to sense the temperature and heartbeat of the patient. More sensors are placed at home to sense the humidity and the temperature of the room and upload the data onto the cloud. Gwen [3] proposed a design for a more ergonomic face mask for more comfort which generates less wastage in terms of production with the materials most suitable for the design of a comfortable yet functional mask. Two reusable 3D-printed components, the face mask and a filter membrane support, and two disposable components, the head band and the filter membrane, make up this 3D-printed mask. Sasilatha et al. [4] proposed a system which uses noninvasive heart rate monitoring technique that uses the variation of light intensity from the skin from each heartbeat used to estimate heart rate. A RGB camera is used to record the video. The region of interest (ROI) is obtained using face detection and tracking algorithms. The mean value is taken across the frame yielding three values per frame, thereby estimating the heartbeats per min. Anoop Kumar et al. [5] proposed a system which deals with scope of design and fabrication of 3D-printed mask that enables us to get a broader perspective of material science for a strong and sturdy yet comfortable build. 3D printer according to its virtual design is proposed at reduced cost. Material used for this project should have good mechanical properties along with being bio-disposable (ecofriendly) in nature so they preferred polylactic acid (PLA). Further, Novak et al. [6] proposed that there are 3D-printed face shields that use fused filament fabrication process most suitable in order to enhance the PPE supply experience through realistic alternatives. Kousalya et al. [7] proposed that the wireless sensor network key management has efficient tracking and energy method of transfer. The proposed scheme attains high connectivity among several sensor nodes and is applied for various routing protocols, and simulation shows greater resilience. Furthermore, Wan et al. [8] proposed a wearable IoT device which adapts a number of interactive sensors to observe the health vitals. Next Prof. Hagargund et al. [9] had given a smart and automatic health monitoring system which is around the concept of wireless sensor network which is essential in the scope of remote monitoring.

2 System Overview

The component setup is as shown in Fig. 1. The basic components of this system include an Arduino LilyPad which is used as a microcontroller as a motherboard of the entire project, and an ESP8266 Wi-Fi module is used for the data communication with the cloud and the mobile monitoring using Virtuino app. Dht11 sensor is used for monitoring the temperature and humidity. Respiratory sensor is used in order to monitor the breath cycles count for every one minute. Heart rate pulse sensor is used

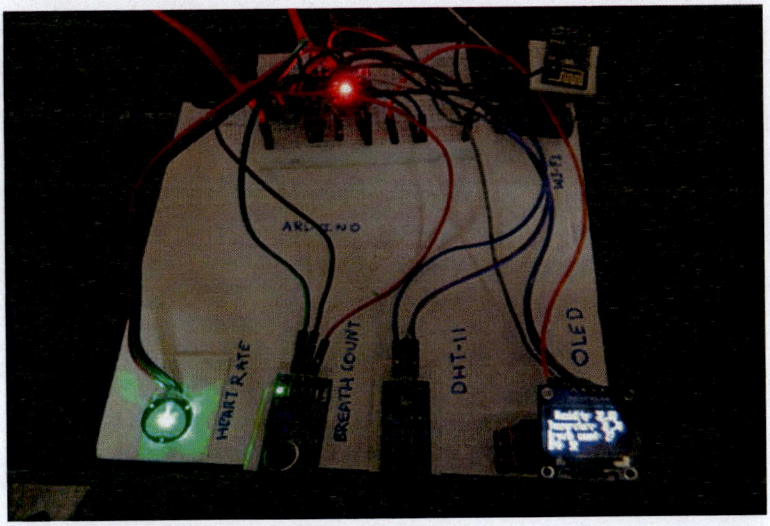

Fig. 1 Complete setup of the smart mask

to monitor the heart rate for every second. OLED display is used to monitor real time. All the vitals are printed on the screen in order to reduce the periodic checking of temperature in public areas. The connections are made as per the circuit diagram shown in Fig. 2 Arduino LilyPad is used as a microcontroller; it has seven analog pins and 13 digital pins along with I2C and UART communication; in this project, we are using five different sensors for monitoring the vitals of human. Firstly, we are using humidity sensor in order to monitor the moisture level inside the mask; it is been connected to pin A0 analog pin and monitors the temperature and humidity present inside the mask. Secondly, we are using infrared thermometer inside the mask in order to monitor the object temperature which uses infrared rays for the measurement. The infrared sensor works on I2C communication which is connected to A4 and A5 pin which act as SCL and SDA pins for data and clock. Thirdly, heart rate pulse sensor is used to measure the heart pulse which is been connected to pin A2 analog pin; it works on optocoupler principle based on the light reflection and absorption; the difference is been converted into variables and measured using microcontroller. Respiratory sensor is used which will calculate the breath cycles for every minute, stores the value in a register and prints the output which is been connected to pin A1 analog output. The output measured is obtained in two different platforms: One is real-time display, and other is on cloud and Virtuino app.

In digital display, we have used is OLED display because of its size, shape and less space consumption. The display we use has a pixel size of 1.3-inch 128 × 64 OLED graphic display. OLED display works on I2C communication where SCL and SDA pins are used for data communication with the microcontroller, where it reduces the pin consumption and less circuit complexity. The entire circuit is power

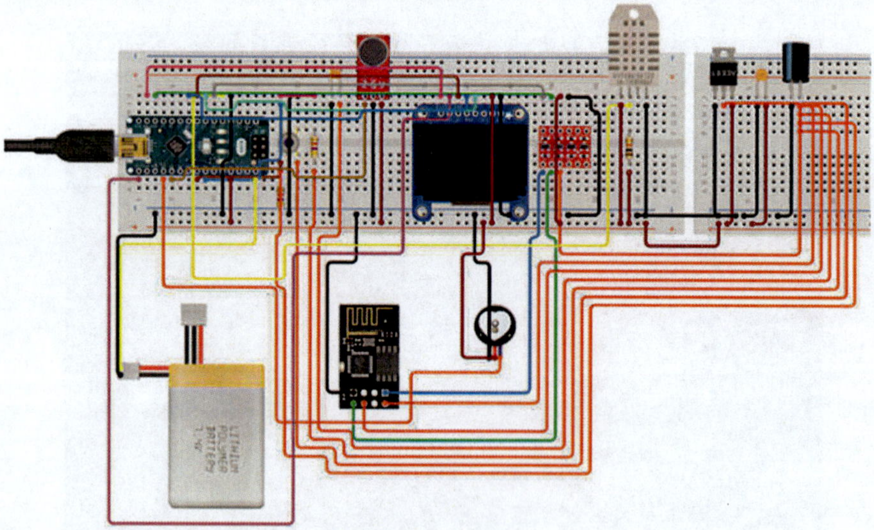

Fig. 2 Circuit diagram

by 7 V li-po 500 mA h battery which is been connected to 1 A power charger, and the battery is rechargeable. Audio amplifier is used inside the mask in order to amplify the audio and gives the output to the speaker. PAM8403 is used as an audio amplifier class D, two-channel non-tuneable amplifier. The circuit is powered by 5 V, the mic is connected to the left in L T R, the speaker is connected to left terminal, and even we can connect two speakers for better audio quality. ESP6266 is connected to the microcontroller to the pins 2 and 3, where pin 2 is Tx and pin 3 is Rx. The chip enable pin is set to high and 3.3 V, and ground is been connected in order to make the module high. Arduino LilyPad is powered by lithium-ion battery. This is connected to a 1 A USB micro charger port which can be used to charge externally.

3 Mask Design

The mask is designed using computer-aided design, there are four major parts, and those are front part, mask, mask cap and motor holder. These parts are printed using 3D printing machine. The material which was used in the printing of mask is acrylonitrile butadiene styrene (ABS) because of its heat resistance and high temperature withstanding capacity up to 100 °C. Figure 3 is the front part of mask which holds the OLED display on the outer part, and the front part is further subdivided into two chambers: one is inlet and outlet air purifier filtrates. The motor holding part is fitted inside the front part of the inlet and outlet of the mask. The charging port along with battery is mounted inside the front part of the mask. Arduino LilyPad and sensors are placed inside the mask. Figure 4 is the main part of the mask which has air purifier filtrates and holds the front part. The inlet and outlet parts of mask are closed by mask cap as shown in Fig. 5. On combining all these parts, the expected view is shown in Fig. 7 and 8 (Fig. 6).

Fig. 3 Front part of mask along with inlet and outlet

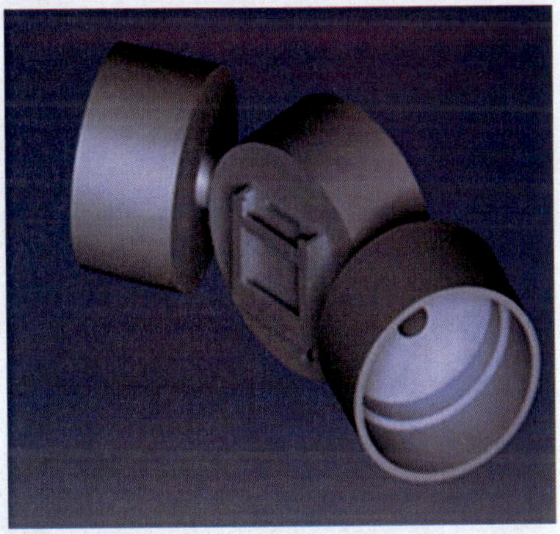

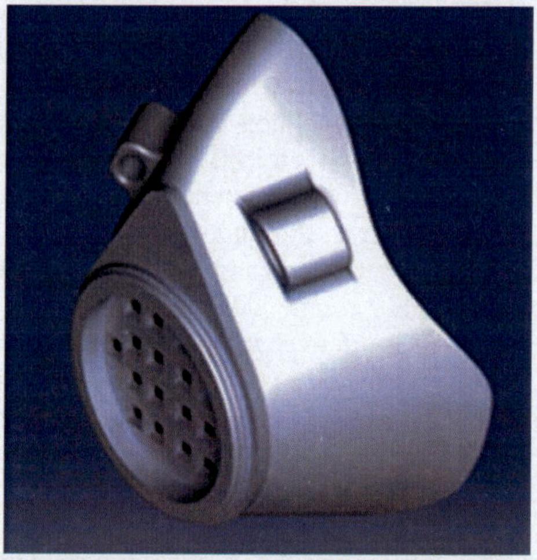

Fig. 4 Mask

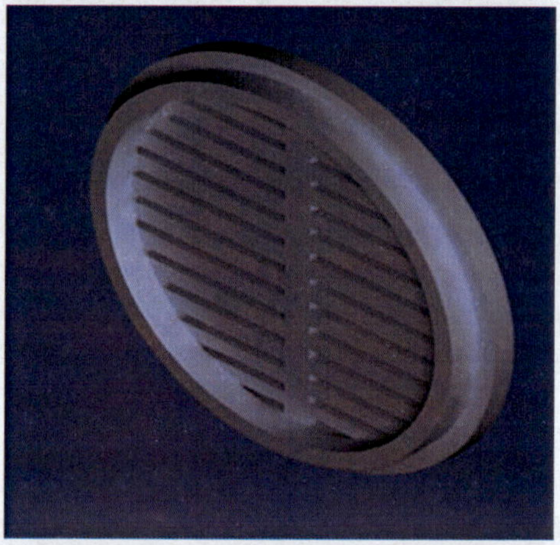

Fig. 5 Mask cap

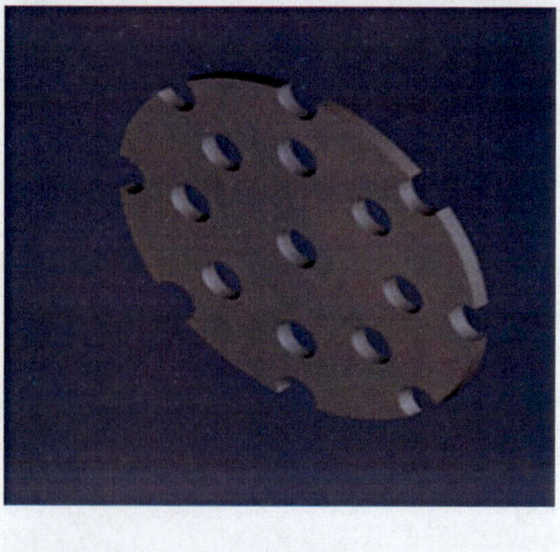

Fig. 6 Motor holder

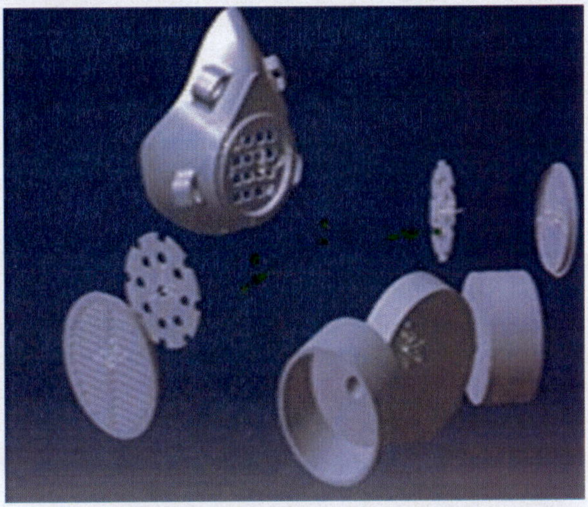

Fig. 7 Assembly of the parts of mask

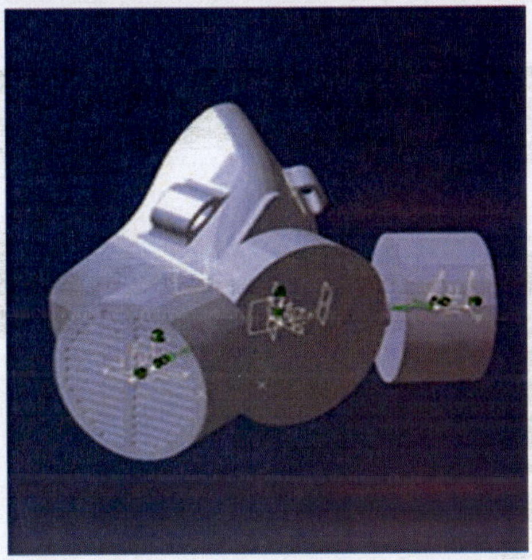

Fig. 8 Smart mask

3.1 Hardware Implementation

A. Microcontroller

Arduino LilyPad is the microcontroller board which is used in our mask because of its circular shape that can fit into the mask. The microcontroller can be programmed using external UART communication using FTDI. The board has 14 digital pins and six analog pins. It has Tx and Rx pins for communicating with Wi-Fi and Bluetooth. The board is the heart of our project which performs arithmetic and logical operations.

The Atmel328P is the on-chip controller present on the board. It has a reset button to reboot the uploaded program.

B. Sensor Integration

The mask has five main sensors, the sensors are used for monitoring the vitals of human that change according to individual body, and these vitals are converted to the standard using appropriate formula.

1. With the aid of ADC, the temperature sensor connecting to the analog pin of the Arduino controller is converted into a digital value. The controller translates this digital data into the real temperature value in degrees Celsius using the **temperature (°C) float mv = (val/1024.0)*5000; float cel = mv/10**;
2. The heart rate pulse sensor works on based on optocoupler where the photo light is transmitted on the skin and reflected back due to the ions present in the blood; this difference in values is calculated using formula. The digital pulses are sent to a microcontroller, which uses the formula to calculate the heartbeat rate: **beats per minute (BPM) = 60*P**, where P is the pulse frequency.
3. Along with the temperature sensor, a humidity sensor is used to detect, calculate and record both moisture and air temperature. Humidity sensors track changes in electrical currents or temperatures in the air to determine humidity levels. The following formula is used to measure relative humidity:

   Float V = (ADC Value/1023.0)*5.0;
   Percent relative humidity = (V − 0.958)/0.0307;

4. The breath sensor, which is built into the front of the mask, detects the amount of breath cycles per minute by detecting breath pressures and variations in variation. A force-sensitive resistor (FSR) based on the piezo-resistive effect is used in the device. The math is as follows:

   Val = map(val,0,1023,0,100)

C. OLED Display

OLED display is used in the smart mask for displaying the sensor output for user visual. We can display a text which will correspond to the required vitals of the patient. This display uses I2C communication to reduce the number of pins and sends data using CLK and data lines.

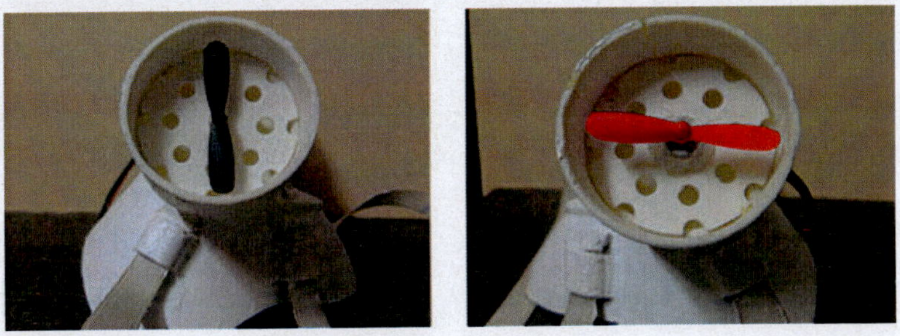

Fig. 9 Inlet and outlet valve of the mask

D. Inlet and Outlet Valve of The Mask

The inlet and outlet valves are attached for filtering in a face mask to provide an exhalation valve and a mouthpiece to direct exhaled air out of the mask, minimizing heat and moisture within the mask. This system can include a filter to clean the exhaled air, making it suitable for use in areas where directly exhaled air is undesirable, such as operating rooms and clean manufacturing environments (Fig. 9).

E. ESP 8266

ESP8266 Wi-Fi module is used for data communication with ThinkSpeak and Virtuino app; the module is set in mode 1. In mode 1, it acts as a Wi-Fi, and in mode 2, it acts as an access point and so on. It has an inbuilt patch antenna for data transmission into electromagnetic radiation and has coverage up to 100 m distance.

F. IoT Integration

ThinkSpeak cloud is used in our project for visualizing the output, plotting the graph, obtaining the outcome and notifying when the threshold limit is crossing. The data is sent through the read key and write key. There are four different channels to store individual vitals. First channel stores the temperature, second channel stores the humidity, third channel stores heart rate BPM for every minute, and fourth channel stores the breath count. This data can be further used for future health analysis.

G. UV Sanitizing

Additionally, we have used UV light to sanitize the internal components and the filtrate of the mask to ensure clean and germ-free interspacing of the mask; this helps the user of the mask to stay safe of the virus that may reside in the mask during its usage. The entire mask can be sanitized using UV sanitization toolkit which is available in the market for commercial use.

3.2 Software Implementation

The above flowchart shown in Fig. 10 represents the communication between the ESP266 and the ThinkSpeak module using AT commands. Firstly, the ESP8266 module is enabled and set as mode 1 which act as a Wi-Fi. There are five different channels which store individual values of each sensors. ThinkSpeak gets data using get commands. The cloud will check 24/7 and store the data; once the threshold limit is crossed alert, message will be sent to the provided number. Secondly, the data will

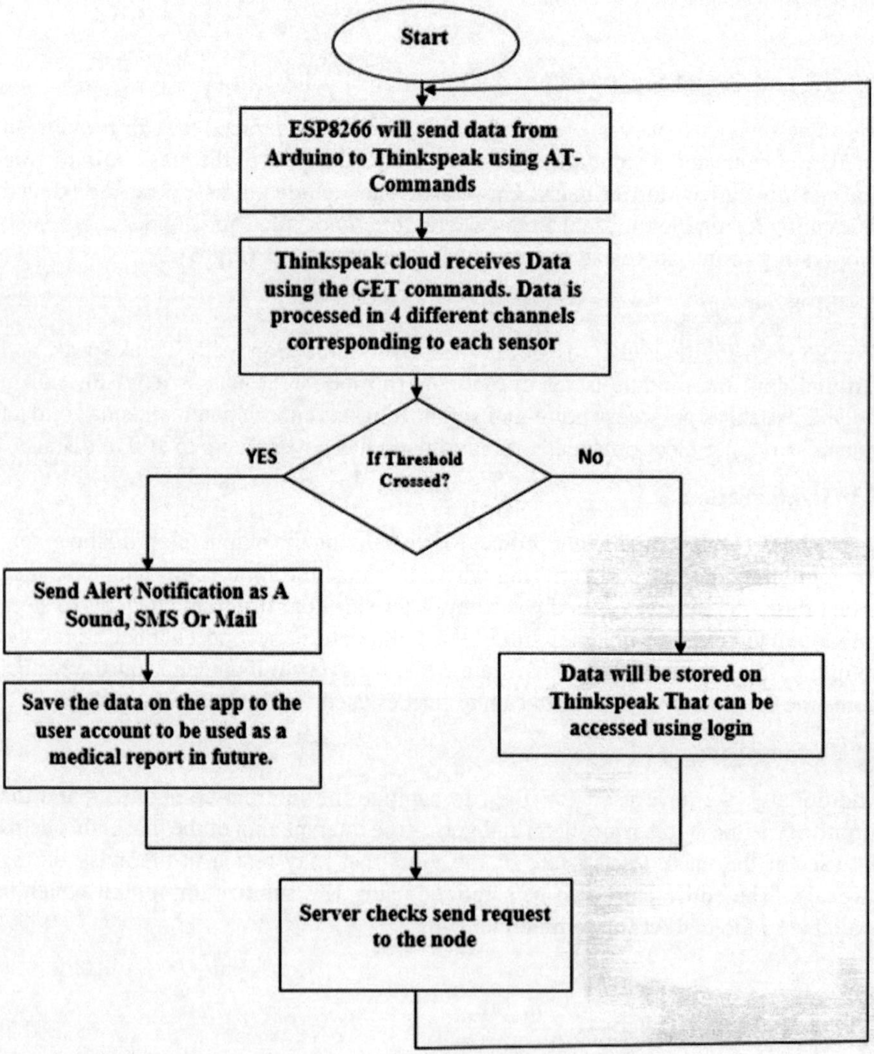

Fig. 10 Flowchart representing the communication with ESP8266 and ThinkSpeak

be accessed using mobile application. Virtuino is the application which is been used in the project which works based on read key and write key. The ThinkSpeak web is used to access the data and stores the values in the app that can be used for future medical application. ThinkSpeak can be accessed using login ID for the personal cloud. The circuit initiation and enabling are made as shown in Fig. 11. Initially, the program runs as the code is set in void loop. In Arduino program, the code runs infinite loop; all the sensor pins are defined in the start of program, and pin mode is set in void setup. Each sensor is allocated a specific time to read and store the data as shown in the flowchart. Heart sensor stores value for every 10 s, and by enabling the A0 pin high for 10 s, the data are read. Similarly, respiratory sensor counts the number of breath cycles for every 60 s and stores the value. Dht11 sensor is enabled for 5 s and stores the value. These values of the sensors are displayed on the OLED display; when the threshold limit is reached, the inlet and outlet motors are enabled; the alert message will be sent, and the data value will be uploaded in the cloud. The values of heart rate, breath count, temperature and humidity will be uploaded in cloud as well as will be displayed on the screen and serial monitor.

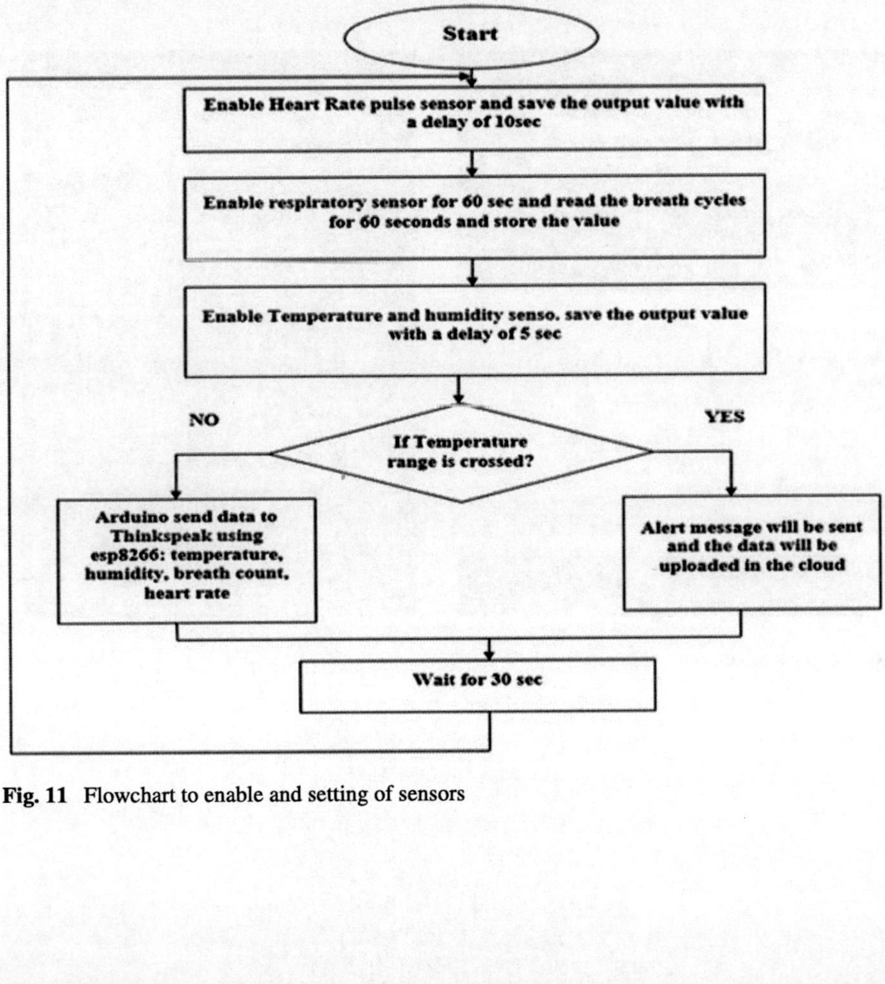

Fig. 11 Flowchart to enable and setting of sensors

4 Result

A product is developed for fighting against the coronavirus. The mask developed is integrated with digitally advanced setup consisting of various biosensors. It includes designing of hardware for mask using CAD, and coding for the required system is done through embedded C in Arduino LilyPad. And interface for IoT is established in ThinkSpeak cloud services and Virtuino app.

4.1 Virtuino Output

The Virtuino app gets the values from various sensors and displays the analog output on the paired mobile device. This output is not constant, and they change periodically. When the threshold limit is crossed, an alert or SMS-based notification on mobile phone will be sent; the data set can be downloaded and sent to the nearest hospital (Fig. 12).

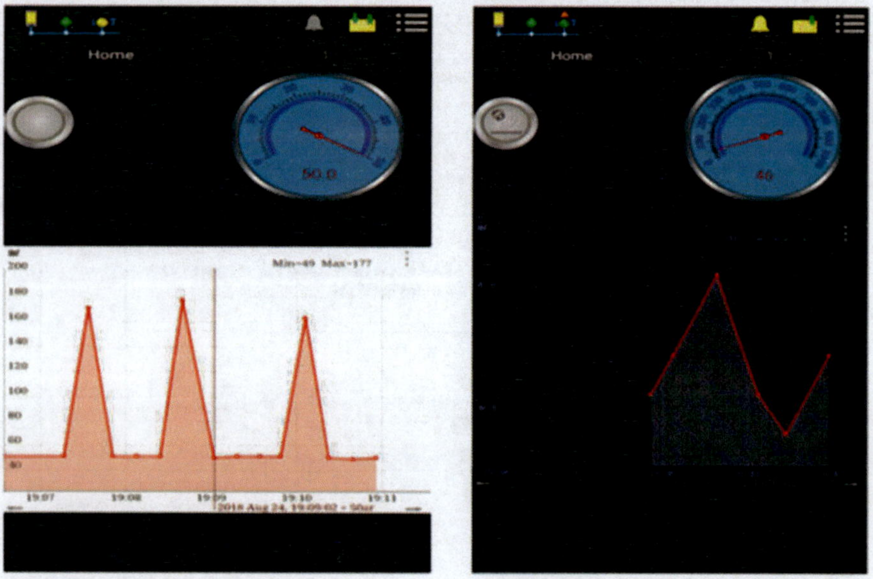

Fig. 12 Virtuino output

4.2 *ThinkSpeak Output*

The ThinkSpeak cloud services are used to continuously update the values of the required biosensors on the cloud, where individual data is uploaded in each field. These fields will update every 1 min; this data set would be used for analysis by the doctor. Totally, five fields are used to store the data of humidity, temperature, heart rate, breath count and body temperature (Fig. 13).

5 Conclusion

By using a wide array of test cases, all possible cases of sensors are tested, and result anomaly is near to nix, and accuracy of the sensors is tested before integrating it in the circuit. The sensors are integrated in the curated mask design as per the requirement, and sensors are then mounted in it for comfortable usage of the mask. The testing loss fluctuates between an acceptable range, and it falls about at less than 2% variance. Table 1 represents the confusion matrix of the testing phase. The developed architecture shows only single sample of our multiple tests. By this proposal system using this kind of E-mask, we can monitor as well as control the spread of corona kind of virus.

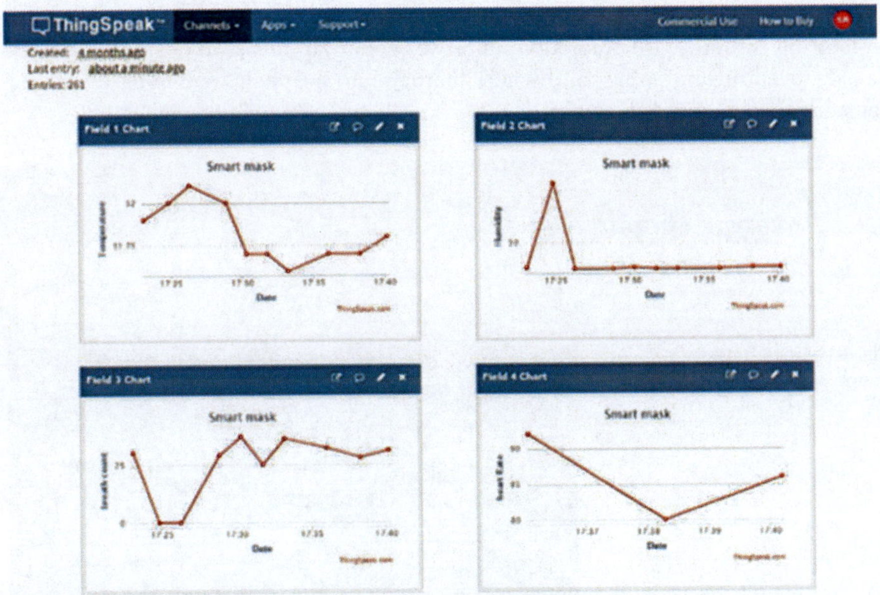

Fig. 13 ThinkSpeak output

Table 1 Expected and tested output

Sl. No	Sensors	Expected outcome	Tested outcome
1.	Temperature	98.6 F	98.3 F
2.	Humidity	86%	82%
3.	Pressure	300 hpa	290 hpa
4.	Heart Rate	64 BPM	60 BPM
5.	Respiratory	0.96 and 1.0 Cycles per min	0.92 Cycles per min
6.	Microphone Amplifier	3db	2.4 db

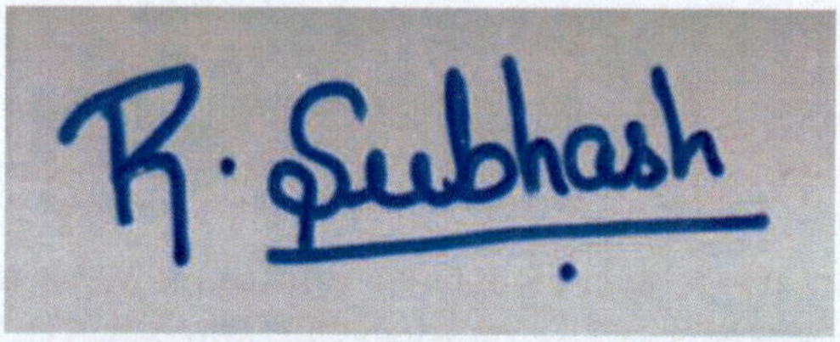

Overall equipment is less bulky with all the required features, it is rechargeable, and the filter can be easily replaced. However, camera module can be implemented, and temperature-based thermal image detection can be made. Cost of the mask can be reduced; machine learning-based spread prediction can be made. Battery is not for life time; regular charging is needed. Component handling is required for long life time. Mobile-based health monitoring system is easy to carry, IoT-based health monitoring is for disease prediction, improves control of this kind of spread and can be used even in rural areas, and where there are no hospitals, online-based doctor consulting can be used (Fig. 14).

5.1 Prototype Output

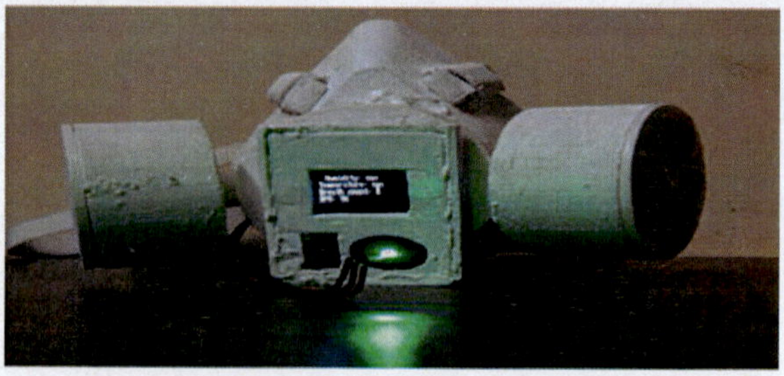

Fig. 14 Smart mask prototype

References

1. Atif I, Cawood FT, Mahboob MA (2020) The role of digital technologies that could be applied for prescreening in the mining industry during the COVID-19 pandemic. Trans Indian Natl Acad Eng 1–12
2. Valsalan P, Baomar TA, Baabood AH (2020) IoT based health monitoring system. J Crit Revi 7(4):739–743
3. Swennen GRJ, Pottel L, Haers PE (2020) Custom-made 3D-printed face masks in case of pandemic crisis situations with a lack of commercially available FFP2/3 masks. Int J Oral Maxillofac Surg
4. Sasilatha T, Kousalya G, Venkatesan G (2019) Non-contact heart rate monitoring using facial video. Int J Eng Adv Technol (IJEAT) 9(2):4087–4089
5. Singh AK, Kumar UA, Laxminarayana P (2020) Design and development of face shield by 3D printing for the COVID-19 epidemics. Int J Res Appl Sci Eng Technol 8(6):380–384
6. Novak JI, Loy J (2020) A quantitative analysis of 3D printed face shields and masks during COVID-19. Emerald Open Res 2
7. Kousalya CG, Mala GA (2012) Secure and energy-efficient traffic-aware key management scheme for wireless sensor network. Int J Wirel Inf Netw 19(2):112–121
8. Wan J, et al (2018) Wearable IoT enabled real-time health monitoring system. EURASIP J Wirel Commun Netw 2018(1):298
9. Hagargund AG, et al (2018) Smart and automatic health monitoring of patient using wireless sensor network. In: 2018 9th international conference on computing, communication and networking technologies (ICCCNT), IEEE

Role of IoT and Machine Learning in Smart Grid

Vijay Kumar Garg and Sudhir Sharma

Abstract The conventional power system is transforming into a new, modern, and digital power system. Integration of Internet of Things (IoT) and machine learning in smart grid improves power system entities' overall performance like load forecasting, data acquisition, fault analysis and system security, etc. Smart grid (SG) takes good decisions according to the requirement, faults, and resolutions to organize power and maximize electrical energy usage. These decisions increase the power and regulation of the grid by keeping stability between power generation and consumption. This paper attempts to focus on IoT and machine learning in the smart grid that help smart grids in the decision-making process. IoT-integrated network system is prone to cyber-attacks and network threat, which needs to be adequately addressed in the near future.

Keywords IoT · Smart grid · Smart meter · Advanced metering infrastructure (AMI) · Machine learning · Supervised learning

1 Introduction

A conventional power system has three parts, i.e., generation, transmission, and distribution. The system has various issues such as large Aggregate Technical and Commercial (AT&C) losses, a gap between availability and electricity demand, network operations, minimum usage of information technology, and one-way communication/information flow. Transformation of centralized controlled traditional power grid into smart, reliable, and self-healing grid is taking place. These new smart/microgrids can efficiently operate generation, transmission, and electricity

V. K. Garg (✉)
Research Scholar, IKG Punjab Technical University, Jalandhar, Punjab, India

Department of Electrical Engineering, UIET, Kurukshetra University, Kurukshetra, Haryana, India

S. Sharma
Department of Electrical Engineering, DAV Institute of Engineering and Technology, Jalandhar, Punjab, India

N. Marriwala et al. (eds.), *Emergent Converging Technologies and Biomedical Systems*, Lecture Notes in Electrical Engineering 841,
https://doi.org/10.1007/978-981-16-8774-7_58

usage to minimize environmental issues [1]. The modern power system appears to be a complex structure with an additional component, e.g., distributed generation (DG), electric vehicle, power electronics interfacing, IoT, and different types of techniques and information. SG provides two-way communication, i.e., servers to consumer and consumer to the server. Smart grid uses different devices to monitor, examine, and manage the grid-like Advanced Metering Infrastructure (AMI), online measurements, fault sufferance, and load management. These decisions increase the power and regulation of the grid by keeping stability between power generation and consumption. Such kinds of devices are kept at power plants, transmission towers, and lines. They also spread customer's offices, and the amount of such devices increases from hundreds of millions. The main task of SG is to provide connectivity, robotization, and tracing these large number of devices. For this, monitoring, examining, and managing by high speed and bidirectional communication are required. The IoT connects any object with the Internet for data transformation and connecting with smart devices [2].

Firstly, the Internet provides connectivity from person to person and person to other objects. But, in 2008, the number of objects linked with the Internet increases. Internet of Things is a nexus of many material objects that are connected with the Internet. These types of things are provided with automation to their environments. These objects notice, examine, control, and decide themselves or discuss with other objects by high speed and bidirectional communication in allocatable, self-governing ways. So, by integrated IoT devices like sensors, switches, and intelligent measure and providing congruency, robotization, and tracing, IoT techniques support SG by providing many network functions in production, storage, and distribution.

Now SG is observed as the extreme application of IoT. Today, we have many household tools utilizing electricity and the Internet. However, there are still many appliances that are not at all linked to the Internet. For instance, devices like washing machine, coolers, AC, fridge, oven, etc., are significantly less in number that uses the Internet. If all the devices are connected to the Internet, we can operate them using remote and can off. So, it saves cost and gives lenience to consumers. So, it is not wrong to assume that the combination of SG and IoT is greater than SG today. SG cannot use alone without the help of IoT techniques. Using IoT as a standard and base for SG, many new ways come out for future revolution. Based on IoT and SG's collaboration, here an attempt is made to assess IoT in smart grid with IoT and machine learning.

2 Internet of Things (IoT)

Internet of Things is a concept where material objects get linked to the Internet with their unique IP addresses and communicate with gateways. These automated communication models tend to make the devices aware of context, organize properly, transmit information, and respond to dynamic circumstances. In a situation where numerous objects and sensors are connected to the Internet, every entity needs its unique identifier to send data frames to other systems or devices. It can be expected that the number of Internet-enabled devices will increase due to the fall of technologies' cost. This considerable growth would create necessary modernizations to the present TCP/IP stack's scalability concerning support for naming, addressing, location, classification, mobility, routing, etc. Due to the massive number of existing and future estimated devices, this becomes possible with IPv6 addresses that provide a significant increase in address space [3].

Using IPv6 addressing proxy and mapping for legacy technologies (that do not cooperate with IPv6) brings traffic management capability in a standardized, flexible, and effective manner via IP-based protocols. As a result, data can be transferred automatically without requiring human interaction. Usage of the Internet and computers for capturing data, instead of human-made analysis, can provide higher accuracy and lower the amount of time needed. Objects connected by IoT communicate and sense the environment and respond swiftly to the current situation due to sensor network technology. A wireless sensor network is seen as a significant part of IoT. It connects to devices (sensors) in an observed area to create a vaulting network system that can read, gather real time, process, and manage figures to send them to the data center. IoT may enable more dynamic energy pricing due to real-time collected data and smart meters installed in households. That gains benefits for power system operator as managing and balancing load demand efficiently. By deploying, the IoT quality of the smart grid's self-healing feature can be improved. Unpredictable conditions or breakdowns can be detected by sensors and can make a rapid response.

3 IoT Technologies

The optimal operation and coordination of various intelligent technologies make the overall power system an intelligent grid. Some of the essential technologies for applying IoT to the smart grid are as follows:

- **Sensor innovation**: The measurement of various pieces of information takes place with the help of sensing devices. Sensors are devices utilized in detecting the material world and give crude data to data preparing, sending, investigating and input, including power, heat, electricity, light, signals, and sound. Installation of sensors can be done at local, station/feeder, and centralized control center or various configurations. In a smart grid, sensors and actuator network (SANETs) systems have used diverse field like renewable penetration, grid monitoring and control, generation dispatch, etc. [4].
- **Information and correspondence innovation**: Based on data and correspondence innovation, the recognition data's transmission and cooperation can be acknowledged; thus, the force lattice devices' condition can be detected.
- **Data combination innovation**: The assets for IoT terminals usually are restricted, involving battery limit, handling capacity, stockpiling limit, and transfer speed.

During the time spent on social affair data, it is not fitting to send all information to the bunch hub since it would squander transfer speed and energy.

- **Reliable correspondence for brilliant lattice under smart grid application condition**: There are a few necessities of IoT applications in various situations, for example, dependability, self-association, signal entrance, mixture correspondence innovation, and self-mending. Since the IoT exhibition exceptionally depends on the actual condition, IoT innovation should be deliberately intended to conquer the unfavorable natural elements. For instance, when a tiny part of devices neglects to communicate information, the course and transmission system would be reselected without anyone else mending innovation; hence, the entire organization's dependability would not be influenced.

4 Machine Learning

Machine learning is managing data by various analytical processes in which computers are trained with artificial techniques. The systems are made smart to take decision automatically as per their training. In an IoT-based lattice framework, colossal data is produced, which needs various operations like data collection, data cleaning, size reduction, reformulation, and data exploration. The analysis of various information is done to produce a decision/prediction. It contains different calculations that dissect the accessible information through many directions to create information-driven expectations and choices [5, 6]. The processes can be load forecasting, price prediction, optimum scheduling, sizing, and contingency analysis. Learning machines go through a complete cycle of planning and programming unequivocal calculations with anticipated execution. Figure 1 shows applications of machine learning in the smart grid. Machine learning can be distinguished into two types [7]:

- **Supervised Learning**: In this learning approach, a mapping is performed between input and the desired output. The tasks can be specific objectives like real-time monitoring of solar energy and battery power for home energy management, demand response system for maintain heating, ventilation and air-condition system, etc.
- **Unsupervised Learning**: The input data is not composed of corresponding output variables information. Unsupervised learning aims to find functional patterns in distribution. It may also model the below structure to enhance the input data's understanding.

5 Applications of IoT and Machine Learning in Smart Grid

A smart grid is an electricity network that uses intelligent appliances, techniques, and digital systems to control and monitor electricity transmission from the source, i.e.,

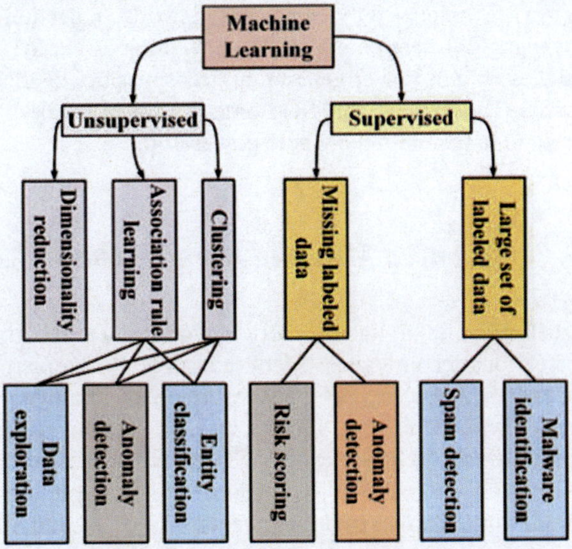

Fig. 1 Application of machine learning in smart grid security

the generating station to the destination, i.e., end users [4]. SG aims to synchronize all the parts of the network as much as possible to increase productivity. In smart grid-layered architecture, there are four types of layers. Layer 1 is a terminal layer consisting of IoT devices installed with many SG functions like generation, transmission, distribution, and consumption. The instruments of IoT possess RTU, intelligent devices, smart electronic devices, and data-gathering devices. The data gathered by this layer from the IoT devices is transferred to the second layer, i.e., field network layer. According to the IoT devices, the framework of the second layer is wired or wireless. Now, the information collected by this layer is transferred to the third layer, i.e., remote communication network layer. This layer connects IoT devices with the master station system layer. This layer works as a control unit for SG, i.e., it manages all SG consequences. IoT techniques are essential in structure formation for sensing information and transferring for SG, help in framework formation, security management, data gathering, tracking, calculation, and is user friendly, etc., for example. In a conventional power grid, the companies know about the disruption of service only when a user informs itself, but in SG, these companies themselves come to know about any disorder as, from the defected part, the signal is not transferred further. So, companies notice the problem and solve it. The IoT helps start the structure in which all SG parts have their unique IP label and give bidirectional communication [8]. The communication system is divided into three layers: the Home Area Network (HAN), which uses powerlines as a wired medium, and ZigBee, Wi-Fi, Bluetooth as wireless mediums; Neighbor Area Network (NAN), which uses various communication medium to cover up to a thousand meters; Wide Area Network (WAN), which transmits data to a more significant distance [9].

IoT techniques provide a better network connection to the consumers and devices by using different communication techniques via IoT intelligent devices. IoT techniques help in power generation, transmission, distribution, and consumption flow in SG. The conventional SG framework mainly works when the power suppliers are needed to maintain the whole power grid.

5.1 Advanced Metering Infrastructure (AMI)

AMI provides a linkage between consumer and utility with the incorporation of various technologies. Many consumers use smart meters by GPRS and other networks. At present, users have already an intelligent framework but not still integrated with the present SG structure. The resolutions for IoT and SG system do not apply directly to IoT-integrated SG system because these resolutions are only for one design, either for IoT or SG system, as these resolutions are made by considering the framework of either of both systems. So, IoT is used in all the techniques to enhance them. In electricity generation, the IoT is used to keep an eye on and manage the electricity used, energy storage, power plants, etc. In power transmission, IoT is used to control transmission lines and intermediate stations and help in the conservation of towers for transmission. In power distribution, IoT is used for the management of devices for distribution. In power utilization, IoT is used for smart appliances and checks the electricity used, managing energy efficiency and controlling the need for energy consumption [9].

Figure 2 illustrates the smart grid architecture used by the electricity board for the use of smart meters. The smart meters are placed in offices, houses, and industries. These smart meters transmit information to Data Controller Unit (DCU) present on an electric pole near the house. These meters give information about the power used by the users. The DCU is located in the surroundings, gathering data about electricity consumption and other things connected to meters' status. The collected data is transferred to data centers utilizing a wired or wireless network. All the complete information of this smart grid can be tracked by web portal using phones, laptops, etc.

These web portals are linked with DCUs to share the data collected and to process it. It maintains the record of electricity consumption, information of bill and loads, etc. The various components of the smart grid are depicted in Fig. 3. The smart grid's main components are smart meter, distribution automation, renewable energy sources, electric storage, and demand response management.

In AMI, IoT is used to gather information, transfer information among all the smart devices, check the quality of electricity, and examine users' power. The power industry is confronting unprecedented changes and difficulties. The solidness and security of the framework can be accomplished by setting up a severe metering standard foundation. The brilliant meter is a significant segment of the AMI. Detailing of principles for intelligent metering hardware should be done to meet the AMI's prerequisites. The foundation of the wise lattice network is its AMI. With the AMI,

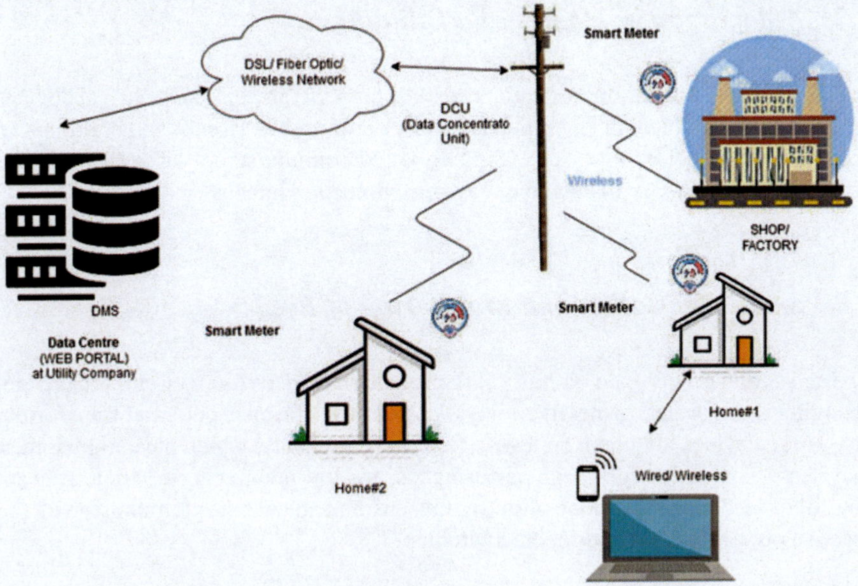

Fig. 2 Architecture of the smart grid with AMI

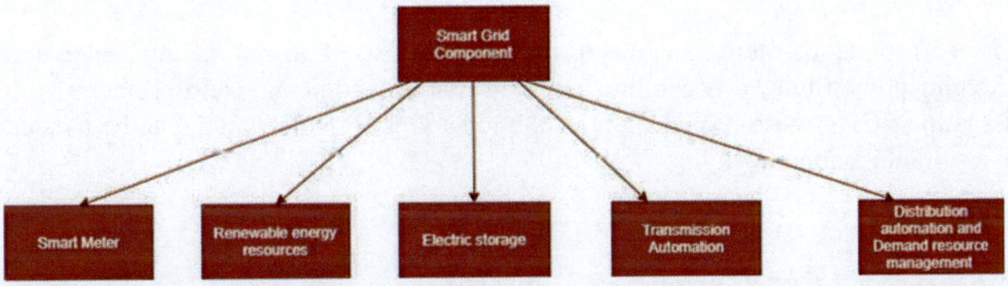

Fig. 3 Components of smart grid

individuals can do some altered control as for the interest reaction. AMI is a framework that gathers, measures, and examines information by speaking with intelligent metering devices [9]. AMI networks should be worked to scale, and significant necessities, for example, transfer speed, inertness throughput and unwavering quality should be met. An AMI comprises the smart meter, two-way correspondence way, meter information obtaining framework, and meter information of the board framework. Advanced Encryption Standard (AES) mechanism and framework confirmation systems of public key are utilized in AMI applications.

5.2 Automation in Homes and Buildings

In smart homes, we use smart appliances like smart meters, digital electrical devices, broadband, etc., which make human life more comfortable. Homes and buildings are equipped with devices that can make two-way communication with utility, central controller, local energy management system, home appliances, and DER [10].

5.3 Smart Substation and Monitoring of Feeder

The substation is equipped with primary protection devices like a circuit breaker, tap changing transformer, protective relays, current transformer, potential transformer, etc. These devices are connected with fiber-based sensors, which have higher accuracy, lesser size and weight, high performance, and low maintenance. Monitoring and control of feeders can be done with digital sensors and switches to monitor voltage, reactive power, outage, and feeder switching.

5.4 Assistant Management System of Electric Vehicle (EV)

The management system of an electric vehicle consists of an EV, tracing center, and charging point. Somebody can find a nearby charging point and parking station with the help of GPS. With GPS's support, the most appropriable station can be located in a suitable manner [4].

5.5 Demand-Side Management (DSM)

DSM is a proactive methodology for arranging, executing, and observing energy utilization during top hours. It essentially depends on the present age with a request by controlling utilization at the client side. The term DSM is first presented by Gelling's, a senior individual from Electric Power Research Institute (EPRI). The DSM's fundamental objectives are top section, valley filling, load moving, critical load development, vital protection, and adaptable load shape. DSM is applied in various locales with various situations [11, 12].

5.6 *Load Forecasting (LF)*

It is used to estimate the requirements of energy consumed by a system based on history and forecast parameters. LF provides a balance between demand and supply energy. LF can predict load around for short and long period, which helps in future planning of power system expansion and load management. It can be performed with several techniques like multiple regression, ANN, GA, fuzzy logic, etc. [13].

5.7 *Wind Energy Forecasting*

Wind power is among the quickest developing sustainable power sources on the planet. Coordination of wind power sources with the network gives a few technological, financial, and ecological advantages. Be that as it may, because of the discontinuous and stochastic nature of wind power, it provides a few snags during the generation of power and dissemination. Variety in wind speed causes uncertainty in the wind power plant yield, which prompts instability in the network. Consequently, legitimate estimating is required for wind energy-based force networks and can help in making operational methodologies.

5.8 *Solar Energy Forecasting*

Sun-powered energy is one of the most noticeable sustainable power sources. Numerous normal and artificial obstructions, such as climatic conditions, occasional changes, geological rise, spasmodic creation, and intra-hour changeability, impact sunlight-based PV framework execution. Subsequently, sunlight-based energy data ought to be gained ahead of time to limit the working expenses brought about by the different snags. There is various algorithm of machine learning, which are having some limitation and benefits. Few of these techniques are presented in Table 1.

6 Energy-Efficient Framework

This section introduced an energy productive structure for the intelligent network. The framework utilizes a blend of GPRS innovation and the Zigbee module for communication with sensors. In this system, one can embrace a two-layer remote organization to give more opportunity and adaptability. The primary level uses IEEE 802.15.4 or Zigbee distance, which is easy, low energy utilization, and has a correspondence run between 100 and 1000 m in every hub [8]. As to Zigbee organizing

Table 1 Taxation of machine learning algorithms with pros and cons

Name of algorithm	Description	Pros	Cons
Linear regression	• Linear regression is used to predict a correlation between one or more independent variables and a dependent variable • A straight-line relationship appears when we plot this on the graph • $Y = mX + b$ • It is the best fit line through all data points. All the predictions are numerical	Easy to understand and good in learning data analysis	Not capable of dealing with nonlinear relationships, complex patterns
Logistic regression	• Used for classification; used for binomial or multinomial classification • It gives output in terms of 0 or 1 based on input values • It is used to evaluate the output of logit functions • Logit function—chances of happening of an event over the prospects of not happening of this event • $p/1-p$ is the logit of p	Simple to implement, efficient, easy regularization, no scaling is required for input features	Unable to solve nonlinear functions, prone to overfitting

(continued)

Table 1 (continued)

Name of algorithm	Description	Pros	Cons
Support vector machine	• Proposed by Vladimir Naumovich Vapnik and Alexey Yakovlevich Chervonenkis • Samples are treated as p-dimensional • Separate these points with a $(p-1)$-dimensional hyper plain	High accuracy	Slow training, computationally expensive
Sequential optimization algorithm (SMO)	• Proposed by John Platt In 1998 • SMO is a fast and straightforward algorithm used for training support vector machine • Dual quadratic optimization problems are solved by optimization of the minimal subset at each iteration	Analytical and straightforward, based on dividing large quadratic problem into small to solve them in less time; fast and time saving	
KNN	• K-nearest neighbor classifies similar instances • In multidimensional space, all neighbors are classified	More time is required for more neighbors	Performance decreased with the increase of neighbors
Decision tree types: ID3 C4.5 CART	• Based on the divide and conquer method • Information gain and splitting used	Simple, easy to implement, speed, accuracy	Space limited, overfitting, intolerance of missing values, sensitivity to noise

(continued)

Table 1 (continued)

Name of algorithm	Description	Pros	Cons
Naïve Bayes (NB)	• Proposed in 1950 and since then researched widely • Derived from Bayes theorem; assuming that all samples are strongly independent • Used for text classification like email classification, etc., with accuracy	Speed of learning and classification	Tolerance of missing values, intolerance of irrelevant attributes
Random forest	• Set of decision tree • Each tree used Bootstrap sample and randomly selected predicators	RF does not overfit; we can run as many trees as we can, fast	–
Neural network	• A neuron is a function $Y = f(X)$; X is input, and Y is output • The neuron can be linear or nonlinear • Four basic learning rules in NN are as follows: error correction rules, Boltzmann rules, Hebbian rules, and competitive learning	More robust to noise, handle complex problems	Needs lots of data to train

ability, work geography is proposed in this framework. The work geography's fundamental advantage is that each hub can speak with some other hub straightforwardly inside the inclusion region.

Moreover, it expands unwavering network quality and supports remote association on the off chance that one of the hubs has a fall flat, misfortune sign, or incapacitated. The subsequent level uses the GPRS module to help the organization in sending information. The GPRS innovation can improvise network execution for continuous information just as it is more proficient and vigorous [5]. GPRS module also bolsters TCP or IP convention that empowers sending information straightforwardly to the worker utilizing a specific hub's location. Figure 4 portrays the sending schematic of the hardware in the appropriation framework-based IoT. The IOT device, network model, correspondence geography, and information handling are like the transmission framework.

Nonetheless, observing the status of substation is of the real worry in the dissemination framework. In this way, the substation should be well outfitted with an intelligent sensor and smart meter. There is a significant boundary; for example, transformer temperature, current and voltage profile, oil level, load profile, shortcoming, and blackout can be checked. Observing transmission and appropriation framework-based IoT is an integral asset to build framework dependability and acknowledges early warning and ongoing checking through the executives' cloud data. The intensity transmission and appropriation framework status can be shown outwardly on PC, cell phone, and laptop.

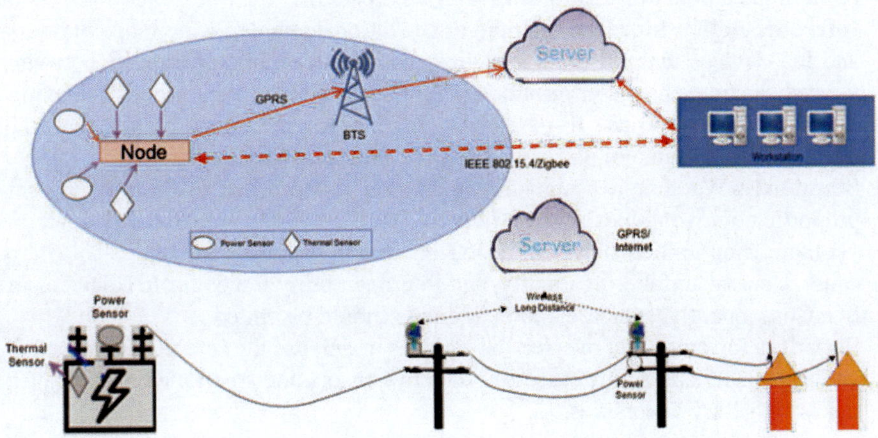

Fig. 4 Load distribution system-based IoT

7 Difficulties and Future Research Directions

IoT devices should work in various conditions like high voltages, high or low temperatures, humid environment, and prolog to electromagnetic waves. Along these lines, they should fulfill requirements at those circumstances, for instance, constancy or likeness.

- **Data fusion**: In different applications, IoT devices and sensors manage batteries like various sensors utilized to screen transmission lines, so appropriate energy procuring methodology should be used or arranged. We have a couple of correspondence networks in different bits of the SG. Accordingly, IoT devices should maintain significant correspondence shows to move data from sharp meters to the central system which is possible and guaranteed. Since IoT devices in SG have limited resources and limits, similar to batteries, dealing with power, storing, or movement speed, data mix cycles should be used to pack and add up to important data to have more capable energy bandwidth use and data combination.
- **Delay**: Deferral and group setback are critical limits that choose the introduction of smart grid. Since blockage causes deferral and bundle hardship, it brings down system execution considering that IoT devices, just as entryways IoT devices, must resend data which causes greater delay and extends the probability of stop up again. Additionally, SG cannot satisfy fated necessities, as most prominent average deferment. Along these lines, it is imperative to restrict delay, improve network plan by finding an ideal number of entries and IoT devices and breaking point in the amount of relationship with each passage.
- **Interoperability**: Since the splendid organization contains a wide scope of doors and IoT devices with different specifics and resources, interoperability between the devices to exchange information is fundamental. One response for achieving interoperability is to use IP-based associations. Another game plan is that IoT devices should maintain particular correspondence shows and structures.
- **Standards**: We should design the smart grid to store and cycle this colossal proportion of assembled data beneficially. There are various separate IoT devices, yet there is no unified standard for IoT devices in the adroit structure. This may cause security, unfaltering quality, and interoperability issues for IoT devices in SG. Consequently, standardization attempts should be united.
- **Security**: To screen and oversee IoT devices in SG, use the Internet unprotected, and aggressors can control assessed data by sensors and smart meters and cause many budgetary adversities.

8 Conclusion

In this paper, an attempt has been made to focus on IoT in smart grid application areas. Smart grid helps to distribute load automatically according to user requirements. The applications, components, architecture, and future issues of the smart grid environment have been discussed. Finally, it provides a proposed mechanism in which IoT devices and machine learning algorithms are used to provide energy-efficient load distribution frameworks for smart grid environments. In future, it is intended to continue working in a smart grid and proposes a more reliable mechanism based on unsupervised learning for handling overloaded grids.

References

1. Kumar D, Zare F, Ghosh A (2017) DC Microgrid technology: system architectures, AC grid interfaces, grounding schemes, power quality, communication networks, applications, and standardisations aspects. IEEE Access 5:12230–12256. https://doi.org/10.1109/ACCESS.2017.2705914
2. Hossain E, Khan I, Un-Noor F, Sikander SS, Sunny MSH (2019) Application of big data and machine learning in smart grid, and associated security concerns: a review. IEEE Access 7:13960–13988. https://doi.org/10.1109/ACCESS.2019.2894819
3. Arya AK, Chanana S, Kumar A (2014) Role of smart grid in power system planning and operation in India. Int J Recent Trends Eng Technol 11(1):456
4. Dileep G (2020) A survey on smart grid technologies and applications. Renew Energy 146:2589–2625. https://doi.org/10.1016/j.renene.2019.08.092
5. Ibrahim MS, Dong W, Yang Q (2020) Machine learning driven smart electric power systems: current trends and new perspectives. Appl Energy 272:115237. https://doi.org/10.1016/j.apenergy.2020.115237
6. Alimi OA, Ouahada K, Abu-Mahfouz AM (2020) A Review of machine learning approaches to power system security and stability. IEEE Access 8:113512–113531. https://doi.org/10.1109/ACCESS.2020.3003568
7. Farhoumandi M, Zhou Q, Shahidehpour M (2021) A review of machine learning applications in IoT-integrated modern power systems. Electr J 34(1):106879. https://doi.org/10.1016/j.tej.2020.106879
8. Ghorbanian M, Dolatabadi SH, Masjedi M, Siano P (2019) Communication in smart grids: a comprehensive review on the existing and future communication and information infrastructures. IEEE Syst J 13(4):4001–4014. https://doi.org/10.1109/JSYST.2019.2928090
9. Sharma K, Saini LM (2015) Performance analysis of smart metering for smart grid: an overview. Renew Sustain Energy Rev 49:720–735. https://doi.org/10.1016/j.rser.2015.04.170
10. Stegner C, Glaß O, Beikircher T (2019) Comparing smart metered, residential power demand with standard load profiles. Sustain Energy Grids Netw 20:1–10. https://doi.org/10.1016/j.segan.2019.100248
11. Sedhom BE, El-Saadawi MM, El Moursi MS, Hassan MA, Eladl AA (2021) IoT-based optimal demand side management and control scheme for smart microgrid. Int J Electr Power Energy Syst 127:106674. https://doi.org/10.1016/j.ijepes.2020.106674
12. Singh P, Dhundhara S, Pal Y, Tayal N (2021) Optimal battery utilisation for energy management and load scheduling in smart residence under demand response scheme. Sustain Energy Grids Netw 26:100432. https://doi.org/10.1016/j.segan.2021.100432
13. Uppal M, Garg VK, Kumar D (2020) Weather biased optimal delta model for short-term load forecast. IET Smart Grid 1–8. https://doi.org/10.1049/iet-stg.2019.0331

A Quantitative Study of Small Dataset Machining by Agglomerative Hierarchical Cluster and *K*-Medoid

Pruthvi Raju Garikapati, K. Balamurugan, T. P. Latchoumi, and G. Shankar

Abstract An attempt has been made to investigate the possibility of applying the advantages of hierarchical and partitioning mechanism methods in a small dataset like machining method such as abrasive water jet machine (AWJM). LM13 alloy with 63% SiC composite was taken as the study material, and it was machined using AWJM for Taguchi's L27 experimental runs. As individual thresholds, water pressure, cutting distance, and cutting velocity are taken as AWJM parameters, and material removal rate (MRR), Kerf angle (KA), and surface profile roughness (Ra) are taken as the output responses. Agglomerative hierarchical clustering (AHC) classifiers classify L27 OA into three groups of nine perceptions each. The test on *K*-medoid esteem is taken as 3 instead of AHC bunch L27 OA in three groups to look at and analyze the distinction between partitional clustering and progressive clustering procedures at a comparable class degree. K's approximation is fixed by three and bundled into three groups of nine impressions each. For the investigation of AHC and *K*-medoid, XLSTAT programming is used. Besides, for each class/arrangement of AHC and *K*-medoid, direct relapse conditions and contrast and test impressions are generated. The analysis shows that the classification of *K*-medoid based on the parceling method suits well with the perceptions of the trial. For all the groups, AHC produces a sole condition, while *K*-medoids create singular conditions for each of its classes.

Keywords Abrasive water jet machine · Support vector machine · Agglomerative hierarchical clustering · *K*-Medoid

P. R. Garikapati · K. Balamurugan (✉)
Department of Mechanical Engineering, VFSTR (Deemed To Be University), Guntur, Andhra Pradesh 522213, India

T. P. Latchoumi · G. Shankar
Department of Computer Science and Engineering, SRM Institute of Science and Technology, Ramapuram campus, Chennai, Tamil Nadu 600089, India

N. Marriwala et al. (eds.), *Emergent Converging Technologies and Biomedical Systems*, Lecture Notes in Electrical Engineering 841,
https://doi.org/10.1007/978-981-16-8774-7_59

1 Introduction

Machining methods for industrial parts have grown quickly in the most recent decade because of new machines arrivals with high bearing load limits, the materials utilized in their designs, and they perpetually progressed control frameworks [1, 2]. This mechanical improvement encourages the machining of segments with higher exactness and better surface quality in a limited time. The limited manufacturing time enhances productivity, and along these lines, more benefits can be acquired. This can bring about a high-income surplus in large-scale manufacturing. In the hour of Industry 4.0, when the origination of PC controlled mechanized plants is being broadened, programmed information assortment and investigation can be used to help in dynamic action [3]. This medoids the time information of creation measures are accessible in a more limited time and at a more significant level of exactness [4]. For a given innovation, the machining time and cost can fundamentally be streamlined by the cutting information (cutting pace, profundity of-cut, feed, and so on), and also, the legitimization of supporting exercises of a creation cycle can diminish the occasions associated straightforwardly or in a roundabout way to the machining. This medoid that diminishes can be made in the planning time or the time required for material taking care of among the working environments. A few plants identified solutions after being developed for late many years, e.g., lean creation, six-sigma, or the hypothesis of imperatives. The surface irregularity of the turned steel is optimized using these methods for an exact surface roughness device. A forecast model instead of normal surface roughness was made by methods for nonlinear relapse assessment with the guide of MINITAB programming. The good machining settings are perceived by Taguchi's strategy and checked with an affirmation preliminary. The outcomes will uncover that machining under micro-lubrication condition displayed lesser temperature at the instrument work interface and the nature of the machined segments likewise shows lesser unpleasantness when contrasted and parts of dry machining condition [5].

Mixture aluminum lattice composites are the second age of composites that improve properties by potentially replace of single reinforced composites. This paper researches the achievability and suitability of growing hybrid composites for car and aviation applications. Further, the manufacturing qualities and mechanical conduct of hybrid composite created by the mix projecting course have additionally been inspected. The optical micrographs of the hybrid composite demonstrate that the strengthening particles are genuinely conveyed in the grid combination and the porosity levels have been discovered to be satisfactory for the casted composites. The thickness, hardness, elastic conduct, and crack durability of these composites have been discovered to be superior to available reinforced composite. In light of the information base for material properties, the application territory of hybrid composite has been proposed in the current survey [6]. It has been argued that in the plan of future segments depending on the support mix and piece, cross-breed composites provide greater adaptability and unwavering consistency.

K-medoid bunching calculation is utilized for gathering the understudies in the college dependent on position and evaluating framework [7]. *K*-medoid calculation was not appropriate for an enormous measure of the dataset, for example, shading pictures, since it requires setting each an incentive as a medoid regardless of whether its recurrence (e.g., number of pixels of same power) is extremely low. As the shading picture has some various powers to set as medoids, it needs more opportunity for the count. The other significant disadvantage of existing calculation is to locate the ideal number of cycles, and in our test result, we show that how many emphases assume a significant part to locate the best ideal arrangement. To overcome this barrier, this paper gives an altered *K*-medoids calculation by utilizing the histogram leveling method. To demonstrate the effectiveness of this new calculation, we give different exploratory outcomes over various pictures with a correlation of the current calculation.

The impacts of cutting apparatus covering material and cutting rate on cutting powers and surface roughness were researched by Taguchi exploratory plan. Primary cutting power, Fz, is considered as a model. The impacts of machining boundaries were explored utilizing Taguchi L18 symmetrical exhibit. Ideal cutting conditions were resolved utilizing the sign-to-commotion (S/N) proportion which is determined for normal surface unpleasantness and slicing power as per the "more modest is better" approach. Utilizing consequences of examination of fluctuation (ANOVA) and sign-to-noise (S/N) proportion, impacts of boundaries on both normal surface roughness and cutting powers were genuinely measured. It was seen that feed rate and cutting rate had a higher impact on cutting power in Hastelloy X, while the feed rate and cutting device had a higher impact on cutting power in Inconel 625. As per normal surface roughness, the cutting device and feed rate had a higher impact in Hastelloy X and Inconel 625 [8].

The focal point of this paper is on cycle getting ready for huge parts to fabricate in frameworks of unequivocal cycle capacities, including the utilization of multi-hub machining focuses. Arrangement ideas applied and activity groupings decided in related cycle plans went through examinations. The paper presents specifically a thinking way to deal with arrangement sequencing and machine task in assembling huge size parts of seaward developments. The applicable thinking component inside a dynamic plan on created measure plan is indicated dependent on a contextual investigation got from the seaward area [9].

The inside and out an investigation of cutting system is a subject exceptionally compelling in assembling productivity because in the enormous scope of creation in the viable utilization for creation limits and to have improved income [10]. The investigation on time and material removal rate, which are in close connection to creation, is significant in arranging a machining technique. In the paper three strategies applied in hard cutting are looked at based on these boundaries and another boundary, the functional boundary of material removal rate, are presented. It estimates the proficiency of cutting since it incorporates the qualities estimated by time investigation. In the examinations, the material removal rate was broken down, first based on mathematical information of the segment. After that diverse machining systems (hard machining) were thought about for some average surfaces. The outcomes can give some valuable signs about machining system choice. Expansion in the hybrid composite is 15.24% more than the base compound. The effect of the strength of the hybrid composite was diminished in contrast with the base combination. In sliding, wear considers, the composite with 1 wt. % B4C has demonstrated less weight reduction and coefficient of erosion [11].

Aluminum-based hybrid matrix composites replace single fortified composites in numerous applications because of their mechanical and tribological properties. Numerous examinations have been done on mechanical conduct on composites mixture; however, so far no examinations have been done with cylinder combination. This examination centers around discovering the impact of graphite (Gr) particulates as an optional fortification on the mechanical conduct of LM 13/Silicon carbide (SiC) composites. Agglomerative bunching was the most commonly known method of multiple level grouping used to assemble objects based on their similarities in classes [12].

Progressive bunching techniques depend on building a chain of groups, which is frequently represented as graphically methods in the form of a tree structure called a dendrogram. This progressive system results from the way that groups of expanding likeness are converged to shape bigger ones (agglomerative calculations) or that bigger clustering are part into more modest ones of diminishing dissimilarities (troublesome methodology) [13]. Such methodologies have the benefit of permitting investigation for the information at various degrees of similitude/difference and giving a more profound knowledge into the connections among tests (or factors, if those are the things to be grouped). Another large bit of scope is that, since they depend on characterizing a comparability record among the clustering, any sort of information (genuine esteemed, discrete, and twofold) can be broken down by these methods [14] which will further increase the interest among the readers.

2 Materials and Methods

LM13 alloy which has excellent strength and toughness is sufficiently heated through an electric furnace to 250° C. Dissolving 63 percent SiC in the LM 13 matrix was accepted as an increase in the composite will lead to the improper dispersion inside the matrix. The heater temperature decreased to 600 °C, which cools the SiC fuse fluid mixture. In the semi-strong lattice mixture with an exceptionally expected stirrer, the optional fortification (SiC) with molecule size varying from 15 to 30 microns was pre-oxidized at 900 °C for 2 h. Under the view of argon gas, the semi-strong composite structure is blended. With the ceaseless blending state, the dissolve is warmed to 750 °C, and the temperature was kept up for 5 min. To attain composite ingots of 25 cm × 25 cm × 1.2 cm, robust iron passes of 8 mm divider thickness are loaded with composite slurry [15]. In Fig. 1, the development courses of action were shown.

Shimadzu's AUX 220 model utilizes high-precision gauging equilibrium to measure the volume of material eliminated during machining. Each moment of MRR

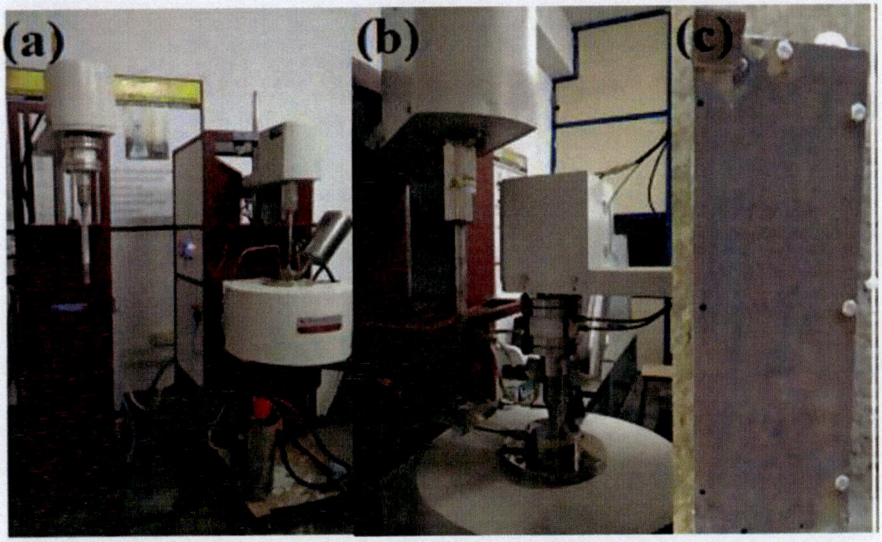

Fig. 1 Fabrication setup

was calculated using the corresponding Eq. (1).

$$\text{MRR} = (W_a - W_b)/t \quad (1)$$

where W_i—Job piece in grams before machining, W_a—Workpiece in grams after machining, and t—Trial time (minute).

Using the AWJM, the machining effect of the composite is carried out. Water pressure, cutting distance, and cutting speed are shifted into three different stages, each calculating the yield output attributes. Machining limits and thresholds are shown in Table 1. Garnet 80 microns of lattice size was used as abrasives. The microstructure of the fabricated composite is seen in

Table 1 Selected factor and levels

S. no.	Parameter	Symbols	Levels			Units
			1	2	3	
1	Water pressure	WP	220	240	260	bar
2	Cutting distance	CD	1	2	3	mm
3	Cutting speed	TS	20	30	40	mm/min

2.1 Support Vector Machine (SVM)

Support vector machine (SVM) is perhaps the most common supervised learning calculations that are used just as regression for classification. It is used in machine learning for classification problems. The goal of the SVM calculation is to establish the best line or option limit that can isolate *n*-dimensional space into classes such that we can later place the new knowledge point in the correct classification without much of a stretch. As a hyperplane, this best choice limit is known. The exceptional focuses/vectors that help make the hyperplane are chosen by SVM.

With the fundamental goal that deeply fits colossal datasets in AI and data disclosure, SVM calculation was developed. It offers answers of greater order precision for organizing both paired and multi-class problems. For the machining period, SVM processes are used which help to understand the fundamental knowledge between different machining boundaries and characterize the perceptions into a limited set of information, i.e., classes.

2.2 Agglomerative Hierarchical Clustering (AHC)

Stage 1: At the underlying level, by fixing its boundaries, an actual data point is a bunch together.

Stage 2: A comparative individual cluster based on comparability is organized into a solitary group.

Stage 3: Check the accessibility of a few clustering.

Stage 4: To get the characterized number of clustering to rehash stage 2.

Stage 5: Clustering yield results.

2.3 K-Medoids Clustering

In 1987, Kaufman and Rousseeuw suggested a measure of *K*-medoids (also known as partitioning around medoid). A medoid may be defined as the party point, whose dissimilarities are least with the broad variety of different focuses in the bunch.

Medoid (Ci) and object (Pi) differences are calculated by the use of $E = |\mathrm{Pi} - \mathrm{Ci}|$

In the *K*-medoids estimate, the cost is given as

$$C = \sum |\mathrm{Pi} - \mathrm{Ci}| \quad (2)$$

Algorithm

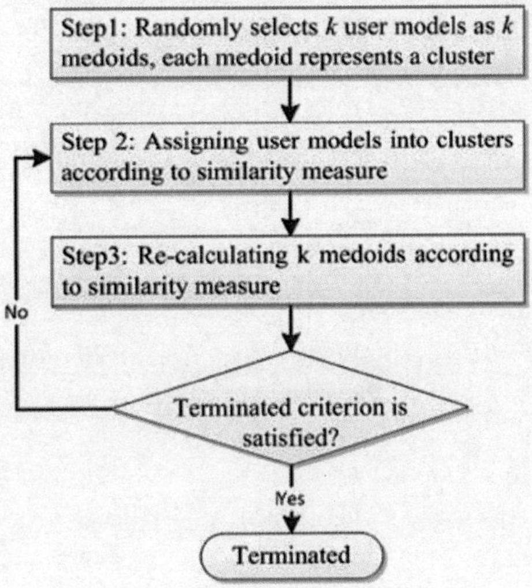

Fig. 2 Step-wise *K*-means algorithm flowchart

1. Initialize: pick *k* random brings up as the medoids from the n knowledge focuses.
2. Each data from the partner highlights the closest medoid by using some standard distance metric strategies.
3. Whereas the cost is decreasing:

For each medoid m, for each data o point that is not a medoid:

1. Trade m and o, partner both data, highlight the nearest medoid, and recalculate the cost.
2. On the off possibility that the absolute cost in the previous advance is greater than that, correct the exchange.

A problem with the classification of *K*-means and *K*-means++ is that the last centroids are not interpretable or all in all, centroids are not the real point, but rather the average emphasis in that bunch. Here are the 3-centroid directions that do not take from the dataset after true emphasis. The probability of *K*-medoids classification is to concentrate on rendering the last centroids as real results. As seen in Fig. 2, this finding makes the centroids interpretable.

3 Results and Discussions

3.1 Abrasive Water Jet Machine

With Taguchi L27 experimental runs, the generated hierarchical composite was machined at an alternate level. The perceptions are shown in Table 2.

Table 2 Experimental observations

Ex No	PR	SOD	TV	MRR	KA	Ra
1	220	1	20	0.0042	0.2376	3.447
2	220	1	30	0.0055	0.1623	3.457
3	220	1	40	0.0070	0.2608	3.097
4	220	2	20	0.0047	0.3147	3.246
5	220	2	30	0.0060	0.2739	3.346
6	220	2	40	0.0083	0.3743	3.525
7	220	3	20	0.0048	0.5602	3.595
8	220	3	30	0.0067	0.6750	3.490
9	220	3	40	0.0081	0.5234	3.586
10	240	1	20	0.0046	0.5736	2.963
11	240	1	30	0.0055	0.2000	3.333
12	240	1	40	0.0084	0.2768	3.401
13	240	2	20	0.0046	0.5021	3.206
14	240	2	30	0.0064	0.3054	3.503
15	240	2	40	0.0086	0.9212	3.622
16	240	3	20	0.0045	0.7042	3.349
17	240	3	30	0.0072	0.7487	3.118
18	240	3	40	0.0099	0.7906	3.757
19	260	1	20	0.0044	0.5881	4.645
20	260	1	30	0.0059	0.5877	4.259
21	260	1	40	0.0078	0.4554	4.915
22	260	2	20	0.0043	0.5554	4.754
23	260	2	30	0.0065	0.3014	3.908
24	260	2	40	0.0083	0.5503	4.093
25	260	3	20	0.0052	0.7393	3.996
26	260	3	30	0.0068	0.3481	3.928
27	260	3	40	0.0090	0.5703	3.780

3.2 K-*Medoids and AHC of MRR*

A line map for the relevant MRR groups for AHC and *K*-medoids is plotted to understand the AHC and *K*-medoids equations working over the expectations of the trial. For both AHC and *K*-medoids, a direct relapse model has been developed. A lone direct condition for MRR is obtained by AHC, and it is seen in Figs. 3, 4, 5, and 6. In *K*-medoids, each class generates its state and is shown separately as classes 1, 2, and 3 in the diagram. From the conditions shown, the close diagram is obtained, and it appears in the figure. It seems to be reasoned, from the perception, that the groups separated by *K*-medoids are considered to be ideal. For *K*-medoid and AHC,

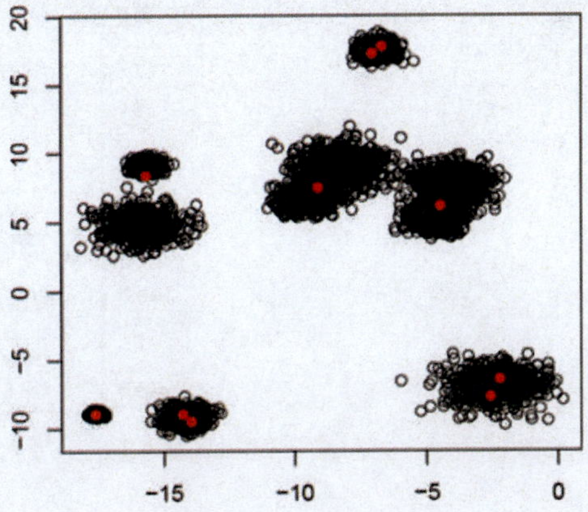

Fig. 3 *K*-Medoid for class 1

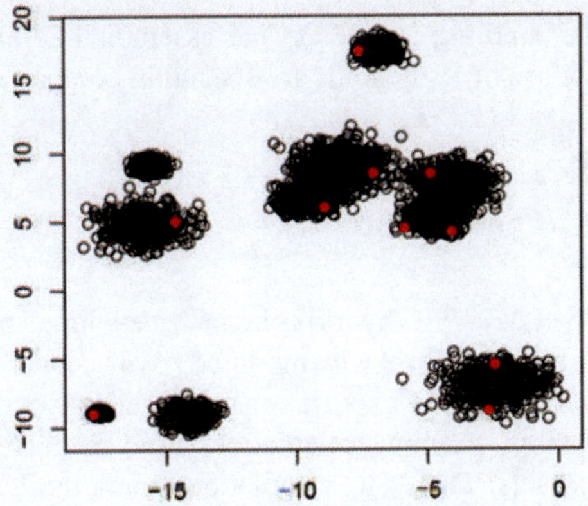

Fig. 4 *K*-Medoid for class 2

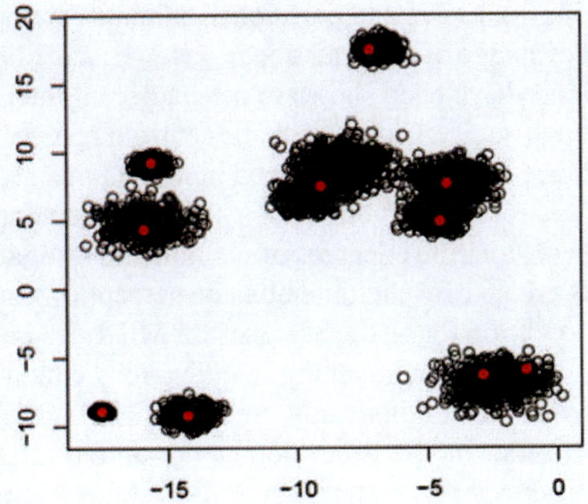

Fig. 5 *K*-Medoid for class 3

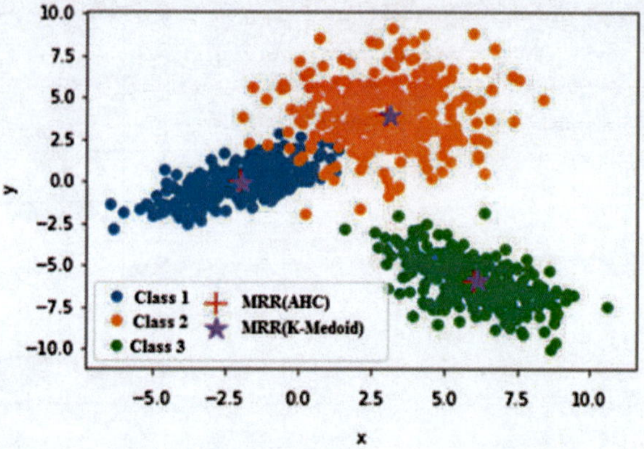

Fig. 6 *K*-Means and AHC of MRR for three classes

the bundling of L27 OA has assembled 27 experiences into three classes where the classes of *K*-medoids are special in comparison with AHC.

4 Conclusion

The LM13/SiC hybrid composite developed by the stir casting process is machined at an alternate level with modified AWJM conditions. For the characterization measurements, AWJM expectations are used as source evidence. AHC and *K*-medoids are notable grouping calculations used to decrease the numerical unpredictability of datasets. The AHC calculation orders the L27 Taguchi array into 3 classes with 9 experiences in each class. Although the value of $K = 3$ to allow a close analysis of progressive and partitional estimates of approaches on machining parameters, the advantage of this equation is reviewed and closed as follows. The expected characteristics have been shown to have a decent interaction with the *K*-medoids exploratory opportunity. Centered on the centroid respect AHC, whereas the degrees of *K* importance can be set to the need in *K*-medoids groups. For the same cause, the degree of *K* is set as 3, although it may have phenomenal alignment with the perceptions of the trial at various degrees of *K*. In this investigation, a straight relapse condition model is created for the quantities of perceptions on each class. AHC builds up a solitary condition for all the 3 classes for MRR, KA, and Ra, while *K*-medoids because of the uniqueness in bunching it age various conditions for all the classes for all the yield reactions. In this study, for the amounts of expectations in class, a straight relapse disorder model is developed. For all the three classes for MRR, KA, and Ra, AHC produces a solo state, while *K*-medoids age for all classes for all the yield reactions due to the uniqueness of bunching it. The conditions created for *K*-medoids are suitable only for the basic perceptions of the class. Because of any vulnerability that occurs in the equations, this situation should not be used by other class experiences.

To solve these challenges, some analysis must be performed later on, whereas no such things will occur within the AHC.

References

1. Bhasha AC, Balamurugan K (2019) Fabrication and property evaluation of Al 6061+ x%(RHA+ TiC) hybrid metal matrix composite. SN Appl Sci 1(9):1–9
2. Balamurugan K (2020) Fracture analysis of fuselage wing joint developed by aerodynamic structural materials. Mater Today: Proc
3. Bhasha AC, Balamurugan K (2020) End mill studies on Al6061 hybrid composite prepared by ultrasonic-assisted stir casting. Multiscale Multidiscip Model, Exp Des, 1–12
4. Singh S, Prakash C, Antil P, Singh R, Krolczyk G, Pruncu CI (2019) Dimensionless analysis for investigating the quality characteristics of aluminium matrix composites prepared through fused deposition modelling assisted investment casting. Mater. https://doi.org/10.3390/ma12121907
5. Tiwari S, Das S, Venkat ANC (2019) Mechanical properties of Al–Si–SiC composites. Mater Res Express 6:076553
6. Ghandvar H, Idris MH, Ahmad N, Moslemi N (2017) Microstructure development, mechanical and tribological properties of a semi-solid A356/xSiCp composite. J Appl Res Technol 15:533–544
7. Choi JH, Jo MC, Lee D, Shin S, Jo I, Lee SK, Lee S (2018) Effects of SiC particulate size on dynamic compressive properties in 7075-T6 Al-SiCp composites. Mater Sci Eng, A 738:412–419
8. Wang G, Tian N, Li C, Zhao G, Zuo L (2019) Effect of Si content on the fatigue fracture behavior of wrought Al–*x*Si–0.7Mg alloy. Mater Sci Forum 941:1143–1148
9. Antil P, Singh S, Manna A (2018) SiCp/glass fibers reinforced epoxy composites: Wear and erosion behavior. Indian J Eng Mater Sci 25:122–130
10. Latchoumi TP, Balamurugan K, Dinesh K, Ezhilarasi TP (2019) Particle swarm optimization approach for waterjet cavitation peening. Meas 141:184–189
11. Antil P, Singh S, Manna A (2019) Experimental investigation during Electrochemical Discharge Machining (ECDM) of hybrid polymer matrix composites. Iran J Sci Technol, Trans Mech Eng. https://doi.org/10.1007/s40997-019-00280-5
12. Pradhan A, Ghosh S, Barman TK, Sahoo P (2017) Tribological behavior of Al-SiC metal matrix composite under dry aqueous alkaline medium. Silicon 9:923–931
13. Antil P, Singh S, Manna A (2019) Analysis on the effect of electroless coated SiCp on mechanical properties of polymer matrix composites. Part Sci Technol 37:787–794
14. Zain AM, Haron H, Sharif S (2011) Genetic algorithm and simulated annealing to estimate optimal process parameters of the abrasive waterjet machining. Eng Comput 27:251–259
15. Garikapati P, Balamurugan K, Latchoumi TP, Malkapuram R (2020) A cluster-profile comparative study on machining AlSi 7/63% of SiC hybrid composite using agglomerative hierarchical clustering and K-Means. Silicon, 1–12

Deep Learning-Based Face Mask Detecting System: An Initiative Against COVID-19

Komal Saini and Nikhil Marriwala

Abstract In this era of pandemic, wearing mask and taking precaution is a must, and this paper provides a way of detecting mask with the help of deep learning. Deep learning is an important part of machine learning. OpenCV, an important part of Python, is used for real-time image detection. This is a very decent system which can be applied at various platforms and can help in slowing down the transmission of coronavirus.

Keywords Deep learning · Python · OpenCV · ROI (region of interest) · Adaboost · Cascade Classifier

1 Introduction

Coronavirus disease 2019 (COVID-19) is an infectious disease transmitted by a newly discovered virus naming coronavirus. Severe acute respiratory syndrome coronavirus 2 (SARS-CoV-2) is the reason for coronavirus disease which is an ongoing global health emergency. Most of the infected people experience mild to moderate scale of respiratory illness, and many may recover without even requiring any unusual treatment. People with some previous disease like cardiovascular disease, cancer, sugar or any elder age disease are more prone to get infected by this virus.

The finest way to stop or sluggish the transmission of this virus is to be well aware about this virus, the sickness it causes and how it may spread. Protecting ourself and others from infection is very essential and can be done by taking precautions using an alcohol-based sanitizer frequently or washing our hands and not touching your face [1].

K. Saini (✉) · N. Marriwala
Department of Electronics and Communication Engineering, University Institute of Engineering and Technology, Kurukshetra University, Kurukshetra, Haryana, India

N. Marriwala
e-mail: nmarriwala@kuk.ac.in

N. Marriwala et al. (eds.), *Emergent Converging Technologies and Biomedical Systems*, Lecture Notes in Electrical Engineering 841,
https://doi.org/10.1007/978-981-16-8774-7_60

This virus is spreading by droplets of sneeze form nose and saliva when any infected person coughs or sneezes, so it is very important to practice respiratory etiquette (e.g. by covering face while sneezing and coughing). This virus can impact the mental health in some cases [2].

COVID hit the world suddenly and left us in a jeopardy. It is very necessary in these times that everyone should follow protocols provided by government. Wearing mask, sanitizing and washing hands is a must. But some people seem to just ignore all these and got infected because of their unresponsible actions.

2 Approach

For this project, the approach followed is very simple. There is a need of some utilities to be installed which will make the task very easy. The data is taken, then, it is preprocessed, and then, training of the convolutional neural network (CNN) with the data is done. A multi-layer neural network serves well for this purpose. A CNN is a system with different layers of convolution kernels that operate with any original dataset, special features according to the need from dataset are extracted, and thus, it is a very powerful tool for computer vision tasks [3]. Then, the trained model attached with a video stream builds a face recognition system. The next step is testing, and the task is done (Fig. 1).

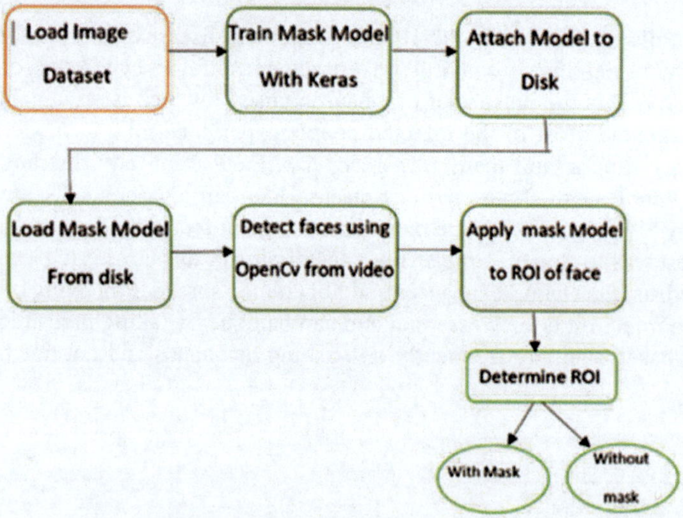

Fig. 1 Flow chart of the face mask detector

3 Deep Learning

Deep learning is a part of machine learning. This system aims at learning the feature extraction from higher levels of the hierarchy, and the extracted features can be used for training the CNN. Automatically the extracted features are used and layer by layer help in building CNN. This method can also be used in complex problems [4]. Therefore, deep learning helps in learning representation of the data (Fig. 2).

Deep learning network is similar to a multilevel information-distillation operation, in this any information that goes through a number of filters and comes out increasingly purified (that is, useful with regard to some task) [5].

Utilities used:

- TensorFlow
- Keras
- Imutils
- OpenCV Python.

3.1 TensorFlow

TensorFlow is an interface that can be used for algorithm of machine learning. This can be used in number of areas like voice recognition, text summarization, information extraction and many more. Using this for our face mask detection system would be a very good choice [6].

Keras

Keras gives a basic reflection, and this is a part of TensorFlow. It has many useful libraries that can ease the task of mask detector model making [7].

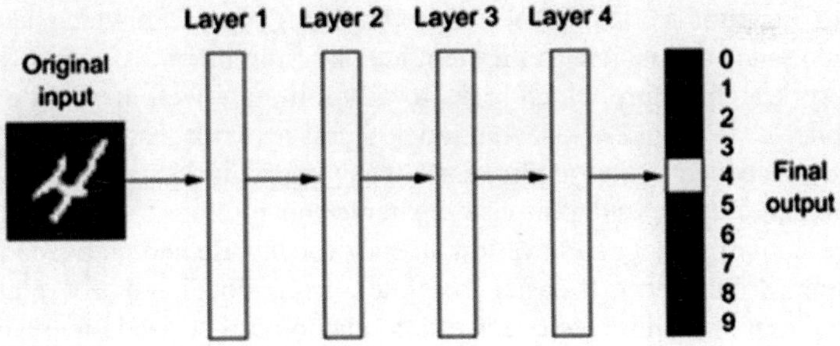

Fig. 2 Deep learning model

3.2 Preprocessing

For preprocessing, some images of people wearing mask and some of people not wearing mask are collected to make dataset. These images can be collected from Google or any other open-source image library. Then, these images split in two folders naming "with mask" and "without mask".

Now in training code, there are two list, i.e. data [] and labels [], the data [] list contain images, and label [] will be having the labels, i.e. "with" or "without" mask. After this, the images are converted into arrays because deep learning model works on arrays only. For converting images to arrays, an image_to_array function from Keras is the best choice. Keras is an open-source library in Python for deep learning. This contains many such functions which can ease the process of working with deep learning.

The images are now in machine understandable form (array), but labels are still in alphabetic order. For labels to be in machine understandable form, a label binarizer function from Sklearn would work well, which have many unsupervised and supervised learning algorithms and which can convert labels in binary form.

Next step is splitting the dataset into two sets, and those are train and test. As dataset is small, so ImageDataGenerator function is used to expand the dataset. This function increases the dataset as it is able to convert many images of a single image, i.e. rotated, flatted, etc. After this, the dataset will be increased and help in making a better model.

4 Training

For training of the model, MobileNet, which is similar to CNN in working but it is faster and uses lesser parameters, is the best choice. MobileNet models are skilled in TensorFlow through using RMSprop with an asynchronous gradient descent which is similar to Inception V3 [8]. CNN is a deep learning algorithm which takes input, assigns importance and is able to differentiate one from other. It is a convolutional neural network architecture which seeks to perform quite well on mobile devices. Here, MobileNet is a kind of convolutional neural network that was designed for mobile and embedded vision applications. They normally hinge on a streamlined architecture that practices a depth-wise separable convolutions to shape lightweight deep neural networks that can have low latency for mobile and embedded devices [9]. By using MobileNet, it is easier to create a head model and a base model for the module, "relu" which is a go to activation function can be used for creating head model.

For training purpose, the code uses the learning rate, the epochs and bit size, and this can be chosen according to the required accuracy, which totally depends on the user. If training rate is less, the system would be more accurate.

The image dataset should be converted into a similar pattern. A desired pixel size can be chosen, and all image data is converted into that size. Like (x, y) can be used for resizing height and width. So that the data is symmetric and is uniform.

After resizing the pixels, max pooling is done, which is nothing but a method of extracting the prominent features and avoiding the unnecessary details. It will extract the necessary details from data. Now, this code is compiled and run, the model will get trained, and a plot of accuracy and loss is plotted.

After training a model which will be able to detect a mask on a human face is generated. But the task is not done yet, this model will only detect mask but for detecting face there is a need to create a program using OpenCV in which can detect a human face and use mask detection model with it to detect face mask.

5 Face Detection

The model generated using Keras for mask detection will be coped with a face detection model using OpenCV. The following shown is the AdaBoost algorithm, which is used to build this system.

5.1 AdaBoost

In AdaBoost, all weights are prepared equally, but with each next round, the weights of imperfectly classified examples are enlarged so that the weak learner in model is forced to focus on the hard examples in the trading set [10].

For m = 1 to M.

1. Hand-pick and abstract km from the pool of classifiers that minimizes

$$W_e = \sum_{yi \neq k_m} \omega_i^{(m)}$$

2. Set the weight of the classifier

$$\alpha_m = \frac{1}{2} ln\left(\frac{1 - e_m}{e_m}\right)$$

3. Apprise the weights of the data points for next iteration
   If $k_m(x_i)$ is a miss, set

$$\omega_i^{(m+1)} = \omega_i^{(m)} e^{\alpha} = \omega_i^{(m)} \sqrt{\frac{1 - e_m}{e_m}}$$

Otherwise

$$\omega_i^{(m+1)} = \omega_i^{(m)} e^{-\alpha} = \omega_i^{(m)} \sqrt{\frac{e_m}{1 - e_m}}$$

5.2 *OpenCV*

Open-source computer vision library (OpenCV) is a useful library, because it has a number of functions which can be helpful for real-time operations, It is established by Intel. It mainly is good with real-time operations because of the libraries it have [11]. OpenCV contains various functions and utilities that appear to be well suited for real-time operations [12].

The architecture of deep learning consists of a number of layers; all are bound to different functions. This layer system is always evolved in the process a system recognition. Hence, deep learning laterally with the face detection can work as the deep layer learning model [13]. Therefore, in face detection area, deep learning usually works in two domains; those are discovering face in a frame and then recognizing it [12].

Python language is a prevailing programming languages and is used all across the world, and this language can be a very decent choice for face recognition task. Python is talented to support a wide variety of third-party tools which make Python a lot more easier to use and motivate the consumers to continue with [14]. Both recognizing and detecting of face can be of ease by using Python and OpenCV [12]. OpenCV practices face detector called "Haar Cascade classifier". It takes an input image, usually from the camera or real-time video frame, and then, it checks whether it is human face or not and also its location [15].

For detecting any human face, OpenCV can be useful with camera function and image display. In Python, there are a number of libraries like FaceNet which can help in detecting a human face. **FaceNet** can be demarcated as a system that directly learns a planning from face images to a Real-time face detection by using OpenCV, Keras and Python (Fig. 3).

The approach for detecting human face follows extracting the ROI of face using NumPy slicing. NumPy can be defined as a Python library that is used for working with array. It is able to provide high performance multidimensional arrays. NumPy is called an open-source library from Python.

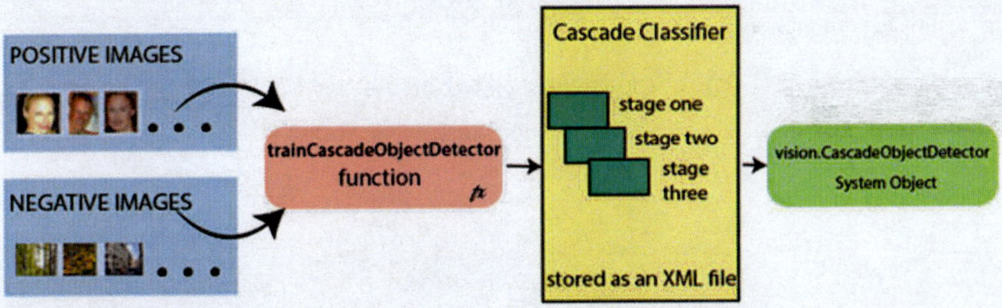

Fig. 3 Cascade classifier

6 Result

After successful completion of training and testing the codes, the result would be amazing. After compilation is done, a frame appears as shown below. The window captures real-time frames and detects face, along with that it shows a box around face with the prediction percentage of surety of a mask or not.

With Mask

These are the results with mask, taken from different angles and distances. The results do not depend on colour of mask. The model works well even in less light. Figures 4 and 5 is taken from a closer distance, but Fig. 6 is taken from a farther distance. Also, it can be seen in Fig. 7 that more than one person can also be detected by this model.

Fig. 4 Image with mask (female)

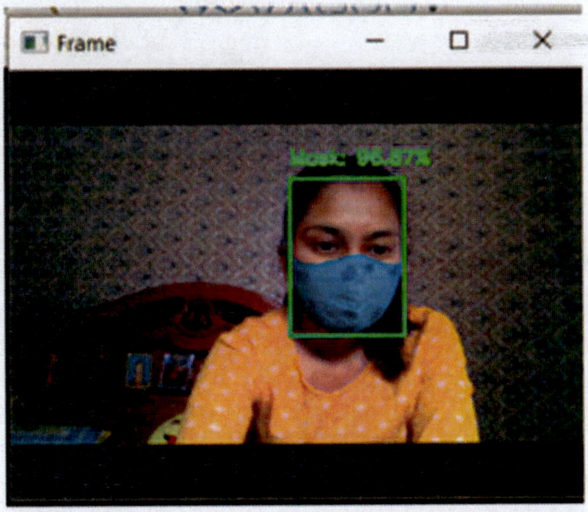

Fig. 5 Image with mask (male)

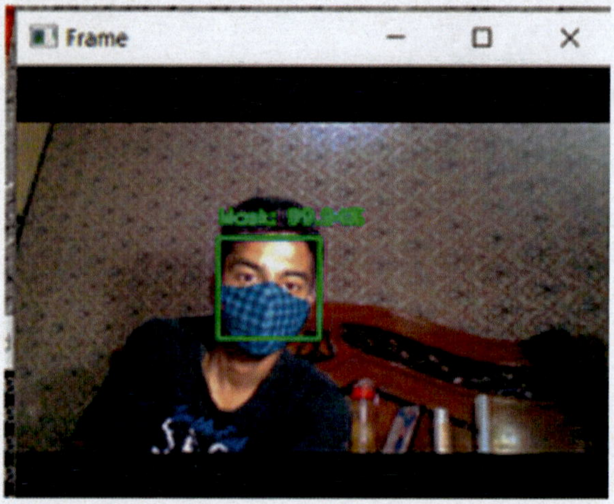

Fig. 6 Image with mask from a distance

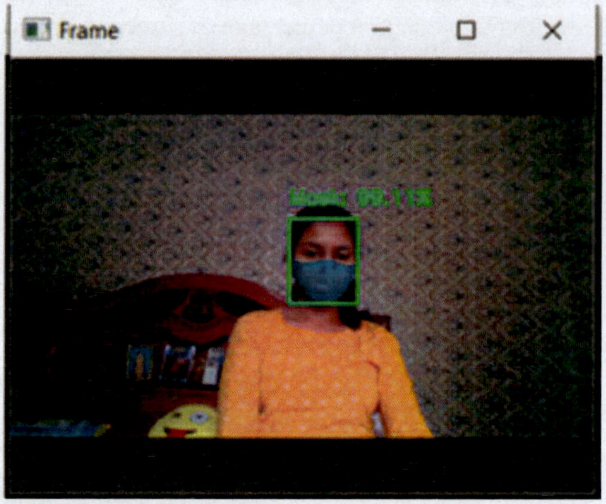

Without Mask

These are the results without mask, taken from different angles, lighting and distances (Figs. 8, 9, 10, 11). This model also works in low lights as shown in Figs. 12 and 13. Also, wearing mask properly is necessary as in Fig. 9 nose is not covered so the model is indicating no mask (Figs. 14 and 15).

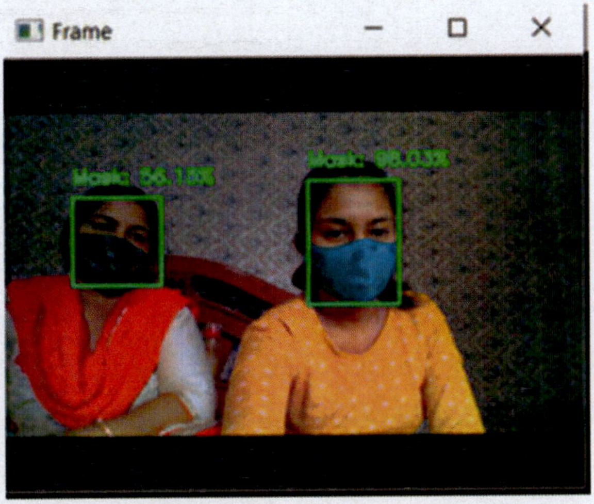

Fig. 7 Image of two people with mask at a time

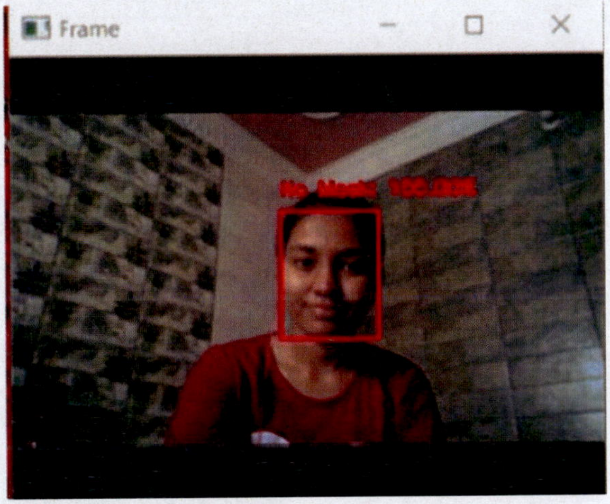

Fig. 8 Image without mask

7 Conclusions

Face mask detection systems can be simply associated with several of the top technological corporations and industries and can make the work of face mask detection a lot relaxed. This tool is convenient because of the presence of python programming language which is very easy to use and OpenCV. The projected system is very convenient and can be proved very much helpful in a number of places, as this system is easy to build and implement.

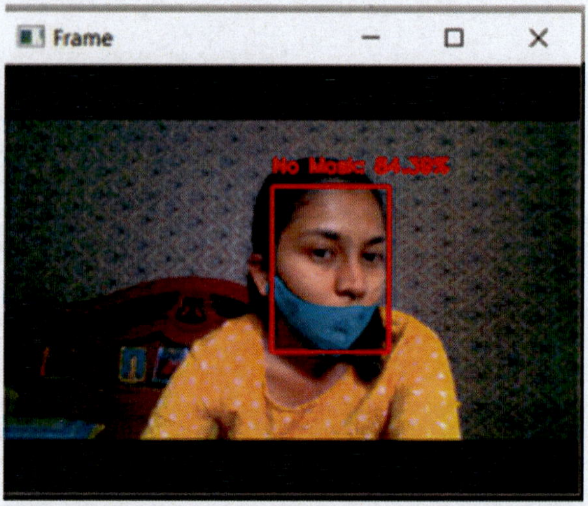

Fig. 9 Image with half mask on

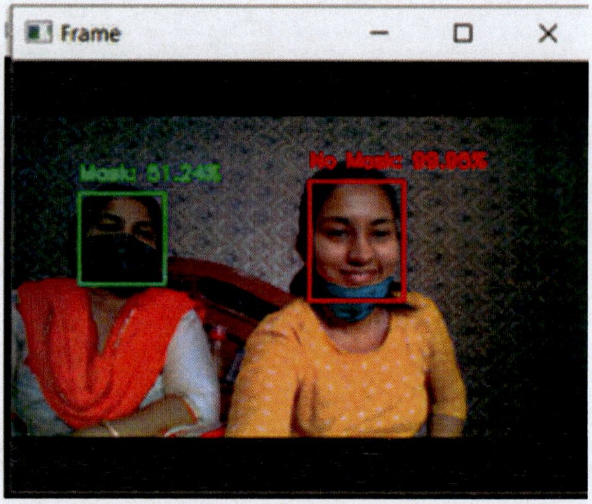

Fig. 10 Image with one person wearing mask and one not at a same time

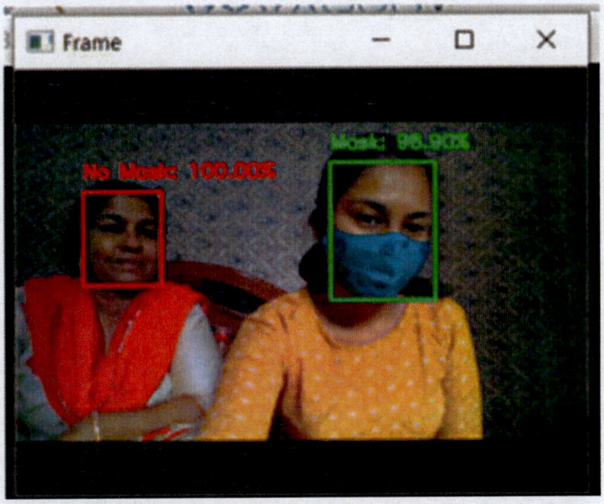

Fig. 11 Image with one person wearing mask and one not at a same time

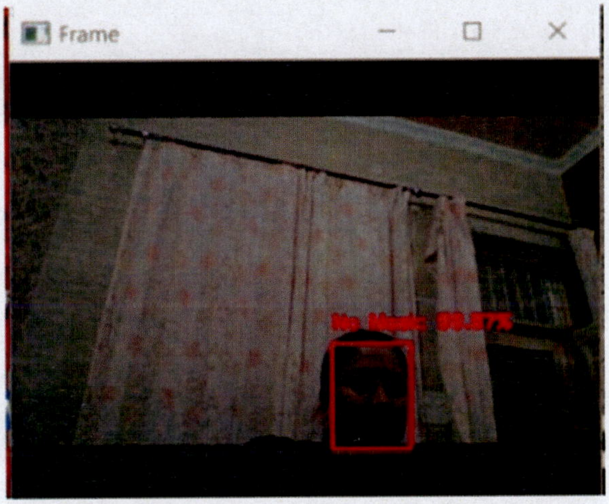

Fig. 12 Image of person not wearing mask at a distance

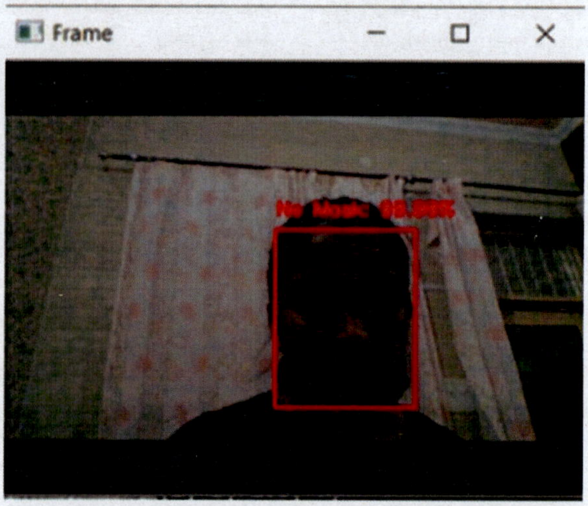

Fig. 13 Image with no mask in less light

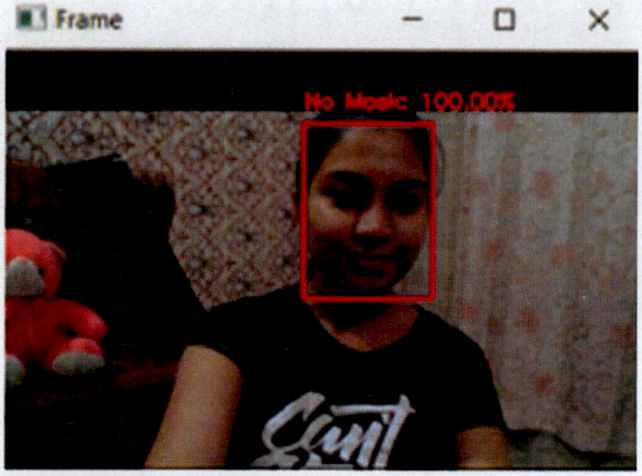

Fig. 14 Image with no mask in proper light

Fig. 15 Image with no mask in proper light

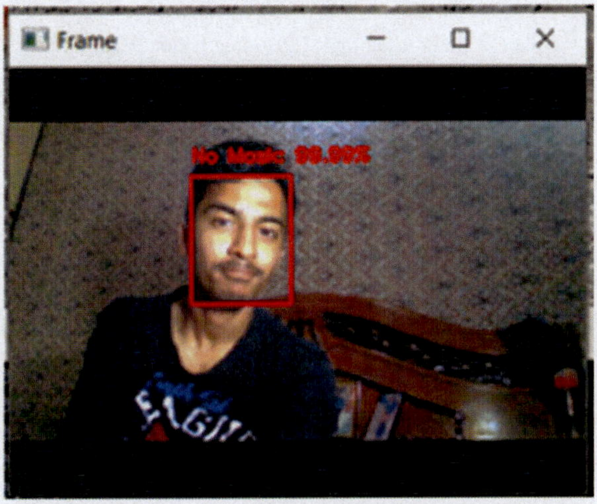

References

1. Yuen KS, Ye ZW, Fung SY, Chan CP, Jin DY (2020) SARS-CoV-2 and COVID-19: The most important research questions. Cell Biosci 10(1):1–5. https://doi.org/10.1186/s13578-020-00404-4
2. Torales J, O'Higgins M, Castaldelli-Maia JM, Ventriglio A (2020) The outbreak of COVID-19 coronavirus and its impact on global mental health. Int J Soc Psychiatry 66(4):317–320. https://doi.org/10.1177/0020764020915212
3. Rahman MM, Manik MMH, Islam MM, Mahmud S, Kim JH (2020) An automated system to limit COVID-19 using facial mask detection in smart city network. IEMTRONICS 2020—Int. IOT, Electron. Mechatronics Conf Proc. https://doi.org/10.1109/IEMTRONICS51293.2020.9216386.
4. Vinitha V, Velantina V (2020) Covid-19 Facemask detection with deep learning and computer vision. Int Res J Eng Technol 7(8):3127–3132
5. Feng S, Shen C, Xia N, Song W, Fan M, Cowling BJ (2020) Rational use of face masks in the COVID-19 pandemic. Lancet Respir Med 8(5):434–436. https://doi.org/10.1016/S2213-2600(20)30134-X
6. Batagelj, Peer P, Štruc V, Dobrišek S (2021) How to Correctly Detect Face-Masks for COVID-19 from Visual Information? Appl Sci 11(5):2070. https://doi.org/10.3390/app11052070.
7. Sinha D, El-Sharkawy M (2019) Thin MobileNet: an enhanced mobilenet architecture. In: 2019 IEEE 10th annual ubiquitous computing, electronics & mobile communication conference UEMCON 2019, pp 0280–0285. https://doi.org/10.1109/UEMCON47517.2019.8993089.
8. Michele A, Colin V, Santika DD (2019) Mobilenet convolutional neural networks and support vector machines for palmprint recognition. Procedia Comput Sci 157:110–117. https://doi.org/10.1016/j.procs.2019.08.147
9. Goswami K, Sowjanya AM (2020) Detection of face mask through machine learning 11:450–4
10. Wang R (2012) AdaBoost for feature selection, classification and its relation with SVM, a review. Phys Procedia 25:800–807. https://doi.org/10.1016/j.phpro.2012.03.160
11. Goyal K, Agarwal K, Kumar R (2017) Face detection and tracking: using OpenCV. In: Proceedings of the International Conference on Electronics and Communication and Aerospace Technology ICECA 2017, vol 2017-Janua, no 4, pp 474–478. https://doi.org/10.1109/ICECA.2017.8203730.

12. Khan M, Chakraborty S, Astya R, Khepra S (2019) Face detection and recognition using OpenCV. In: Proceedings of 2019 International Conference on Information and Communication Technology and Systems ICCCIS 2019, vol 2019-Janua, pp 116–119. https://doi.org/10.1109/ICCCIS48478.2019.8974493.
13. Kota VM, Manoj Kumar V, Bharatiraja C (2020) Deep Learning—a review. IOP Conf Ser Mater Sci Eng 912(3). https://doi.org/10.1088/1757-899X/912/3/032068.
14. Sharma A, Khan F, Sharma D, Student FY, Area SI (2020) Python : the programming language of fut Int J Innov Res Technol 6(12):115–118
15. Naveenkumar M (2016) OpenCV for Computer Vision Applications, no. March 2015, 2016